THESAURUS OF MEDICAL TERMS

Key Word	Adjective	Study	Specialist	Major Disorders
immunization	immunologic, immunological	immunology	immunologist	poliomyelitis, measles, smallpox
internal medicine			internist	
joints and muscles		rheumatology	rheumatologist	rheumatoid arthritis, osteoarthritis
kidney	renal, nephric	nephrology	nephrologist	nephritis, kidney failure
law and medicine		forensic medicine, forensic pathology		
liver	hepatic	hepaticology	hepaticologist	hepatitis
lung	pulmonary	internal medicine	internist	emphysema, lung cancer, tuberculosis
medicine *See* general medicine, internal medicine, osteopathic medicine, rehabilitation.				
mental illness	psychiatric	psychiatry	psychiatrist	neurosis, psychosis, psychosomatic disease
muscles *See* joints and muscles.				
nervous system	neural, neurologic, neurological, neuropathological	neurology, neuropathology	neurologist, neuropathologist, neurosurgeon	epilepsy, cerebral palsy, brain tumors, meningitis
nose *See* ear, nose, and throat.				
osteopathic medicine	osteopathic	osteopathy	osteopath	
plastic surgery		plastic surgery, cosmetic surgery	plastic surgeon, cosmetic surgeon	scars, burns, cosmetic improvements
radiology	radiologic, radiological, X-ray	radiology, roentgenology	radiologist, roentgenologist	
rectum *See* colon and rectum.				
rehabilitation		physical medicine	physical therapist	
reproductive system (female)	obstetric, obstetrical, gynecologic, gynecological	obstetrics, gynecology	obstetrician, gynecologist, ob-gyn specialist	pregnancy and its complications, infertility, fibroid tumors, dysmenorrhea, birth control, ovarian cysts
reproductive system (male) *See* urinogenital tract (male).				
skin and hair	dermal	dermatology	dermatologist	dermatitis, acne, psoriasis
surgery	surgical	surgery	surgeon	
throat (*See also* ear, nose, and throat.)	laryngologic, laryngological	laryngology	laryngologist	laryngitis, upper respiratory infections
tooth	dental, orthodontic, periodontal	dentistry, orthodontics, orthodontia, oral or dental surgery, periodontics, periodontia	dentist, oral or dental surgeon, orthodontist, periodontist, pediatric dentist	caries (tooth decay), periodontal disease, malocclusion, children's dental needs
tumor	oncologic	oncology	oncologist	cancer, benign tumors
urinary tract (female)	urologic, urological	urology	urologist	cystitis, nephritis
urinogenital tract (male)	urologic, urological	urology	urologist	kidney stones, nephritis, prostate problems
X ray *See* radiology.				

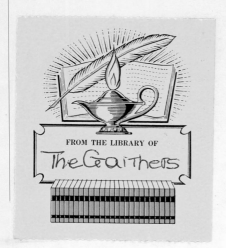

The Complete Illustrated Book of

BETTER HEALTH

The Complete Illustrated Book of
BETTER HEALTH

EDITED BY

Richard J. Wagman, M.D.

Assistant Clinical Professor of Medicine
Downstate Medical Center
New York, New York

AND BY

the J. G. Ferguson Editorial Staff,

Sidney I. Landau, *Managing Editor*

CONSULTING EDITOR

N. Henry Moss, M.D., F.A.C.S.

Associate Clinical Professor of Surgery
Albert Einstein Medical Center and
Temple University Health Sciences Center

J. G. FERGUSON PUBLISHING COMPANY / CHICAGO

Distributed to the book trade by Doubleday & Company, Inc. / New York

Portions of this book have been previously published
under the title of *The New Concise Family Health and
Medical Guide,* edited by Richard J. Wagman, M.D.

Contributors to
The Complete Illustrated Book of Better Health

EDITOR
Richard J. Wagman, M.D.
Assistant Clinical Professor of Medicine
Downstate Medical Center
New York, New York

CONSULTING EDITOR
N. Henry Moss, M.D., F.A.C.S.
Associate Clinical Professor of Surgery
Albert Einstein Medical Center and
Temple University Health Sciences Center;
Past President
American Medical Writers Association;
Past President and Member, Board of Governors
New York Academy of Sciences

CONSULTANTS IN PSYCHIATRY
Julian J. Clark, M.D.
Rita W. Clark, M.D.
Department of Psychiatry
Downstate Medical Center
New York, New York

EXECUTIVE EDITOR
Thomas C. Jones
J. G. Ferguson Publishing Company

KENNETH N. ANDERSON (KNA)
Formerly Editor
Today's Health

PETER B. BARLOW, M.D. (PBB)
Assistant Professor of Internal Medicine
Case-Western Reserve University
Cleveland, Ohio

CHARLES H. BAUER, M.D. (CHB)
Clinical Associate Professor of Pediatrics
and Chief of Pediatric Gastroenterology
The New York Hospital–Cornell
Medical Center
New York, New York

BRUCE O. BERG, M.D. (BOB)
Assistant Professor
Departments of Neurology and Pediatrics
University of California
San Francisco, California

JULIAN J. CLARK, M.D. (JJC)
Clinical Assistant Professor of Psychiatry
Downstate Medical Center
New York, New York

RITA W. CLARK, M.D. (RWC)
Clinical Assistant Professor of Psychiatry
Downstate Medical Center
New York, New York

D. Jeanne Collins (DJC)
Assistant Professor
University of Detroit School of Dentistry
Detroit, Michigan

Anthony A. Davis (AAD)
Assistant Professor
Department of Allied Health Professions
College of Medicine
Howard University
Washington, D. C.

Peter A. Dickinson (PAD)
Editor Emeritus
Harvest Years/Retirement Living

Gordon K. Farley, M.D. (GKF)
Assistant Professor of Child Psychiatry
Chief, Children's Diagnostic Center
University of Colorado Medical Center
Denver, Colorado

Arthur Fisher (AF)
Group Editor of
Science and Engineering
Popular Science Monthly

Edmund H. Harvey, Jr. (EHH, Jr.)
Editor
Science World

Helene MacLean (HMacL)
Free-lance medical writer

Ben Patrusky (BP)
Science Editor
American Heart Association

Douglass S. Thompson, M.D. (DST)
Clinical Associate Professor of Obstetrics and
Gynecology, and of Community Medicine
University of Pittsburgh School of Medicine
Pittsburgh, Pennsylvania

Stanley E. Weiss, M.D. (SEW)
Attending Physician, Renal Service
Long Island College Hospital
Brooklyn, New York

Jeffrey S. Willner, M.D. (JSW)
Chief Resident, Radiology Department
Mount Sinai Hospital
New York, New York

CONTRIBUTORS' INITIALS

AAD	Anthony A. Davis	DST	Douglass S. Thompson, M.D.	KNA	Kenneth N. Anderson
AF	Arthur Fisher	EHH, Jr.	Edmund H. Harvey, Jr.	PAD	Peter A. Dickinson
BOB	Bruce O. Berg, M.D.	GKF	Gordon K. Farley, M.D.	PBB	Peter B. Barlow, M.D.
BP	Ben Patrusky	HMacL	Helene MacLean	RWC	Rita W. Clark, M.D.
CHB	Charles H. Bauer, M.D.	JJC	Julian J. Clark, M.D.	SEW	Stanley E. Weiss, M.D.
DJC	D. Jeanne Collins	JSW	Jeffrey S. Willner, M.D.		

EDITORIAL STAFF

Managing Editor: Sidney I. Landau

Editors: Dorothy Dunbar, Katharine Milton, Elaine Murray,
Diane S. Williams, Rita P. Wolfson

Contributing Editors: Ronald Bogus, Simon Dresner, Jo Ann Miller

Editorial Assistants: Gail Longinetti, Dorothy Mobley

Design and Production: Marian Hurd Manfredi

Assistant Designer: Abigail Moseley

Illustrator: Neil O. Hardy

Indexer: Dee Atkinson

Contents

Acknowledgments

Grateful acknowledgment is made of the courtesy of the following organizations and individuals:

Mayo Medical Museum, Mayo Clinic, Rochester, Minnesota, for granting permission to the publishers to photograph its medical exhibits in color for the purpose of illustration in this book;

Parke, Davis & Company, Detroit, Michigan, for permission to reproduce original oil paintings in color from its distinguished *Great Moments in Medicine* series;

Victor W. Sidel, M.D., for permission to reproduce his own color transparencies demonstrating the use of acupuncture;

A. J. Nystrom & Company, Chicago, Illinois, for permission to reproduce in color a number of anatomical and health-related charts.

Color Illustrations

Introduction

The American public has in the past few years focused increasing attention on the deficiencies of our current health care delivery system. Excessive fragmentation of medical care from overspecialization, the rising cost of hospitalization, the maldistribution of physicians, and the lack of adequate primary care have received copious comment in both the public and professional press.

Also receiving increasing recognition is the preventive approach to our health needs. Whereas our present health care delivery system concentrates over 90% of its effort in curing the sick, many of the new health insurance proposals, numerous articles, and recent health messages by the President and members of Congress aim to devote a larger share of our health resources to preventive measures. Thus the next few years will undoubtedly result in efforts to build a true health system, including a major preventive component and not a sickness system of curative medicine alone. Such a system would attempt to detect illness much earlier and when it is relatively inexpensive to be treated. It would also aim to encourage those health habits in daily living to minimize the risk of becoming ill.

It is therefore most timely that a new and up-to-date encyclopedia of health care has been written for the use of the public by a distinguished group of medical experts. The emphasis has been placed on preventive approaches to illness and the development of proper advice and guidance for better health. Many of the topics included in this volume are not found in previous medical encyclopedias for the public.

The opening chapter offers a comprehensive review of the structure and functions of the body. It allows the reader to understand the roles that the organs and organ systems play in the day-to-day functioning of his body. Chapter 2, *Staying Healthy and Attractive Through the Years*, places heavy emphasis on proper methods of maintaining good health. Chapter 3, dealing with the emotional and intellectual development of the individual at various age levels, covers a broad gamut of topics that go beyond the traditional boundaries of medicine, yet are of unquestionable importance to health. Other subjects that are covered in depth include leisure activities, nutrition and weight control, and care of the skin and hair.

The chapters on alcohol and drugs deal with subjects that pose increasingly significant social and medical problems to our society. A greater number of physicians than ever before are now beginning to face difficult diagnostic and therapeutic problems in these social diseases and are learning how to cope with the realities of their impact. Parents of involved children are facing issues never before encountered by middle-class America. It is most useful to have a candid presentation of the problem and helpful guidance in meeting some of the issues brought on by the use and abuse of alcohol and drugs.

The chapter *Medical Emergencies* has special importance in a medical encyclopedia; its red-edged pages identify it for rapid access at the time of an emergency. It provides the urgent information and advice that in many instances are so vital to survival before a physician arrives on the scene or before the patient can be taken to the nearest hospital.

Despite preventive efforts, any person may become sick with any one of a myriad of diseases. Any one of the numerous systems or organs in the body may become afflicted. It is therefore important to have a ready reference available for an individual to learn about a malady involving himself, a member of his family, or a friend. A systematic review of such illnesses is presented in *The Complete Illustrated Book of Better Health* and covers the cause when known, symptoms, diagnostic measures, and the latest in treatment.

The *Information Key* is innovative in that it gives much more information than the traditional type of index. This is achieved by the use of ten major subindexes organized according to organ or system, and one according to age group. All of the subindex entries are repeated, often with definitions, in the general index; thus the reader has a much better chance of finding the reference he seeks. The *Information Key* as a whole contains well over 7,000 items, including 2,000 glossary items, and is introduced by a *Thesaurus of Medical Terms,* by which means the reader can find the appropriate medical term applying to a subject and look up the term in the index.

The illustrations are clear, pertinent to the text, and abundant in number. The anatomical drawings of Neil O. Hardy are especially fine, and succeed in accurately illustrating the body's systems without superfluous detail.

This ready reference will make a most useful addition to any home library and will prove useful to any member of the family, regardless of age.

N. Henry Moss, M.D.

The Complete Illustrated Book of

BETTER HEALTH

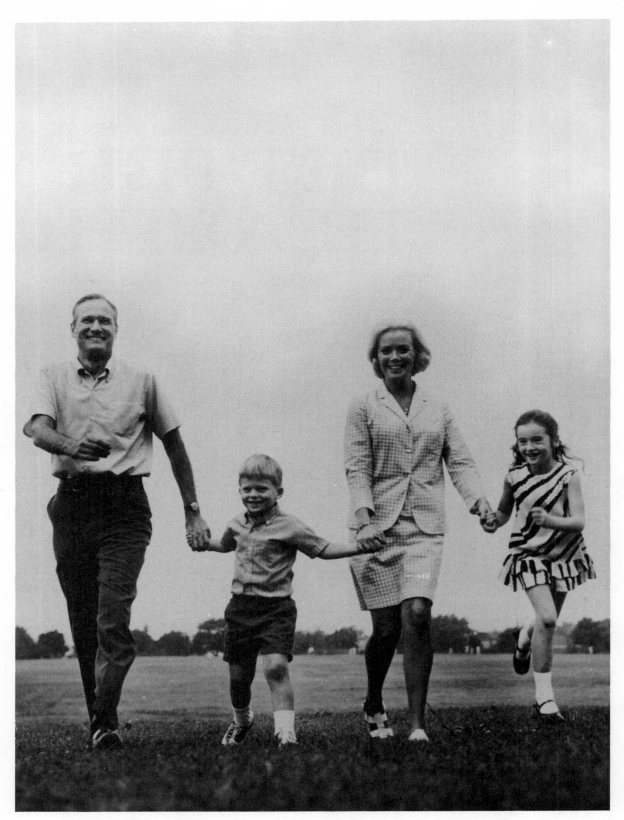

"He who has health has hope," says an Arabian proverb, "and he who has hope, has everything."

CHAPTER 1

Your Body

THE SKELETON

Say "skeleton" to children and you probably conjure up in their minds a rickety structure of rigid sticks, or, to the more fanciful child, a clickety-clacketing collection of rattling bones cavorting under a Halloween moon. A look at almost any anatomical drawing of the human skeletal system bears out the child's image: dry sticks of bones, stripped of skin and flesh, muscle and tendon—a grotesque caricature of a living human being.

Our living bones are something quite different. They are rigid, yes, but not entirely so: they also may bend a little and grow and repair themselves; and they are shaped and fitted together so that—rather than the herky-jerky motions of a wooden puppet—they permit the smooth grace and coordinated power displayed by an accomplished athlete or a prima ballerina.

Our bones do not do just one thing but many things. Some bones, like the collarbone or *clavicle*, mainly give support to other body structures. Others, like the skull and ribs, encase and protect vulnerable organs. Still others, like the *metacarpus* and

phalanges that make up our hands and fingers, give us mechanical advantages—leverage and movement. There are even bones, the tiny *ossicles* in the middle ear, whose vibrations enable us to hear.

Finally, to think of bone simply as a structural member, like a solid steel girder in a skyscraper, ignores the fact that bone is living tissue. It is one of the busiest tissues in our bodies, a chemical factory that is continually receiving, processing and shipping a wide variety of mineral salts, blood components, and a host of other vital materials.

How the Bones of the Skeletal System Fit and Work Together

Medical textbooks name a total of 206 bones making up the skeletal system of the normal, adult human being. The words "normal" and "adult" are significant. A newborn baby normally has 33 vertebrae making up its backbone (also called spinal column or simply spine); but by the time a person reaches adulthood, the number of

3

individual vertebrae has shrunk to 26. The explanation: during the growth process, the nine bottom vertebrae fuse naturally into just two. In like fashion, we "lose" some 60 bones as we grow up. Some otherwise perfectly normal adults have "extra" bones or "missing" bones. For example, although the normal number of ribs is 12 pairs, some adults may have 11; others may have 13 pairs.

Even a practicing doctor might be hard-pressed to identify each of our 200-plus bones and describe its function. An easier way to gain a general understanding of the various functions, capabilities—and weaknesses, too—of our bones is to visualize the skeletal system as a standing coatrack, say, about six feet high.

Call the central pole the backbone. About ten inches down from its top (the top of your skull) is a horizontal cross-bar (your shoulders—collarbones and shoulder blades), approximately a foot-and-a-half across. Sixteen or so inches below the bottom of the top cross bar is another, shorter cross bar, broader and thicker—the *pelvic girdle*. The coatrack with its two cross bars is now a crude model of the bones of the head and trunk, collectively called the *axial skeleton*. Its basic unit is the backbone, to which are attached the skull at the top, then the bones of the shoulder girdle, the ribs, and at the bottom, the bones of the pelvic girdle.

By hanging down (or appending) members from the two ends of the top cross bar, and doing the same at the lower cross bar, we would simulate what is called the *appendicular skeleton*—arms and hands, legs and feet.

Now, make the coatrack stand on its new legs, cut off the central pole just below the lower bar (if you wish, calling it man's lost tail), and you have the two main components of the skeletal system, joined together before you. Let us look at each more closely.

The Axial Skeleton

Within the framework of the axial skeleton lie all the most vital organs of the body. People have gone on living with the loss of a hand or a leg—indeed, with the loss of any or all of their limbs. But nobody can live without a brain, a heart, a liver, lungs, or kidneys—all of which are carried within the framework of the axial skeleton.

The Skull

The bones of the skull have as their most important function the protection of the brain and sense organs. There are also, of course, the jawbones that support the teeth and gums and which enable us to bite and chew our food.

Most of the skull appears to consist of a single bone—a hard, unbroken dome. Actually, the brain cage or *cranium* consists of eight individual platelike bones which have fused together in the process of growth. At birth, these bones are separated, causing the soft spots or *fontanelles* we can readily feel on a baby's head. As the baby's brain enlarges, the bones grow along their edges to fill in the fontanelles, finally knitting together in what are called *suture lines*, somewhat resembling inexpertly mended clothes seams. Along the suture lines, the skull bones continue to grow until the individual's mature skull size is reached.

Teeth: The hardest substance in the human body is the *enamel* that covers the exposed surface of a tooth. Below the gum, the tooth's outside surface is composed of somewhat softer *cementum*. Beneath enamel and cementum is a bonelike substance, called *dentin*, which covers the soft interior of the tooth, called *pulp*. Pulp is serviced by blood vessels and nerves through the root or roots of the tooth. The passageway of nerves and blood vessels that lead up through the tooth from the gum sockets is called a *root canal.* Tooth

THE STRUCTURE OF A TOOTH

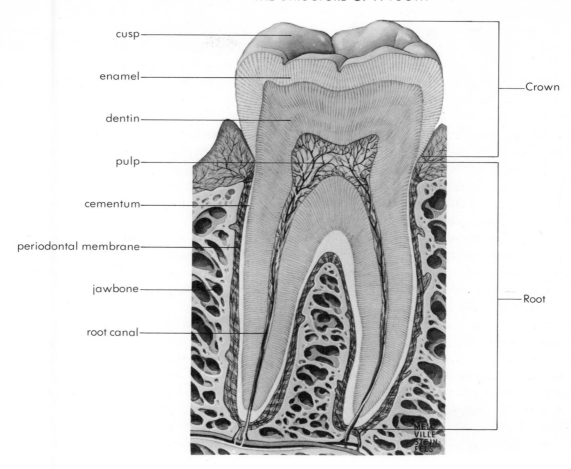

cusp
enamel
dentin
pulp
cementum
periodontal membrane
jawbone
root canal

Crown

Root

MEL VILLE STEIN FELS

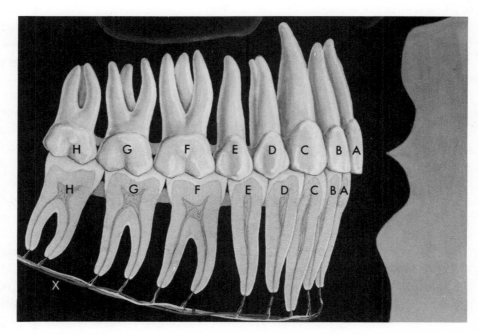

THE ADULT
TEETH

A. central incisors
B. lateral incisors
C. cuspids
D. first bicuspids
E. second bicuspids
F. first molars
G. second molars
H. third molars
X. artery, vein,
   and nerve

and gum are stuck to each other by a tough, adhesive tissue called *periodontal* (or peridental—"surrounding the tooth") *membrane.*

The Backbone

At the base of the skull, the backbone begins. The skull is supported by the topmost *cervical* (neck) vertebra. The curious thing about a backbone is that the word has come to suggest something solid, straight, and unbending. The backbone, however, just isn't like that: it consists of 26 knobby, hollowed-out bones—*vertebrae,* rather improbably held together by muscles, ligaments, and tendons. It is not straight when we stand, but has definite backward and forward curvatures; and even some of its most important structures (the disks between the vertebrae) aren't made of bone, but of cartilage.

All in all, however, the backbone is a fairly well designed structure in terms of the several different functions it serves—but with some built-in weaknesses. For a discussion of backache, see under *Aches, Pains, Nuisances, Worries, p. 409.*

The vertebrae: Although they all have features in common, no two of our 26 vertebrae are exactly alike in shape, size, or function. This is hardly surprising if we consider, for example, that the cervical vertebrae do not support ribs, while the *thoracic vertebrae* (upper trunk, or chest) do support them.

But for a sample vertebra, let us pick a rib-carrying vertebra, if for no other reason than that it lies about midway along the backbone. If viewed from above or below, a thoracic vertebra, like most of the others, would look like a roundish piece of bone with roughly scalloped edges on the side facing inward toward the chest and on the side facing outward toward the surface of the back, and would reveal several bony projections. These knobby portions of a vertebra—some of which you can feel as

bumps along your backbone—are called *processes.* They serve as the vertebra's points of connection to muscles and tendons, to ribs, and to the other vertebrae above and below.

A further conspicuous feature is a hole, more or less in the middle of the typical vertebra, through which passes the master nerve bundle of our bodies, the spinal cord, running from the base of the skull to the top of the pelvis. Thus, one of the important functions of the backbone is to provide flexible, protective tubing for the spinal cord.

Between the bones of one vertebra and the next is a piece of more resilient cartilage that acts as a cushion or shock absorber to prevent two vertebrae from scraping or bumping each other if the backbone gets a sudden jolt, or as the backbone twists and turns and bends. These pieces of cartilage are the intervertebral disks—infamous for pain and misery if they become ruptured or slipped disks.

Regions of the backbone: The backbone can be divided into five regions, starting with the uppermost, or *cervical* region, which normally has seven vertebrae. Next down is the *thoracic* (chest) section, normally with 12 vertebrae. From each vertebra a rib extends to curl protectively around the chest area. Usually, the top ten ribs come all the way around the trunk and attach to the breastbone (or *sternum*); but the bottom two ribs do not reach the breastbone and are thus called floating ribs. The thoracic section also must support the shoulder girdle, consisting of the collarbones (*clavicles*) and shoulder blades (*scapulas*). At the end of each shoulder blade is a shoulder joint—actually three distinct joints working together—where the arm connects to the axial skeleton.

Below the thoracic vertebrae come the five vertebrae of the *lumbar* section. This area gets a good deal of blame for back miseries: lower back pain often occurs

THE HUMAN SKELETON

Front View

Rear View

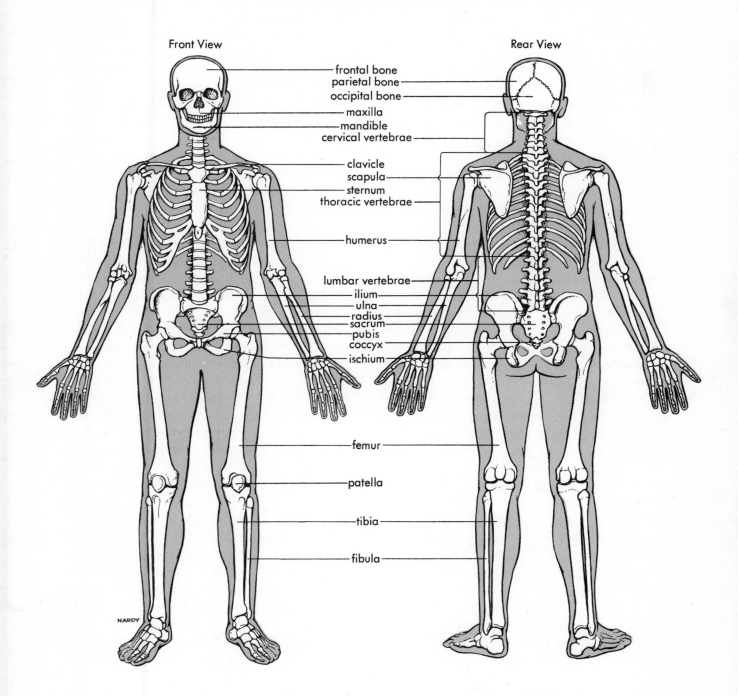

frontal bone
parietal bone
occipital bone
maxilla
mandible
cervical vertebrae

clavicle
scapula
sternum
thoracic vertebrae

humerus

lumbar vertebrae
ilium
ulna
radius
sacrum
pubis
coccyx
ischium

femur

patella

tibia

fibula

HARDY

around the area where the bottom thoracic vertebra joins the top lumbar vertebra; furthermore, the lumbar region or small of the back is also a well-known site of back pain; indeed, from the word "lumbar" comes *lumbago*, medically an imprecise term, but popularly used to describe very real back pain.

Below the lumbar region are two vertebrae so completely different from the 24 above them—and even from each other— that it seems strange they are called vertebrae at all: the *sacrum* and the *coccyx*. These two vertebrae are both made up of several distinct vertebrae that are present at birth. The sacrum is a large bone that was once five vertebrae. The coccyx was originally four vertebrae—and, incidentally, is all that remains of man's tail in his evolution from the primates.

The pelvic girdle: The sacrum is the more important of these two strange-looking vertebrae. It is the backbone's connection to the *pelvic girdle*, or pelvis. On each side of the sacrum, connected by the sacroiliac joint, is a very large, curving bone called the *ilium*, tilting (when we stand) slightly forward and downward from the sacrum toward the front of the groin. We feel the top of the ilium as the top of the hip—a place mothers and fathers often find convenient for toting a worn-out toddler.

Fused at each side of the ilium and slanting toward the back is an *ischium*, the bone we sit on. The two *pubis* bones, also fused to the ilium, meet in front to complete the pelvic girdle. All the bones of the pelvis—ilium, ischium, and pubis—fuse together so as to form the hip joint (*acetabulum*), a deep socket into which the "ball" or upper end of the thighbone fits.

The Appendicular Skeleton

The bones of the appendages—arms, hands, and fingers; legs, feet, and toes—allow human beings to perform an astonishing array of complex movements, from pushing themselves through the physical rigors of the Olympic decathlon to creating an elaborate piece of needlework. The key points in the appendicular skeleton, as indeed, in the axial skeleton, are where the ends or edges of bones lie close together and must work with or against one another in order to achieve coordinated movement. These key points are the *joints*. They are, of course, not really bones but the nonbony spaces between bones.

The Joints

A typical joint consists of several different structures. First, there are the bones themselves—two, three, four, or more almost touching in the area of the joint—with their ends or edges shaped to fit in their respective niches. Between the bones of an appendage joint (as between the vertebrae of the back) is the smooth, resilient material called *cartilage* which allows the bones to move over one another without scraping or catching. At the joint, the bones, with their layer of cartilage between them, are held together by tough bonds of muscle. *Bursas*, tiny sacs containing a lubricating fluid, are also found at joints; they help to reduce the friction between a joint's moving parts.

The hip and knee: The hip joint must not only support the weight of the head and trunk, but must allow for movement of the leg and also play a part in the constant balancing required to maintain upright posture. Similar stresses and strains, often literally tending to tear the joint apart, are placed on every joint in the body.

The notoriety of athletes' bad knees attests to the forces battering at the knee joint, the largest in the human body. However, the fact that there are not more disabled sports heroes also speaks well for the design of the knee joint. The same can be said of the ankle joint and the joints of the foot and toes.

The shoulder, elbow, and wrist: The counterpart of the hip joint in the upper trunk is the shoulder joint. Free of weight-bearing responsibilities, the shoulder has a system of three interconnected joints that allow it and the arm far more versatile movements than the hip and leg.

The elbow connects the upper arm bone (*humerus*) with the two bones of the lower arm (*radius* and *ulna*). Like the knee, it is basically a hinge joint, which allows the lower arm to be raised or lowered. The elbow is also constructed to allow some rotation by the hand; likewise, the knee joint allows us to waggle the foot.

Of all our bony parts, the wrist, hand, and fingers are perhaps the most elegantly and finely jointed—witness the performance of a concert pianist—and our ankles,

feet, and toes probably the most subject to everyday misery.

Bone As Living Tissue

Our bones, like all our tissues, change as we grow up, mature, and finally grow old. There are changes in the chemical activity and composition of bone representative of each stage of life.

In young children, the ends and edges of bones are mainly cartilage, forming a growing surface on the bone that is gradually replaced by hard bone as full size is attained. The bones of a child are more pliable and less likely to break than those of a full-grown adult.

Similarly, as an adult ages, the bones turn from a resilient hardness to a more

BONES OF THE HAND AND FOOT

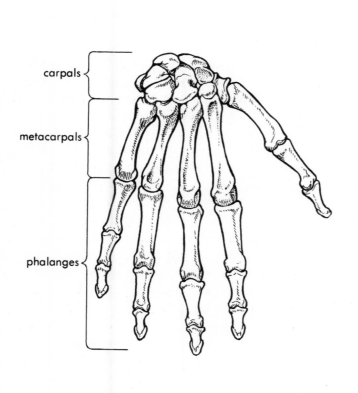

carpals

metacarpals

phalanges

Right Hand

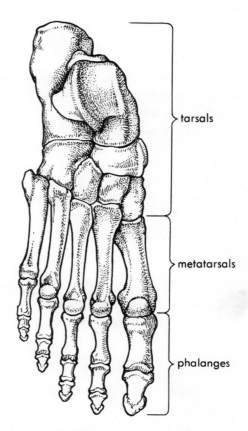

tarsals

metatarsals

phalanges

Right Foot

THE STRUCTURE OF THE FEMUR

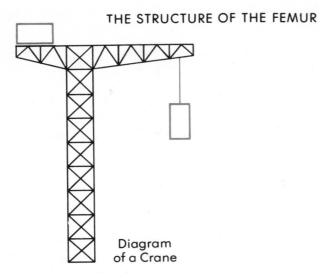

Diagram
of a Crane

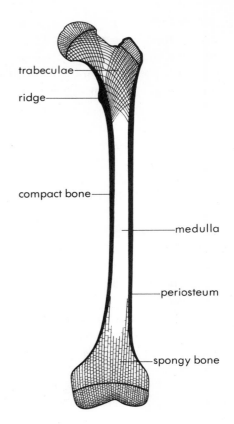

trabeculae

ridge

compact bone

medulla

periosteum

spongy bone

The femur, the large bone of the upper leg, combines strength and lightness better than all but the strongest materials. The minimum of substance is used by having the bone shaft hollow, like the girders of a crane. This is feasible because most of the stress on a long structure occurs at the outside. Within the head of the femur are *trabeculae* (strands of connective tissue) that crisscross roughly at right angles. They correspond to the main lines of the compression and tension when a bone is bearing weight. A similar device is used in the crisscross girders of the crane. Ridges provide areas for muscle attachment and reinforce bones against the pull of muscles.

brittle hardness. This accounts for the much greater danger of broken bones in older people.

These changes with age are an indication of the great amount of chemical activity going on within bone. We sometimes forget that our bones are amply supplied and penetrated by blood vessels. There is a constant building up and breaking down, an interchange of materials between blood and bone.

The Composition of Bone

A living bone does not have a single uniform composition, but instead is composed of several different kinds of tissue. To begin with, there are actually two types of bone tissue in the same bone: compact and spongy. In addition, bone is sheathed in a tough membranous tissue called the *periosteum*, interlaced with blood vessels.

Finally, within most of the larger and longer bones of the body, as well as in the interior of the skull bones and vertebrae, are two more kinds of tissue: red marrow and yellow marrow.

Marrow: Within the spongy bone areas, *red marrow* produces enormous numbers of red blood cells, at a rate of millions per minute. These are needed for growth as well as for replacement of red cells, which also die in enormous numbers. Children's bones contain greater proportions of red marrow than adults'. With age, *yellow marrow*, composed mainly of fat cells, begins to fill the interior bone cavities formerly occupied by red marrow.

Calcium: Bone also serves as a storage and distribution center for one of the most important elements in our body. Calcium, in the form of *calcium phosphate*, is the basic chemical of bone tissue, but this element also must always be present in the bloodstream at a certain level to insure normal heartbeat, blood clotting, and muscle contraction. When the calcium level in the blood is deficient, the bones release some calcium into the bloodstream; when the blood has a surplus of calcium, the bones reabsorb it.

Fractures

Like most other tissues, broken bone can repair itself, and it is a remarkable process to observe. It is a process, however, that will proceed even if the ends are not aligned or set—an important reason why any suspected fracture should be checked by a doctor.

A break in a bone causes a sticky material to be deposited by the blood around the broken ends. This material begins the formation of a kind of protective, lumpy sleeve, called a *callus,* around the broken ends. Mainly cartilage, the callus hardens into spongy bone, normally within a month or two. Then, the spongy bone begins to be reduced in size by bone-dissolving cells produced in the marrow, while at the same time the spongy bone in the area of the break is beginning to be replaced by hard bone.

Depending on the particular bone involved and the severity of the fracture, the broken bone can be completely healed within four to ten months.

Potential Trouble Spots

Essentially there are two kinds of things that can go wrong with the skeletal system and cause trouble.

Mechanical Difficulties

A healthy bone's mechanical functions —support, movement, protection—can be impaired. This can happen as a result of a physical injury resulting in a fracture or dislocation.

The stack of vertebrae called the backbone is vulnerable to a number of painful conditions from top to bottom, especially in the region of the lower back. Unfortunately, man seems to have evolved relatively quickly from a four-footed creature, and his backbone is not ideally suited for standing and walking on two feet. Back troubles become increasingly common with age.

Areas where bones interact are also very susceptible to injury because of the stresses and strains they undergo even in people who are not especially active. Normal wear and tear also takes its toll on our bones and joints; for example, the bones' structure or their alignment at a joint may be altered slightly with age, making one bone or another prone to slipping out of the joint, causing a dislocation. In any case, it is not advisable to make the same demands on our skeletal system at 40 as we did at 20. (Pole vaulting, for example, is not recommended for the middle-aged.) Joints are also the site of arthritis.

Disease

Second, and generally more serious if untreated, the interior bone tissues themselves may become infected and diseased. This, of course, can lead as a secondary effect to impairment of the bones' mechanical functions. *Osteomyelitis,* for example, a bacterial infection of bony tissues, can destroy large portions of bone unless antibiotics are started at once.

Fortunately, disorders of the skeletal system generally reveal themselves early and clearly by pain. Any severe or lingering pain of the joints or bones should be reported to a doctor. For example, some people may feel that aching feet are unavoidable—and a little undignified. But a foot is not meant to hurt, nor is any part of the skeletal system. Consulting a doctor could prevent much present and future misery. See also *Diseases of the Skeletal System,* p. 448.

EHH, Jr.

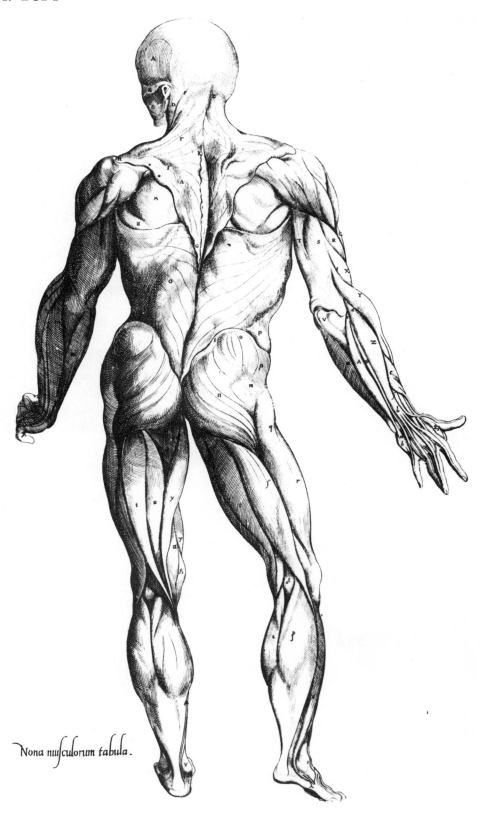

Nona musculorum tabula.

This masterful drawing is by Vesalius (1514–1564), the father of modern anatomy.

THE MUSCLES

Some 600 muscles of all sizes and shapes are attached to the framework of the skeletal system. Altogether these muscles make up nearly half of a normal adult's weight. They hold the skeleton together and, on signals originating in the brain, empower its various parts to move. Everywhere throughout the skeletal system, muscles work together with bones to protect the body's vital organs and to support and move its parts.

Skeletal Muscle

Such muscles are called, collectively, *skeletal muscle*. They are also called *voluntary muscles* because, for the most part, we can choose when 'we want them to act and what we want them to do—drive a car, kick a football, turn a page, jump a brook, toss a baseball. Skeletal muscle also goes by two other names, based on its appearance under a microscope—striped and striated.

Skeletal, voluntary, striped, striated—all refer to the same general type of muscle. To avoid confusion, the term used throughout this section is skeletal muscle.

Smooth Muscle

There are two other general types of muscle. One is called *smooth muscle* because, under the microscope, it lacks the clearly defined stripes of skeletal muscle. Smooth muscle has another name, *involuntary muscle,* so called because the brain does not voluntarily control its actions. Smooth muscle is responsible for movements such as the muscular action that moves food and waste along the digestive tract, or the contraction and dilation of the pupil of the eye, as well as countless other involuntary movements of the sense and internal organs—with the exception of the heart.

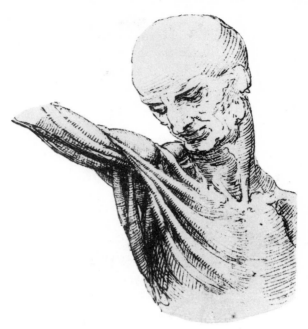

This drawing by Leonardo da Vinci (1452–1519) illustrates the anatomy of the shoulder muscles.

Cardiac Muscle

The third and last general type of muscle is confined to the heart area, and is called *cardiac muscle.* (Cardiac means having to do with the heart). It is involved in the rhythmic beating and contractions of the heart, which are not under conscious control, and cardiac muscle is therefore termed involuntary.

Structure of the Muscles

Each of the three kinds of muscle shares certain structural similarities with one or both of the others. All are made up of bundles of varying numbers of hair-thin fibers. In skeletal and smooth muscles, these fibers are lined up side by side in the bundle, while in cardiac muscle the fibers tend more to crisscross over one another. Skeletal muscle and cardiac muscle are both striped, that is, they show darker and lighter bands crossing over a group of adjacent fibers, while smooth muscle lacks these distinct cross-bands.

Both involuntary muscle types, smooth and cardiac, are controlled by signals carried by the autonomic nervous system. Signals that result in movements of the skeletal muscles are carried by a different nerve network, the central nervous system. The individual fibers in a muscle bundle with a particular function all react simultaneously to a signal from the nervous system; there is no apparent time lag from fiber to fiber.

How the Skeletal Muscles Work

The great range and variety of functions served by skeletal muscles can be suggested by naming just four: the diaphragm, used in breathing; the muscles that make the eye wink; the deltoid muscle that gives the shoulder its shape; and the tongue.

As with the bones, the body tends to make its greatest demands on muscle tissue in the area of the joints and the backbone. A smoothly functioning joint requires that bone, cartilage, and muscle all be sound and able to work together effectively.

TENDON

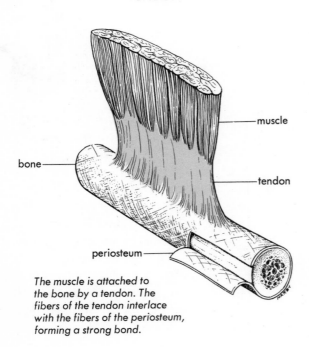

bone

muscle

tendon

periosteum

The muscle is attached to the bone by a tendon. The fibers of the tendon interlace with the fibers of the periosteum, forming a strong bond.

Tendons and Ligaments

We often hear the words tendon and ligament used in the description of the knee or another joint. These are actually two types of skeletal muscles, distinguished as to their function.

A *tendon* can be described as a tight cord of muscle tissue that attaches other skeletal muscle to bone. For example, the Achilles tendon running down the back of the calf, the strongest tendon in the body, connects the muscles of the calf with the bone of the heel. A *ligament* is a somewhat more elastic band of muscle fibers that attaches bone to bone.

A tendon is not always evident in the connection of muscle to bone. Various groups and shapes of muscle fibers may be similarly employed, forming connective tissue without the formation of a tendon.

Various associated tissues between or around skeletal muscles serve to reduce the wear and tear of friction in areas such as a joint, where muscle, bone, and cartilage may rub against one another. For example, the tendons that pass along the back of the hand from the wrist to the fingertips, as well as many other muscle groups throughout the body, are enclosed in lubricated sheaths. The muscle-sheathed *bursas*, lined inside with lubricating fluid, are also found in areas subject to friction, such as where a tendon passes closely over a bone.

Man's upright posture and two-legged locomotion subject the backbone to heavy stresses. It is buttressed, however, with scores of tightly packed bundles of muscle, attached to either side of the spinal column, which ease the burden of standing and walking erect.

Flexors and Extensors

Most of us probably first used the word "muscle" when, as children, we watched an older child or adult flex an arm and proudly display the bump of muscle between the

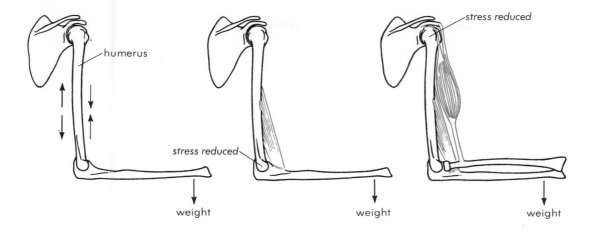

humerus

stress reduced

weight   weight   weight

stress reduced

Bones are prevented from bending under normal stress by a system of braces, in which ligaments play an important role. But the main braces are the muscles. The diagrams above show the arm attached to the shoulder blade with the hand supporting a weight. Without muscles (*left*), the weight would pull unevenly on the humerus, which would bend, thus compressing one side of the bone and stretching the other side. (*Middle*) Addition of a single-jointed muscle (as the brachialis) reduces the stress on the lower end of the humerus. (*Right*) Addition of a two-jointed muscle (as the biceps) also reduces the stress on the upper part of the humerus. There is now no shearing stress that is liable to break the bone, only a compression.

crook of elbow and shoulder. This biceps muscle works together with the triceps muscles on the underside of the arm. The arm is bent at the elbow by contraction of the biceps, which makes this muscle get shorter and thicker; in this position, called *flexion*, the triceps muscle is relaxed. To return the arm to its normal straight position, called *extension*, the biceps relaxes and the triceps contracts. In this bit of muscle teamwork, the biceps, which bends the arm at the elbow joint, is called the *flexor*, while the triceps straightens the arm and is called the *extensor*. Similar flexor-extensor action can be observed at many body joints, including the fingers.

Smooth Muscle

Beginning about midway down the esophagus, layers of smooth muscle line the walls of the 25 feet of digestive tract, extending into the stomach and through the intestines. These muscles keep the stomach and intestinal walls continually in motion,

MUSCLE ACTION IN FOREARM MOVEMENT

Muscles usually work in pairs to produce movement of a part of the body.

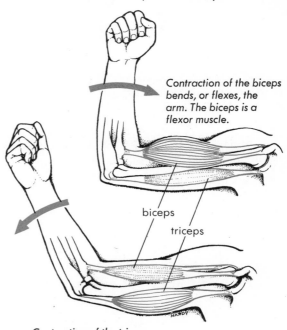

Contraction of the biceps bends, or flexes, the arm. The biceps is a flexor muscle.

biceps

triceps

Contraction of the triceps extends the arm. The triceps is an extensor muscle.

constricting and relaxing to push food along. Smooth muscle also effects the opening and closing of important valves, called *sphincters,* along the digestive tract.

Trouble Spots

The functions and failures of the skeletal muscles are closely allied to those of the skeletal system. The same areas are vulnerable—joints and back—and the same rule holds: severe or persistent muscle pain is a cause to consult your doctor.

Hernia: One type of disorder associated exclusively with a weakness or abnormality of muscle is a rupture or *hernia.* This is the protrusion of part of another organ through a gap in the protective muscle. A likely area for a hernia to appear is in the muscles lining the abdomen, although hernias may occur in any other part of the body where there is pressure against a muscle wall that is not as strong as it should be. Weight control and a sensible program of exercise—abdominal muscles being particularly liable to slackness—are good preventive measures against hernia.

All our muscles, in fact, benefit from regular exercise; but you don't have to exhaust yourself physically every day in order to reach and maintain the desirable plateau doctors describe as good muscle tone.

Atrophy of muscle tissue: Muscle tissues are likely to *atrophy* (shrink and weaken) if they are not used for too long a time. Thus, illness or injuries that cause paralysis or an extended period of immobility for the body or a part of it must be followed by a medically supervised program of physical therapy to rebuild the weakened muscles. See also *Diseases of the Muscles and Nervous System,* p. 469.   EHH, JR.

SKIN, HAIR, AND NAILS

Perhaps no other organ of the human body receives so much attention both from its owner and the eyes of others, as the skin and its associated structures—hair and nails.

Vanity is hardly the issue. The simple facts are that skin is the last frontier of our internal selves, the final boundary between our inside and outside, and our principal first line of defense against the dangers of the outside world. It shows, not always clearly, evidence of some internal disorders; and it shows, often quite clearly, the evidence of external affronts—a bump, a cut, a chafe, an insect bite, or an angry reaction to the attack of germs.

In personal encounters, the unclothed portion of our skin is one of the first things other people observe, and—if we happen to have some unsightly scratch, rash, or blemish—the last thing by which we wish to be remembered. Of all our organs, the skin is the most likely candidate for a program of self-improvement.

The Organ Called Skin

It is always a little surprising to hear, for the first time, the skin referred to as a single organ. This is not to say it is a simple organ; on the contrary, it is an exceedingly complex and varied one. However, despite variations in appearance from part to part of the body, our entire outer wrapper (the more technical word is *integument*) is similarly constructed.

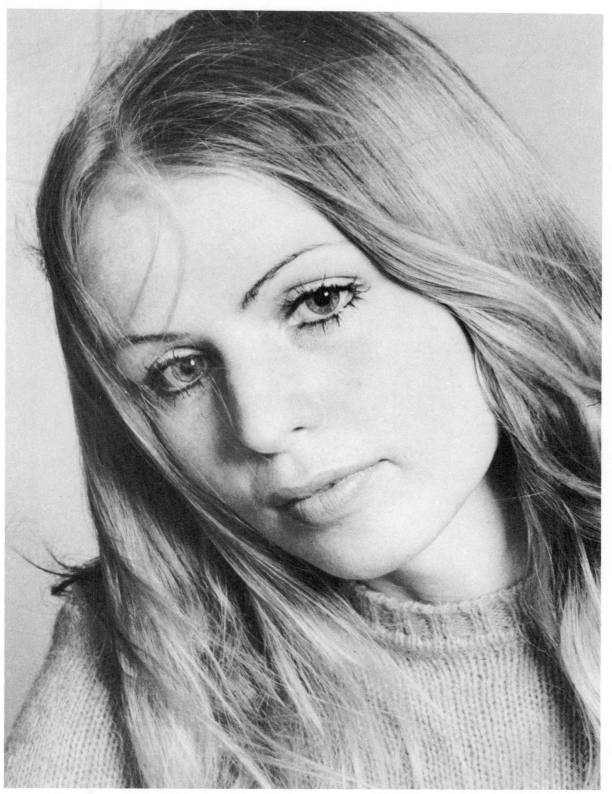

Proper care of the skin, hair, and nails is essential to good health and good looks. This attractive young woman illustrates how becoming a well-groomed appearance can be.

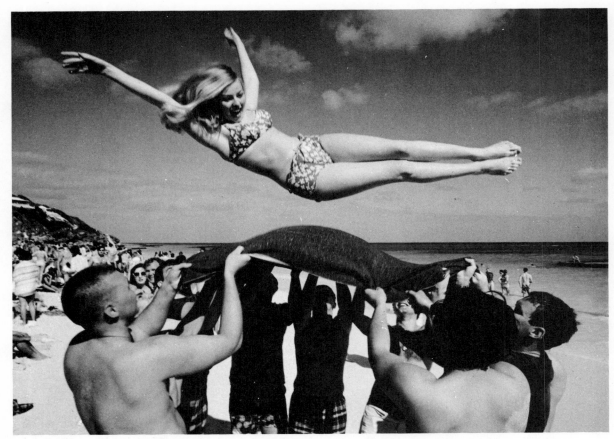

It's obvious that these college students have other things on their mind than exposure to sun, and indeed, at 18 years of age they have little immediate cause for concern. But prolonged exposure to sun ages the skin and can cause other, more serious conditions.

One might object: "But my nails and hair certainly look different from the skin on my nose!" This is perfectly true, but nails and hair are extensions of the skin, and wherever they occur are composed of similar tissues: the nail on a little toe is made of the same material as the hair.

Functions of the Skin

The skin has three main functions, and its different outward appearance on different parts of the body reflects to some extent which of these functions a certain area of skin primarily serves. The three main functions are protection (from germs or blows), temperature control (e.g., through perspiration, to aid in keeping the body's internal organs near our normal internal temperature of 98.6 degrees F.), and perception. Nerve endings in the skin give us our sensations of touch, pain, heat, and cold. Associated with the skin's important role in temperature regulation is its function as an organ of excretion—the elimination, via perspiration, of water and other substances. Skin is also the site of the body's natural production of vitamin D, stimulated by exposure to sunlight.

Composition of the Skin

Skin has three more or less distinct layers. The outermost is called the *epidermis;* the middle, the *dermis;* and the innermost, *subcutaneous* (underskin) tissue. The epidermis may also be called *cuticle;* and the dermis either *corium* or *true skin.*

The subcutaneous layer: The subcutaneous layer is really a rather vague border zone between muscle and bone tissues on one side, and the dermis on the other, a kind of springy, fatty padding that gives bounce and a look of firmness to the skin above it. With age, the fatty cells of the subcutaneous layer are not continually replaced as they die, and this layer tends to thin out. The result is wrinkles, which form where the outer layers of skin lose their subcutaneous support, much like the slip-cover of a cushion that has lost some of its stuffing.

The dermis: The dermis is serviced by the multitude of tiny blood vessels and nerve fibers that reach it through the subcutaneous tissue. In addition, many special structures and tissues that enable the skin to perform its various functions are found in the dermis: *sebaceous* (skin oil) glands and sweat glands; minuscule muscles; and the roots of hairs encased in narrow pits called *follicles.*

The topmost layer of the dermis, interconnecting with the epidermis above it, resembles, under a microscope, nothing so much as a rugged, ridge-crossed landscape carved with valleys, caves, and tunnels. The basic forms of this microscopic terrain are cone-shaped hills called *papillae;* between 100 and 200 million of them are found in the dermis of an adult human being.

Since the dermal papillae serve as the bedrock for the surface layer of skin, the

ANATOMY OF THE SKIN

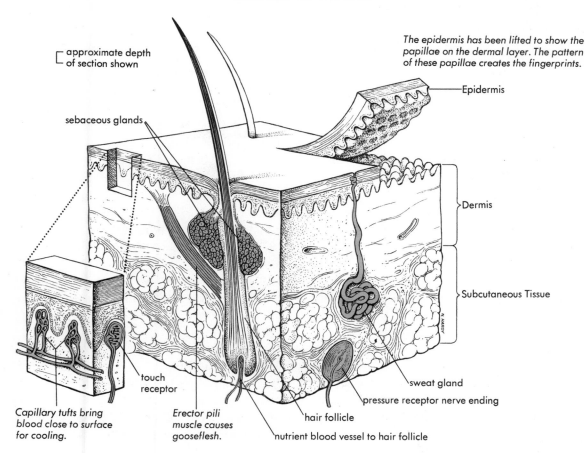

approximate depth of section shown

The epidermis has been lifted to show the papillae on the dermal layer. The pattern of these papillae creates the fingerprints.

Epidermis

sebaceous glands

Dermis

Subcutaneous Tissue

touch receptor

sweat gland

pressure receptor nerve ending

Capillary tufts bring blood close to surface for cooling.

Erector pili muscle causes gooseflesh.

hair follicle

nutrient blood vessel to hair follicle

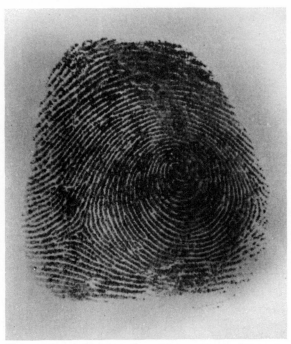

The pattern of ridges in a fingerprint reflects the contours of the papillae (conelike bumps) of the upper layer of the dermis, just below the epidermis.

epidermis, we can understand why there is really no such thing as smooth skin; even the smoothest patch of a baby's skin appears ridged and cratered under a magnifying glass.

The distribution of papillae in the skin falls into certain distinctive patterns which are particularly conspicuous on the soles of babies' feet and on the fingertips, and give each of us our unique finger, toe, and foot prints. The mathematical possibility of one person having the same fingerprints as another is thought to be about one in 25 billion. The papillae ridges on the fingertips also make it easier for us to pick up and handle such things as needles or pencils or buttons.

Finally, because there are relatively more papillae concentrated at the fingertips than on most other areas of the body, and because papillae are often associated with dense concentrations of nerve endings, the fingertips tend to be more responsive to touch sensations than other parts of the body.

The epidermis: The bottom layer of the epidermis, its papillae fitted into the pockets of the layers of the dermis beneath it, is occupied by new young cells. These cells gradually mature and move upward. As they near the surface of the skin, they die, becoming tough, horny, lifeless tissue. This is the outermost layer of the epidermis, called the *stratum corneum* (horny layer), which we are continually shedding, usually unnoticed, as when we towel off after a bath, but sometimes very noticeably, as when we peel after a sunburn.

A suntan, incidentally, is caused by the presence of tiny grains of pigment, called *melanin,* in the bottom layers of epidermis. Sunlight stimulates the production of melanin, giving the skin a darker color. A suntan fades as the melanin granules move to the surface and are shed with dead skin cells.

Hair and Nails

Certainly the most noticeable of the specialized forms of skin are our hair and nails. What we see of them is really a dead tissue, called *keratin,* similar to the dead skin cells that are continually being shed by our bodies, but much more firmly packed together. However, hair and nails both originate in cells that are very much alive—as anyone who has plucked a group of hairs or suffered the pain of a torn-out nail knows very well. Growth occurs in this living region, with new cells pushing the dead, hard, hair and nail stalks upward, then dying themselves and being replaced from below.

The bottom end or root of a hair is lodged, as noted above, in a *follicle,* a hollow resembling a rounded bottle with a long, narrow neck slanting toward the skin's surface. Each follicle is supported by the little hummock of a papilla, and is serviced by tiny oil glands that lubricate the shaft (or neck) through which the hair pushes toward the surface.

The follicles of the long hairs of the scalp, groin, and armpits may be found deep in the subcutaneous layers of the skin; others are no deeper than the top layers of dermis. Attached to a follicle are microscopic muscle fibers that, if stimulated by cold or emotional factors, can contract around the follicle; the result is goose flesh or sometimes even the sensation that our hair is standing on end.

A nail's living, growing part is found beneath the whitish half moon, or *lunula*, at its base. The lunula is sometimes obscured because a layer of epidermis (cuticle) has grown over it. Except at its very top (the part we can trim without pain), the nail is firmly attached to the ridged upper layer of the dermis, a region richly laced with tiny blood vessels.

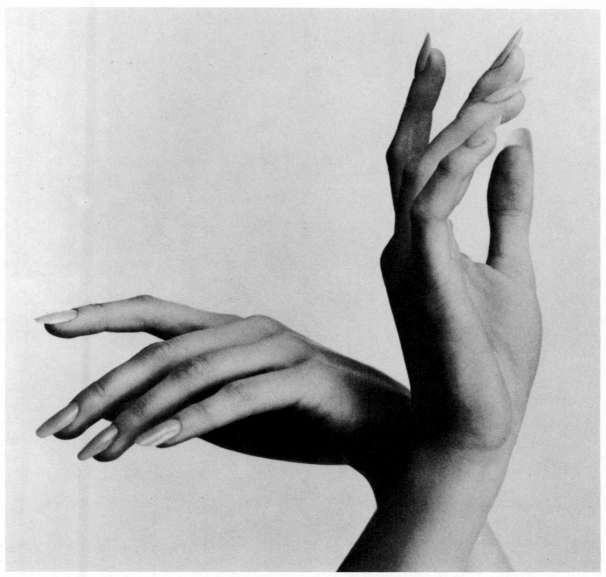

Nails, like hair, are composed of keratin, which is dead tissue. Growth occurs in the living tissue at the base of the nail under the skin, which pushes the dead cells outward.

Oil Glands

The skin's oil-producing (or *sebaceous*) glands are almost always associated with hair follicles, into which they seep their oils (or *sebum*). The oily substance works its way up toward the surface, lubricating both the hair and outer layers of epidermis, which need continual lubrication in order to stay soft and flexible. Also, skin oils serve as a kind of protective coat against painful drying and chapping.

Sweat Glands and Blood Vessels

While everybody is aware that the amount we perspire is related to the temperature around us, not everybody is aware that the countless tiny blood vessels in our skin—some 15 feet of them coursing beneath every square inch of skin—also react to changes in outside temperatures. Working together, and both controlled by an automatic "thermostat" in our brain, sweat glands and blood vessels have the all-im-

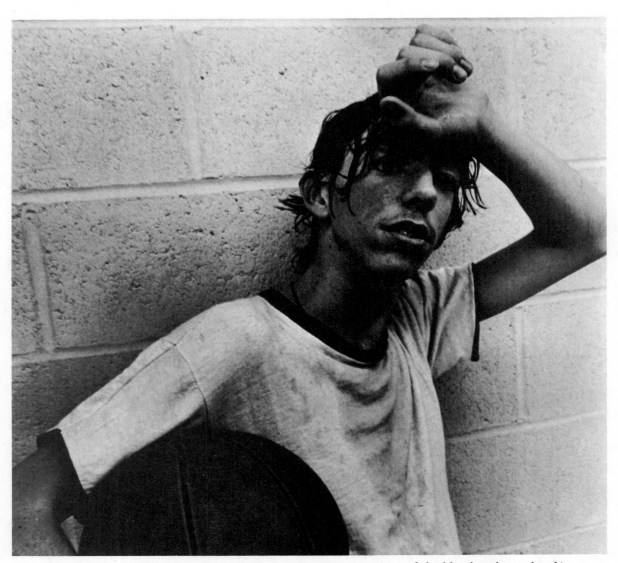

After a hard workout the skin's blood vessels dilate to expose more of the blood to the cooler skin. If the sweat does not evaporate, however, the skin's surface, hence the blood, is not cooled.

portant role of keeping our internal organs near their normal 98.6° Fahrenheit temperature.

The trick in maintaining an internal body temperature near normal is to conserve body heat when it is colder outside and to lose heat when it is warmer. Blood circulating near the surface of the skin is warmed (gains heat) or cooled (loses heat) according to the outside temperature.

The skin's myriad blood vessels constrict when the outside temperature is colder. This means that less blood can come into contact with the colder temperatures, and therefore the overall temperature level of the blood remains warmer than if the blood vessels had not become constricted. On the other hand, when the body needs to lose heat—for example, during and after a vigorous tennis match—the skin's blood vessels dilate. This accounts for the "heat flush" or reddening of skin that light-skinned people exhibit when very heated.

Sweat glands aid in temperature regulation by secreting moisture, which, evaporating on the skin's surface, cools the skin and therefore the blood flowing beneath it. Moisture that does not evaporate but remains as liquid on the skin or runs off in rivulets is not efficient in cooling. Humid air tends to prevent evaporation, while moving air or wind aids it. Sweat that evaporates as soon as it reaches the skin's surface usually goes unnoticed. Fresh sweat has no odor; but if it remains without evaporating, bacteria begin to give it the odor known medically as *bromidrosis.*

There are some two million sweat glands in the skin. Each consists of a coiled, corkscrewlike tube that tunnels its way up to the surface of the skin from the dermis or from the deeper subcutaneous layer.

Potential Trouble Spots

All of us are very conscious of the condition of our skin and worry when something seems to be wrong with it. The temptations to worry too much, to overtreat, to take the advice of a well-meaning friend, to use the wrong (but heavily advertised) product are very great. Knowing about the properties of the skin and what medical knowledge has to say about skin problems can help to avoid mistakes in caring for it. See *Skin and Hair,* p. 377. For a discussion of adolescent skin problems, see also under *Puberty and Growth,* p. 122.   EHH, Jr.

THE NERVOUS SYSTEM AND THE BRAIN

Most of us have heard often enough that the brain, acting as control center for a communication network we call our nervous system, is an incredible computer, weighing a mere three pounds. Its form and functions, however, are often described as being so much more intricate and complex than any existing or imagined computer that thorough knowledge of the brain seems very remote. This is certainly true. But it doesn't prevent us from knowing some general things about the brain and nervous system, or what its most significant parts are and how they work.

Basically, the nervous system has just two functions: first, getting information (impulses, signals, messages) from outside or inside the body to where it can be acted upon, usually in the brain; and secondly, feeding back information (for example, to the muscles) so that the indicated action can be taken. Thus, nerves can be divided by their function into two general types, each following a separate pathway: those that receive information— for example, from our senses—and pass it along, are called *sensory*, or *afferent* (inward-traveling). Those that relay information back, with a directive for action, are called *motor*, or *efferent* (outward-traveling).

The brain and the spinal cord can be considered as the basic unit of the *central nervous system*. All sensory and motor information comes or goes from this central core. The spinal cord is the master nerve tract (or nerve trunk) in our body and consists of millions of nerve fibers bundled together, somewhat like many small threads making up a large rope.

Like the spinal cord, all the lesser nerves, shown as single cords in a typical anatomical drawing, are made up of hundreds of thousands of individual fibers. Each fiber is part of a single nerve cell, or *neuron*. Neurons—there are 12 to 15 billion of them in our brain alone—are the basic structural units of the brain and nervous system, the tubes and transistors and circuits of which our personal computer is built.

The Brain

The appearance of the brain within the skull has been described as a huge gray walnut and a cauliflower. The inelegance of such descriptions is the least of many good reasons why we should be happy our brains are not exposed to public view.

Brain tissue—pinkish gray and white— is among the most delicate in our body, and the destruction of even a small part may mean lasting impairment or death. Its protection is vital and begins (if we are so fortunate) with a mat of hair on the top,

back, and sides of our skull. Next comes the resilient layer of padding we call the scalp, and then the main line of defense— the rounded, bony helmet of skull.

The brain's armor does not stop with bone. Beneath are three strong, fibrous membranes called *meninges* that encase the brain in protective envelopes. Meninges also overlie the tissue of the spinal cord; infection or inflammation of these membranes by bacteria or viruses is called *cerebrospinal meningitis*.

Between two of the meninges is a region laced with veins and arteries and filled with *cerebrospinal fluid*. This fluid-filled space cushions the brain against sudden blows and collisions. The cerebrospinal fluid circulates not only about the brain but through the entire central nervous system. Incidentally, chemical analysis of this fluid, withdrawn by inserting a hypodermic needle between vertebrae of the spinal column (a spinal tap), can provide clues to the nature of brain and nervous system disorders.

The cerebrum: What we usually mean by "brain" is that part of the brain called the *cerebrum*. It is the cerebrum that permits us all our distinctly human activities —thinking, speaking, reading, writing. Only in man does the cerebrum reach such size, occupying the interior of our entire dome above the level of the eyes.

The surface of the cerebrum is wrinkled, furrowed, folded and infolded, convoluted, fissured—anything but smooth. This lavishly wrinkled outer layer of the cerebrum, about an eighth of an inch thick, is called the *cerebral cortex*. From its grayish color comes the term "gray matter" for brain tissue. There is a pattern among its wrinkles, marked out by wider or deeper fissures, or furrows, running through the brain tissue. The most conspicuous fissure runs down the middle, front to back, dividing the cerebrum into two halves, the left hemisphere and the right hemisphere. The nerves

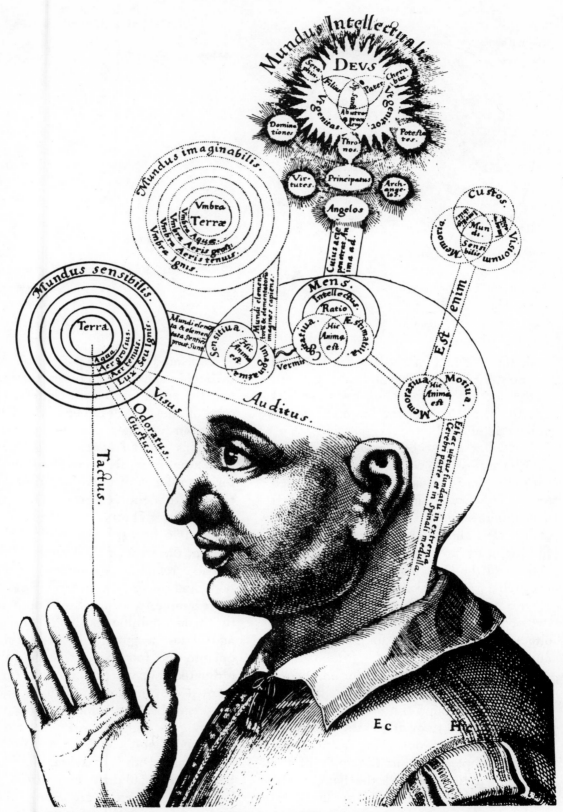

This 17th-century view of the mind recognizes the intellect, imagination, and the senses.

THE BRAIN

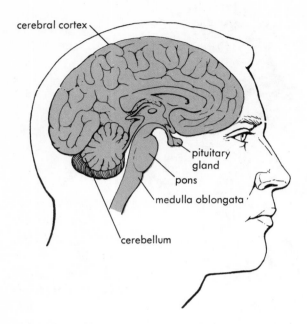

FUNCTIONAL AREAS
OF THE CEREBRAL CORTEX

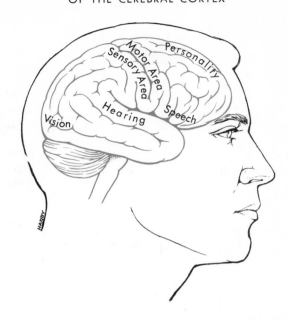

from the left half of the body are served by the right hemisphere, and the right half of the body by the left hemisphere, so that damage to one side of the brain affects the other side of the body.

The lobes of the cerebrum: Smaller fissures crisscross the cerebrum and mark out various specific areas of function called *lobes.* The frontal lobes, one on the left hemisphere and one on the right in back of our eyes and extending upward behind the forehead, are perhaps the most talked about and the least understood by medical researchers. The specific functions of most other lobes in the cerebrum, such as the two occipital lobes (centers for seeing) and olfactory lobes (centers for smelling) are much better known.

The brain stem: The cerebrum, like a large flower obscuring part of its stalk, droops down around the *brain stem.* Thus, while the brain stem originates just about in the middle of our skull, it does not emerge completely from the folds of the cerebrum until it reaches the back of the neck. Then it soon merges into the spinal cord.

Associated with this portion of the brain —roughly speaking, between the cerebrum and the spinal cord—are centers that take care of the countless necessary details involved in just plain existing, and structures (such as the *medulla oblongata* and the *pons*) that serve also as traffic control points for the billions of nerve impulses traveling to and from the cerebrum. The largest of these "lesser brains" is the *cerebellum,* whose two hemispheres straddle the brain stem at the back of the head.

The cerebellum is the site of balance and body and muscle coordination, allowing us, for example, to "rub the tummy and pat the head" simultaneously, or tap the foot and strum a guitar, or steer a car and operate the foot pedals. Such muscle-coordinated movements, though sometimes learned only by long repetition and practice, can become almost automatic—like reaching for the light switch as we enter a darkened room.

But many other activities and kinds of behavior regulated by the part of the brain below the cerebrum are more fully automatic: the control of eye movement and focusing, for example, as well as the timing of heartbeat, sleep, appetite, and metabolism; the arousal and decline of sexual drives; body temperature; the dilation and constriction of blood vessels; swallowing; and breathing. All these are mainly functions of the *autonomic nervous system*, as opposed to the more voluntary actions controlled by the *central nervous system*.

The Body's Nervous Systems

Simply speaking, the human body has only one nervous system, and that is all the nerve cells, nerve cords, nerve centers, voluntary and involuntary, in the body. It is helpful, however, though quite arbitrary, to divide our nerves into the central and autonomic nervous systems. This division tends to obscure the countless interconnections and interplay between the two systems. For example, where do you place the control of breathing, or blinking? Such actions are automatic except when we choose to regulate them.

The Central Nervous System

The central nervous system, as noted above, includes the brain and the spinal cord. It also includes all the nerves of conscious response and voluntary action that link up with the brain and spinal cord.

Twelve pairs of *cranial nerves* originate within the brain and emerge at its base. These include the very important nerves that connect with our sense organs, nerve bundles that control the facial and neck muscles, and the *vagus* (or tenth cranial nerve) that serves the heart, lungs, stomach, intestines, esophagus, larynx, liver, kidneys, spleen, and pancreas. The vagus nerve, although anatomically part of the central nervous system, controls bodily functions that are mainly automatic.

Spinal nerves branch out from the spinal cord as it snakes its way through the vertebrae of the spinal column. All the major nerve cords that wrap around the trunk and reach the arms and hands, legs and feet, originate from spinal nerves.

THE BRAIN AND THE CRANIAL NERVES

Cranial Nerves

1. olfactory: smell
2. optic: vision
3. oculomotor: muscle of eyes
4. trochlear: muscle of eyes
5. trigeminal: sense of touch in face
6. abducens: muscle of eyes
7. facial: muscles of face
8. acoustic: hearing and balance
9. glossopharyngeal: taste
10. vagus: heart, lungs, abdomen
11. hypoglossal: tongue muscles
12. accessory: neck muscles, eyeball

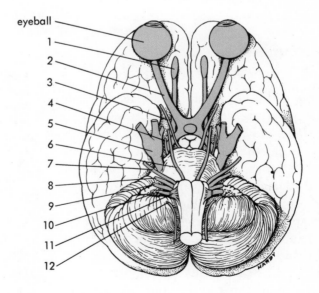

View of the Underside of the Brain

The cranial nerves and the spinal nerves, together with all those nerves lying outside the confines of the brain and spinal cord, are sometimes referred to as the *peripheral nervous system*. This term can be confusing, however, because it is also used to include all the nerves of the autonomic nervous system, next discussed.

The Autonomic Nervous System

The muscles served by the central nervous system are all of one general type (striated), while the muscles served by the autonomic system are called involuntary or smooth. The autonomic nerves regulate body activity without our conscious control—for example, as we sleep. They are rather elegantly divided into two categories: *sympathetic* and *parasympathetic* nervous systems. These are distinguishable primarily by their opposite effects on the body organs. For example, impulses along parasympathetic nerve trunks dilate blood vessels, slow the heartbeat rate, and increase stomach secretions, while the sympathetic system constricts blood vessels, increases rate of heartbeat, and inhibits stomach secretions.

The Neuron—
What Nerves Are Made Of

A nerve cell is a grayish blob of tissue from which protrude several short gray fibers, *dendrites*, and one longer whitish fiber, an *axon*. Both the dendrites and the axon resemble ropes with their ends splayed and frayed. Dendrites register impulses coming into the central blob of the neuron (perhaps from a neighboring neuron's axon); an axon picks up the incoming impulses and carries them away.

Both units are equally important for normal nerve functioning, but the axon is far more showy as an anatomical structure. All nerve cords are made up of the single

THE AUTONOMIC NERVOUS SYSTEM

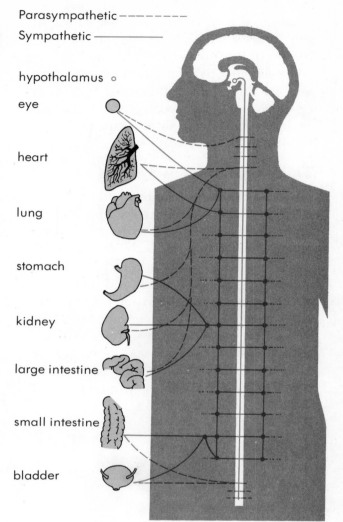

Parasympathetic ---------
Sympathetic ————

hypothalamus ○

eye

heart

lung

stomach

kidney

large intestine

small intestine

bladder

Emotional stress can cause sympathetic nerves automatically to dilate the pupils of the eyes, affect breathing and digestion, quicken heartbeat, increase blood supply to the muscles, stimulate sweat glands, etc. In contrast, parasympathetic nerves relax internal organs and glands. The tiny hypothalamus above the pituitary gland controls and balances the workings of the two sets of nerves.

strands of many axons, which may reach lengths of several feet. In other words, if we could stretch out certain neurons in our body—for example, those making up the sciatic nerve that runs from the small of the back to the toes—their axon "tails" would make them three or four feet long.

Myelin: A normal axon usually has a fatty coating of insulation called *myelin.* An axon severed into two pieces cannot grow together again; but if the myelin sheath is pretty much intact, a surgeon can sometimes restore nerve function by sewing the two ends together, or replace the nerve with one from another part of the body. The part of the severed axon connecting to the central portion usually remains alive in any case—which is why a person can often still retain the sensation of feeling in an amputated part.

Certain serious and progressively disabling diseases involve the gradual loss (*demyelination*) of this coating, causing paralysis, numbness, or other loss of function in an organ; a demyelinated nerve fiber is not able to carry impulses to and from the brain. Two such diseases are multiple sclerosis and "Lou Gehrig's disease" (amyotrophic lateral sclerosis).

Effects of aging: Once we reach maturity, the number of our nerve cells begins to decrease, because our bodies cannot manufacture new neurons to replace the ones that die in the normal process of living. (Other kinds of tissue are continually replenished with new cells.) This has some relation to senility, but the loss of a few million out of many billions of brain and nerve cells has little effect on mental powers unless the losses are concentrated in one area.

THE NEURON

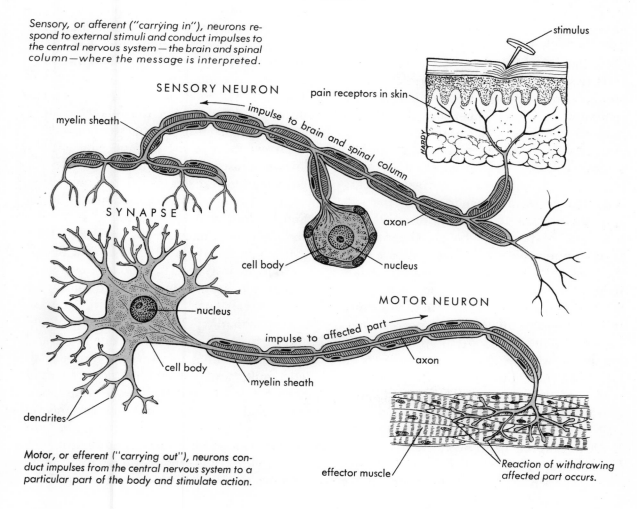

Sensory, or afferent ("carrying in"), neurons respond to external stimuli and conduct impulses to the central nervous system — the brain and spinal column — where the message is interpreted.

stimulus

SENSORY NEURON

myelin sheath

impulse to brain and spinal column

pain receptors in skin

SYNAPSE

axon

cell body

nucleus

nucleus

MOTOR NEURON

impulse to affected part

cell body

myelin sheath

axon

dendrites

Motor, or efferent ("carrying out"), neurons conduct impulses from the central nervous system to a particular part of the body and stimulate action.

effector muscle

Reaction of withdrawing affected part occurs.

Synapse, Ganglion, and Plexus

When a nerve impulse, traveling away from the neuron's central part, reaches the ends of an axon, it meets a gap which it must jump to get to the tentaclelike dendrites of the next neuron. This gap is called a *synapse*.

At certain points in the body a great many nerve cell bodies and branches are packed closely together, with a resulting profusion of interwoven axons, dendrites, and synapses. Such a concentration of nervous tissue is called a *ganglion,* or *plexus*. A blow or jolt to such an area can be extremely painful and even stupefying—affecting as it does a whole network of nerves —as anyone who has been hit in the solar plexus or learned the pressure points of karate knows.

The Movement of Impulses Along Nerve Fibers

There is really no exact counterpart in the mechanical world for how an impulse moves along a nerve fiber and then jumps across a synapse to the next nerve. Nor is this movement completely understood by scientists. Suffice it to say that it is somewhat like an electrical current moving along in a chemical environment that allows the impulse to travel, in discreet little jumps, at a speed of about 200 miles per hour—quite slowly when we compare it to the speed of light or electricity: 186,000 miles per second. This speed serves us quite well in most situations, but there are times when we wish human beings' nerves could act more quickly—on the highway, for example, or when a cherished vase starts to topple off the mantelpiece.

One of the simplest and quickest kinds of reactions to an outside stimulus is one that bypasses the brain. We don't really think to pull our hand away from a piping hot radiator. This is called a *spinal reflex*. What happens is that the sensory nerve endings in the finger pick up the "too hot" impulse from the radiator; the impulse then travels to the spinal cord where it activates the motor nerve pathway back to the burned finger, carrying the message, "Jerk your finger away!"

When to Suspect Trouble

Our entire existence as human beings depends so much on the normal functioning of our brain and nervous system that any real brain or nervous disorder or disease is a very serious matter. A sprained joint or cut foot can spell doom for an animal that depends on speed and mobility for survival; but the same injury is often not much more than a painful inconvenience to us. Impairment of our brain or nervous system is far more of a threat to our survival.

Multiple sclerosis and meningitis have been mentioned as serious disorders affecting the nerves; others are Parkinsonism, shingles, encephalitis, and brain tumors. These are six good reasons why we should never shrug off any of the following signs and symptoms of nervous-system disorders: recurrent headaches, intense pain of unknown cause, tremors, numbness, loss of coordination, dizziness, black-out, tics, cramps, visual difficulties, and loss of bowel and bladder control. Also, any person who has remained unconscious for more than a few minutes should be taken to a doctor as soon as possible. This applies even when the person has regained consciousness and says he feels fine.

Our complex emotions, of course, are linked to the functioning of our brain and nervous system. A mind free of undue anxiety, guilt, and frustration functions better than a mind racked with worries and conflicts, and is a much more efficient and reliable leader of the body. See also *Diseases of the Muscles and Nervous System*, p. 469. For a discussion of emotional maturation and health, see Chapter 3, p. 216. EHH, Jr.

THE CIRCULATORY SYSTEM, THE HEART, AND BLOOD

When the heart stops beating—that is to say, stops pumping blood—for longer than a couple of minutes, we stop living. But the heart, fortunately, is extremely sturdy. It is also simple in construction, capable of operating at a great many different speeds, in many cases self-repairing if damaged, and probably the one continuously operating automatic pump that we could, with any confidence, expect to last 60 or 70 years or longer.

These simple facts tend to be forgotten today, in what is probably the most heart-conscious era in history. True, heart disease, along with cancer, is statistically one of today's major killers. But we should remember two circumstances: not until about 50 years ago did deaths from heart disease begin to be accurately recognized and reported; second, with longer and longer life spans, it becomes more likely that a non-stop vital organ like the heart will simply wear out. Heart transplants, open heart surgery, and artificial heart parts—often reported sensationally in the public media—have also conditioned us to think of our hearts as terribly vulnerable, rather delicate, a bit inadequate to their tasks, and quite open to improvement.

Advances in heart surgery do, indeed, hold great promise for persons whose hearts had been considered, until now, irreversibly damaged or diseased. But the great attention accorded such miracles of medicine tends to obscure the humdrum, day-in-day-out, low-key drama performed for a lifetime by a healthy, uncomplaining heart.

The Heart and Circulatory Network

Perhaps the best way to put the heart in perspective is to place it where it belongs, at the hub of the body's circulatory system. This hollow, fist-sized lump of sinewy tissue is located behind the breastbone, centered just about at the vertical mid-line of our chest. It is connected into a closed system of flexible tubes, called blood vessels, ranging down from finger-thick to microscopically slender, that reach into every cavern, crevice, and outpost of our body—a network of some 70,000 miles.

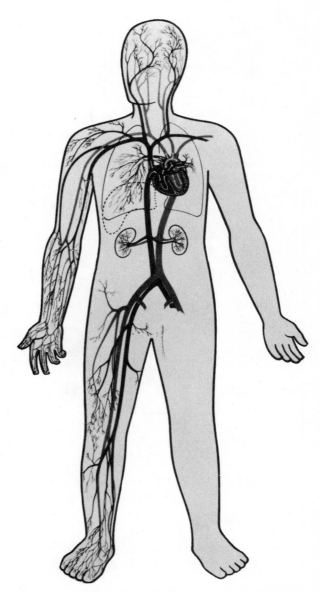

The positions of the heart, lungs, liver, and kidneys are shown in relation to the circulatory system.

THE CIRCULATORY SYSTEM

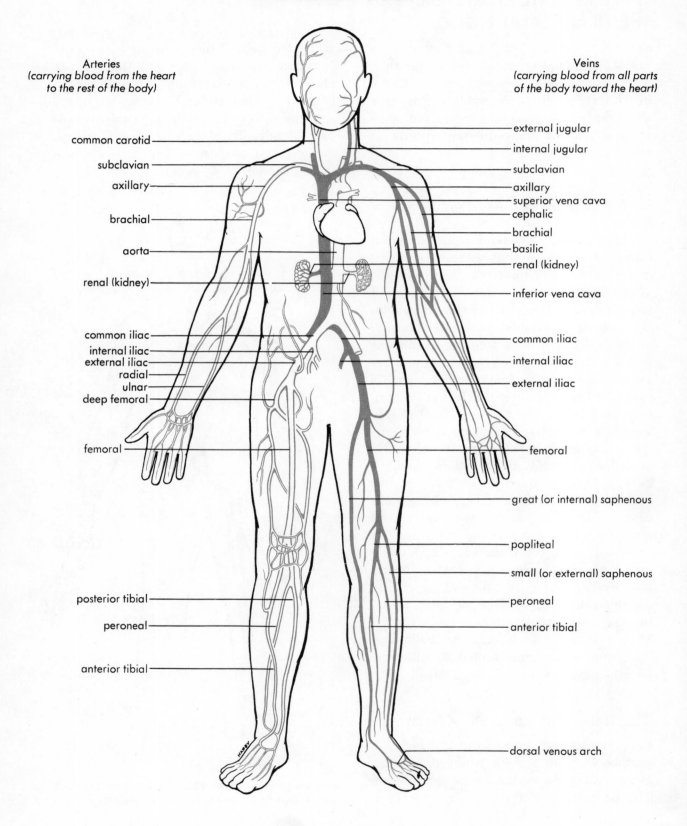

Arteries
*(carrying blood from the heart
to the rest of the body)*

Veins
*(carrying blood from all parts
of the body toward the heart)*

common carotid

subclavian

axillary

brachial

aorta

renal (kidney)

common iliac
internal iliac
external iliac
radial
ulnar
deep femoral

femoral

posterior tibial

peroneal

anterior tibial

external jugular

internal jugular

subclavian

axillary

superior vena cava

cephalic

brachial

basilic

renal (kidney)

inferior vena cava

common iliac

internal iliac

external iliac

femoral

great (or internal) saphenous

popliteal

small (or external) saphenous

peroneal

anterior tibial

dorsal venous arch

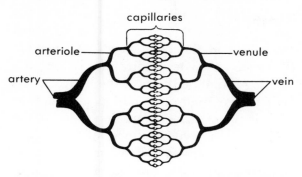

Diagram of Artery-Capillary-Vein Sequence

Blood

What makes this fairly rudimentary collection of plumbing so absolutely indispensable to life is the fluid it pumps—blood. If any part of the body—cell, tissue, or major organ—is denied circulating blood and the substances it carries with it for longer than a few minutes, that part will fail. It is the job of the heart and the blood vessels to get blood to all the body's far-flung tissues, where it both picks up and deposits substances.

The heart has essentially one function—to push blood, by pumping action, through this 70,000-mile network of blood vessels. We have about six quarts of blood in our body, pumped at the rate of about five ounces every time the heart beats (normally about 72 times a minute), which we feel as our pulse. The blood circulates and recirculates through the blood vessels, pushed along by the pumping of the heart.

Arteries and veins: The blood vessels are generally described as *arterial,* referring to the *arteries* that carry blood away from the heart; or *venous,* referring to the *veins* through which blood seeps and flows back toward the heart to be repumped. A large artery such as the *aorta* branches into smaller arteries, and these eventually into still smaller vessels called *arterioles,* and the arterioles, finally, into the smallest blood vessels, the *capillaries.* These in turn open onto other capillaries, which are the starting point for the return of blood to the heart.

The microscopic capillaries typically form a kind of cat's cradle connection, sometimes called a capillary bed, at the transition zone where arterial blood becomes venous blood. The returning blood moves from the capillaries to small veins called *venules* (the counterparts of arterioles) and through successively larger veins back to the heart.

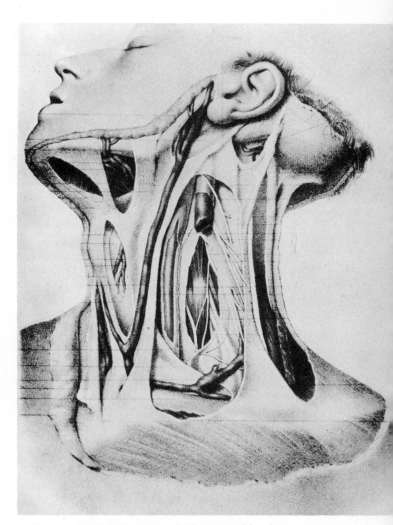

In this anatomical drawing of the major blood vessels of the neck, the long vessel running in front of the ear is the carotid artery. The large vessel in cross-section directly below the ear is the jugular vein.

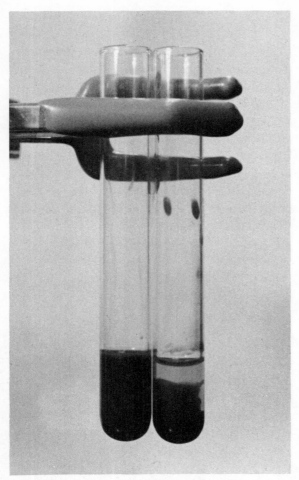

The right test tube shows a retracted clot of whole blood. Left standing for two hours, the plasma's clotting factors combined with red cells, leaving a clear fluid (serum) above. The blood in the left tube was treated with an anticoagulant to prevent clotting.

by oxygen starvation of vital tissues. Before a unit of blood is pumped out by the heart to the body, it picks up in the lungs the oxygen that we have inhaled and which every cell in the body needs to function. The blood then transports the oxygen, delivering it to other parts of the body. By the time a given unit of blood has made a tour of the blood vessels and returned to the lungs, it has given up most of its oxygen and is laden instead with carbon dioxide, the principal waste product of living processes. The venous blood releases its carbon dioxide, to be exhaled by the lungs.

Distributor of nutrients: Food, or more accurately the nutrient molecules needed by cells, are also transported throughout the body by the blood. In the digestive tract, food is broken down into tiny submicroscopic pieces that can pass through the tract's walls (mainly along the small intestine) and be picked up by the blood for distribution around the body.

One of the specialized, small-volume transportation jobs handled by the blood is to pick up hormones from the endocrine glands and present these chemical messengers to the organs they affect.

Blood and Our Internal Fluid Environment

Blood is a distinctive and recognizable type of tissue, but this does not mean it is a stable, uniform substance with a fixed proportion of ingredients. Quite the opposite is true: its composition is ever changing in response to the demands of other body systems. Other organs are constantly pouring substances into the blood, or removing things from it. Blood in one part of the body at a given moment may be vastly different in chemical make-up from blood in another part of the body.

Despite its changing make-up, blood does have certain basic components. A sample of blood left to stand for an hour

Blood is really a kind of fluid tissue. About 80 percent of its volume is water, and blood's indispensable, life-sustaining power is owed in great part to its watery base, which permits it both to flow and to take up and carry materials in solution. All our tissues and organs have a kind of give-and-take arrangement with the circulating blood.

Carrier of oxygen: Perhaps the most critical of these give-and-take transactions occurs in the lungs; it is this transaction that if interrupted by heartbeat stoppage for more than a very few minutes causes death or so separates into a clear, watery fluid with a yellowish tinge and a darker, more solid clump. The clear yellow liquid is called *plasma,* and accounts for about 55 percent of the volume of normal blood. The darker clump is made up mainly of the blood's most conspicuous and populous inhabitants, the red cells that give blood its color.

Plasma: It is the plasma that enables our blood to carry out most of the transportation tasks assigned it. Being over 90 percent water, the plasma has water's property of being able to carry substances both in solution and in suspension. (A substance in solution is one, like salt, that must be removed from water by chemical or physical action, such as boiling; while a substance in suspension—such as red blood cells within whole blood in a standing test tube—separates out more readily, particularly when its watery carrier has been contained and its flow stilled.)

Red blood cells: Red blood cells (or *erythrocytes*) numbering in the trillions are carried in suspension by the plasma. In turn, the red blood cells carry the single most important substance needed by the body's cells—oxygen. For such an important task, the red blood cell looks hardly adequate. As it matures, this cell loses its nucleus. Lacking a nucleus, it is sometimes not even called a cell but a red blood *corpuscle.* What gives red blood cells their special oxygen-carrying ability, and also their color, is their possession of a complex iron–protein substance called *hemoglobin.*

Hemoglobin: Molecules of hemoglobin have the property of loosely combining with oxygen where it is plentiful, as in the lungs. They can then hold on to oxygen until they reach an area where oxygen has been depleted by the demands of living processes. There—usually in the fine tubes of the capillaries—hemoglobin's hold on oxygen is challenged by the demands of other cells, and the red blood cells give up their

oxygen. The hemoglobin of red cells develops an immediate affinity for carbon dioxide, the waste product of cell metabolism, and the red blood cells then carry this carbon dioxide back to the lungs for exhalation.

Hemoglobin's ability to carry oxygen is not unique. Water, and therefore plasma, also have this ability. Hemoglobin's specialness lies in how much oxygen it can carry. Hemoglobin increases by more than 50 times the oxygen-carrying capacity of our blood.

White blood cells: White blood cells have many different shapes and sizes, all going

This three-dimensional model of the hemoglobin molecule is about 127,000,000 times its actual size.

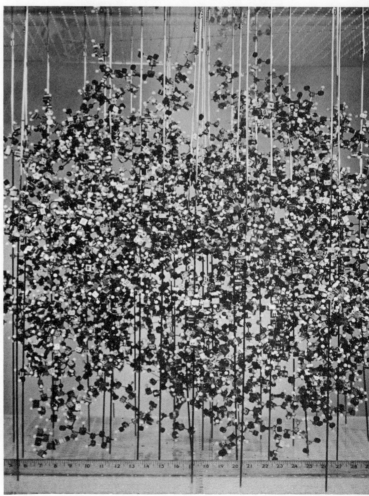

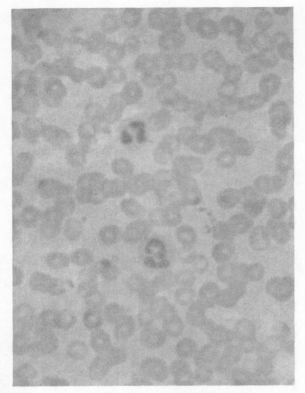

In this normal blood smear, red corpuscles, which are really biconcave disks, look like doughnuts. The two larger, darker shapes near the center are white blood cells; the specks nearby are platelets.

under the general scientific name of *leukocytes.* They are typically larger than red blood cells, but far less numerous. If we accept an estimate of 25 trillion as the number of living red blood cells in our body, then the number of white blood cells might be generously estimated at around 40 billion, a ratio of one white cell to about 600–700 reds.

According to their shape, size, and other characteristics, white blood cells have been divided into various categories such as lymphocytes, monocytes, and granulocytes. But as a group these blood cells are distinguished by their common propensity for attacking foreign bodies that invade our tissues, whether these invaders be sizable splinters or microscopic bacteria. White blood cells move in force to the site of an infection, do battle with the intruding

agents, and frequently strew the area with the wreckage of the encounter—a collection of dismantled alien bacteria and dead white cells which we know as pus.

Platelets: Platelets, also called *thrombocytes,* initiate some of the first steps in the complex biochemical process that leads to the clotting of blood. They thus help to spare us from bleeding to death from a slight injury. Platelets are the most rudimentary and diminutive of the major blood components. Like mature red blood cells, they lack nuclei, but are only one-quarter as big. By no stretch of the imagination can they be called blood cells. Rather, they are blood elements—bits of cell substance with a recognizable size and shape, circulating with the blood.

The proportions of blood cells: All the several types of blood cells and subcells in a healthy body occur in proportions that, though never precisely fixed and unchanging, are recognized as having normal upper and lower limits. If a particular type of cell shows a sudden increase or decrease in population, so that its proportion relative to other blood cells shows a variation markedly outside its normal range, some infection, disease, or disorder must be suspected.

In addition to occurring in certain normal-range proportions, each type of cellular blood component has a typical shape, appearance, and set of chemical and physical properties. Variations from these norms occur in many diseases.

The analysis of blood samples (usually taken from the finger or arm) and their inspection under a microscope have proved invaluable in diagnosing illness and disease, often before a person feels any symptoms whatsoever. This is why a thorough medical check-up should always include taking a sample of your blood. It is then up to the doctor to decide which of the dozens of tests should be made on your blood in the medical laboratory. One common test is a *blood count,* in which the number of a certain type of cell in a given unit of your blood can be estimated, and then compared to the normal number in the same amount of blood.

Blood groups and Rh factors: The identification of *blood groups* and *Rh factors* is another aspect of blood analysis. The four most common blood groups are called A, B, AB, and O, classifications based on chemical differences that may be incompatible if one group is mixed with another. Thus, it is absolutely essential before a person receives a blood transfusion to know both his own blood type and the type of the blood he is to be given. Blood group "O" is considered the safest for transfusion, and people with type O blood are sometimes called "universal donors." It is a wise practice to carry, along with your other important cards, a card giving your own blood type. The blood of a donor, however, is always *cross-matched* (checked for compatibility) with the blood of the person who is to receive it in order to avoid transfusion reactions.

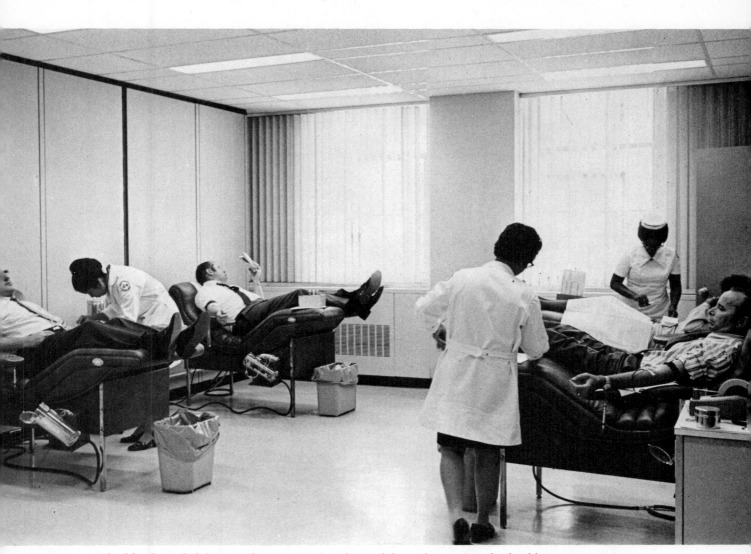

The blood needed for transfusions must be obtained from donors. For the healthy person, giving blood is painless and safe, and modern donor centers provide a cheerful, efficient atmosphere.

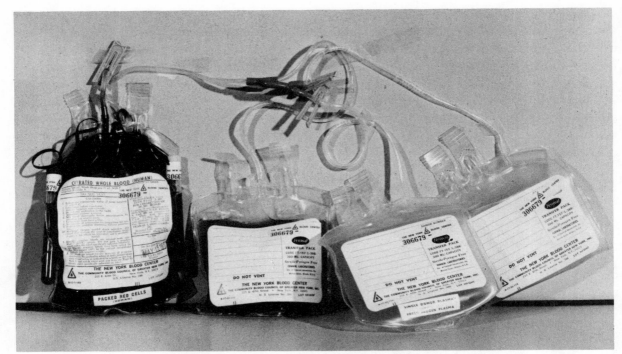

The blood from a single donor can help five people get well by being separated into five components. Shown here is a "quad pack" used for the fractionation of whole blood into red cells,
white cells, platelets and plasma. The plasma will yield clotting factors used in treating hemophilia.

Blood Cell Manufacture and Turnover

Most types of blood cells, both red and white, are manufactured in the red marrow of bones. The rate and quantity of total production is staggering; estimates range from one to five million red blood cells per second. This prodigious output is necessary because blood cells are disintegrating, having served their useful lives, in the same enormous numbers every second. The normal lifespan of a red blood cell is about four months, which means that four months from now every blood cell in your body will have died and been replaced with new cells.

The liver as a producer of red blood cells: The red bone marrow is backed up by several other tissues that can, if called upon, turn out blood cells in quantity or serve as specialized producers of certain blood cells and blood elements. One such organ is the liver, which, before and after birth and into childhood, is a site of red blood cell production. In an emergency, such as severe internal hemorrhage, the liver sometimes reverts to its earlier function of manufacturing red cells. The liver also serves as a kind of salvage yard for the iron from dead red cells. It stores the iron for later combination into hemoglobin, and passes off the rest of the red blood cell fragments as part of the bile pigments that empty into the duodenum of the small intestine.

The spleen as a producer of blood cells: Certain white blood cells, in particular the lymphocytes, are produced at a variety of locations in the body—for example, by the lymph nodes, by little clumps of tissue called Peyer's Patches in the intestinal tract, and by the spleen.

The spleen plays a number of interesting secondary roles in blood cell production. Like the liver, it can be pressed into service as a manufacturer of red blood cells and serve as a salvage yard for iron reclaimed from worn-out red blood cells. A newborn baby is almost totally dependent on its spleen for the production of red blood cells, with a little help from the liver. In an adult, however, a damaged or diseased spleen can be surgically removed, with little or no apparent effect on the health or lifespan of the person, provided the patient's bone marrow is in good functioning order.

Movement of blood cells through the capillaries: A blood cell must be able to slip through the microscopic, twisting and turning tunnels of the capillaries that mark the turn-about point in the blood cell's round-trip voyage from the heart. Blood cells, therefore, must be small (the point of a pin could hold dozens of red blood cells), and they must be jellylike in order to navigate the tight, tortuous, capillary channels without either blocking the channel or breaking apart themselves. A red blood cell is further adapted to sneaking through the capillaries by its concave-disk shape, which allows it to bend and fold around itself. Nevertheless, so narrow are the passageways within some of the capillaries that blood cells must move through them in single file.

Lymph and the Lymphatic System

Of all our body systems, perhaps the most ignored is the lymphatic system, although it forms a network throughout our body comparable to the blood vessels of our circulation system.

Lymph is a whitish fluid that is derived from blood plasma. As plasma circulates through the body, some of it seeps through the walls of capillaries and other blood vessels. This leakage is of the utmost importance, because the leaked fluid, lymph, supplies the liquid environment around and between individual cells and tissues that is essential for their survival.

The presence of lymph requires a drainage system to keep the fluid moving. If there were no drainage system, two things could happen: the dammed-up lymph could create areas swollen with water in which cells would literally drown, or stagnant pools of lymph could become breeding grounds for infection.

As it moves through the vessels of the lymphatic system, lymph carries away from the tissues the bits and pieces of cells that have died and disintegrated, and also potentially harmful bacteria and viruses.

Lymph and lymphocytes: Confusion often arises about the connection between the white blood cells called lymphocytes and the lymph itself. Lymph is not made up of lymphocytes, although it often carries them; lymph is simply a watery vehicle moving through the lymphatic network. At certain points along this network, the vessels enlarge into clumpy structures called *lymph nodes* (or, misleadingly, lymph glands). Lymph nodes are major manufacturing sites for lymphocytes.

Lymph nodes: Swollen glands are actually swollen lymph nodes, where a small army of lymphocytes is doing battle against invading bacteria or other harmful microscopic organisms. The lymph nodes, more than a hundred of them distributed around the body, serve as defense outposts against germs approaching the interior of the body. Those in the neck, groin, and armpits most frequently exhibit the pain and swelling that may accompany germ-fighting.

Circulation of lymph: Lymph circulates without any help from the heart. From the spaces between cells, it diffuses into lymph capillaries which, like the venous capillaries, merge into larger and larger vessels moving inward toward the heart. The lymph moves—even upward from the legs and lower part of the body—because the muscles and movements of the body are constantly kneading and squeezing the lymph vessels. These vessels are equipped with valves that prevent back-flow. This is not so very different from the way venous blood makes its way back to the heart.

Eventually, master lymph vessels from the head, abdomen, and torso join in the thoracic lymph duct, which then empties into large neck veins that carry lymph and venous blood, mixed together, back to the heart.

HOW BLOOD CIRCULATES THROUGH THE HEART

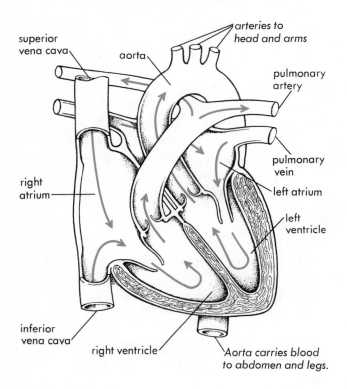

superior vena cava

aorta

arteries to head and arms

pulmonary artery

pulmonary vein

left atrium

left ventricle

right atrium

inferior vena cava

right ventricle

Aorta carries blood to abdomen and legs.

Blood from the head and arms enters the right atrium from the superior (i.e. upper) vena cava. Blood from the torso and legs enters from the inferior (i.e. lower) vena cava. The blood, controlled by a valve, passes to the right ventricle. It is then pumped into the pulmonary artery, which divides into two vessels, one leading to each lung. After being enriched with oxygen, the blood is brought back to the left atrium via the pulmonary veins, is admitted by a valve into the left ventricle, and is pumped through the aorta to be distributed to all parts of the body.

Both atria contract at the same time, forcing blood into the ventricles. Then both ventricles contract (while the atria relax), forcing blood into the great arteries. This period of contraction is called systole, and is followed by a period of relaxation called diastole.

The Heart at Work

The structure and performance of the heart, at first glance rather complicated, assume a magnificent simplicity once we observe that this pulsating knot of hollow, intertwining muscle uses only one beat to perform two distinct pumping jobs.

The heart has a right side (your right) and a left side (your left), divided by a tough wall of muscle called a *septum*. Each side has two chambers, an upper one called an *atrium* (or *auricle*), and a lower one called a *ventricle*.

How the Heart Pumps the Blood

Venous blood from the body flows into the right atrium via two large veins called the *superior vena cava* (bringing blood from the upper body) and the *inferior vena cava* (bringing blood from the lower part of the body). Where the blood enters the right atrium are valves that close when the atrium chamber is full.

Then, through a kind of trap-door valve, blood is released from the right atrium into the right ventricle. When the right ventricle is full, and its outlet valve opens, the heart as a whole contracts—that is, pumps.

To the lungs: The blood from the right ventricle is pumped to the lungs through the pulmonary artery to pick up oxygen. The trap-door valve between the right atrium and ventricle has meanwhile closed, and venous blood again fills the right atrium.

Having picked up oxygen in the lungs, blood enters the left atrium through two pulmonary veins. (They are called veins despite the fact that they carry the most oxygen-rich blood, because they lead *to* the heart; just as the pulmonary artery carries the oxygen-poorest blood away from the heart, to the lungs.) Like the right atrium, the left atrium serves as a holding reservoir and, when full, releases its contents into the left ventricle. A valve between left atrium and ventricle closes, and the heart pumps.

To the body: Blood surges through an opening valve of the left ventricle into the aorta, the major artery that marks the beginning of blood's circulation throughout the body. The left ventricle, because it has the job of pumping blood to the entire body rather than just to the lungs, is slightly larger and more muscular than the right ventricle. It is for this reason, incidentally, that the heart is commonly considered to be on our left. The organ as a whole, as noted earlier, is located at the center of the chest.

The Heart's Own Circulatory System

Heart tissue, like that of every other organ in the body, must be continually supplied with fresh, oxygen-rich blood, and used blood must be returned to the lungs for reoxygenation. The blood inside the heart cannot serve these needs. Thus the heart has its own circulation network, called *coronary arteries and veins,* to nourish its muscular tissues. There are two major arteries on the surface of the heart, branching and rebranching eventually into capillaries. Coronary veins then take blood back to the right atrium.

Structure of the Heart

The musculature of the heart is called cardiac muscle because it is different in appearance from the two other major types of muscle. The heart muscle is sometimes considered as one anatomical unit, called the *myocardium.* A tough outer layer of membranous tissue, called the *pericardium,* surrounds the myocardium. Lining the internal chambers and valves of the heart, on the walls of the atria and ventricles, is a tissue called the *endocardium.*

These tissues, like any others, are subject to infections and other disorders. An infection of the endocardium by bacteria is called *bacterial endocarditis.* (Disease of the valves is also called *endocarditis,* although it is a misnomer.) An interruption of the blood supply to the heart muscle is called a *myocardial infarction,* which results in the weakening or death of the portion of the myocardium whose blood supply is blocked. Fortunately, in many cases, other blood vessels may eventually take over the job of supplying the blood-starved area of heart muscle.

Heartbeat

The rate at which the heart beats is controlled by both the autonomic nervous system and by hormones of the endocrine system. The precise means by which the chambers and valves of the heart are made to work in perfect coordination are not fully understood. It is known, however, that the heart has one or more natural cardiac pacemakers that send electrical waves through the heart, causing the opening and closing of valves and muscular contraction, or pumping, of the ventricles near the normal rate of about 72 times per minute.

One particular electrical impulse (there may be others) originates in a small area in the upper part of the right atrium called the *sinus node.* Because it is definitely known that the contraction of the heart is electrically activated, tiny battery-powered devices called *artificial pacemakers* have been developed that can take the place of a natural pacemaker whose function has been impaired by heart injury or disease. Through electrodes implanted in heart tissue, such devices supply the correct beat for a defective heart. The bulk of the device is usually worn outside the body or implanted just under the skin. For illustrations of pacemakers, see pp. 520–521.

The fact that both ventricles give their push at the same time is very significant. It allows the entire heart muscle to rest between contractions—a rest period that adds up to a little more than half of a person's lifetime. Without this rest period,

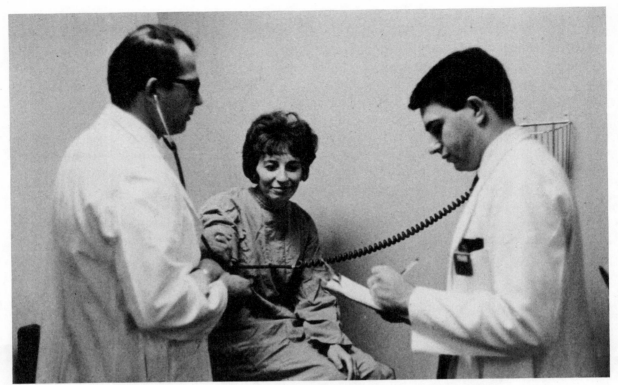

Blood pressure measures the response of the walls of major blood vessels to the force of the blood pumped through them by the heart. Pressure is greatest at systole and least at diastole.

it is more than likely that our hearts would wear out considerably sooner than they do.

Blood pressure: A doctor's taking of blood pressure is based upon the difference between the heart's action at its period of momentary rest and at the moment of maximum work (the contraction or push). The split-second of maximum work, at the peak of the ventricles' contraction, is called the *systole*. The split-second of peak relaxation, when blood from the atria is draining into and filling up the ventricles, is called the *diastole*.

Blood pressure measures the force with which blood is passing through a major artery, such as one in the arm, and this pressure varies between a higher *systolic* pressure, corresponding to the heart's systole, and a lower *diastolic* pressure, reflecting the heart's diastole, or resting phase. The device with which a doctor takes your blood pressure, called a *sphygmomanom-*

eter, registers these higher and lower figures in numbers equivalent to the number of millimeters the force of your arterial blood would raise a column of mercury. The higher systolic force (pressure) is given first, then the diastolic figure. For example, 125/80 is within the normal range of blood pressure. Readings that are above the normal range—and stay elevated over a period of time—indicate a person has high blood pressure, or hypertension.

Hypertension has no direct connection with nervous tension, although the two may be associated in the same person. What it does indicate is that a heart is working harder than the average heart to push blood through the system. In turn, this may indicate the presence of a circulatory problem, or suggest that the heart or circulation system might eventually endanger health. See also *Diseases of the Circulatory System,* p. 484, and *Heart Disease,* p. 500. EHH, Jr.

THE DIGESTIVE SYSTEM AND THE LIVER

A doctor once remarked that a great many people seem to spend about half their time getting food into their digestive tracts and the other half worrying about how that food is doing on its travels. The doctor was exaggerating, but he made his point.

The digestive tract has essentially one purpose: to break down food, both solid and fluid, into a form that can be used by the body. The food is used as energy to fuel daily activities or to nourish the various tissues that are always in the process of wearing out and needing replacement.

A normally functioning digestive tract, dealing with a reasonable variety and quantity of food, is designed to extract the maximum benefit from what we eat. Urine and feces are the waste products—things from which our body has selected everything that is of use.

Our digestive system's efficiency and economy in getting food into our bodies, to be utilized in all our living processes, can be attributed basically to three facts.

First, although the straight-line distance from the mouth to the bottom of the trunk is only two or three feet, the distance along the intestinal tract is about 10 times as great—30 feet—a winding, twisting, looping tunnel that has more than enough footage to accommodate a number of ingeniously constructed way-stations, check-points, and traffic-control devices.

Second, from the moment food enters the mouth, it is subjected to both chemical and mechanical actions that begin to break it apart, leading eventually to its reduction to submicroscopic molecules that can be absorbed through the intestinal walls into the circulatory system.

Finally each of the three main types of food—carbohydrates, fats, and proteins—receives special treatment that results in the body deriving maximum benefit from each.

Sensing the Right Kind of Food

Lips, eyes, and nose are generally given scant notice in discussions of the digestive process. But if we consider digestion to include selection of food and rejection of substances that might do us harm, then all three play very important roles.

The sensitive skin of our lips represents one of our first warning stations that food may be harmful if taken into the mouth. It

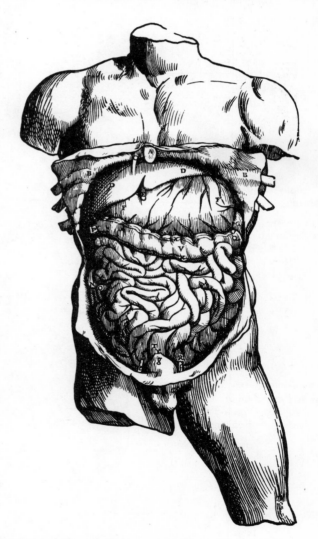

This 16th-century drawing shows the relative positions of the liver (marked D), stomach (F), and intestines.

THE DIGESTIVE SYSTEM

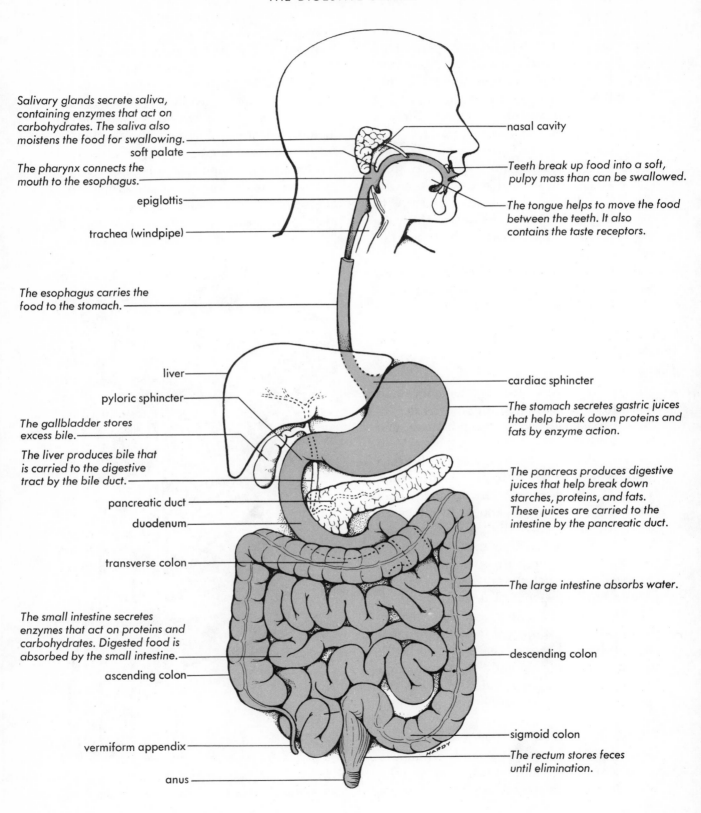

Salivary glands secrete saliva, containing enzymes that act on carbohydrates. The saliva also moistens the food for swallowing.

soft palate

The pharynx connects the mouth to the esophagus.

epiglottis

trachea (windpipe)

The esophagus carries the food to the stomach.

liver

pyloric sphincter

The gallbladder stores excess bile.

The liver produces bile that is carried to the digestive tract by the bile duct.

pancreatic duct

duodenum

transverse colon

The small intestine secretes enzymes that act on proteins and carbohydrates. Digested food is absorbed by the small intestine.

ascending colon

vermiform appendix

anus

nasal cavity

Teeth break up food into a soft, pulpy mass than can be swallowed.

The tongue helps to move the food between the teeth. It also contains the taste receptors.

cardiac sphincter

The stomach secretes gastric juices that help break down proteins and fats by enzyme action.

The pancreas produces digestive juices that help break down starches, proteins, and fats. These juices are carried to the intestine by the pancreatic duct.

The large intestine absorbs water.

descending colon

sigmoid colon

The rectum stores feces until elimination.

may tell us if a forkful of food is too hot or warn us of a concealed fishbone.

Our eyes, too, are important selection-rejection monitors for food. What else keeps us from sitting down to a crisp salad of poison ivy? Or, less facetiously, popping a moldy piece of cake into our mouth?

As mammals' noses go, man's is a very inferior and insensitive organ. Nevertheless, we probably make more use of our sense of smell in the selection and enjoyment of foods than in any other activity. The nose adds to our enjoyment of favorite food and drink not only before they enter the mouth, but also after, because stimulation of the olfactory cells in the nasal passages combines with the stimulation of the taste cells on the tongue to produce the sensation and discriminating gradations of taste.

The Mouth: Saliva, Teeth, and Tongue

By the time food leaves the mouth and is pushed down into the gullet (or esophagus), it has already received a sampling of all the kinds of punishment and prodding that will be provided by the 30-foot tube that lies ahead of it. The chances are slim that any piece of food will end that journey in the same condition it started, but if it did it would have traveled those 30 tortuous feet at the rate of something less than two feet per hour. Normally, the elapsed time is between 17 and 25 hours.

As in the rest of the digestive tract, the mouth puts both chemical and mechanical apparatus to work on a bite of food. Saliva supplies the chemical action. Teeth and tongue, backed up by powerful sets of muscles, are the mashers, crushers, and prodders.

Saliva

The mere presence of food in our mouth —or even the smell, memory, or anticipation of it—sends signals to our brain, and our brain in turn sends messages back to a system of six salivary glands: one pair, called the *sublingual glands,* located under the tongue toward the front of the mouth; another pair, the *submaxillary* (or *submandibular*) glands, a bit behind and below them; and the largest, the *parotid glands,* tucked in the region where jaw meets neck behind the ear lobes.

Saliva is mainly composed of water, and water alone begins to soften up food so that it can pass more smoothly down the esophagus toward encounters with more powerful chemical agents.

There is also a very special substance in saliva, an enzyme called *ptyalin,* whose specific job is to begin the breakdown of one of the toughest kinds of food our digestive system has to handle—starches. Starch is a kind of carbohydrate, the group of foods from which we principally derive energy; but in order for our body to utilize carbohydrate, it must be broken down into simpler forms, which we call sugars. Ptyalin, then, begins the simplification of carbohydrate starch into carbohydrate sugar.

Saliva also does a favor or two for the dominating structures of the mouth—the tongue and teeth. Without its bathing action, the tongue's taste cells could not function up to par; and because it has a mild germicidal effect in addition to a simple rinsing action, saliva helps protect our mouth and teeth from bacterial infection.

Teeth

The role of the teeth in digestion can be summed up in one word: destruction. What the wrecker's ball is to a standing building, our teeth are to a lump of solid food. They do the first, dramatic demolishing, leaving smaller fragments to be dealt with and disposed of in other ways.

Starting from the center of the mouth, we have two incisors on either side, top and bottom, followed by a canine, a couple of premolars, and three molars, the most

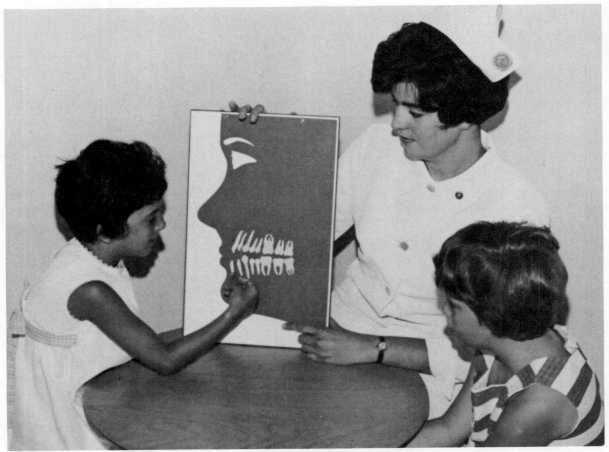

A dental assistant shows the positions of the teeth to two young patients and explains
the functions of the incisors, canines, and molars—cutting, tearing, and grinding.

backward of which (it never appears in some people) is the curiously named "wisdom" tooth, so called because it commonly appears as physical maturity is reached, at about 20 years of age.

Our teeth equip us for destroying chunks of food by a gamut of mechanical actions ranging from gripping and puncturing to grinding and pulverizing. The teeth in front —canines and incisors—do most of the gripping, ripping, and tearing, while the premolars and molars at the back of the jaws do the grinding.

The Tongue

The surface of the tongue is not smooth, but has a finely corrugated look and feel. This slightly sandpapery surface is due to the presence of thousands of tiny papillae, little pyramid-shaped bumps. When we are young, the walls of a single papilla may contain up to 300 taste cells, or buds. As we get older, the maximum number of taste buds per papilla may decline to under 100.

There are four kinds of taste cells, distinguished by the type of taste message each sends to the brain: salty, sweet, sour, and bitter. Each of the four types is a narrow specialist in one type of taste. However, simultaneous or successive stimulation of all four types (combined almost always with information picked up by our sense of smell) can produce a tremendous variety of recognizable tastes—although perhaps not so many as some gourmets or wine-tasters might have us believe.

All four types of taste buds—salty, sweet, sour, and bitter—are found associated with papillae in all areas on the surface of the tongue; but there tend to be denser populations of one or the other kinds of taste cells in certain places. For example, salty and sweet cells predominate at the tip of the tongue and about halfway back along its sides; sour cells are more numerous all the way back along the sides; bitter buds are densest at the back of the tongue.

In addition to its tasting abilities, the tongue is a very versatile, flexible, and admirably shaped bundle of muscle. Not only can it flick out to moisten dry lips and ferret out and dislodge food particles in the oral cavity, but it also performs the first mechanical step in the all-important act of swallowing.

Swallowing

Swallow. You'll find that you feel the top of your tongue pressing up against the roof of your mouth (*hard palate*). You may never have thought about it consciously, but the pressing of the tongue against the hard palate prevents food from slipping to the front of your mouth—and also gives the food a good shove up and to the back of your mouth. At this point, the *soft palate* (from which the teardrop-shaped piece of tissue called the *uvula* hangs down) slips up to cover the passageway between mouth (oral cavity) and nasal cavity, nicely preventing the food from being misdirected toward your nose.

Once past the soft palate, the food is in the *pharynx,* a kind of anatomical traffic

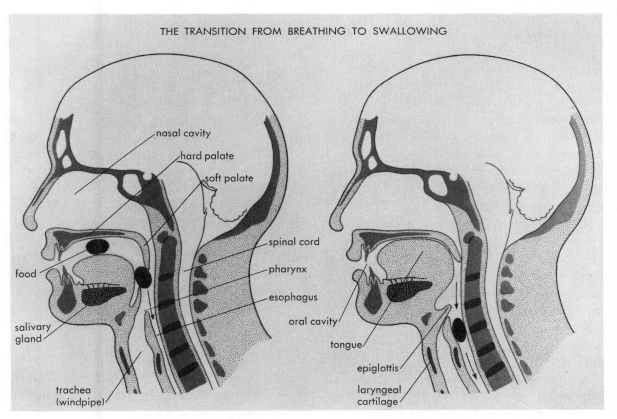

THE TRANSITION FROM BREATHING TO SWALLOWING

nasal cavity

hard palate

soft palate

spinal cord

pharynx

esophagus

oral cavity

food

salivary gland

tongue

epiglottis

laryngeal cartilage

trachea (windpipe)

(Left) The soft palate begins to move upward to close off the nasal cavity, and the epiglottis to move downward to close off the trachea. *(Right)* By the time the food has passed into the esophagus, the trachea and the nasal cavity are completely shut off.

circle with two roads entering at the top, those from the mouth and nasal cavity, and two roads leading away from the bottom, the *trachea* (windpipe) and the *esophagus* or food tube.

The epiglottis: A wedge of cartilage called the *epiglottis* protrudes from the trachea side, the side toward the front of the neck. When we are breathing, the epiglottis is flattened up against the front wall of the pharynx, allowing free movement of air up and down the trachea. Simultaneously, the epiglottis helps to close off the entrance to the esophagus; a good part of the esophagus-closing work is done by a bundle of sinewy, stretchy tissue we associate primarily with speech—the tissue of the vocal cords, otherwise known as the voice box or *larynx*. The laryngeal tissue is connected to the epiglottis above it, and supplies the epiglottis with most of its muscle for movement.

During the movement of a swallow, the larynx exerts an upward force against the epiglottis that serves to block off the trachea. At the same time, the larynx relaxes some of its pressure on the esophagus. Result: food enters the esophagus, where it is meant to go, and not the windpipe, which as we all know from having had something "go down the wrong way," produces an immediate fit of coughing.

Once we have swallowed, we lose almost completely the conscious ability to control the passage of food along the intestinal tract. Only when wastes reach the point of elimination do we begin to reassert some conscious control.

Peristalsis

The mechanical action called *peristalsis,* effected by muscles in the walls of all the organs of the gastrointestinal tract, first comes into play in the esophagus. Two layers of muscles intermesh in the intestinal walls: the inner layer encircles the esopha-

gus in a series of rings; the outer layer stretches lengthwise along the tube. These two sets of muscles work in tandem to produce the basic action of peristalsis, called a *peristaltic wave.*

The alternate contraction and relaxation of the muscles—closing behind swallowed food and opening in front of it—combine to move both liquid and solid food (medical term, *bolus*) along the digestive tract. Gravity, in a sense, is left behind once food enters the esophagus. Because of peristalsis, we can swallow lying down or even standing on our heads; and astronauts are able to eat in near zero-gravity or under weightless conditions.

Peristalsis has another important function besides moving food through the body. The constricting and relaxing muscles serve also to knead, churn, and pummel the solid remains of food left after our teeth have done their best.

Digestive Sphincters

If you think about it, the gastrointestinal tract has to be equipped with a number of gates that can open or shut, depending on the amount of food that is passing through. Otherwise, the food might push through so fast that little nourishment could be extracted from it: we would feel hungry one minute and glutted the next. The gastrointestinal tract is thus equipped at critical junctures with a number of muscular valves, or *sphincters*, which, usually under the direction of the autonomic nervous system, can regulate the movement of food through the digestive tube. Another function of a sphincter is to prevent backflow of partially digested food.

The muscles of a sphincter are often described as "pursestring muscles" because the way they draw together the sides of the digestive tube is roughly similar to drawing up the pursestrings of a purse. The first of these pursestring valves occurs at the *cardia,* the opening where the esophagus meets the stomach, and is called the *cardiac sphincter,* from its location almost directly in front of the heart. (But there is no physical connection.)

Another important muscle ring is the *pyloric sphincter,* at the opening called the *pylorus,* located at the other end of the stomach, at the connection between stomach and small intestine. The release of waste from the rectum is controlled, partly voluntarily, by an *anal sphincter,* located at the *anus,* which marks the end of the tract.

The Stomach

About ten inches down the esophagus, the food we swallow must pass the cardiac sphincter. Then the food, by now fairly well diced and mashed, passes into the stomach.

Inelegant as it sounds, the stomach is best described as a tough, leather-skinned balloon. When empty, its skin shrivels around itself like a deflated balloon; but when "pumped up" by a hearty meal, the stomach becomes a plump, J-shaped bag about a foot long and six inches wide, holding about two quarts of food and drink.

The Passage of Food Through the Stomach

Although its food-processing function tends to get more attention, the stomach's role as a storage reservoir is equally important. A moderate, well-rounded meal with a good blend of carbohydrates, proteins, and fats takes usually a minimum of three hours to pass out of the pyloric sphincter into the small intestine—more if the meal is heavy in fats and rich foods. Thus, a meal that might take us 15 minutes to eat, may take up to 20 times as long to pass from the stomach into the small intestine. This decelerating of food's rate of passage has two very significant results: first, it allows time for the food-processing activities within the stomach; and second, it releases food (in a mushy form called *chyme*) in small, well-

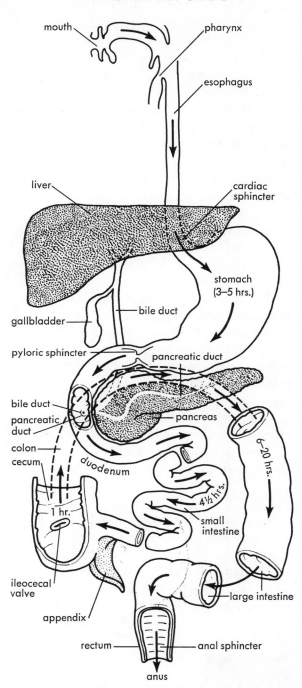

THE PASSAGE OF FOOD THROUGH THE ALIMENTARY CANAL

mouth — pharynx — esophagus — liver — cardiac sphincter — stomach (3–5 hrs.) — bile duct — gallbladder — pyloric sphincter — pancreatic duct — bile duct — pancreatic duct — pancreas — colon — cecum — duodenum — 4½ hrs. — 6–20 hrs. — small intestine — 1 hr. — ileocecal valve — large intestine — appendix — rectum — anal sphincter — anus

This drawing indicates the duration of each digestive process. Food enters the mouth and is passed through the pharynx and esophagus into the stomach, where it is partly digested. The small intestine completes digestion and absorbs digested food. The large intestine absorbs excess water. Indigestible residue collects in the rectum for later disposal.

spaced amounts that can be efficiently handled by the small intestine.

Although the stomach is not an absolutely essential organ—a person can live a full life with part or even all of it removed—it is a tremendous convenience. Without a stomach, frequent, carefully selected, well-chewed small feedings rather than "three square meals a day" are necessary so as not to overburden the small intestine, which can handle only a small quantity of food, well-mashed, at one time. If too much food goes directly to the small intestine, only so much nourishment (carbohydrates, proteins, fats) per meal can be supplied to the body, with the result that we would be weak from hunger after going a few hours without eating.

It will come as no surprise to know that the food processing done in the stomach is both mechanical and chemical. The three layers of crisscrossing muscles in the stomach walls are rarely still. They contract and relax continually, squeezing, pummeling, and mixing the stomach's contents into chyme. So active and relentless is the stomach's muscular activity that it actually "chews up" pieces of food that have been swallowed too hastily.

Stomach Chemicals

The various chemicals found in the stomach are produced and secreted into the stomach cavity by some 40 million gland cells that line the interior stomach walls. The constant wiggling and jouncing of the stomach helps to mix these chemicals thoroughly into the food. Each of the chemicals is secreted by a special type of cell and has a specific function. They include the digestive enzymes pepsin, rennin, and lipase; hydrochloric acid; and watery mucus.

A look at the special assignments of rennin, pepsin, hydrochloric acid, and mucus—and how they interact with and depend upon one another—provides a good glimpse into the elegant and complex chemical events that occur when the stomach encounters a swallow of food.

Rennin and pepsin: Rennin, well known to cheesemakers, has essentially one task: to turn milk into milk curds. But the curds are not ready to pass on to the small intestine until they are further dismantled by *pepsin.* Pepsin has other duties as well: one of them is to begin the breakdown of proteins. But pepsin can only begin to split up protein foods after they have been worked on by *hydrochloric acid.*

Hydrochloric acid: Hydrochloric acid is a corrosive substance and, except in very dilute strengths, could quite literally eat away the lining of the stomach. (This is apparently what happens in cases of gastric ulcers.) Mucus secretions, with the help of fluids in the food itself, dilute the hydrochloric acid to a point where (in a normal stomach) it is rendered harmless. Even so, the normal, healthy condition inside our stomach is slightly acid. The slight acidity of the stomach serves to inhibit the growth of organisms such as bacteria.

The Small Intestine

By the time food-turned-chyme gets through the pyloric sphincter, it has already traveled about two-and-a-half feet: about 6 inches from lips to epiglottis; 10 or 12 inches down the esophagus; and about a foot through the stomach. But at this point it has actually traveled less than one-tenth of the gastrointestinal (GI) tract, and the longest stretch lies just ahead: the 20-plus feet of the small intestine, so named because of its relatively small one-to-two inch diameter. The preparation of food particles to pass through the walls of the GI tract is completed in the small intestine—almost completed, in fact, before the chyme has traveled the first foot of the small intestine. By the time it leaves the small intestine, chyme has given up virtually all its nutrients. In other words, the process called *absorption* or *assimilation* has taken place: the nutrients have left the GI tract for other parts of the body via the circulating blood and lymph. What passes on to the large intestine is principally waste and water.

The small intestine is somewhat arbitrarily divided into three sections: the *duodenum,* the *jejunum,* and the *ileum.*

The Duodenum

Within this horseshoe loop, eight to ten inches long and about two inches in diameter, more chemical interactions are concentrated than in any other section of the GI tract. One of the first jobs in the duodenum is to neutralize the acidity of the chyme. The final steps of digestion, and the absorption of food through the intestinal lining, proceed best in a slightly alkaline environment.

The alkaline juices needed to neutralize the acidity of the chyme come mainly from the liver in the form of bile. Bile produced by the liver but not needed immediately in the duodenum is stored in concentrated form in the gallbadder, a pouch-like, three-inch long organ. On signal from the autonomic nervous system, the membranous muscular walls of the gallbladder contract, squeezing concentrated, highly alkaline bile into a short duct that leads to the duodenum. Bile components are indispensable for the digestion and absorption of stubborn fatty materials.

Through a duct from the pancreas, a host of pancreatic enzymes, capable of splitting apart large, tough molecules of carbohydrate, protein, and fat, enters the duodenum. These digestive enzymes manufactured by the pancreas are the most powerful in the GI tract.

What triggers the production of bile and pancreatic juice for the duodenum? Apparently, it is a two-step process involving hormones. When the stomach walls secrete hydrochloric acid on the arrival of food,

hormones are released; they travel to the liver and pancreas with instructions to step up their production of digestive juices.

Still other strong enzymes are secreted by the walls of the duodenum and join the bile and pancreatic enzymes in the duodenum.

Thus, in the not quite foot-long tube of the duodenum, the final breakdown of food —digestion—reaches a dramatic climax. The nutrients in the food eaten some hours ago have almost all been reduced to molecules small enough to be absorbed through the intestinal walls into the bloodstream. Carbohydrates are reduced to simpler sugars; proteins to amino acids; and fats to fatty acids and glycerol.

Some absorption of these nutrients occurs in the duodenum, but the far greater proportion takes place in the next two, longer sections of the small intestine: the eight- to ten-foot jejunum and the twelve-foot ileum. Likewise, some oversize food molecules that get past the duodenum may be digested further along the small intestine.

The Jejunum

As peristalsis pushes the nutrient broth out of the duodenum and into the first reaches of the jejunum, a gradual change in the appearance of the intestinal lining is evident. Greater and greater number of *villi*—microscopic, hairlike structures— sprout from the already bumpy walls of the intestinal lining into the GI tube.

The villi: The villi (singular, *villus*) have the primary responsibility for absorbing amino acids (from protein), sugars (from carbohydrates), and fatty acids and glycerol (from fats) from the digested contents of the small intestine, and starting them on their way to other parts of the body. What the villi do not remove from the chyme—such as the cellulose fragments of fruits and vegetables—passes on to the large intestine in a thin, watery soup almost completely lacking in nutritional value.

Gland cells near the bottom of a villus secrete various enzymes, mucus, and other substances that perform digestive "mop-up operations" along the whole length of the small intestine.

The Ileum

In this third and final 12-foot section of the small intestine, villi line the walls in such profusion that the intestinal lining resembles, under moderate magnification, nothing so much as a plush, velvety carpet. The greatest numbers of the estimated five or six million villi in the small intestine are found along the lining of the ileum, making it the primary absorption site of the GI tract.

Also adding to the ileum's absorption efficiency is its gradually narrowing diameter (just one inch at its junction with the large intestine), which helps to keep the chyme always in close contact with the swishing villi. The end of the ileum is marked by the *ileocecal valve,* beyond which lies the first bulge of the large intestine, the *cecum.*

Principally because of vigorous peristaltic contractions and relaxations, the walls of the small intestine are always moving like the walls within some spasmodically flexing, nightmarish tunnel. Attached to the intestinal walls, the villi, too, are always in restless motion: waving and thrashing, protracting and retracting, even growing thinner or fatter.

Although the entire distance through the small intestine, from the pyloric sphincter to the ileocecal valve at the junction with the large intestine, is only a bit over 20 feet, the villi give the small intestine's internal lining a relatively gigantic surface area—over 100 square feet. This is about five times the surface area of our body's skin. Of course, the greatly enlarged surface area gives the small intestine lining that much more space in which to absorb nutrients.

The small intestine is supported in the abdomen by a fan-shaped web of tissues called the *mesentery.* Attached at the back of the abdomen, the mesentery connects to the small intestine at various points, and yet allows it some freedom to squirm and sway—much like the V network of ropes that attaches either end of a hammock to a tree. Nerve fibers and blood vessels also reach the small intestine via the mesentery.

The Liver, Gallbladder, and Pancreas

These three organs all share a common function—sending digestive substances to the duodenum—although, except in the case of the gallbladder, it is not their only function. Lying outside the GI tract proper, they nevertheless are indispensable in the processes of digestion and absorption. Digestive fluids from all three converge like tributaries of a river at the common bile duct, and their flow from there into the duodenum is controlled by a sphincter muscle-ring separating the duodenum and common bile duct.

From the liver, bile drips into the *hepatic duct,* which soon meets the *cystic duct* arriving from the gall bladder. Converging, they form one duct, the *common bile duct,* which meets the *pancreatic duct,* carrying enzymatic fluid from the pancreas. Like a smaller river meeting a larger one, the pancreatic duct loses its own name at this confluence and becomes part of the common bile duct, which empties on demand into the duodenum. When the sphincter of the bile duct is closed, bile from the liver is forced to back up into the cystic duct, and eventually into the gallbladder. There it is stored and concentrated until needed, when it flows back down the cystic duct.

The Liver

Four pounds of highly efficient chemical-processing tissues, the liver is the largest solid organ in the body. You can locate it

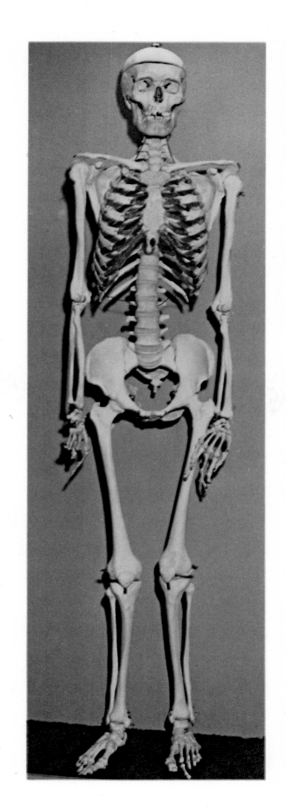

SKELETON OF THE HUMAN BODY

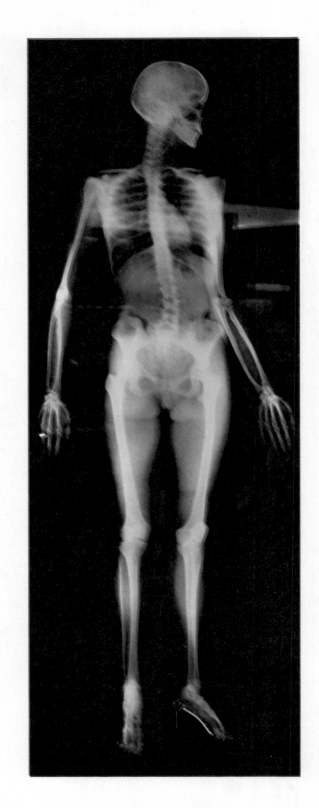

X-RAY OF THE HUMAN BODY
SHOWING THE
BONE STRUCTURE

MUSCULAR SYSTEM

Muscles are composed of special tissue in the form of bands or rings. This tissue by contracting and relaxing produces movement. These movements are under nervous control, some voluntary and some involuntary. Tendons are strong cords of tissue which attach some muscles to bones. Through their metabolic processes, muscles are responsible for a considerable share of the body's heat.

Important Muscles and Some of Their Functions

1. **Masseter** —moves the lower jaw upward.
2. **Sterno-mastoid** —bends and rotates the head.
3. **Trapezius** —raises the shoulders.
4. **Deltoid** —raises the upper arm.
5. **Pectoralis major** —pulls in the upper arm.
6. **Latissimus dorsi** —pulls back the shoulders.
7. **Biceps** —flexes the forearm.
8. **Triceps** —extends the forearm.
9. **Flexors** —of the hand and fingers.
10. **Extensors** —of the hand and fingers.
11. **Rectus abdominis** —bends the trunk forward.
12. **External oblique** —bends the trunk sideways.
13. **Sartorius** —flexes and rotates the upper leg.
14. **Gluteus maximus** —keeps the body erect.
15. **Quadriceps femoris** —extends the lower leg.
16. **Biceps femoris** —flexes the lower leg.
17. **Tibialis anterior** —flexes the foot upward.
18. **Gastrocnemius** —extends the foot downward.
19. **Peroneus longus** —flexes the foot sideways.

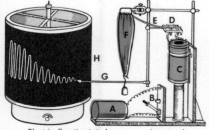

Electrically stimulated nerve causing muscle contraction and fatigue.
A. Battery B. Switch C. Inductorium D. Electrodes
E. Nerve F. Muscle G. Tracing lever H. Kymograph

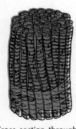

Cross section through a bundle of Muscle Fibers.

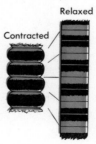

Relaxed

Contracted

Single Muscle Fiber

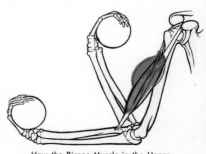

How the Biceps Muscle in the Upper Arm moves the Lower Arm.

CIRCULATORY SYSTEM

Normal Heart

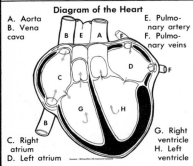

A. Aorta
B. Vena cava superior
C. Right atrium
D. Left atrium
E. Pulmonary artery
F. Coronary blood vessels

Diagram of the Heart

A. Aorta
B. Vena cava
C. Right atrium
D. Left atrium
E. Pulmonary artery
F. Pulmonary veins
G. Right ventricle
H. Left ventricle

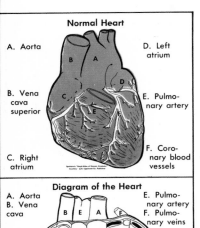

Action of the Heart

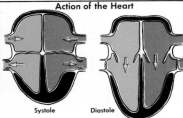

Systole   Diastole

In systole, the atria relax and fill with blood from the vena cava and pulmonary vein. The ventricles contract and force blood out through the pulmonary artery and aorta. In diastole, the atria contract, filling the relaxed ventricles.

Output of the Heart

(gallons of blood per minute) when man is

Resting

Walking

Running

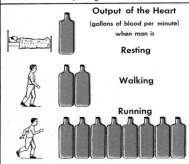

Velocity of the Blood

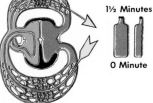

1½ Minutes

0 Minute

It takes about 1½ minutes for the total blood volume of 1½ gallons to traverse the entire Circulatory System.

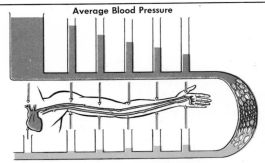

Average Blood Pressure

Illustrating diagrammatically the gradual decrease in arterial blood pressure (Red) and the continuance of the decrease in veins (Blue) after the blood has flowed through the capillaries (Purple).

A Capillary

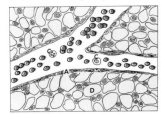

A. Capillary Wall
B. Red Blood Corpuscles
C. White Blood Corpuscles
D. Reticular Tissue

Capillary Response

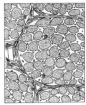 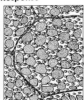

In 1/5 sq. in. of resting muscle, about 5 capillaries are open.

In 1/5 sq. in. of working muscle, about 190 capillaries are open.

Capillary Bed

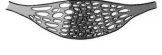

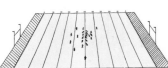

The total surface of the capillaries in the normal man amounts to an area equal to that of a football field.

The Blood Vessels

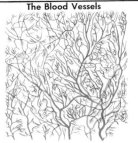

The minute network of Arteries, Veins, and Capillaries in muscle tissue.

Work of the Heart

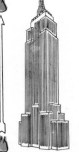

15 Minutes

The work performed by the heart in 15 minutes would be sufficient to lift its own weight to the height of the Empire State Building in the same length of time.

0 Minute

Edited by Ervin and Gordon

BLOOD

Production of Blood

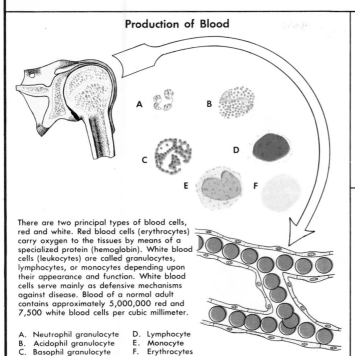

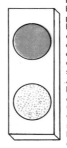

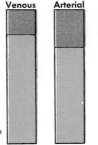

There are two principal types of blood cells, red and white. Red blood cells (erythrocytes) carry oxygen to the tissues by means of a specialized protein (hemoglobin). White blood cells (leukocytes) are called granulocytes, lymphocytes, or monocytes depending upon their appearance and function. White blood cells serve mainly as defensive mechanisms against disease. Blood of a normal adult contains approximately 5,000,000 red and 7,500 white blood cells per cubic millimeter.

A. Neutrophil granulocyte   D. Lymphocyte
B. Acidophil granulocyte   E. Monocyte
C. Basophil granulocyte   F. Erythrocytes

Clotting of Blood

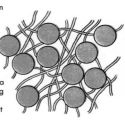

When blood is released from a blood vessel it forms a clot. This is caused by one of the blood proteins changing into tough fibers (fibrin) which form a lacy network around the blood cells.

Illustrated in the cylinder is a blood clot which by shrinking has squeezed out much of the blood liquid. At the right is a microscopic diagram showing the protein fibers wrapped around the blood cells.

Typing of Blood

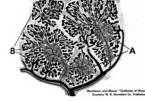

Because of differences in the blood cells and plasma, it is possible to divide all human blood into four types. When certain of these blood types are mixed together no harm occurs, but with other combinations, the blood cells stick together in tiny clots. Anyone can give or receive blood from a person of his own blood type. Blood is typed by mixing an unknown with known types on a glass slide and observing if the blood cells form clots. The arrows at the right indicate which type can safely donate to another.

(Moss System)

Chemistry of Blood

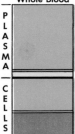

Whole Blood

PLASMA

CELLS

Venous   **Arterial**

Whole blood is composed of cells and a liquid called plasma. Plasma contains 50% water (blue), 0.5% salt (green) and 4.5% protein (yellow) as related to the whole blood. The cells contain 27% water (blue), 0.5% salt (green), and 17.5% hemoglobin and other proteins (red).

Venous blood carries approximately 18% oxygen (red) and 82% carbon dioxide (blue), while arterial blood carries 27% oxygen and 73% carbon dioxide.

The Spleen

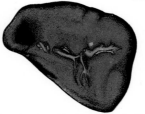

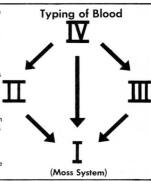

The spleen is an important organ in the circulation of blood. Among its functions are storage of blood, disposal of old blood cells, and production of lymphocytes.

Diagrammatic cross section of the spleen showing the production centers of lymphocytes (A) and the sinuses where blood is sorted (B).

LYMPH

Lymphatics

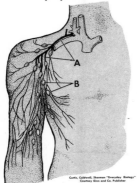

A typical distribution of the lymph vessels in one region of the body. (A) Lymph vessel, (B) Lymph node.

Production of Lymph

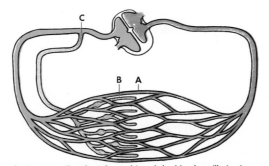

The lymphatic system (lymph and vessels) and the blood capillaries insure even distribution of liquid in the tissues, and assist in the transportation of food and waste. Lymph filters out into the tissues from the blood capillaries (A), collects in lymph vessels (B), passes through several lymph nodes, and finally flows into the large veins (C).

A Lymph Node

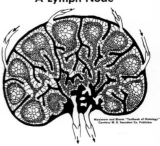

As lymph flows through the lymphatic system it is filtered through lymph nodes. These nodes remove bacteria and other foreign particles from the lymph. The diagram above shows the maze through which the lymph is filtered. Arrows indicate direction of flow.

RESPIRATORY SYSTEM

The Nasal Cavity

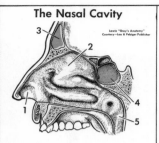

Lewis "Gray's Anatomy"
Courtesy—Lea & Febiger Publisher

Sagittal Cross Section
1. Nasal orifice
2. Nasal conchae
3. Frontal sinus
4. Sphenoidal sinus
5. Pharynx with opening of Eustachian tube.

Frontal Cross Section

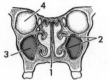

Lewis "Gray's Anatomy" Courtesy—Lea & Febiger Publisher

1. Nasal septum   3. Maxillary
2. Nasal conchae   4. Orbitae

The Sinuses

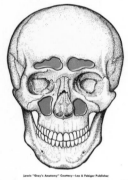

Lewis "Gray's Anatomy" Courtesy—Lea & Febiger Publisher

The sinuses are air-containing cavities in the skull which, as far as it is known, perform no function. Above, the relative positions of some sinuses are shown.

- ▬ Frontal Sinuses
- ▬ Maxillary Sinuses

The Larynx

1. Tongue
2. Epiglottis (cover of larynx)
3. Vocal cords
4. Trachea
5. Esophagus
6. Thyroid

The upper figure shows a cross section of the larynx in relation to other organs. The lower figure presents the larynx as seen from above. The slit in the center is the opening between the two vocal cords.

(Central Figure)

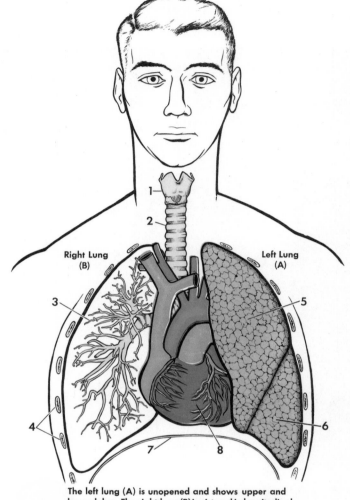

Right Lung (B)   **Left Lung (A)**

1
2
3
4
5
6
7
8

The left lung (A) is unopened and shows upper and lower lobes. The right lung (B) is pictured in longitudinal cross section with outlines of bronchial ramifications.

1. Larynx   5. Upper lobe
2. Trachea   6. Lower lobe
3. Bronchial tree 7. Diaphragm
4. Ribs   8. Heart

Respiratory Movements

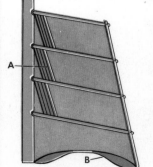

A
B

Contraction of intercostal muscles (A) and diaphragm (B) increases the volume of the chest cavity (shown in gray color) and causes inspiration.

Relaxation of intercostal muscles and diaphragm decreases chest cavity volume, causing expiration.

Alveoli

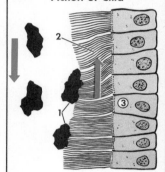

Jordan "A Textbook of Histology"
Courtesy D. Appleton-Century Co. Publisher

This is a slightly diagrammatic and greatly enlarged picture of the final ramification of the bronchi called alveoli. The gas exchange between the blood and the inspired air takes place through the wall of these little chambers (blood vessels are not shown in this picture).

Action of Cilia

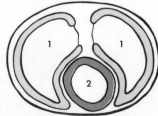

2
1
3

The respiratory canals, mainly the trachea and bronchi, are lined with ciliary epithelia. The continuous movement of the cilia shifts anything deposited on them, such as dust particles, toward the larynx.

1. Dust particles   2. Cilia
3. Ciliary epithelia

Chest Cavities

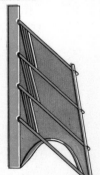

1   1
2

The above diagram shows in a cross section how the lungs and the heart are wrapped up in the pleura and the pericard and how the duplication of these membranes forms the pleural and pericardial cavities.

1. Lungs   2. Heart
   Pleural   Pericardial
   cavity   cavity

RESPIRATION

Transportation of Oxygen from air to the tissues and removal of Carbon dioxide from the tissues to the air.

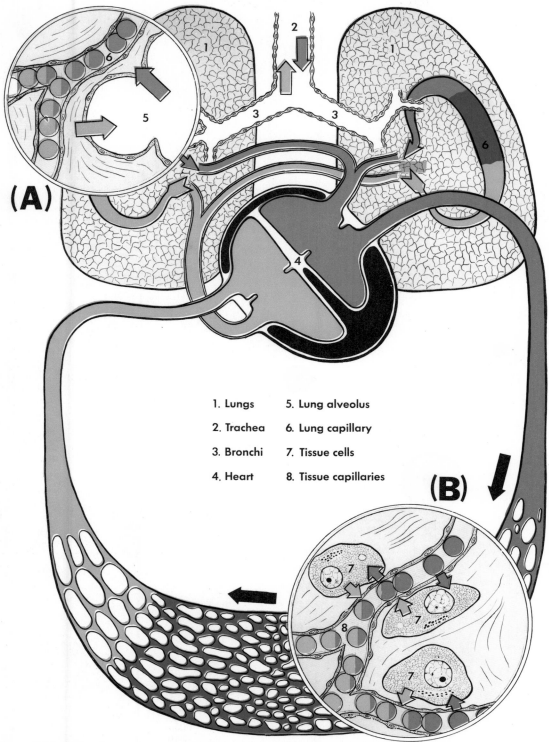

1. Lungs
2. Trachea
3. Bronchi
4. Heart
5. Lung alveolus
6. Lung capillary
7. Tissue cells
8. Tissue capillaries

Diagram showing the respiratory and circulatory systems in their common function of transporting oxygen and carbon dioxide through the body. (A) is a microscopic diagram showing the gas exchange between the alveoli and blood capillaries in the lung. (B) is a microscopic diagram showing the gas exchange between blood capillaries and tissue cells. Red arrows represent oxygen flow, blue arrows carbon dixoide flow. Blood cells in the capillaries are shown as red-blue circles in order to indicate the proportional gas content (red-oxygen, blue-carbon dioxide).

URINARY SYSTEM

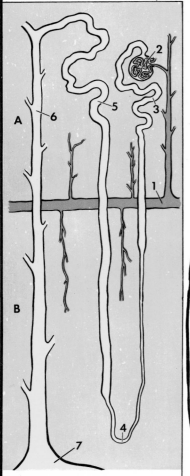

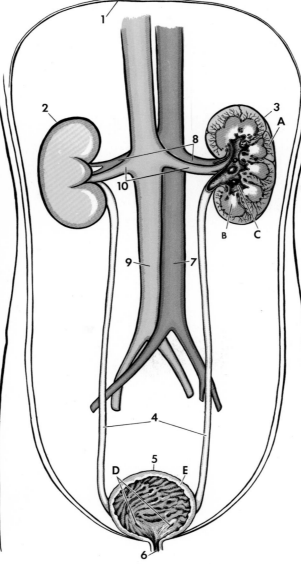

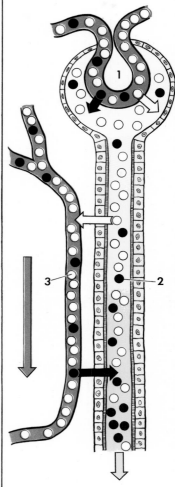

Diagrammatic cross section of the cortical (A) and medullary (B) substance showing an individual renal tubule and its blood supply. The location of the cortical and medullary substance is shown in the opened kidney of the large central figure. Production of urine in the glomerulus (2) is explained in the drawing on the right-hand side of this chart.

1. Arterial blood supply
2. Glomerulus
3. 1st convoluted tubule
4. Henle's loop
5. 2nd convoluted tubule
6. Collecting tubule
7. Pelvis

This figure illustrates the principal organs and blood supply of the urinary system and their relative positions in the human body. Urine, continuously formed in and eliminated from the kidneys through the ureters, is stored for a while in the bladder until excreted from the body through the urethra.

1. Diaphragm
2. Right kidney (unopened)
3. Left kidney (opened)
   A. Cortical substance
   B. Medullary substance
   C. Kidney pelvis
4. Ureters

5. Urinary bladder
   D. Orifices of ureters
   E. Muscular wall
6. Urethra
7. Abdominal aorta
8. Renal arteries
9. Inferior vena cava
10. Renal veins.

Production of Urine

The material to be eliminated from the blood (red) is water (white circles and arrows) and waste (black circles and arrows). In the glomerulus (1) water and waste are filtered from the blood into the initial part of the renal tubule (2). As this filtrate moves along the tubule, water is reabsorbed into the capillaries (3) surrounding the tubule. This process concentrates the filtrate. The filtrate becomes even more concentrated by the passage of additional waste material from the capillary (3) into the renal tubule. Thus urine is produced which eventually flows into the urinary bladder through the pelvis and ureters.

by placing your left hand over your right, lowermost ribs; your hand then just about covers the area of the liver. More than any other organ, the liver enables our bodies to benefit from the food we eat. Without it, digestion would be impossible, and the conversion of food into living cells and energy practically nonexistent. Insofar as they affect our body's handling of food—all the many processes that go by the collective name of nutrition—the liver's functions can be roughly divided into those that break down food molecules and those that build up or reconstitute these nutrients into a form that the body can use or store efficiently.

Breaking down food molecules: Bile, as we have seen, assists in the destruction of large food molecules in the small intestine, enabling absorption of nutrients by the villi. Bile acts to increase alkalinity, breaking down big fat molecules; stimulates peristalsis; and prevents food from putrefying within the digestive tract. Unusable portions of the bile, destined to be eliminated as waste, include excess cholesterol, fats, and various components of dead disintegrated cells. Pigments from dead cells in bile give feces their normal, dark, yellow-brown color. Other cell fragments in bile, especially iron from disintegrated red blood cells, are reclaimed from the intestines and eventually make their way via the bloodstream to other parts of the body, where they are built into new cells.

Reconstituting nutrients: Oddly enough, the liver rebuilds some of the proteins and carbohydrates that the bile has just so effectively helped to break down in the digestive tract. But this is really not so strange as it sounds. The types of proteins and carbohydrates that can be used by man for cell-rebuilding and energy are usually somewhat different in fine structure from those in his food. Thus, the liver receives the basic building blocks of proteins and carbohydrates—amino acids and sugars—

and with them builds up molecules and cells that can be utilized by the human body. The amino acids and sugars reach the liver through the *portal vein,* which is the great collection tube for nutrient-carrying blood returning from capillaries along the stomach and small intestine.

Glycogen and glucose: In the liver, sugars from the small intestine are converted into a special substance called *glycogen;* amino acids are made available as needed for building new cells to replace the cells that are always naturally dying in a healthy, normal body. Glycogen, simply speaking, is the liver's solution to a difficult space and storage problem. The form of carbohydrate the body can use best is a sugar called *glucose,* but the liver isn't large enough to store the necessary amount of glucose. The answer is glycogen, a tidy, compact sugar molecule that the liver can store in great quantities. When a call comes from any part of the body for glucose, the liver quickly converts some glycogen to glucose and releases it into the bloodstream. By this mechanism, healthy blood-sugar levels are maintained.

The liver also builds up human fats from fatty acids and glycerol, packs them off to storage, then reverses the process when necessary by breaking down body fats into forms that can serve as fuel to be burned by the body for energy.

Other functions: In addition to its functions closely related to digestion and nutrition, the liver also serves as a storehouse and processor of vitamins and minerals— it is, in fact, the manufacturer of vitamin A. It can remove many toxic substances from the blood and render their poisons harmless. It picks up spent red blood cells from the circulation and dismantles them; and it continually manufactures new blood elements.

The liver is also a manufacturing site for *cholesterol,* a substance belonging to the class of body chemicals called steroids.

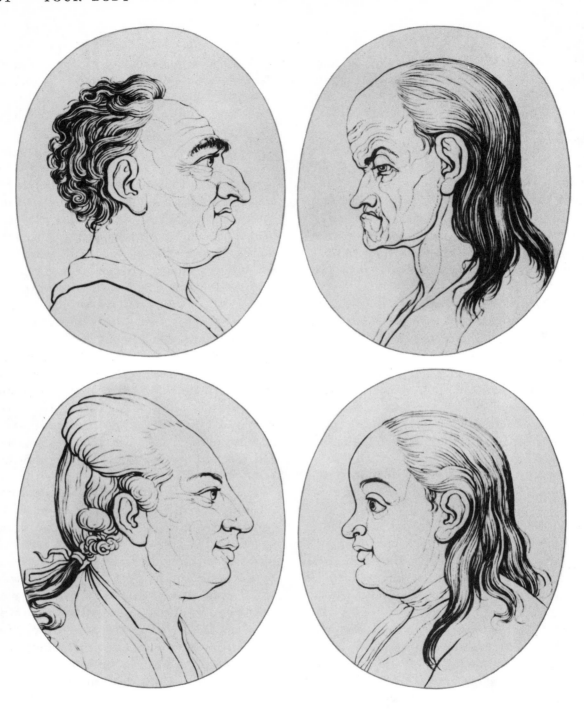

In medieval times, temperament was believed to be determined by the predominance of one or the other of four basic body liquids, or *humors:* yellow bile, black bile, blood, and phlegm. These 18th-century drawings depict representatives of each type. The person with an excess of yellow bile, thought to be secreted by the liver, was said to have a *choleric* disposition (*upper left*), characterized by a hot temper and irritability. Too much black bile was supposed to cause a *melancholic* temperament (*upper right*), marked by gloominess and depression. An excess of blood resulted in a *sanguine* disposition (*lower left*)—associated then as now with a ruddy complexion and cheerful temperament. Finally, an excess of phlegm caused one to be *phlegmatic* (*lower right*), marked by a slow or sluggish disposition.

Above-normal levels of cholesterol in the blood have been linked to hardening of the arteries and heart disease; but cholesterol in the proper amounts is needed by almost every tissue in the body. Some brain and spinal tissues, for example, have cholesterol as one of their main structural components.

With all these vital chemical activities and more, the liver might be expected to be a most delicate and fragile organ. In a sense it is: minor liver damage from one cause or another is thought to be fairly common. But what saves our liver (and us) is that we have a great deal more of it than we need for a normal healthy life. Before symptoms of a liver deficiency appear, over 50 percent of the liver cells may be destroyed. Furthermore, the liver has a great capacity for regeneration, rebuilding diseased tissues with new liver cells.

The Gallbladder

Bile stored in the gallbladder is much more concentrated and thicker than bile that is fresh from the liver. This allows the three-inch gallbladder to store a great deal of bile components. But the thickening process can also create problems in the form of extremely painful gallstones, which are dried, crystallized bile. Fortunately, the entire gallbladder can be removed with little or no lasting ill-effect. All that is missing is a small storage sac for bile.

The Pancreas

This manufacturer of powerful digestive enzymes, only six inches long, resembles a branchlet heavily laden with ripe berries. Its important role in digestion is often overshadowed by the fact that it also manufactures the hormone *insulin*. The pancreas cells that manufacture digestive enzymes are completely different from those that manufacture insulin. The latter are grouped into little clusters called the *islets of Langerhans*, which are discussed under *The Endocrine Glands*, p. 64.

The Large Intestine

The large intestine, also called the large bowel, is shaped like a great, lumpy, drooping question mark—arching, from its beginning at the ileocecal valve, over the folds of the small intestine, then curving down and descending past more coiled small intestine to the anus, which marks the end of the GI tract. From ileocecal valve to anus, the large intestine is five to six feet in length.

The junction between the ileum and the *cecum,* the first section of the large intestine, occurs very low in the abdomen, normally on the right-hand side. The cecum is a bowllike receptacle at the bottom of the colon, the longest section of the large intestine.

Just below the entrance of the ileum, a dead-end tube dangles down from the cecum. This is the *appendix vermiformis* (Latin, "worm-shaped appendage") commonly known as the appendix. Three to six inches long and one-third inch in diameter, the appendix may get jammed with stray pieces of solid food, become infected, swell, and rupture, spewing infection into the abdominal cavity. This is why early diagnosis of *appendicitis* and removal (*appendectomy*) are critically important.

Sections of the colon: The colon is divided into three sections by pronounced *flexures,* or bends, where the colon makes almost right-angle changes of direction. Above the bowl of the cecum, the *ascending colon* rises almost vertically for about a foot and a half.

Then there is a flexure in the colon, after which the *transverse colon* travels horizontally for a couple of feet along a line at navel height. At another flexure, the colon turns vertically down again, giving the name of *descending colon* to this approximately two feet of large intestine. At the end of the descending colon, the large intestine executes an S-shaped curve, the *sigmoid flexure,* after which the remaining several inches of large intestine are known as the *rectum.*

Some people confuse the terms rectum and anus: the rectum refers specifically to the last section of the large intestinal tube, between sigmoid flexure and the anal sphincters, while the anus refers only to the opening controlled by the outlet valves of the large intestine. These valves consist of two ring-like voluntary muscles called anal sphincters.

Any solid materials that pass into the large intestine through the ileocecal valve (which prevents backflow into the small intestine) are usually indigestible, such as cellulose, or substances that have been broken down in the body and blood in the normal process of cell death and renewal, such as some bile components. But what the cecum mainly receives is water.

Functions of the large intestine: The principal activity of the large intestine—other than as a channel for elimination of body wastes—is as a temporary storage area for water, which is then reabsorbed into the circulation through the walls of the colon. Villi are absent in the large intestine, and peristalsis is much less vigorous than in the small intestine.

As water is absorbed, the contents of the large intestine turn from a watery soup into the semisolid feces. Meanwhile, bacteria—which colonize the normal colon in countless millions—have begun to work on and decompose the remaining solid materials. These bacteria do no harm as long as they remain inside the large intestine, and the eliminated feces is heavily populated with them. Nerve endings in the large intestine signal the brain that it is time for a bowel movement.

The peritoneum: Lining the entire abdominal cavity, as well as the digestive and other abdominal organs, is a thin, tough, lubricated membrane called the *peritoneum.* In addition to protecting and supporting the abdominal organs, the peritoneum permits these organs to slip and slide against each other without any harm from friction. The peritoneum also contains blood and lymph vessels that serve the digestive organs. See *Diseases of the Digestive System,* p. 522.

EHH, Jr.

THE RESPIRATORY SYSTEM AND THE LUNGS

The heart, by its construction and shape, tells us a great deal about the lungs and respiration.

Interaction Between Heart and Lungs

The heart is divided vertically by a wall called a septum into right (your right) and left parts. The right part is smaller than the left: its muscles only have to pump blood a few inches to the lungs, while the muscles of the left half have to pump blood to the whole body.

The apparent reason why we have a right half of our heart, in fact, is to receive oxygen-poor blood from the veins of the body. Venous blood empties into the top-right chamber, or right atrium, of the heart, and the right ventricle pumps that oxygen-poor blood (via the pulmonary artery) to the lungs, where the blood, passing through minute capillaries, picks up oxygen.

From the lungs, the oxygen-rich blood flows back into the heart's left atrium via the pulmonary veins; and from the left atrium, the oxygen-rich blood drains into the left ventricle, from whence it is pumped via the aorta to the body.

The blood pumped to the lungs by the right ventricle is oxygen-poor blood: it has given up its oxygen to the cells that need it around the body. But this "used blood" is rich in something else—carbon dioxide. As the body's cells have taken oxygen, they have given up carbon dioxide to the circulating blood. For both oxygen and carbon dioxide, the "carrier" has been *hemoglobin*, a complex iron-protein substance that is part of our red blood cells.

Capillaries and alveoli: The pulmonary artery carrying this lung-bound blood soon branches into smaller and smaller vessels, and eventually into microscopic capillaries which reach in to every crook and crevice of the lungs.

In the lungs, the walls of the capillaries touch the walls of equally microscopic structures called *alveoli* (singular, *alveolus*). The alveoli are the smallest air sacs of the lungs. These tiny, expandable air cells are the destination of every breath of air we take. Estimates of the total number of alveoli in both our lungs vary between 300 million and a billion—in any case, we normally have several hundred million of them.

Carbon dioxide and oxygen exchange: Where they meet, the membranous walls of both a capillary and an alveolus are both about as thin as any living tissue can be— a thickness that is only the width of one cell. Under such conditions, the carbon dioxide carried by the hemoglobin in our blood to the lungs diffuses (as tiny gaseous "bubbles") across both the wall of a capillary and the wall of an alveolus.

Once inside the sac of the alveolus, carbon dioxide is ready to be exhaled from the body by "breathing out." One indication of just how efficient this system is:

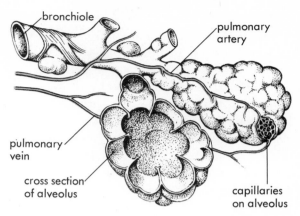

THE ALVEOLI

bronchiole

pulmonary artery

pulmonary vein

cross section of alveolus

capillaries on alveolus

The branches of the pulmonary tree terminate in the alveoli, grapelike clusters of air sacs covered by capillaries, where the gaseous exchange occurs.

the air we exhale has roughly 100 times more carbon dioxide than the air we breathe in.

At the same time that hemoglobin dumps carbon dioxide at the interface of the capillary and alveolus walls, it picks up the oxygen made available from inhaled fresh air that has reached the alveoli. The molecular oxygen bubbles cross the membranes in the same way—but in the opposite direction—as the carbon dioxide.

Hemoglobin in the capillaries picks up the oxygen and carries it via veins leading away from the lungs, to the left atrium of the heart.

Essential role of moisture: The alveolar membranes are supplied with a thin film of moisture that is absolutely indispensable to the exchange of gases in the lungs. As in so many of our body's reactions, our evolutionary descent from water-dwelling ancestors is revealed by the wet environment demanded if our lungs are to supply our body with oxygen.

Respiration at the One-Cell Level

Oxygen molecules, then, are carried to the body's cells by the hemoglobin of the arterial blood pumped by the heart's left ventricle. But how does a cell take oxygen from the blood and use it?

The transfer of oxygen from blood to cell is accomplished in much the same way as the exchanges that take place in the lungs. The circulating arterial blood has a surplus of oxygen; the cells have a surplus of carbon dioxide. When the oxygen-rich blood reaches the finest capillaries, only the very thinnest membranous walls (of cell and capillary) separate it from the carbon-dioxide-rich cells. As in the lungs, both these gases (dissolved in water) diffuse through these thinnest of membranes: the oxygen into the cell, the carbon dioxide into the blood for eventual deposit in the alveoli, and exhalation.

Within the cell, the oxygen is needed so that food, the body's fuel, can be burned to produce energy. At the cellular level, the most convenient and common food is a fairly simple carbohydrate molecule called glucose.

Energy is locked into a carbohydrate molecule such as glucose in the form of chemical bonds between its atoms. If one of these bonds is broken—say, a bond holding together a carbon and a hydrogen atom —a bit of pent-up energy is released as if, in a stalemated tug of war, the rope suddenly broke and both teams went hurtling off a few feet in opposite directions. This is precisely the effect of respiration within a cell: the cell "breaks the ropes" holding together a carbohydrate molecule. The result is the release of energy—either as body heat or to power other activities within the cell.

It is useful—but a somewhat misleading oversimplification—to consider cellular respiration as a type of burning, or combustion. When a typical cell burns food, a carbohydrate molecule (glucose) together with molecules of oxygen are changed into carbon dioxide and water. During this change, chemical energy is released—energy that has been trapped, as we have seen, in the carbohydrate molecule. That complex, energy-rich molecule has been dismantled into the simpler molecules of carbon dioxide (CO_2) and water (H_2O). Oxygen is necessary here just as it is in fiery combustion. But the energy released here, instead of rushing out as heat and flame, is used to power the living activities of the cell.

This description of cellular respiration is all right in principle, but the trouble is this: if it all happened at once—if carbohydrate was so abruptly dismantled, split up at one stroke to water and carbon dioxide—such a great amount of energy would be released that the cell would simply burn itself up. As one biologist has said, the cell would be in exactly the same position as a wood furnace built of wood.

Role of enzymes: What protects the cell is its army of enzymes. These remarkable protein molecules combine briefly with energy-containing food molecules, causing them to break down bit by bit, so that energy is released gradually rather than all at once.

Carbon Dioxide—Precious Waste

In most of our minds, oxygen tends to be the hero of respiration and carbon dioxide the villain or at least the undesirable waste gas. This isn't really a fair picture. While it is true that too much carbon dioxide would act as a poison in our body, it is also true that we must always have a certain amount of the gas dissolved in our tissues. If we did not, two potentially fatal events could occur. First, our blood chemistry, especially its delicate acid-alkali balance, would get completely out of control. Second—and something of a paradox—the body's whole automatic system of regulating breathing would be knocked out.

It is the level of carbon dioxide in the bloodstream that controls our breathing. This level is continuously being monitored by the autonomic nervous system, specifically by the lower brain's "breathing center" in the medulla at the top of the spinal cord. When the level of carbon dioxide in our body goes above a certain level, signals from the medulla force us to breathe. Almost everybody has played, "How long can you hold your breath?" and knows that, past a certain point, it becomes impossible *not* to breathe. When you are holding your breath, the unexhaled carbon dioxide rapidly builds up in your system until the breathing center is besieged with signals that say "Breathe!" And you do.

Our Big Breathing Muscle: The Diaphragm

What gets air into and out of our lungs? The answer may seem as obvious as breathing in and breathing out. But except for those rare instances when we consciously regulate our breathing pattern—which doctors call "force breathing"—we do not decide when to inhale and when to exhale. And even when we do force-breathe, it is not primarily the action of opening the mouth and gulping in air, then blowing it out, that gets air down the windpipe and into the alveoli of the lungs. The main work of inhaling and exhaling is done by the contraction and relaxation of the big helmet-shaped muscle on which the lungs rest and which marks the "floor" of the chest or thoracic cavity and the "ceiling" of the abdominal cavity. This muscle is the *diaphragm.*

It is the diaphragm that causes the lungs to swell and fill with fresh air, then partially collapse to expel used gases. The muscles and tendons of the sinewy diaphragm are attached at the back to the spinal column, at the front to the breastbone (*sternum*), and at the lower sides to the lower ribs.

The diaphragm contracts and relaxes on orders from the brain's breathing center, orders that are carried along the pathways

THE DIAPHRAGM

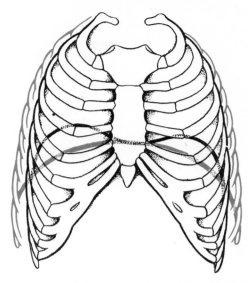

The positions of the rib cage and diaphragm are shown during inspiration of breath (in color) and expiration (in black). Thoracic volume increases during inspiration as the diaphragm is stretched.

of the autonomic nervous system. When the medulla sends messages to the breathing muscles to contract, the diaphragm is pulled downward, enlarging the space filled by the lungs. This creates a temporary partial vacuum, into which air rushes, inflating and expanding the lungs. When the diaphragm relaxes, the lung space is reduced, pushing air out.

Other breathing muscles: The diaphragm muscle's leading role in breathing is supported by several other muscles that play minor parts. Among these are the *intercostal muscles* between the ribs that give the rib cage a slight push upward and outward, enlarging the thoracic cavity, and the *serratus muscles,* which are mainly muscular sheaths along the ribs, to which other muscles attach.

The Trachea and the Lungs

The right lung (your right) is somewhat bigger than the left. The lungs hang in the chest attached to the windpipe or *trachea.*

THE RESPIRATORY SYSTEM

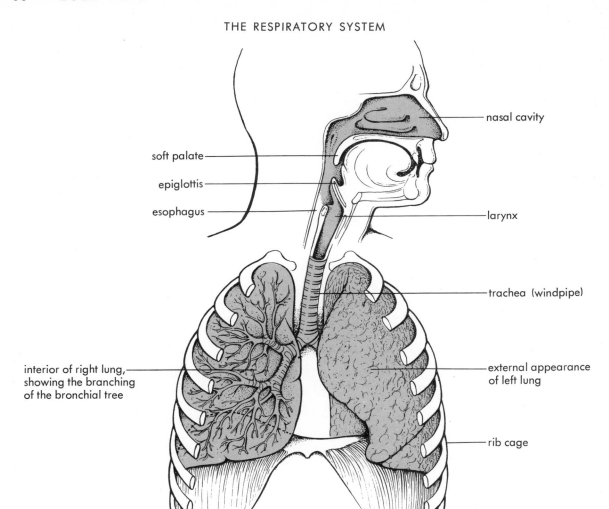

soft palate

epiglottis

esophagus

nasal cavity

larynx

trachea (windpipe)

interior of right lung, showing the branching of the bronchial tree

external appearance of left lung

rib cage

diaphragm

The Trachea

The trachea itself branches off at the back of the throat, or *pharynx*, where the epiglottis prevents food from entering the trachea and channels swallowed food along its proper route, the esophagus. The top part of the trachea forms the voice box or *larynx*, made up of vocal cords—actually two flaps of cartilage, muscle, and membranous tissue that protrude into the windpipe—whose vibrations in response to air exhaled from the lungs give us our voice.

Below the larynx, the trachea descends five or six inches to a spot just about directly behind your breastbone, where the first of many thousands of branchings into *bronchi*, *bronchioles*, and alveoli occurs. C-shaped rings of cartilage give the trachea both support and flexibility. Running your finger down the front of your neck, you can feel the bumps made by the cartilage rings.

Above the base of the trachea in midchest the lungs arch on either side like giant butterfly wings, then fall to fill out the bottom of each side of the thoracic cavity.

The Pleural Membranes

Both lungs are encased in moist, clinging, tissue-thin membrane called the *pleura,* which also lines the inside of the thoracic cavity where it comes into contact with the pleural coating of the lungs. The slippery pleural membranes hold tightly to each other, because there is an air lock or vacuum between them, but at the same time are free to slide over each other. The principle is the same as when you moisten the surfaces of two pieces of plate glass and place the moistened surfaces together: the two pieces of glass will slide over each other but will resist being pried apart, because a partial vacuum exists between them.

The pleural cavity: The vacuum space between the pleura of the lung and the pleura of the thoracic cavity—although it is normally not a space at all—is called the *pleural cavity.* Each lung has its own pleural membrane: that of one lung does not interconnect with the other, so that one pleura may be injured without affecting the other.

It is extremely fortunate for us that the pleural linings both stick fast and can slide along each other's surfaces. Although the lungs are virtually without muscle, they are extremely elastic and in their natural condition are stretched fairly taut, held to the sides of the thoracic cavity by the suction of the pleura.

Collapsed lung: Should this suction be broken and the pleural linings pull apart, the lung would shrink up like a deflated balloon. Such a condition, caused by the rush of outside air into the pleural cavity, is known medically as *pneumothorax* and causes a lung collapse. Violent injuries such as gun and stab wounds, various lung diseases, and obstructions of the breathing tubes can cause a lung or portion of a lung to collapse.

In the surgical procedure called *artificial pneumothorax,* a physician deliberately injects air between the pleural linings to collapse a portion of a lung. This is done to rest a lung in severe diseases such as tuberculosis, or to control heavy bleeding within the thoracic cavity.

Pleurisy: The intense chest pains called *pleurisy* are caused by inflammation of the pleura. The pleural linings lose their slipperiness and the increased friction stimulates pain receptors in the pleural lining of the chest. There are, however, no pain receptors in the lungs' pleural linings nor in the lungs themselves: this is why pain is not an early warning signal of lung cancer.

Structure of the Lungs

The bronchi: Just behind the breastbone and just in front of the heart, the trachea divides into the right bronchus and the left bronchus, leading respectively to the right and left lungs. These are the primary two *bronchi* or *bronchial tubes.* Each is the main trunk of a bronchial tree that serves its respective lung.

Soon after leaving the trachea, each bronchus branches repeatedly into smaller tubes called *bronchioles,* which in turn branch into alveolar ducts, which terminate finally with the hundreds of millions of microscopic air sacs called alveoli, discussed at the beginning of this section. The alveoli are the site of the all-important exchange of carbon dioxide and oxygen.

Lobes and segments: The larger right lung has three distinctive sections, or *lobes* —upper, middle, and lower. The left lung has only an upper and lower lobe. The lobes. themselves are divided into smaller segments. Medically, these lobes and segments are important because they are somewhat independent of each other and can be damaged or removed surgically, as in operations for lung cancer, usually without damaging the function of adjacent, healthy segments or lobes.

The fact that a lung segment, lobe, or even an entire lung can be removed implies

Oxygen Requirements

How much air do we breathe, and how much oxygen do we absorb into our body from the air? A normal, moderately active person breathes in and out (a complete respiration or breath cycle) about 18 times a minute; that is, the diaphragm contracts and relaxes 18 times a minute, or something over 25,000 times every day. At about four-fifths of a pint of air per breath cycle, this means that we inhale and exhale about 20,000 pints, or 10,000 quarts, or 2,500 gallons of air every day.

Only a very small proportion of this volume is oxygen that finds its way into our bloodstream: about a pint every minute in normal, quiet breathing, a little over 1,400 pints, or 700 quarts, or 175 gallons of oxygen every day. The amount of oxygen our lungs are capable of delivering to our body, however, varies tremendously: a sleeping man may need only a half-pint of oxygen per minute, half the average, while the lungs of a hard-driving athlete striving to break the mile record can deliver up to five quarts to the bloodstream: ten times the average.

At any given time, there are about two quarts of oxygen circulating in our blood. This is why a stoppage of breathing has an upper time limit of about four minutes before it causes irreversible damage or death. With our body needing about a pint of oxygen every minute for normal functioning, we have about four minutes before we use up the oxygen dissolved in our blood and other tissues.

Pollution Control in the Respiratory System—Filters, Cleaners, and Traps

Air pollution being what it is these days, it is fortunate that we have several natural devices that serve to filter out and wash away most of the impurities in the air we inhale.

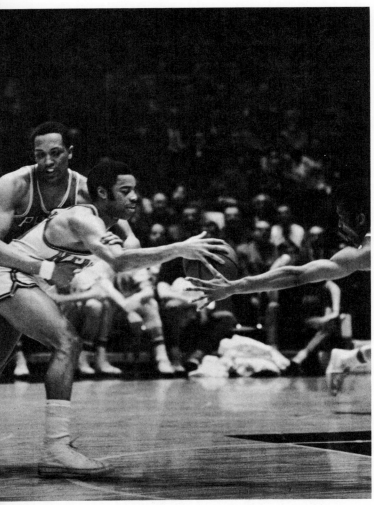

The lungs of an athlete in all-out competition can deliver up to ten times the normal amount of oxygen to the bloodstream. Good blood circulation aids the rapid exchange of oxygen and carbon dioxide.

that we have plenty of reserve lung tissue, and this is indeed the case. When we are at rest, we use only about one-tenth of our total lung capacity. The total surface area exposed within our lungs to outside air is a staggering 600 square feet. This compares to a mere 20 square feet of skin surface. To appreciate the incredibly intricate, lacelike finery of the lungs' structure, we need only know that those 600 square feet of surface area are contained within two organs that together weigh only two-and-a-half pounds.

Air gets into the lungs from outside about equally well via the nose or mouth. The mouth offers the advantage of getting more air in at a faster rate—absolutely a must if we have to push our body physically. But the nose has more and better equipment for cleaning air before it reaches the trachea. Via the mouth, air must only pass over a few mucous membranes and the tonsils, which can collect only so many germs and impurities.

Nose filter system: Air taken in through the nose, however, first meets the "guard hairs" (*vibrissae*) of the nostrils, and then must circulate through the nasal cavity, a kind of cavern framed by elaborate scroll-shaped bones called *turbinates,* and lined with mucus-secreting membranes and waving, hairlike fibers called *cilia.* Foreign particles are caught by the cilia and carried away by the mucus, which drains slowly down the back of the throat.

It would be nice to be able to ascribe an important function to the eight *paranasal sinuses,* four on either side of the nose: the headache and discomfort of sinusitis might then be more bearable. But these "holes in the head" seem to exist simply to cause us trouble; for example— swelling to close the nasal air passages, making it impossible to breathe, as recommended, through the nose.

Filter system beyond the nose: The cleansing and filtering action started in the nose and mouth does not stop there, but is repeated wherever air travels along the air passages of the lungs. Cilia project inward from the walls of even the tiniest bronchioles of the lungs, and impurities are carried from the alveoli on films of mucus that move ever back toward the trachea for expulsion—as when we cough. See also *Diseases of the Respiratory System,* p. 539, and *Lung Disease,* p. 555. EHH, JR.

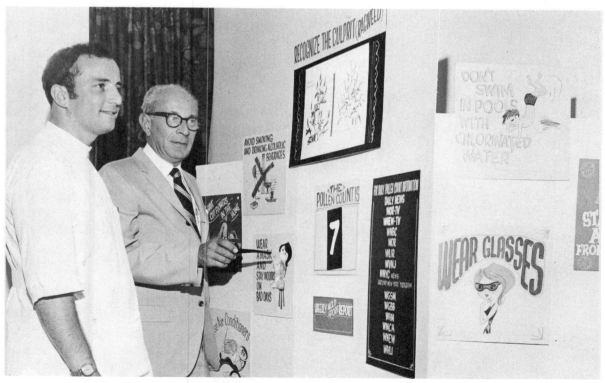

Hay fever sufferers had best adopt extra precautions to augment their natural filter systems. Here an allergist points out some recommended steps.

THE ENDOCRINE GLANDS

Technically speaking, a gland is any cell or organ in our bodies that secretes some substance. In this broad sense, our liver is a gland, since one of its many functions is to secrete bile. So too, is the placenta that encloses a developing baby and sup-

plies it with chemicals that assure normal growth. Even the brain has been shown by modern research to secrete special substances. But lymph glands are not considered true glands and are more correctly called lymph nodes.

THE ENDOCRINE GLANDS

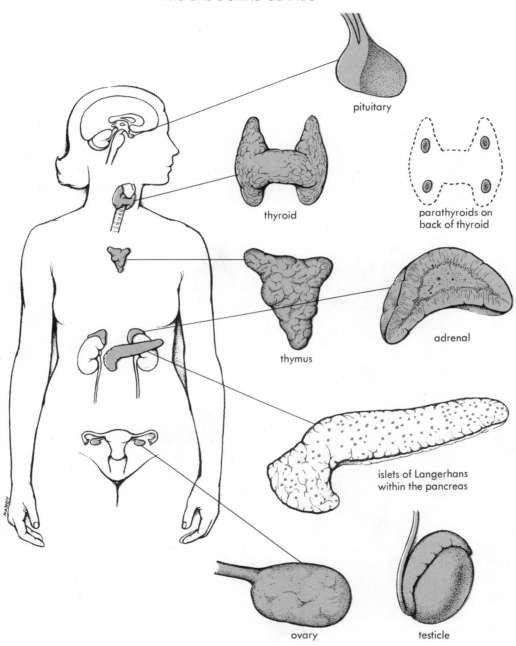

pituitary

thyroid

parathyroids on
back of thyroid

thymus

adrenal

islets of Langerhans
within the pancreas

ovary

testicle

Doctors divide the glands into two categories. *Endocrine glands* are also known as *ductless glands,* because they release their secretions directly into the bloodstream. *Exocrine glands,* by contrast, usually release their substances through a duct or tube. Exocrine glands include the sebaceous and sweat glands of the skin; the mammary or milk glands; the mucous glands, some of which moisten the digestive and respiratory tract; and the salivary glands, whose secretions soften food after it enters the mouth. The pancreas has both an endocrine and an exocrine function and structure.

The Role of the Endocrine Glands

The *endocrine glands* have the all-important role of regulating our body's internal chemistry. The substances they secrete are complex compounds called *hormones.*

Together with the brain and nerves, the system of endocrine glands controls the body's activities. The nervous system, however, is tuned for rapid responses, enabling the body to make speedy adjustments to changing circumstances, internal and external. The endocrine glands, with some exceptions, like the adrenal, are more concerned with the body's reactions over a longer period of time—from season to season, as it were. They regulate such processes as growth, levels of metabolism, fertility, and pregnancy.

For a group of tissues that exercise awesome power over our body's well-being, the endocrine glands are surprisingly small and inconspicuous—all of them together would weigh less than half a pound. Nor are they placed with any particular prominence in our body. They tend to be little lumps of tissue attached to or tucked behind grander bodily structures. Their power comes from the hormones they release into the bloodstream.

Scientists have discovered the exact chemical make-up of a number of these complex substances, have extracted several in pure form from living tissue, and have succeeded in making a few synthetically in the laboratory. This avenue of research, called *endocrinology,* has enabled doctors to treat persons suffering from certain endocrine gland disorders.

Hormones have been aptly described as chemical messengers. Their action, while still not completely understood, is that of catalysts. This means that the presence of a hormone (the name comes from a Greek word meaning "arouse to activity"), even in very small quantities, can affect the rate at which a chemical change occurs or otherwise stimulate a reaction, and without itself being affected. The hormone is a promoter, either of a positive or negative sort; it speeds up a process or slows it down.

The endocrine glands form an interdependent family. The functioning or malfunctioning of one can affect all the others.

The Pituitary—Master Gland

The *pituitary* is often called the master gland, because the hormones it secretes play an active part in controlling the activities of all the other endocrine glands. This impressive power is wielded from two little bumps at the base of the brain, about midway between the ears at eye level. The two parts, or lobes, are connected by a tiny bridge of tissue, the three structures together being about the size of a small acorn. The lobe lying toward the front of the head is the *anterior lobe;* the one at the back, the *posterior lobe.* Each lobe is really an independent gland in itself, with its own quite distinct activities.

The Posterior Lobe and the Hypothalamus

The posterior lobe, so far as is known, does not make any of its own hormones, but serves as a storehouse for two hormones manufactured by the *hypothalamus,* located in the brain's cerebellum. The hypothala-

THE PITUITARY GLAND

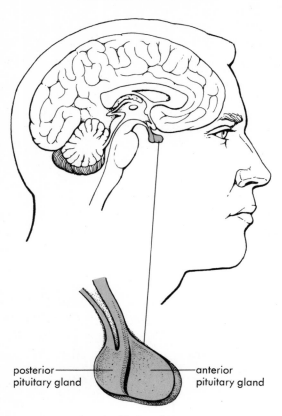

posterior pituitary gland

anterior pituitary gland

Anterior Pituitary Secretes:

Adrenocorticotrophic hormone (ACTH), acting on the adrenal cortex

Follicle-stimulating hormone, acting on the ovaries or the testes

Thyrotrophic hormone, acting on the thyroid gland

Luteotrophin, stimulating milk production in the female

Luteinizing hormone, stimulating testosterone production in the male and estrogen in the female

Growth hormone, stimulating skeletal and visceral growth

Posterior Pituitary Secretes:

Vasopressin, or antidiuretic hormone, raising blood pressure and acting on the kidneys

Oxytocin, causing contractions of the pregnant uterus

mus, apart from having a role in controlling the body's autonomic nervous system, also functions as an endocrine gland, secreting its own hormones, and as a connecting link between the brain's cerebral cortex and the pituitary gland. See the illustration of *The Autonomic Nervous System,* p. 28, for the location of the hypothalamus.

The posterior lobe of the pituitary releases the two hormones it receives from the hypothalamus, called *vasopressin* and *oxytocin,* into the bloodstream. Vasopressin plays a role in the fluid balance of the body; oxytocin is thought to pace the onset and progress of labor during childbirth.

The Anterior Lobe

The anterior lobe secretes no less than six known hormones, five of which act as stimulators of hormone production by other endocrine glands. The sixth, identified as *somatotrophin* in medical textbooks, is more popularly known as the *growth-stimulating hormone* or simply as the growth hormone. It controls the rate of growth and multiplication of all the cells and tissues in our bodies—muscle, bone, and all our specialized organs.

Gigantism: In rare instances, during childhood, the pituitary releases too much or too little somatotrophin. If too much is secreted, the result is an overstimulation of growth processes, causing a disorder known as *gigantism.* Victims of this disorder have been known to grow nine feet tall and weigh 500 pounds.

Dwarfism: If too little somatotrophin is secreted, *dwarfism* results. This pituitary-type dwarf, of which Tom Thumb was one, is different from a dwarf suffering from a disorder of the thyroid (another endocrine gland, discussed below). The pituitary dwarf is usually well-proportioned despite a miniature size, while the thyroid dwarf typically has short, deformed limbs.

Neither pituitary gigantism nor dwarfism affects basic intelligence. If oversecretion of somatotrophin occurs after full size has been reached—as, for example, because of a tumor affecting the pituitary, the condition known as *acromegaly* occurs. The bones enlarge abnormally, especially those of the hands, feet, and face.

Anterior pituitary hormones: Of the five anterior pituitary hormones that regulate other endocrine glands, one affects the adrenal glands, one the thyroid, and the remaining three the sex glands or gonads (the testicles in men and the ovaries in women). Each is identified by a set of initials derived from its full name, as follows:

• *ACTH*, the *a*drenocorticotrophic *h*ormone, affects the production of hormones by the outer "bark" of the adrenal glands, called the *adrenal cortex*.

• *TSH*, the *t*hyroid-*s*timulating *h*ormone, also known as *thyrotrophin,* causes the thyroid gland to step up production of its hormone, *thyroxin.*

• *FSH*, the *f*ollicle-*s*timulating *h*ormone, spurs production in women of estrogen, a sex hormone produced by the ovaries; and in men, of sperm by the testicles. Follicle here refers to the *Graafian follicles* in the ovary, which contain developing female egg cells whose growth is also stimulated by FSH. Graafian follicles have approximate counterparts in the male—tiny pouches (seminal vesicles) on either side of the prostate gland that store mature sperm cells.

• *LH*, the *l*uteinizing *h*ormone, transforms a Graafian follicle, after the follicle has released a ripened egg cell, into a kind of tissue called *corpus luteum*. The corpus luteum, in turn, produces *progesterone*, a hormone that prepares the mucous membrane lining the uterus (the endometrium) to receive a fertilized egg.

• *LTH*, the *l*actogenic *h*ormone, or *luteotrophin,* stimulates the mother's mammary glands to produce milk; LTH also joins with LH in promoting the production of progesterone by the sex glands.

The last three hormones mentioned—follicle-stimulating, luteinizing, and lactogenic—are sometimes called the *gonadotrophic* hormones because they all stimulate activity of the gonads.

The Adrenal Glands

Resting like skull caps on the top of both kidneys are the two identical *adrenal glands*. Each has two distinct parts, secreting different hormones.

Adrenaline

The central internal portion of an adrenal gland is called the *medulla*. Its most potent contribution to our body is the hormone *adrenaline* (also called *epinephrine*). This is the hormone that, almost instantaneously, pours into our bloodstream when we face a situation that calls for extraordinary physical reaction—or keeps us going past what we think to be our normal limit of endurance.

A surge of adrenaline into the bloodstream stimulates our body to a whole array of alarm reactions—accelerating the conversion of stored foods into quick energy; raising the blood pressure; speeding up breathing; dilating the pupils of the eyes

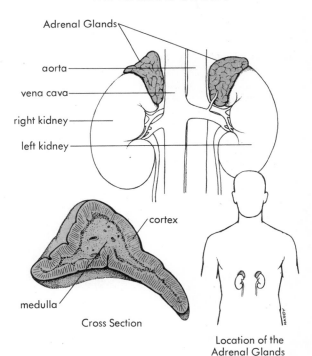

THE ADRENAL GLANDS

Adrenal Glands
aorta
vena cava
right kidney
left kidney

cortex

medulla

Cross Section

Location of the
Adrenal Glands

for more sensitive vision; and constricting the blood vessels, making them less vulnerable to bleeding.

Adrenaline provides a good example of the interdependence of the endocrine system. Its production stimulates the secretion of ACTH by the pituitary gland. And ACTH, as noted above, causes the adrenal cortex to accelerate production of its hormones. Some of these adrenal cortex hormones enable the body to call up the reserves of energy it does not normally need. For example, body proteins are not usually a source of quick energy, but in an emergency situation, the adrenal cortex hormones can convert them to energy-rich sugar compounds.

The Corticoids

There are some 30 different hormones, called the *corticoids*, manufactured in the adrenal cortex—the outer layer of the adrenal. A few of these influence male and female sexual characteristics, supplementing the hormones produced in the gonads. The others fall into two general categories: those that affect the body's metabolism (rate of energy use), and those that regulate the composition of blood and internal fluids. Without the latter hormones, for example, the kidneys could not maintain the water-salt balance that provides the most suitable environment for our cells and tissues at any given time.

THE PANCREAS

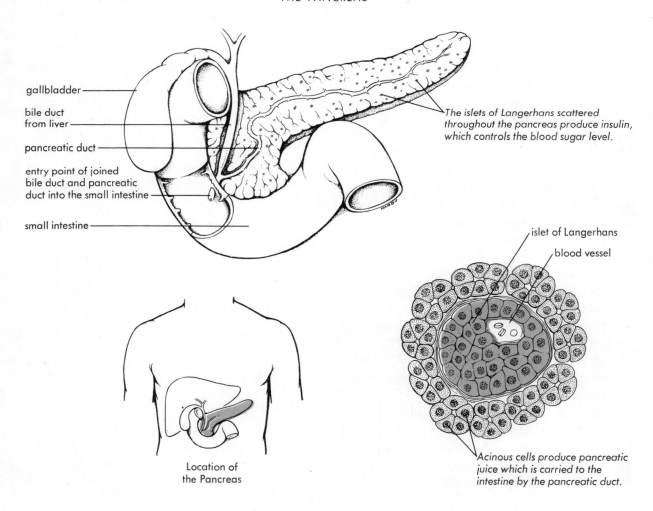

gallbladder

bile duct from liver

pancreatic duct

entry point of joined bile duct and pancreatic duct into the small intestine

small intestine

The islets of Langerhans scattered throughout the pancreas produce insulin, which controls the blood sugar level.

islet of Langerhans

blood vessel

Location of the Pancreas

Acinous cells produce pancreatic juice which is carried to the intestine by the pancreatic duct.

Corticoids also influence the formation of antibodies against viruses, bacteria, and other disease-causing agents.

Extracts or laboratory preparations of corticoids, such as the well-known cortisone compounds, were found some 20 years ago to be almost "miracle" medicines. These substances work dramatically to reduce pain, especially around joints, and hasten the healing of skin inflammations.

The Islets of Langerhans

Strewn at random throughout the pancreas are hundreds of thousands of tiny clusters of cells. Each of them, when seen under a powerful microscope, forms an "islet" of its own, similar to the other distinct islets, but markedly different from the pancreatic tissue surrounding it. These are the *islets of Langerhans,* named after the German scientist who first reported their existence in 1869. Each of these little cell clumps— up to two million or more of them—is a microscopic endocrine gland.

They secrete the hormone *insulin,* and the disease that occurs if they are not functioning properly is *diabetes mellitus.*

Actually, the islets of Langerhans produce not only insulin, but also a related hormone called *glucagon.* Both regulate the amount of sugar (glucose) that is present in the bloodstream and the rate at which it is used by the body's cells and tissues. Glucose supplies the energy for life and living processes.

When insulin and glucagon are not in sufficient supply, the cells' ability to absorb and use blood sugar is restricted, and much of the sugar passes unutilized out of the body in urine. Since the body's ability to obtain energy from food is one of the very foundations of life, diabetes calls for the most careful treatment.

One of the great advances of 20th century medicine has been the pharmaceutical manufacture of insulin and its wide avail-

ability to diabetics. With regulated doses of insulin, a diabetic can now lead a normal life. See *Diabetes Mellitus* p. 573 for a full discussion of this disease.

The Thyroid Gland

The *thyroid gland* folds around the front and either side of the trachea (windpipe), at the base of the neck, just below the larynx. It resembles a somewhat large, stocky butterfly facing downward toward the chest. See the illustration of *The Endocrine Glands,* p. 64.

Thyroxin

The thyroid hormone, *thyroxin,* is a complex protein-type chemical containing, along with various other elements, a large percentage of iodine. Like a number of other hormones manufactured by the endocrine glands, thyroxin affects various steps in the body's metabolism—in particular, the rate at which our cells and tissues use inhaled oxygen to burn the food we eat.

Hypothyroidism: A thyroid that is not producing enough thyroxin tends to make a person feel drowsy and sluggish, put on weight (even though his appetite is poor), and in general make his everyday activities tiresome and wearying. This condition is called *hypothyroidism.*

Hyperthyroidism: Its opposite—caused by too much secretion of thyroxin—is *hyperthyroidism.* A hyperthyroid person is jumpy, restless, and may eat hugely without gaining weight. The difference between the two extremes can be compared to environments regulated by two different thermostats, one set too high and the other set too low.

Although a normally functioning thyroid plays a significant part in making a person feel well, doctors today are less willing than in former years to blame a defective thyroid alone for listlessness or jittery nerves. Twenty or thirty years ago, it was quite fashionable to prescribe thyroid pills (containing thyroid extract) almost as readily as vitamins or aspirin; but subsequent medical research, revealing the interdependence of many glands and other body systems, made thyroxin's reign as a cure-all a short one.

Of course, where physical discomfort or lethargy can be traced to an underfunctioning thyroid, thyroxin remains an invaluable medicine.

Goiter: One disorder of the thyroid gland —the sometimes massive swelling called *goiter*—is the direct result of a lack of iodine in the diet. The normal thyroid gland, in effect, collects iodine from the bloodstream, which is then synthesized into the chemical makeup of thyroxin. Lacking iodine, the thyroid gland enlarges, creating a goiter. The abnormal growth will stop if iodine is reintroduced into the person's diet. This is the reason why most commercial table salt is iodized—that is, a harmless bit of iodine compound has been added to it.

The Parathyroid Glands

Four small glands, each about the size of a small pea, cling to the base of the thyroid gland, two on each of the thyroid's lobes curving back of the trachea. These are the *parathyroids*, whose main role is to control the level of calcium—as well as other elements needed in carefully regulated amounts by the body—in the bloodstream and tissues. The parathyroids secrete two hormones: *parathormone* when blood calcium is too low; *calcitonin* when the calcium level is too high. These hormones work by controlling the interchange of calcium between bones and blood.

The most common symptom of defective parathyroids is *tetany*—a chronic or acute case of muscle spasms, which can be controlled by administration of synthetic parathyroidlike chemicals or concentrated vitamin D preparations.

The Gonads

The *gonads* refer to both the two male testicles and the two female ovaries. See the illustration of *The Endocrine Glands,* p. 64.

There are four hormones secreted by the gonads: the female sex hormones, *estrogen* and *progesterone;* and the male hormones, *testosterone* and *androsterone.* Each sex merely has a predominance of one or the other pair of hormones. Men have some of the female hormones, and women some of the male hormones.

In both sexes, puberty is signaled by the release of the gonadotrophic hormones (or *gonadotrophins*) of the pituitary gland. These stimulate the production of sex hormones by the sex glands and the subsequent appearance of secondary sexual characteristics. In men, these include the enlargement of testicles and penis, growth of facial, axillary (armpit) and pubic hair, and enlargement of the larynx, resulting in deepening of the voice. Pubescent women also experience pubic and axillary hair growth, in addition to breast growth and changes in the genital tract that give it childbearing capability.

Estrogen and progesterone control the cyclic changes within the uterus that involve the development, ripening, and discharge of the egg (ovulation) to be fertilized; the preparation of the lining of the uterus to receive a fertilized egg; and this lining's subsequent dismantling—all the complex biochemical events that occur as part of every woman's menstrual cycle.

The Thymus and Pineal Glands

These are the least-known of the endocrine family; in fact, doctors do not know the function of one of them—the *pineal*—and are not even agreed that it is an endocrine gland. Situated near the hypothalamus, at the base of the brain, this tiny, pine-cone-shaped body has follicles that suggest a glandular function and some calcium-containing bits that medical researchers have dubbed "brain sand."

The *thymus,* only slightly better understood, has the intriguing characteristic of shrinking in size as a person grows up. It is located in the middle of the chest, about midway between the base of the neck and the breast line. There is some evidence that the secretions of the thymus play a role in the body's natural immunity defenses. See also *Diseases of the Endocrine Glands,* p. 566.   EHH, JR.

THE SENSE ORGANS

Once upon a time, a grade-school teacher would ask, "How many senses do we have?" And his pupils would confidently chorus back, "Five!" People who displayed a knack for predicting future events, or whose quick reactions seemed to give them a jump over most everybody else, were credited with having a "sixth sense."

Scientists now recognize about twice that number—12 or 13 or more. Man, of course, has not grown a number of new senses in addition to the traditional five: sight, hearing, touch, smell, and taste. What has happened is that scientists have discovered many more specific kinds of sense receptor cells. For example, whereas touch was formerly thought of as just one sense, it has now been divided into no less than five different senses, each having its own special kind of receptor cell in the skin.

We can talk with a little more justification of the five sense organs, the five anatomical structures we associate with our senses—the eyes, ears, nose, tongue, and skin. But here, too, it does seem to be oversimplifying things to thus equate the nose—having only a tiny patch of olfactory (sense of smell) receptor cells—with the marvelously complex arrangement of sensing structures that make up the eye. Moreover, the other sense organs are not nearly so specialized as the eye. For example, a good case could be made for the nose being more valuable as an air purifier than as an organ of smell, or for the tongue being more valuable as an aid in digestion than as a source of the taste sensation.

Suppose we accept the proposition that pain is one of the senses of the skin; how then do we explain a pain from inside our bodies—say, a stomach ache or a deep muscle pain? The answer, of course, is that there are pain receptors in many other places besides the skin.

What Is a Sense?

A sense is a nerve pathway, one end of which (the receptor end) responds in a certain way to a certain condition affecting our bodies, and whose other end reaches to a part of our brain that informs our conscious mind of what has happened or is happening. A sense is thus distinguished from the body's countless other nerve pathways by the fact that our brain *consciously* registers its impulses, although the impulses themselves are no different from those of the autonomic nervous system.

While remaining aware of the limitations of the traditional list of five sense organs, let us now analyze what they can do and how they operate:

• The eye (vision): Nerve impulses to the brain are stimulated by light waves, from which the brain forms visual images.

• The ears (hearing): Nerve impulses to the brain are stimulated by sound waves, out of which the brain forms meaningful noise, such as speech. Deep within the ear, also, are structures that give us balance.

• The nose (olfaction): Nerve impulses to the brain are stimulated by airborne chemical substances, moistened within the nasal cavity, from which the brain elicits distinctive smells.

• The tongue (taste): Nerve impulses to the brain are stimulated (in presence of water) by chemical substances in food, from which the brain forms sensations of sweet, salty, sour, bitter, or combinations of these tastes.

• Skin (touch): Nerve impulses to the brain are stimulated by the presence of outside physical forces and changes in the physical environment, including varying temperatures, which the brain registers as feelings of contact, pressure, cold, heat, and pain. (Some medical texts add traction, as when the skin is pulled or pinched, as well as the sensation of tickle.)

The Eye

Rather than take a name-by-name anatomical tour of the eye, let's instead take just three programmed tours of the eye to explore:

• The transformation of light energy into vision

• Focusing, or how the structure of the eye prepares light for transformation into vision

• The supporting structures and service units of the eye.

Transforming Light Energy Into Vision

If you could look through the opening in the front of your eye (the *pupil*), and see to the very back surface of your eye (as if you could see through the needle valve opening to the inside skin of a basketball), you would see your own *retina*. On your retina are located all the sense receptor cells that enable us to see. There are none anywhere else in the body.

Rods and cones: A good argument can be made that man's vision is really *two* senses. For on the paper-thin retina are two quite anatomically distinct sense receptors (nerve endings) named, for their appearance under high magnification, *cones* and *rods*. The cones are concentrated at a tiny spot on the retina called the *fovea*.

If the focusing machinery of the eye (cornea, lens, etc.) is working just right, light rays from the outside have their sharpest focus on the fovea. Surrounding the fovea is a yellowish area called the *macula lutea* (Latin, "yellow spot"). Together, the fovea and macula lutea make a circle not much bigger than the head of a pin.

All our seeing of colors and fine details is accomplished by the cones of the fovea and the macula lutea. Beyond the yellowish circumference of the macula lutea, there are fewer and fewer cones: rods become the dominant structures on the retina. It has been estimated that there are something less than 10 million cones on the retina of each eye, but more than 10 times as many rods—100 million of them or more.

Although the tight circle of cones in each eye gives man his ability to do close, detailed work (including reading) and to discriminate colors, the cones are virtually useless in detecting objects that are a bit off center from our direct focus, and furthermore operate only in good lighting conditions or in response to bright light sources.

The rods make up for the specialized limits of the cones. They take over completely in dim light, and also give us the ability to detect peripheral objects and movements—"out of the corner of the eye." Because the rods are not sensitive to colors, our seeing at night is almost completely in black-and-white.

You can give yourself an interesting demonstration of the interacting functions

THE EYE

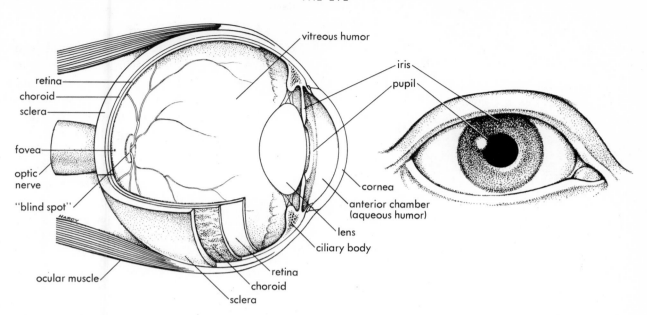

of your own cones and rods if you walk from bright, sunny daylight into a dimly lit theater. In the bright light, your cones have been picking out sharp images and colors. But once in dimness, the cones become inoperative. For a few moments, in fact, you may see almost nothing at all.

Visual purple: The momentary interval after the cones stop working but before the rods begin to function is explained by a curious pigment present in the eye called *visual purple.* This substance is manufactured constantly by the rods, and must be present for the rods to respond to dim light—but it is destroyed when exposed to bright light. Thus, after entering a darkened room, it takes a few moments for visual purple to build up in the retina. One of the principal constituents of visual purple is vitamin A, which is why this vitamin (present in carrots and other yellow produce) is said to increase our capacity to see in the dark.

The optic nerve: Every nerve ending is part of a larger unit, a neuron or nerve cell, and the sense receptors called rods and cones are no exception. Like all nerve cells, each rod and cone sports a long nerve

fiber or *axon* leading away from the site of reception. In each eye, fibers serving the hundred-million-plus rods and cones all converge at a certain spot just behind the retina, forming the *optic nerve*. There are no rods and cones at the point where the optic nerve exits from behind the retina at the back of the eyeball: that is why everybody has a "blind spot" at that point. An image passing through that spot completely disappears.

From the retina, both optic nerves set a course almost directly through the middle of the brain. Right and left optic nerves converge, their individual fibers partially intertwining a short distance behind the

THE BLIND SPOT

The blind spot can be demonstrated by holding the book about 5 inches in front of the right eye. Close the left eye. Focus eye on the plus sign and move the book slowly toward or away from the eye until the fly disappears. At this point the image of the fly is falling on the "blind spot." This is the point where the optic nerve enters the eye.

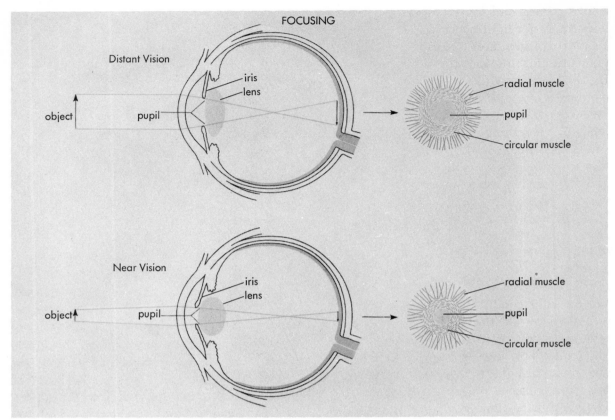

FOCUSING

Distant Vision

iris
lens

object

pupil

radial muscle

pupil

circular muscle

Near Vision

iris
lens

object

pupil

radial muscle

pupil

circular muscle

When viewing a distant object (over 20 feet away), the lens flattens and the pupil dilates, allowing more light to enter the eye. The pupil is dilated by the action of the outer radial muscles of the iris, which contract and thus stretch the previously contracted circular muscles. When viewing a near object, the lens becomes more oval and the pupil contracts as more light enters the eye. This prevents overstimulation of the retina. The pupil is reduced in size by the contraction of the inner circular muscles, which serve to stretch the previously contracted radial muscles.

eyes. Then this joint optic nerve trunk proceeds toward the rear of the head, where the *occipital lobes,* the brain's "centers for seeing," are located. Just before reaching the occipital lobes, the optic nerve splits again into thousands of smaller nerve bundles (called *visual radiations*) that disappear into the visual cortex or "outer bark" of the occipital lobes. Only at this point are the bits of light energy that have stimulated our rods and cones transformed into images that our brain can "see."

Focusing and Light Control

Lacking the structures of the retina and their connection to the brain via the optic nerve, we could not see. Lacking reasonably normal functioning of the cornea, lens, and iris, we do not see well.

Good vision depends upon the eye being able to bend incoming light rays in such a way that the image being observed falls directly on the retina—in other words, upon proper focusing. The bending or *refraction* of light rays is the joint work of two curved, transparent slivers of specialized tissue through which light passes on its way to the retina. These are the *cornea* and the *lens.* Broadly speaking, the degree of curvature and thickness of these two structures determines whether we see well or poorly, are nearsighted or farsighted.

The cornea and lens: The cornea, which does the major light-bending, has a virtually fixed curvature and thickness. The lens puts the finishing touches on the focusing. Its thickness and curvature are adjustable —more or less without our conscious awareness—depending on whether we wish to focus on something nearer or farther away. The lens is made thicker or thinner, a process called *accommodation,* by the relaxing and contracting of tiny, attached *ciliary muscles.* Normally, these muscles do not have to work at all if we are looking at objects more than 20 feet away: but they often are overworked by a great deal of close work.

The pupil and iris: Effective focusing in various light conditions also depends upon the diameter of the hole through which light enters the eye. This hole is the *pupil.* Its diameter is controlled automatically— wider in dim light, narrower in bright light —by the muscles of the surrounding *iris.* The iris muscle contains pigment that gives our eyes color (brown, blue, green, etc.). The pupil, opening into the dark interior chamber of the eye, is black. A fully dilated (widened) pupil, as would occur in the dimmest light, illuminates over 15 times more

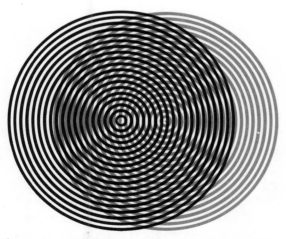

The apparent flickering of the circles is caused by contractions of the ciliary muscles, which control the accommodation (or change in thickness) of the lens for accurate focusing of objects at a variety of distances.

retinal surface than the tiny "pinhole" pupil of an eye exposed to very bright light.

Supporting Structures and Service Units of the Eye

Structural support and protection: Two outer layers protect the eye. The tough outermost layer is the *sclera,* the white of the eye. Underlying the sclera is another layer, the *choroid,* which contains numerous tiny blood vessels that service the sclera and other structures on the eyeball. Both sclera and choroid have concentric openings that allow for the hole of the pupil. The cornea is really a specialized extension of the sclera, and the iris of the choroid.

Two trapped reservoirs of fluid within the eye are important in maintaining the eye's shape as well as the frictionless operation of its moving parts. These two reservoirs contain fluids called the *aqueous humor* and *vitreous humor.* The tiny space between the cornea and lens, corresponding to the pupil, is called the anterior chamber and is filled with the clear, watery, aqueous humor. The larger interior space behind the lens is called the posterior chamber, and is filled with the vitreous humor.

Muscles for movement: In addition to the tiny muscles within the eye that control the opening of the pupil and the shape of the lens, we also have a number of elegant muscles that control the movements of each eyeball, and make both eyeballs move together in unison.

The movements of each eyeball are effected by six muscles attached to its top, bottom, and sides. The teamwork between these muscles—some contracting while others relax—allows the eye to move from side to side, up and down, and at all intermediate angles (obliquely). One of our eyes is always a dominant or leading eye; that is, its movements are always followed by the other eye.

Our protective eyelids, of course, are controlled by opening and closing muscles that lie outside the eye proper. These muscles can function both voluntarily and involuntarily.

Lubrication and hygiene: Without the moisture provided by tears, our eyeball would scrape excruciatingly on the inside lining (the *conjunctiva*) of the eyelid. In addition to lubrication, tears also have a cleansing action, not only because they supply water for washing and rinsing but also because they contain a mild germicide called *lysozyme* that kills bacteria and other potentially harmful microbes.

Tears are produced by the *lacrimal glands* above the eyeball, just under the eyebrow, a bit further toward the temple side than the nose side. They are discharged from several short ducts and spread over the surface of the eyeball by

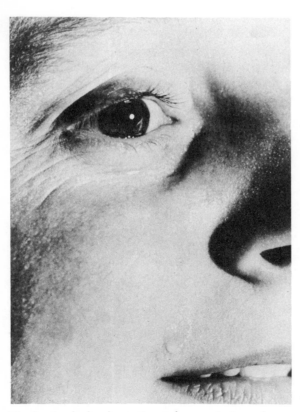

The lacrimal glands continuously secrete tears in response to the suction caused by blinking. Emotional distress or laughter can cause the muscles around the glands to contract and squeeze out excess fluid.

blinking. The *conjunctival sac* at the bottom inner (nose) side of the eye—visible in the mirror as a pinkish flap of tissue—serves as a collecting pool for tears; from there, they drain down a duct into the nasal cavity. This is why somebody who is crying also snuffles and must blow his nose.

There is another tiny drainage network in the eye, located at the interconnection of the cornea and iris, which serves to keep the fluid pressure of the space filled by the aqueous humor within normal limits. Drainage of this area is through microscopic conduits called the *canals of Schlemm.* Improper drainage can cause build-up of pressure, such as occurs in glaucoma, and impairment or loss of vision.

The Ear

Within the tunnels and chambers of the ear lie the two special types of sense receptors that give us, respectively, the sense of hearing and the sense of balance.

The Outer Ear

The *outer ear* includes that rather oddly shaped and folded piece of flesh and cartilage from which earrings are hung, and more important, the external *auditory canal,* a tunnel leading from the ear's opening to the *tympanic membrane,* or *eardrum.*

The Middle Ear

The *middle ear* includes the inner surface of the eardrum and the three tiny, bony *ossicles,* named long ago for their shape (apparently by some blacksmithing anatomist), *the hammer, the anvil,* and *the stirrup;* or in Latin: *the malleus, the incus,* and *the stapes.* These bones respond to the vibrations in the air that are the basis of sound, vibrate themselves, and transmit their vibrations to the inner ear, where the sense receptors for hearing are located, and the *auditory* (or *acoustic*) *nerve* to the brain begins.

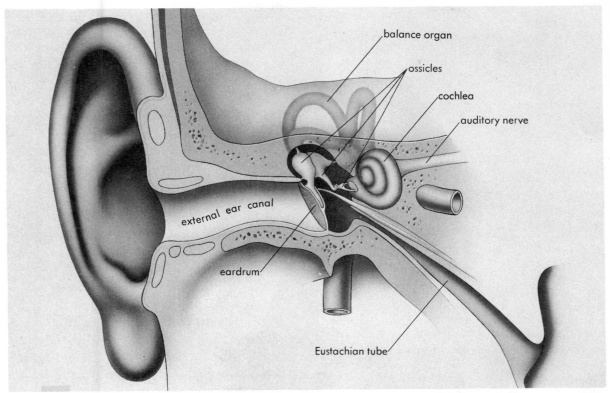

balance organ

ossicles

cochlea

auditory nerve

external ear canal

eardrum

Eustachian tube

The spatial relationships of the parts of the ear are illustrated in this drawing. For a more detailed drawing of the ear and the perception of sound, see page 79.

The middle ear is connected to the back of the throat (pharynx) by the Eustachian tube. This tunnel between throat and middle ear makes the pressure on the inside of the eardrum, via the mouth, the same as the pressure of the atmosphere on the outside of the eardrum. (Thus yawning helps to equalize pressure.) Without it, or if the Eustachian tube becomes clogged, the taut membrane of the eardrum would always be in imminent danger of bursting.

The Inner Ear

The chambers of the *inner ear* are completely filled with fluid, which is jostled by the ossicles "knocking" on a thin membrane called the oval window, separating the middle from the inner ear. Another flexible membrane, the round window, serves to restrict the motion of the inner ear fluid when the movement is too stormy.

Organ of hearing: Within the inner ear is a bony structure coiled like a snail shell about the size of a pea. This is the *cochlea,* the actual Latin word for snail or snail shell. Following the internal spiral of the cochlea is the *organ of Corti,* the true sense receptor for hearing.

The organ of Corti is made up of thousands of specialized nerve endings that are the individual sense receptors for sound. These are in the form of tiny hairs projecting up from the internal membrane lining the cochlea; they wave like stalks of underwater plants in response to the oscillating currents of the inner ear fluid. There are some 20,000 of these hairs within the cochlea, responsive to almost as many degrees of movement of the fluid. These thousands of nerve endings merge at the core of the cochlea and exit from its floor as the nerve bundle of the *auditory nerve.*

THE SEMICIRCULAR CANALS

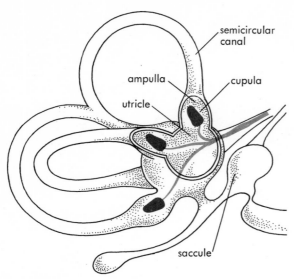

semicircular canal

ampulla

cupula

utricle

saccule

The semicircular canals are swollen at their bases into three ampullae in which receptors are located. When the head moves or accelerates, the fluid within the canals (endolymph) tends to move slower than the head, and the cupula is displaced. This is communicated to the hairlike nerve receptors. Soon the endolymph catches up to the head movement and the cupula returns to its normal position. When movement stops, the endolymph continues to move, the cupula is again displaced, and the nerve receptors are activated until the endolymph ceases to move.

Organ of balance: The organ of balance, or equilibrium, is also behind the oval window that marks the beginning of the inner ear. The principal structure consists of three fluid-filled *semicircular canals* arranged, like the wheels of a gyroscope spinning on a perfectly flat plane or surface, at right angles to each other. When we are in a normal, upright position, the fluid in the canals is also in its normal resting state. But when we begin to tilt or turn or wobble, the fluid runs one way or another in one or more of the canals. This fluid movement is picked up by crested, hairlike nerve endings lining the inside of the canals and relayed as nerve impulses along the *vestibular nerve* to the brain. Then, the brain sends messages to the muscles that can restore our equilibrium.

The term *labyrinth* is sometimes used to refer collectively to the cochlea, semicircular canals and associated structures of the inner ear. The space or cavity within the labyrinth is called the *vestibule,* which gives its name to the vestibular nerve.

How We Hear

Just as our eye has certain special equipment—its focusing apparatus—to prepare light for the retina, so our ear has special equipment to prepare vibrations for reception by the organ of Corti.

This equipment consists of structures that amplify the vibrations reaching the ear, or, more rarely, damping (decreasing) the vibrations caused by very loud or very close occurrences.

Sound waves are really vibrations in the air that reach the eardrum at the narrow end of the funnel-shaped auditory canal. These vibrations set the membrane of the eardrum vibrating ever so slightly. Behind the eardrum, the first ossicle encountered is the hammer, which is attached to the eardrum by a projection descriptively called the hammer-handle.

From the eardrum, vibrations travel up the handle and set the hammer vibrating. The hammer, in turn, sets the anvil vibrating; and the anvil, the stirrup. The stirrup then knocks like an impatient caller on the oval window of the inner ear, and the then vibrating oval window stirs the fluids within the cochlea. This chain of events can account for a tremendous amplification of vibrations—so that we are literally able to "hear a pin drop."

Tiny muscles in the middle ear relax or tighten the eardrum and adjust to changing volumes of sound. For example, a muscle connecting the stirrup and the eardrum relaxes when the stirrup is vibrating violently in the presence of very loud noises. A lax eardrum is less likely to rupture and transmits fewer vibrations to the delicate mechanisms of the middle and inner ear than a taut one. Thus we have to some degree built-in, automatic protection against the assaults of noise pollution—but not nearly enough, according to doctors who are convinced that more and more cases of deafness are caused by the incessant battering of the modern world against our eardrums. Human eardrums are not made to withstand the sound of jet planes taking off, for example. See *Noise Pollution* under *The Environment and Health*, p. 369.

The Nose and Tongue

Taste: The sense receptors on the tongue and within the nasal cavity work very closely together to give us our sense of taste. These five kinds of receptors—the olfactory cell in the nose and the four special cells or taste buds on the tongue for discriminating salty, sweet, sour, and bitter tastes—also have a functional similarity. All are chemical detectors, and all require

THE EAR AND THE PERCEPTION OF SOUND

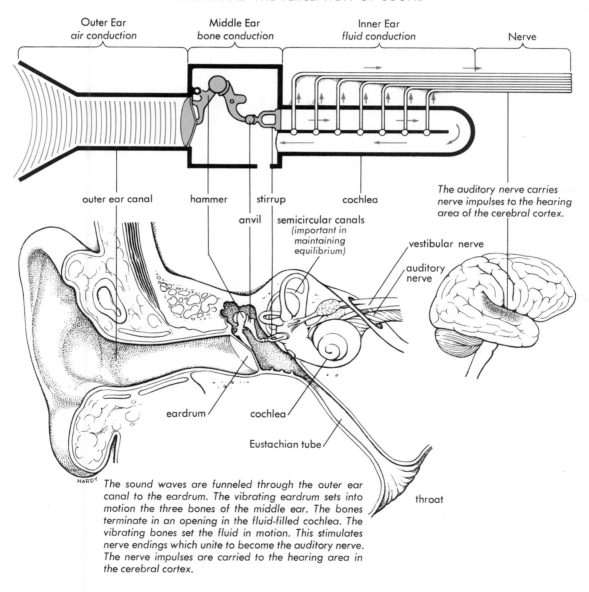

Outer Ear
air conduction

Middle Ear
bone conduction

Inner Ear
fluid conduction

Nerve

outer ear canal   hammer   stirrup   cochlea

anvil   semicircular canals
(important in maintaining equilibrium)

The auditory nerve carries nerve impulses to the hearing area of the cerebral cortex.

vestibular nerve

auditory nerve

eardrum   cochlea

Eustachian tube

throat

HARDY   The sound waves are funneled through the outer ear canal to the eardrum. The vibrating eardrum sets into motion the three bones of the middle ear. The bones terminate in an opening in the fluid-filled cochlea. The vibrating bones set the fluid in motion. This stimulates nerve endings which unite to become the auditory nerve. The nerve impulses are carried to the hearing area in the cerebral cortex.

moisture in order to function. In the nose, airborne substances must first be moistened by mucus (from the olfactory glands) before they can stimulate olfactory cells. In the mouth, the saliva does the wetting.

The general number and distribution of the four types of taste receptors are described under *The Digestive System and the Liver,* p. 43. These nerve endings, numbering in the hundreds of thousands, merge into two nerve bundles traveling away from the tongue to the brain's "taste center." The receptors toward the rear of the tongue collect into the *glossopharyngeal nerve;* those at the front and middle are directed along the *lingual nerve.*

The sense of smell: Our smell receptors are clustered in an area about a half-inch wide on the ceiling of the nasal cavity. This is called, appropriately enough, the smell patch. The nerve endings pass upward through the sievelike *ethmoid bone,* separating the nasal cavity from the brain, and connect to the olfactory bulb, which is the "nose end" of the *olfactory nerve.* At the other end of the olfactory nerve is the "nose brain" or *rhinencephalon*—a tiny part of the cerebrum in man, but quite large in

dogs and other mammals whose sense of smell is keener than man's.

Although man's sense of smell is probably his least used sense, it still has a quite remarkable sensitivity. With it we can detect some chemicals in concentrations as diluted as one part in 30 billion—for example, the active ingredient in skunk spray. Also, man's ability to smell smoke and to detect gas leaks and other warning scents has prevented many a tragedy.

Skin

The sensations stimulated by the various types of sense receptors in the skin are described at the outset of this section. It is worth noting, however, at the end of our tour of the sense organs that the senses associated with the skin are really in a class by themselves. Perhaps the most telling indication of their unique place in the hierarchy of senses is the fact that practically our entire central nervous system (see *The Nervous System and the Brain,* p. 23) is given over to handling the impulses transmitted by these receptors. See also *Diseases of the Eye and Ear,* p. 584.   EHH, Jr.

THE URINOGENITAL SYSTEM AND THE KIDNEYS

In large part our good health depends on the quality of the body's internal environment. There is a kind of ecological principle at work within us—if one chain threatens to break, one system becomes polluted, one balance is tilted, then the whole environment is in imminent danger of collapsing. The major responsibility for keeping our internal environment clean and unclogged lies with our two kidneys. They

are the filters and purifiers of body fluids: the body's pollution-control stations, its recycling plants, and its waste-disposal units.

The Kidneys

The kidneys are located just behind our abdominal cavity on either side of the spinal cord, their tops usually tucked just under the bottommost rib. Each of our kidneys is four to five inches long and weighs about half a pound. The right kidney is normally placed a bit below the left, to accommodate the bulky liver lying also on the right side above it. Neither kidney is fixed rigidly; both can shift position slightly. Lying outside the muscular sheath of the abdominal cavity, the kidneys are more vulnerable than most internal organs to outside blows, but good protection against all but the severest jolts is afforded by surrounding fatty cushions, the big back muscles, and the bone and musculature associated with the spinal column.

As it has with the lungs, the liver, and most other vital organs, nature has supplied us with a large reserve capacity of kidney tissue—a life-giving overabundance in the event of kidney disease or injury. Indeed, normal function of only one-half of one kidney can sustain a person's life.

The kidneys' task of purifying our internal environment—that is, our circulating blood—is really a double task. Each kidney must purify the blood that passes through it, sending back into circulation only "clean blood"; and it must dispose of the impurities it has taken from the blood. The latter is accomplished by the urine draining down a tube, or *ureter*, leading from each of the two kidneys to one common urinary *bladder*. Urine is discharged from the bladder down another tube called the *urethra* to the external opening for urination.

How the Kidneys Process Body Fluids

Blood is brought to the kidney by a renal artery, is treated in the kidney's unique microscopic structures, and exits via the renal vein. (*Renal* means associated with the kidneys.) The sheer volume of blood processed by both our kidneys is prodigious: between 400 and 500 gallons are processed every day.

Internal structure: Within each kidney are over a million microscopic units called

THE ANATOMY OF THE KIDNEY

The cortex is the darker, outer part of the kidney. The medulla, the inner part, includes the renal pyramids and the straight tubules associated with them.

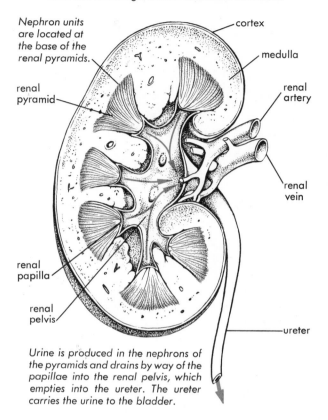

Urine is produced in the nephrons of the pyramids and drains by way of the papillae into the renal pelvis, which empties into the ureter. The ureter carries the urine to the bladder.

nephrons. The nephron is the basic functional unit of the kidney—a little kidney in itself—and is really a superbly engineered and coordinated arrangement of many smaller structures, all working together.

Blood arriving at the kidney from the renal artery is quickly channeled into finer and finer vessels, until finally it flows into a kind of cat's cradle or "ball of wool" structure called a *glomerulus* (composed of intertwining, microscopic vessels called glomerular capillaries). The entire structure of the nephron is built around the microscopic glomerulus (Latin, "tiny ball"). Surrounding the glomerulus, like a hand lightly cupping a ball of wool, is another structure called *Bowman's capsule.* Fluid and dis-

NEPHRON

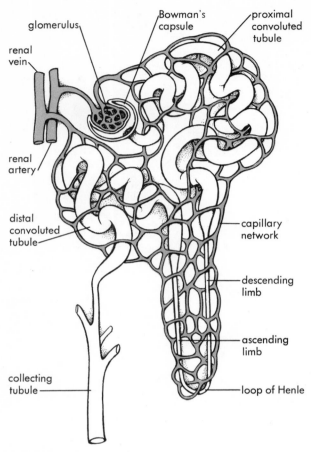

glomerulus

renal vein

renal artery

Bowman's capsule

proximal convoluted tubule

distal convoluted tubule

capillary network

descending limb

ascending limb

collecting tubule

loop of Henle

The nephron is a microscopic unit that filters out certain products from the blood. Useful products are reabsorbed by the capillary network. What remains is the waste product called urine. It is carried to the collecting tubule, which empties into the renal pelvis.

solved materials filter out of the blood from the glomerular capillaries through the membranes into Bowman's capsule.

Substances in Bowman's capsule: The fluids and dissolved materials filtering into Bowman's capsule are by no means all wastes and impurities. In fact, some of the substances must soon be reclaimed. Among the waste substances captured by Bowman's capsule and destined for excretion in urine are various nitrogen salts and other waste products of cellular metabolism, as well as actual or potential poisons that have entered or accumulated in the bloodstream.

Nonwaste substances include needed sugars and salts, and water.

Reclaiming essential substances: Before we leave the glomerulus altogether behind, it should be noted that like any capillary bed, this small ball of blood vessels has not only an inflow from the renal artery but also outflow vessels leading eventually back to the renal vein.

From the cupped lips of Bowman's capsule, fluid and dissolved substances from the blood trickle into a single tube called a kidney *tubule.* The outflow vessels from the glomerulus wind closely over and around the tubule, forming a capillary network around it. By this means the nonwaste substances are reclaimed and returned to refresh the blood moving away from the nephron.

The tubule itself makes many twists and turns—including one hairpin turn so stunning that it has its own medical name—*Henle's loop.* So much twisting and turning gives the tubule a great deal more surface area than a simple, straight tube would have within the same space, thus increasing the amount of water and dissolved substances that can be recaptured by the encircling capillaries.

If there were no recapturing system in the kidneys, death would probably result from dehydration. Even if that could be avoided, the loss of essential salts and other substances would prove fatal in a short time.

The arithmetic of the situation goes something like this: every day, an estimated 42 gallons of fluid filter out of the glomeruli and into the two kidneys' approximately two and a half million tubules. Dissolved in this 42 gallons—representing about three times the body's weight—are about two-and-a-half pounds of common salt, just one of the many substances in the fluid that our body needs in sufficient amounts. The loss of either water or common salt at a rapid rate would prove fatal in a matter of hours.

But so efficient is the tubule-capillary re-capturing system that only an average of less than two quarts of fluid, containing just one-third ounce of salt, pass daily out of the kidneys into the ureter and are excreted as urine. In other words, over 99 percent of both the water and common salt removed from the blood at Bowman's capsules is returned to the blood.

The Kidneys and Blood Pressure

A surprising insight into the critical role played by our kidneys in almost every body function is provided by the relation of blood pressure to kidney function. The blood in the glomerular capillaries must be at higher pressure than the fluid around them, so that the fluid and its dissolved substances can push through the capillary membranes to-ward Bowman's capsule. If blood pressure in the body falls too low (severe *hypoten-sion*) the formation of urine ceases.

On the other hand, if a portion of the kid-ney is suffering from anemia due to some disorder, kidney cells secrete *pressor hor-mones,* which serve to elevate the blood pressure. Thus, high blood pressure (*hyper-tension*) may be a sign of kidney disorder.

The Urinary Tract

From the ends of the million or so tubules in each kidney, urine drains into larger and larger collecting basins (called *calyces,* singular *calyx*) which drain in turn into the kidney's master urine reservoir, the *kidney pelvis*. Then, drop by drop, urine slides down each ureter to the urinary bladder.

Urine is held in the bladder by the con-traction of two muscle rings, or *sphincters,* one located just inside the bladder before it meets the urethra, and the other encircling the urethra itself. When about a half-pint has accumulated, nerves convey the urge to urinate to the brain, and a person volun-tarily causes the sphincters to relax, empty-

ing the bladder. (In exceptional circum-stances, the elastic-walled bladder can hold two or three quarts of urine.) Up to the point where the bladder drains, the male and female urinary tracts are very similar, but after the bladder, any similarity stops.

Female urethra: The female's urethra, normally about one and a half inches long, is not much more than a short channel by which urine is eliminated from the blad-der. Its very shortness often gives it an undesired significance, because it repre-sents an easy upward invasion route for bacteria and other infection-causing mi-crobes from the outside. Acute and painful inflammations of the urethra (*urethritis*) and bladder (*cystitis*) are thus common in women. These lower urinary tract infec-tions, however, can usually be halted before spreading further up the urinary tract by

THE FEMALE URINARY SYSTEM

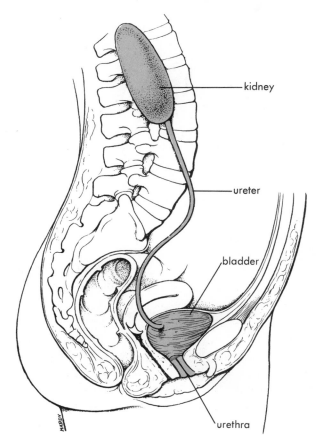

kidney

ureter

bladder

urethra

the administration of any of several anti-microbial drugs.

Male urethra: In contrast to the female, the male's urethra is involved with reproductive functions. So closely connected are the male's lower urinary tract and genital organs that his urethra (from bladder to the outside) is properly called the urino-genital (or genito-urinary) tract. This is the reason why the medical specialty known as *urology* deals with both the urinary and genital apparatus of men; but with only the urinary tract of women. The urologist's specialty does not extend to the female genital and childbearing organs, which are the concern of the *gynecologist* and *obstetrician.*

However, all the distinctly male sex glands and organs are linked more or less directly into the eight- or nine-inch length of the male urethra.

The Genitals

The Female Reproductive System

As indicated above, the urinary and genital systems of women are dealt with by two different medical specialties. For this reason, the female genitals are discussed elsewhere. For a description and illustration of the female reproductive system, see p. 235 under *Social and Sexual Maturation.*

The Male Reproductive System

From its emergence below the bladder, the male urethra serves as a conduit for all the male sexual secretions.

THE MALE URINARY SYSTEM

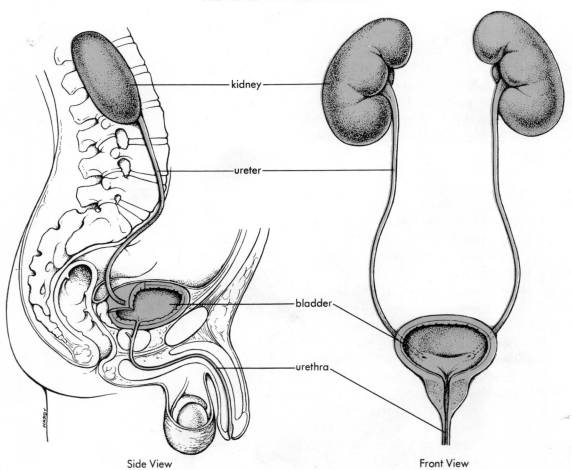

kidney

ureter

bladder

urethra

Side View   Front View

THE MALE REPRODUCTIVE SYSTEM

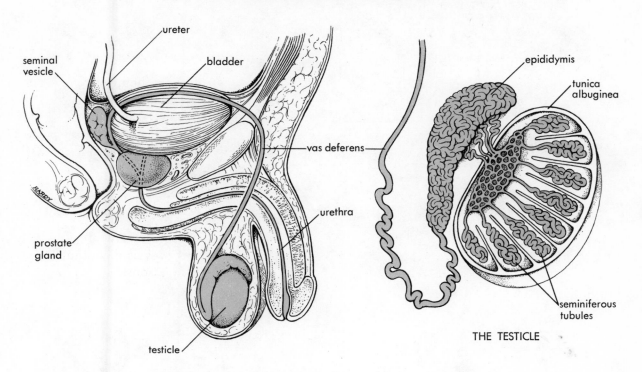

THE TESTICLE

Prostate gland: Directly below the bladder outlet, the *prostate gland* completely enwraps the urethra. The prostate secretes substances into the urethra through ejaculatory ducts; these substances are essential in keeping alive the spermatazoa that arrive from their manufacturing sites in the *testicles* (or *testes*).

Testicles: The two testicles hang down within a wrinkled bag of skin called the *scrotum*. Although the vulnerable position of the testicles remains something of an evolutionary mystery, one clue is that the optimum production of spermatazoa takes place at a temperature some degrees lower than the normal internal body temperature.

Spermatazoa produced in the testicles travel upward toward the urethra through a seminal duct or tube called the *vas*

deferens (one from each testicle). (These are the ducts, incidentally, that are tied and cut in the male sterilization procedure known as a vasectomy.) The sperm cells are then stored, until ejaculation, in little reservoirs called *seminal vesicles* which are situated on either side of the urethra in the area of the prostate gland.

The portion of the male urethra from the bladder to where it emerges from the encircling prostate, having received the emission of both the prostate and the testicles, is called the prostatic or posterior urethra. The remainder, mainly consisting of the conduit running down the middle of the shaft of the penis, ending in the external opening called the *meatus*, is known as the anterior urethra. See also *Diseases of the Urinogenital System*, p. 595.   EHH, JR.

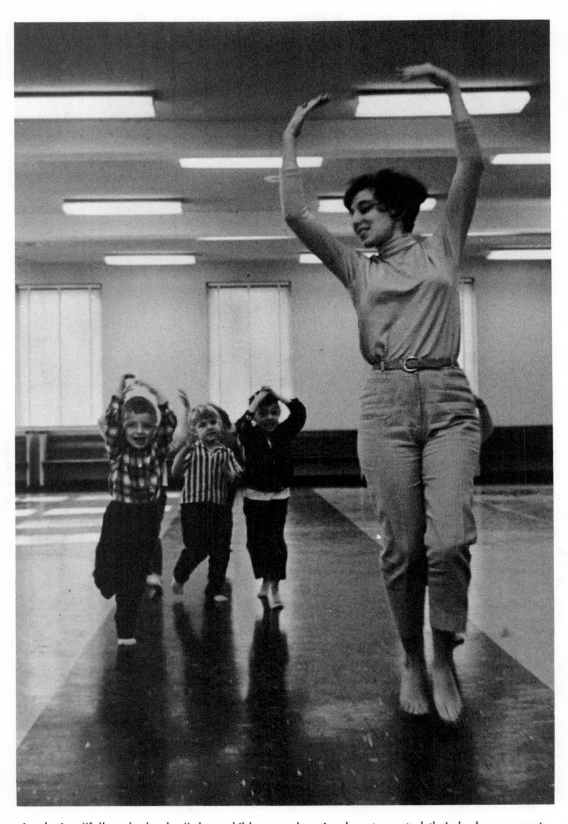

In playing "follow the leader," these children are learning how to control their body movements.

CHAPTER 2

Staying Healthy and Attractive Through the Years

Maintaining good health is far simpler, less expensive, and more comfortable than restoring health that has become poor. Since some diseases cannot be cured after they are contracted, it is only logical to try to prevent all possible health problems. The techniques of modern preventive medicine are available to every American of every age. This chapter deals with the physical development of human beings at various ages. The following chapter (Chapter 3) is devoted to emotional and intellectual development at these age levels.

All people are not beautiful or handsome, but nearly everyone can have the kind of attractiveness and vitality that comes from good health. The health of an individual depends upon the kind of body he inherits and the care he gives it. Good health can be thought of as a state of social, physical, and mental well-being, a goal almost all can attain—if the responsibility for maintaining one's own health with help from the health experts is accepted.

Medical Checkups

The first necessary step in maintaining good health is the periodic medical checkup. The physician can best advise his patients on how frequently they should have checkups. Annual checkups are desirable for most adults, particularly those over 35. For information on the frequency and timing of checkups for children, see *Checkups and Immunization*, p. 113.

The physician giving the checkup has three main objectives. He tries to assess the patient's present state of health, predict possible future problems, and recommend ways of caring for present problems and avoiding future ones.

A checkup can usually be divided into three stages. First, the doctor reviews the patient's health history, asking questions about previous illnesses and operations, illnesses and diseases of other family members, including parents, and allergies, health habits, and the like.

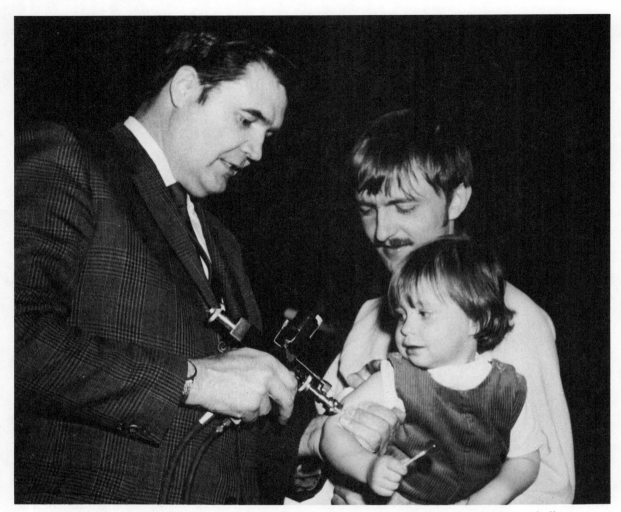

This child is receiving vaccine against rubella (German measles). Immunization against rubella is recommended for young children to prevent the spread of the disease to women of child-bearing age. The disease can cause birth defects in the babies of women who contract it early in pregnancy.

Secondly, he performs a physical examination by observation and various tests, including simple ones such as tapping the back and chest. He will assess vitality, coordination, skin, weight in relation to height and body build, hearing, eyesight, heart, lungs, and blood pressure. He may also include a rectal examination in order to check the condition of certain internal organs, such as the male's prostate gland. Women are often given a Pap test.

Finally, the physician may order certain laboratory tests or procedures to complete his assessment. He may, for example, order chest X rays of blood tests. When the test results are in, the physician will review them in conjunction with examination results and the patient's medical history to obtain a complete and accurate picture of the patient's health. See *Disease*, p. 437, for a fuller discussion of medical checkups.

Immunizations: At the time of the checkup, the physician will also determine what immunizations are required. Immunizations are of great help in maintaining good health. Older readers will recall the threat that polio once presented. During the summer months, people avoided all public meeting places—theaters, beaches, even large stores —from fear of contracting this disabling disease. Today, with widespread polio immunization, we are protected from this disease.

The individual—adult or child—benefits personally from immunization, as does the community, since there is one less susceptible person who might contract and then spread disease. Common immunizations protect against polio, tetanus (lockjaw), smallpox, measles, diphtheria, whooping cough, influenza, mumps, and (for children and certain adults) German measles.

Why Have a Checkup?

Even people who feel healthy should follow the checkup schedule advised by the physician. Many diseases do not give any warning signals until they are fairly far advanced. How one feels is not, therefore, always an adequate gauge of how one really is. Even if the physician says that all is well, it is still important to have had the checkup. What could be more important to peace of mind than receiving word that one is free of detectable disease and advice on how to stay that way?

In addition, there are practical benefits that result from a checkup of a person who feels well. He will have established himself as a particular physician's patient. This relationship will be very important if serious illness does strike, because the physician will have his health history over a period of years. He will know how the patient's health status has changed over the years. Of course, he will also know more about his individual patient and how he prefers to be treated. Should the problem be better treated by a specialist, the physician will be able to recommend one who is not only competent, but whose personality will be compatible with the patient's.

If some problem is detected during the routine checkup, the physician will outline how he proposes to treat it. He may prescribe a medication or a slight change in daily activities or diet. If checkups are regular, problems detected are generally mild. When they are promptly corrected, many years of tiring emotional and physical discomfort can be avoided. Periodic checkups and early detection of disease have saved a great many people from untimely deaths.

Personal Hygiene

Disease germs can enter the body only in a limited number of ways. One of the major ways is through the skin. The skin is a protective covering which, when broken, can admit harmful bacteria or viruses easily.

Simple precautions are very effective. The hands come into contact with disease germs more than any other part of the body. Therefore, they should be washed whenever they are dirty, prior to preparing food or eating, and after using the lavatory.

The rest of the body must also be kept clean, since adequate bodily cleanliness will remove substances which, by irritating the skin, make it more susceptible to infection. Bathing also improves the muscle tone of the skin. For the same reason, hair should be washed often enough to prevent accumulation of dust and dead skin cells.

Openings in the body are also paths by which disease germs can enter the body. The nose and ears should be carefully cleaned only with something soft, for instance, a cotton swab. Genital orifices should be kept clean by frequent bathing. Any unusual discharge from a body opening should be promptly reported to a physician. He can then treat a problem at its earliest stage—the easiest time to solve the problem.

Personal hygiene includes care of the nails. They should always be kept clean and fairly short. Hangnails can be avoided by gently pushing back the cuticle with a towel after washing the hands.

Proper Diet

Proper diet is another contribution an individual can make to his good health, because foods build body tissues and provide energy for the body to work. Adequate diet planning is not difficult. The basic rules of good nutrition must be learned. See *Basic Nutritional Requirements,* p. 295, for a full treatment of diet and nutrition. Applying these rules to a daily diet will take only a few minutes of planning when the menu is decided upon, and will reap enormous rewards in good health and appearance. The hardest part of planning a balanced diet is avoiding the selection of food solely on the basis of taste or convenience, and ignoring nutritional value.

Vitamins: Eating a proper, balanced diet will fulfill vitamin and other nutritional requirements. Therefore, there is no need for a healthy person who eats nutritious foods to take vitamin pills. Vitamins and other food supplements should be taken only on the advice of a physician or dentist. If a person decides he is deficient in some dietary element and purchases a patent medicine to treat the problem, he may only make it worse. It is rare to find someone deficient in only one element, and by trying to treat himself, he may delay seeking the advice of a doctor.

Breakfast: Many Americans neglect breakfast, an important contribution to good diet. Studies prove that men, women, and children need an adequate breakfast. A good breakfast can provide a start in obtaining the day's vitamin and mineral requirements. It is also a help to dieters and those trying to maintain a stable weight, since those who have eaten a good breakfast are able to avoid mid-morning snacks such as sweet rolls, cakes, and the like, which are usually high in carbohydrates and calories.

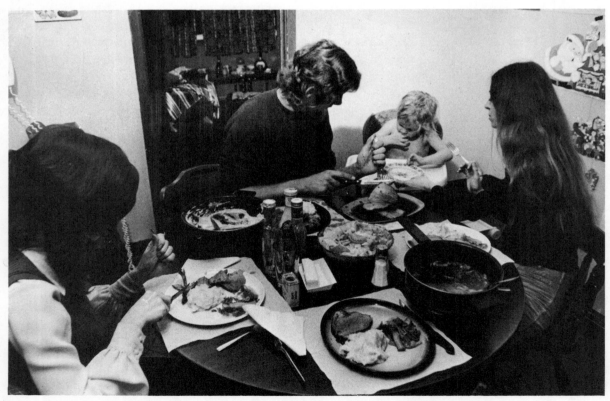

Meat, potatoes, a vegetable, salad—nothing fancy, but a good, nutritious, tasteful meal nonetheless.

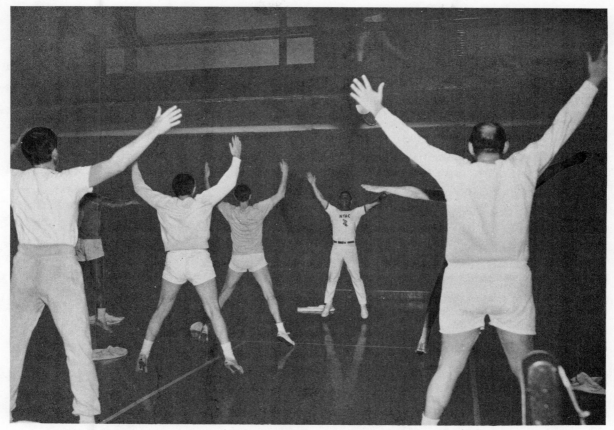

Regular calisthenics supervised by a trained health specialist can improve muscle tone and posture.

Overweight: Overweight is often the result of an unbalanced diet, and should be carefully avoided by those who are concerned with good health and appearance. Obesity is not considered attractive in our society. More important, obesity is a killer. Heart disease, hardening of the arteries, diabetes, and high blood pressure are a few examples of the problems overweight persons develop more often than those who manage to control their weight.

Even those who have not been conscious of the crucial role an adequate diet plays in maintaining good health will find it is never too late to reform. By studying the four basic food groups and making adjustments where necessary, health and well-being can be improved and maintained. Those who are unable to lose weight should seek medical advice.

Exercise

Exercise provides health dividends which will be evident in improved appearance—as seen in vitality, posture, muscle tone, strength, and ease of movement. Increased ability to combat fatigue can be developed only with adequate exercise. The respiratory, circulatory, muscular, and digestive systems function better with exercise. Exercise helps to prevent some of the major killer diseases—for example, hardening of the arteries. Physical activity can make an important contribution to the preservation of health.

In the average person, the fitness which comes from exercise can mean doing everything in daily life better, since every task requires some degree of endurance to resist fatigue and to sustain effort. Those with higher endurance often do better, whether it be studying, cleaning the house, or selling a product.

Exercise is also related to mental health. Life creates unavoidable stresses, but a moderate amount of exercise helps reduce them. When the exercise chosen is enjoyable and absorbs one's attention, tension is lessened and worries are forgotten. There are so many kinds of exercise that it should be easy to choose a few that will prove especially enjoyable. Some type of exercise, though not necessarily the same each time, should be performed daily. For information about particular exercises, see *Keeping Fit*, p. 165.

Since capacity for exercise in the later years depends to a great extent upon the degree of activity a person has followed in earlier years, it is wise to choose the kind of exercises when young that can be carried on in the middle and later years. Tennis, golf, handball, cycling, swimming, and walking are some exercises which can be enjoyed after the individual is no longer young. A physician can guide those with special conditions or problems in the selection of appropriate exercise.

Rest and Sleep

Rest and sleep adequate for one's personal needs are another vital component of good health and good appearance. They also influence human relationships and mental alertness. Scientists believe that during sleep the body replaces tissue cells and eliminates waste products created by fatigue at a faster rate than when awake.

Sleep also rests the heart and blood system, since heart muscle contractions and blood pressure are slower then. Excessive fatigue from lack of sleep increases susceptibility to a number of ailments, including the

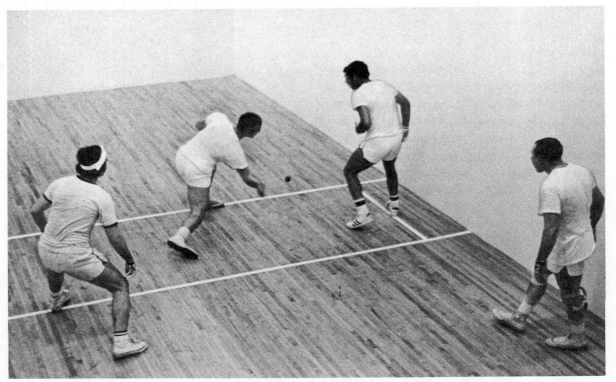

The keen competition in active sports like handball may be the chief reason for playing, but the vigorous exercise, often continued well beyond middle age, is an important health by-product.

common cold. If an individual gets an adequate amount of sleep (usually seven to eight hours for an adult), he will feel ready to meet the day's activities. If not, his memory may not be sharp, and he may be irritable because his nervous system has had inadequate rest.

A quiet, dark, ventilated room, a fairly firm mattress, and performance of a moderate amount of exercise during the day will aid sleep. When worry, frustration, or anxiety make it difficult to sleep, a conscious attempt to relax will help. Sedatives or sleeping pills should not be taken unless they are prescribed or recommended by a physician.

Skin and Hair Care

Skin protects the internal structures of the body. Often taken for granted, it is one of the body's major defenses against the invasion of disease organisms. The skin is also important in the regulation of body temperature and in the excretion of wastes through perspiration. In addition, its ability to sense pain, touch, heat, and cold warns the body of possible danger.

Healthy, attractive skin and elimination of body odors can be achieved by thorough soaping and rinsing of every part of the body. Special care should be taken to wash the groin, armpits, and feet thoroughly.

Frequent hair washing is also necessary, both for the sake of appearance, and for the health of the scalp. Since the root of a hair is beneath the surface of the skin, and since oil (*sebaceous*) glands open into the root area, the secretion of the glands can plug up the *follicle*, the shaft which contains the root. Vigorous brushing and finger-tip massage of the scalp will stimulate circulation of blood, which brings nutrients to the scalp, and helps distribute sebaceous gland secretions. For a more complete discussion of skin and hair care, see *Skin and Hair*, p. 377.

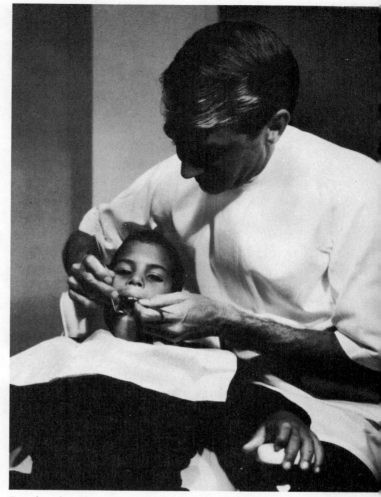

Regular dental examinations are a must for children.

Teeth and Gum Care

An attractive smile is often the first thing that one notices about others. In addition to creating an attractive appearance, healthy teeth and gums are a basic requirement for good overall health. One cannot have a healthy body without a healthy mouth, and vice versa. The dentist should be visited at whatever intervals he recommends, usually every six months.

The dentist will take a general health and dental health history at the first appointment. He will then examine the teeth, gums, bite, and all oral tissues—both visually and with X rays. X rays constitute a vital part

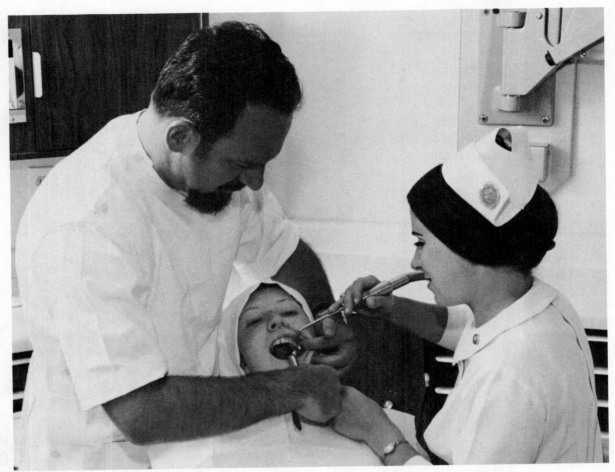

Oral surgery is sometimes necessary to treat diseases of the teeth or gums, or to correct an injury or defect. Here a youngster is having a tooth extracted.

of his examination. Without them, the dentist cannot examine the surfaces between teeth or the three-fifths of the tooth beneath the gums. Other diagnostic tests may be made, such as a test of nerve response. Sometimes it is necessary to take impressions of the teeth. Models made from these impressions are used to study the *occlusion*, the way the teeth meet. Such knowledge is often crucial for deciding the selection of treatment and materials.

After the examination, the dentist will present and explain any proposed treatment. After oral restoration is completed, he will ask the patient to return at particular intervals for a checkup and *prophylaxis*, a cleaning and polishing of the teeth.

Why Have a Dental Checkup?

Because the rate of tooth decay decreases after adolescence, some people discontinue regular dental checkups, and thus do not receive prophylaxis. This in turn can lead to *periodontal diseases*, diseases affecting the gum tissue and underlying bone.

Regular checkups and prophylaxis help prevent these conditions, because a professional cleaning will remove all hard deposits from the teeth, and a polishing will remove stains and soft deposits.

Without this professional help, it would be impossible for anyone to keep his own mouth clean at home. The hard deposits, or *calculus*, have a very rough surface that traps bacteria. The combination of bacterial action and roughness injures the surrounding gum tissue and makes it susceptible to infection and recession. The irritation causes bleeding into the crevice between the tooth and gum, one of the early signs of impaired tissue health. If these irritants are not removed regularly, the bone under the gum can actually be destroyed. Since the bone is what holds teeth in place, its loss will cause loosening of the teeth. Unless complex treatment is undertaken at this point, the teeth will be lost.

Even if the teeth are lost, a problem can still exist. Replacement teeth, or *dentures,* are made to fit over the ridges of the jaws. If the top edge of the ridge has been destroyed by periodontal disease, it is difficult to fit the denture so that it can be held firmly in place. The only way to avoid such a disastrous chain of events is to have the teeth checked and cleaned regularly.

Extra Checkups

If a woman should become pregnant, it is advisable that she see her dentist as well as her obstetrician. Many changes take place in a pregnant woman's body, among them, increased hormone production. A checkup by the dentist during the first three months of pregnancy is needed to assess the oral effects of such changes, and to make sure that all dental problems are examined and corrected.

To avoid the problem of toxic substances or poisons circulating in the mother's bloodstream, all sources of infection must be removed. Some of these sources can be in the mouth. An absessed tooth, for example, which may not yet be severe enough to signal its presence with pain, is directly connected to the bloodstream and can send toxic substances and harmful bacteria through the mother's body.

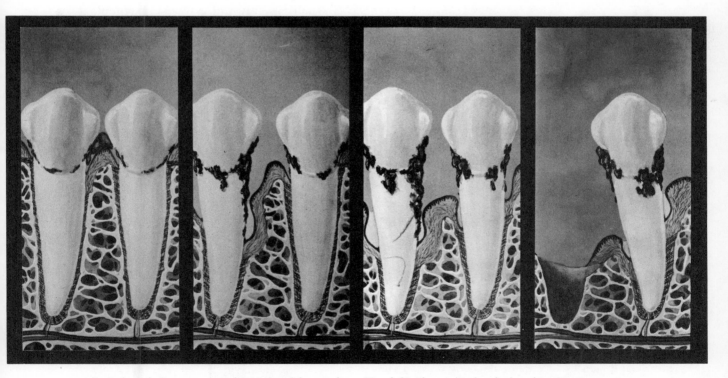

Periodontal diseases are often caused by neglect. (*Far left*) Plaque and calculus deposits accumulate. (*Left*) The irritated, swollen gums bleed easily and have begun to retract. (*Right*) Most of the bony support for the teeth has been destroyed. (*Far right*) One tooth is lost; another weakened.

What To Do Between Checkups

There are three general rules to follow in protecting dental health between checkups. If anyone in the family is under age 15 and lives in an area without adequate fluoride in the water supply, fluoride should be provided. Fluoride provides benefits by strengthening the *enamel,* or outer surface, of the tooth. Those who drink fluoridated water from birth have 60 percent fewer cavities than those who drink nonfluoridated water.

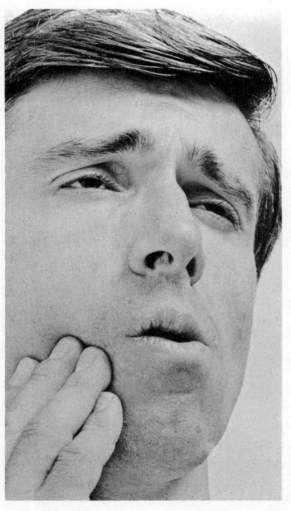

"Ooh! It hurts!" Don't ignore the early warning signs of tooth decay. It's far better to visit the dentist at the first sign of discomfort than to postpone seeing him until the pain—and the decay—are very severe.

Use of fluorides: There are many ways to supplement fluoride deficiency. The dentist can advise the best combination of methods. The most common are adding fluoride to some liquid consumed daily, such as water, applying fluoride to the teeth, and brushing with a fluoride toothpaste. Unless an adult has a severe problem with cavities, fluorides are not widely used after adolescence. Although they would not be harmful, effectiveness is not as great.

Diet and teeth: The second rule to follow for good dental health is proper diet. Nutrition affects cavities, and periodontal and other diseases of the mouth. Although a good diet for total health provides all of the elements of a good diet for dental health, several precautions on sweets and starches must be added. Some of the bacteria normally present in the mouth combine with sugars and starches to produce dental *plaque,* a substance which holds the bacteria tightly against the tooth. The bacteria in the plaque produce the acid which causes cavities. Hard or sticky sweets should be avoided. Such highly refined sweets as soft drinks, cookies, pies, cakes, syrups, jams, jellies, and pastries should be limited. One's intake of starchy foods (potato, bread, macaroni, etc.) should also be controlled.

Obviously, one cannot eliminate all starches and sugars from the diet. They should, however, be avoided between meals. If they are eaten with the meal, damage to the teeth can be lessened by brushing afterwards. In situations where it is impossible to brush, either rinse the mouth or finish the meal with a detergent food. Hard, crunchy, fibrous foods (i.e., carrots, apples, celery) are detergent foods, so named because they clean teeth by removing softer food particles. Those who chew gum should use sugarless gum. Regular gum may remove food particles, but it deposits sugar.

Sweets and starches can also be restricted by substitution. Sugarless and artificially sweetened foods can be used as substitutes,

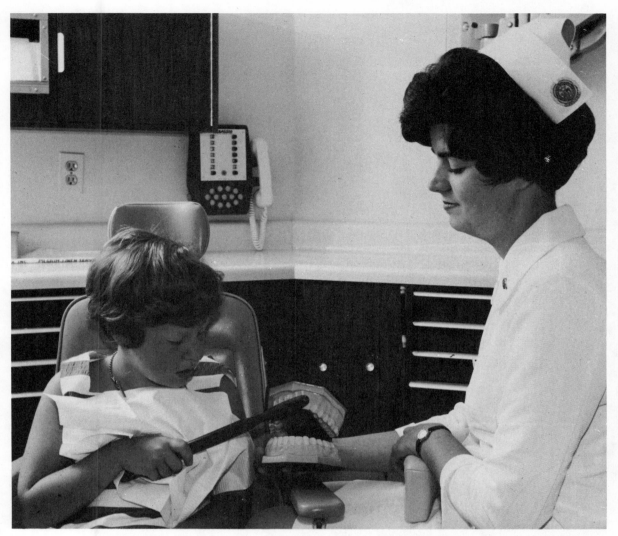

With the aid of an oversize toothbrush and model of the jaws, a dental assistant explains to a young patient the proper method of brushing the teeth.

as suggested by a physician. Such naturally sugarless snacks as meat or cheese, raw vegetables, or popcorn can be substituted for high-sugar snacks.

Brushing: The third rule for proper home care of the teeth is personal oral hygiene, including whatever methods are necessary for the individual. Brushing the teeth is the first essential, since this rids the mouth of the food debris and dental plaque which encourage bacterial growth. Bacterial action is most intense 20 minutes after eating. Therefore, teeth should be brushed as soon

as possible after a meal. There is no one best kind of toothbrush or method of brushing for every mouth. Commonly, however, a multi-tufted, medium-stiff toothbrush is recommended.

If the dentist has not advised a specific brushing method, a good general method is the following. Brush the biting surfaces, or tops, of the back upper and lower teeth. The lines and grooves on these surfaces make them prone to decay. They should be brushed first, before the saliva softens the brush. The cheek and tongue surfaces of

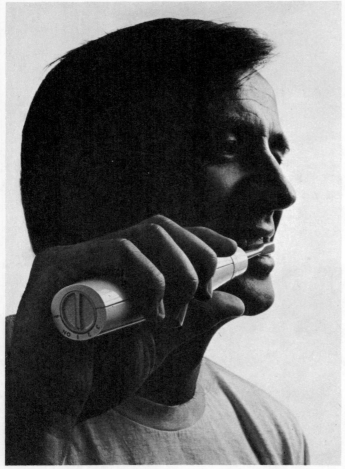

Some people prefer electric toothbrushes because they work much faster and with less effort than an ordinary toothbrush. Regular brushing, however, is more important than the kind of toothbrush selected.

the lower teeth are brushed next. Hold the brush parallel to the teeth with the bristle edges touching the gums. Roll the brush up with the wrist. Repeat the same procedure on the upper teeth, but roll the brush down. This method will also massage the gums to keep them healthy.

Some people prefer electric toothbrushes, which require less pressure to use than ordinary toothbrushes. These are available with two basic motions—up-down and back-forth. Your dentist is the best judge of which kind will serve your needs. Brushes in electric devices tend to wear out quicker than do regular toothbrushes, generally re-quiring replacement every three or four months. The American Dental Association evaluates electric brushes and classifies as acceptable those which meet certain tests of safety and usefulness. Check its most up-to-date ratings before buying an electric toothbrush.

Removing debris: Brushing often does not clean debris from between teeth, an area which traps food and for this reason is prone to decay. Food that sticks between teeth can be removed with dental floss. The floss should be grasped between the thumb and forefinger of each hand and pushed gently between the teeth, then pulled out gently. If floss is snapped in and out, the gums will become irritated. After brushing and flossing the teeth, loosened food particles should be rinsed out with water. Mouthwash is unnecessary and will not prevent bad breath, but it may be used for its temporary good taste.

On the other hand, the dentist may recommend one of the many brands of oral irrigating devices now on the market. Generally, these units create a pulsating stream of water which is used to flush debris from in between teeth. They are commonly recommended for use by people who have had recession of the gums, thus creating a larger space between teeth, or by those wearing such orthodontic appliances as bands. The irrigating device does not replace brushing the teeth, but is usually used after the teeth are brushed.

The effectiveness of brushing, flossing, or oral irrigating for removing plaque can be checked at home by using *disclosing tablets.* After chewing the tablet, a temporary harmless stain will be deposited on any remaining plaque. The tablets facilitate a very thorough and efficient cleaning of the teeth. Many dentists advise that they be used every time one brushes for two weeks or until effectiveness is achieved. Thereafter they can be used weekly to maintain thorough cleaning techniques.   DJC

BIRTH, INFANCY, AND MATURATION: THE FIRST DOZEN YEARS

Before the Baby Arrives

When a husband and wife decide to have a baby they should both undergo complete physical examinations. This will make it possible to detect and treat abnormalities like diabetes and anemia that might affect the future pregnancy. A pregnant woman should have periodic checkups so that her physician can observe both her progress and that of the growing fetus. Such observation will help to assure a pregnancy and delivery which are free from troublesome complications.

What the Newborn Baby Looks Like

At birth the baby's skin is wrinkled or scaly, and may be covered by a cheesy substance called *vernix caseosa*. During the first two weeks the skin will become quite dry to the touch. The skin of white newborns is red,

The feet look more complete than they are. X ray would show only one real bone at the heel. Other bones are now cartilage. The skin is quite commonly loose and wrinkly.

A deep flush spreads over the entire body if the baby cries hard. Veins on the head swell and throb. You will notice no tears, because the tear ducts do not function yet.

The hands, if you open them out flat from their characteristic fist position, have finely lined palms, tissue-paper-thin nails, dry, loose-fitting skin, and deep bracelet creases at the wrist.

The skin is thin and dry. You may see veins through it. Fair skin may be rosy red temporarily. Downy hair is not unusual. Some *vernix caseosa* (white, prenatal covering) remains.

Eyes appear dark blue and have a blank stary gaze. You may catch one or both of them turning or turned to a crossed or wall-eyed position. The lids are characteristically puffy.

Head usually strikes you as being too big for the body. It may be temporarily out of shape—lopsided or elongated—due to pressure before birth or during the birth process.

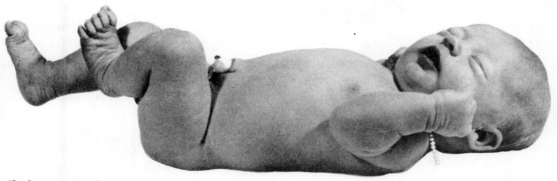

The legs are most often seen drawn up against the abdomen in prebirth position. Extended legs measure shorter than you'd expect compared to the arms. The knees stay slightly bent and legs are somewhat bowed.

Weight unless well above the average of six or seven pounds will not prepare you for how really tiny newborn is. Top to toe measure: anywhere between 18 inches to 21 inches.

Genitals of both sexes will seem too large (especially the scrotum) in comparison with the scale of the hands, for example, to adult size.

The trunk may startle you in some ways: short neck, small sloping shoulders, swollen breasts, large rounded abdomen, umbilical stump (future navel), slender, narrow pelvis and hips.

On the skull you will see or feel the two most obvious soft spots, or *fontanels*. One is above the brow; the other is close to the crown in the back.

The face will disappoint you unless you expect to see pudgy cheeks, a broad, flat nose with only the merest hint of a bridge, a receding chin, and an undersized lower jaw.

and sometimes turns yellow during the first few days. Black newborns often are not as dark as they might be later. Their skin becomes just as yellow as that of white babies, but the change is more difficult to observe.

The newborn's head is large in proportion to the rest of its body. The genitals too may seem large, especially in girls. Newborn girls may have swollen genitalia due to *edema* (fluid in the tissues, causing puffiness), but the swelling is present for only a few days after birth.

The eyes, slate blue in color, can open and react to light, but are unable to focus. Noises produce a *startle response,* a complex

Courses in infant care, often free, give prospective parents the chance to prepare for the new baby with the aid of a life-sized doll and a watchful instructor.

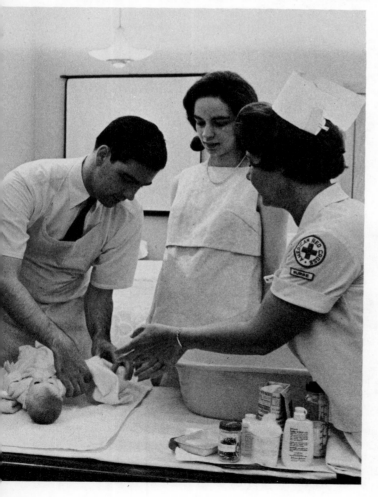

involuntary reaction marked by a sudden, jerky, arm and leg movement. The newborn cries a great deal, sucks, and may sneeze.

The infant's stomach may look rather large and protuberant, and, of course, it has the stump of the umbilical cord dangling from it. The umbilical cord has been cut and tied near the navel, and will eventually fall off.

If you feel the front and back of the baby's head, you will notice one or two soft spots, called the *anterior* and *posterior fontanels.* The posterior fontanel usually closes at the baby's second month of life, the anterior at 18 months or earlier.

You also may feel many different ridges in the baby's head. These are the borders of the different skull bones, which fuse as the baby gets older. They are present so that the skull can grow as the baby's brain and head continue to grow.

Soon after birth, you may detect a swelling on the baby's head just under the scalp. This is called *caput succedaneum.* It is nothing to worry about, as it dissolves a day or two after birth. Occasionally, another swelling known as *cephalhematoma* may also be present. This, too, usually disappears within a few weeks.

The baby's weight will, of course, vary. Most full-term babies weigh between six and eight pounds. Babies of diabetic mothers are often heavier, and may weigh up to twelve pounds.

Some Advice to New Mothers

Unless the new father and mother are really prepared to change some of the conditioned patterns of their relationship, both can be in for a very difficult time. The father suddenly finds himself taking second place in his wife's attentions and affection. The new mother is tired physically and mentally. In-laws and other relatives may infringe on the couple's privacy and interfere with their right to make their own decisions. The

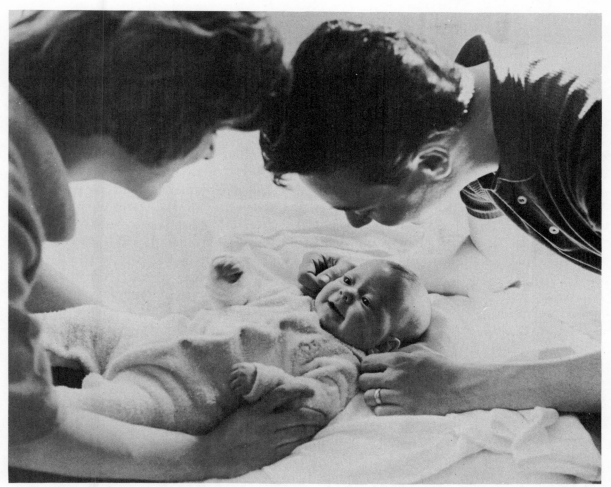

From the beginning of their lives, babies should be exposed to the attention and love of both parents. The father should be encouraged to take an active role in holding and caring for the baby.

new mother may find it hard to reconcile her maternal instinct with her desires as a woman and wife.

All of these problems can be minimized if the mother follows a few common-sense guidelines:

• The new baby is a shared responsibility. Do not shut your husband out of the experience of parenthood. Let him learn to feed the baby, diaper the baby, hold him, get acquainted with him. Make your husband feel just as important to the baby as you are, and just as important to you as he was before the baby was born.

• Arrange for some kind of assistance in your home, and don't wait until the day you

bring the baby home to do it. Plan ahead. You will be physically and emotionally tired after childbirth, no matter how marvelous you may feel when you leave the hospital. During the hospital stay the baby was cared for by a trained staff. At home the burden will fall mainly on you, unless you take steps to get help. If you cannot get your mother or another relative to stay with you, engage a housekeeper or some other trained person. The investment will pay off for you, the baby, and your husband.

• If it is at all possible, arrange to have a separate area for the baby. It is best for a baby not to be kept in the parents' room. Parents must have privacy. If you do not have a bedroom for the baby, section off some spot where you can put a crib and a dressing table to hold the supplies you will need when you feed, change, bathe, and dress him.

• Don't make the baby the focus of attention 24 hours a day. If he fidgets and fusses at times, try not to get nervous. Don't run to him at every whimper so long as you know he has been fed, is dry, and nothing is really wrong. Relax. The baby will be very sensitive to your emotional responses, particularly when you hold him. Through your physical contact you will develop a kind of communication with your baby which he will sense when you pick him up or feed him.

• As important as it is for you and your husband to avoid overhandling the baby, it is more important that family and friends be made to follow a "hands off" policy except at your discretion. A new baby should not be subjected to excessive stimulation. For example, you may notice that if you pick him up and put him back in his crib, and then let someone else hold him a few minutes later, the baby may cry. If you slam a door, the baby's body reacts in the startle reflex, the involuntary reaction previously described. A baby needs a quiet, organized home, free from the kind of upsetting distraction that comes from being surrounded and fussed over by too many people. You and your husband must decide when you want the baby to have visitors and how those visitors are to behave. You must do this even if it causes hurt feelings among your friends and relatives. When the baby is a little older there will be time enough for friends and relatives to admire and play with him.

Feeding the Baby

One of the first questions a mother-to-be must ask herself is how she will feed her baby.

Breast feeding is certainly the simplest method, and many women believe that both mother and child get more emotional satisfaction from it than from bottle feeding. It is also, obviously, less expensive.

Breast Feeding

Almost any healthy woman who wants to breast-feed her baby can do so. All she needs is the desire and motivation. No special preparation is necessary except, perhaps, some stimulation of the breasts, as prescribed by her doctor during pregnancy.

On the other hand, a variety of different factors might necessitate a change from breast to bottle feeding. Although breast feeding may be discontinued at any time, some mothers may feel a sense of failure or frustration at being unable to continue having the intimate relationship that so many other mothers enjoy. No harm will come to the baby by being switched to a formula. Once started on a formula, however, it may be difficult to go back to breast feeding on a regular basis. For a while, at least, the mother will have to stimulate her breasts artificially to increase their milk-producing capacity.

The first few days: When a mother first starts to breast-feed, she may be worried that she won't have sufficient milk for the baby. Her breasts are just beginning to fill up with a creamy, yellowish substance called *colostrum.* Transitional and then regular breast milk will not come in for three to five days or longer. Colostrum contains more protein and less fat than breast milk. Secretions of colostrum are small, but during this time the baby does not need very much fluid, and the colostrum will give him adequate nutrition.

Actually, it is important that the milk does not fill the breasts right away because engorgement would be so severe that the baby would not be able to suck well or strongly enough to empty them. During engorgement, the mother's breasts feel ex-

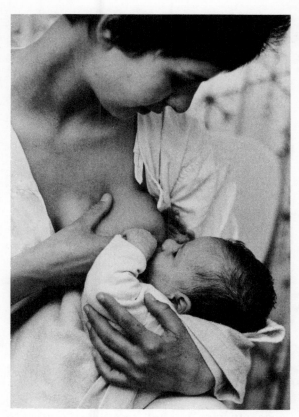

Breast feeding should be begun gradually. The baby should be allowed to suck for only a few minutes at a time on each breast until the nipples have toughened enough to sustain feedings of 15 or 20 minutes.

Be sure to use both breasts. By emptying the breasts, milk production is stimulated; thus an adequate milk supply is dependent upon using both breasts. To avoid any soreness or tenderness, use one breast longer than the other during each nursing period.

Let us assume, for example, that at the first feeding of the day you nurse the baby on the left breast for a long period, then on the right for a short period. During the next feeding the right breast will become the first one on which the baby nurses (for the long period), and the left will be nursed second (for the short period). After a few weeks you should be nursing the baby on the first breast for twenty minutes and on the other for ten minutes.

The feeding schedule: Depending on how often the baby wants to feed, you will be wise to adhere to a modified demand schedule. Don't watch the clock and feed the baby every four hours on the dot. You might feed at approximately every fourth hour, which means that you could start a second feeding early—at a three-hour interval—or late—at a five-hour interval. And, needless to say, never wake your baby up at night. He will awaken you.

Bottle Feeding

New parents nowadays have a choice between prepackaged formulas and the home-made variety. Either provides the same basic nutritional requirements that the infant needs.

The basic home-made formula for newborns consists of evaporated milk, water, and sugar or one of the sugar derivatives. Twice as much water as evaporated milk is used with one to two tablespoons of sweetening. A similar formula can be made with whole milk in somewhat different proportions. As the baby gets older, the formula will be changed from time to time by your physician.

If one formula does not agree with the baby, it will not help to put him on a similar

tremely tender and full. A good nursing brassiere will lift and support the breasts and alleviate the tender sensation during the day-or-two period of the engorgement.

Some advice to nursing mothers: If you do not have enough milk for the first few days, don't worry about it. Let the baby suck on your nipples for three, five, or even ten minutes. Don't keep him on your breasts for twenty or thirty minutes right from the beginning. Start with three minutes the first day, five minutes the second, and so on until you work up to fifteen or twenty minutes. In this way you will toughen your nipples so that your breasts will become accustomed to the baby's sucking. A bland cream may be used to massage the nipple area, particularly if the nipples become sore or cracked.

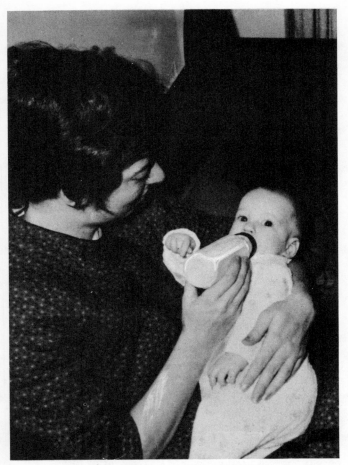

Just how much formula the bottle-fed infant needs varies from child to child. As long as the baby is healthy, it's best to let him decide when he's had enough.

him, you are not only providing nutritional nourishment for his growing body but giving him emotional and mental food for his evolving personality.

The First Six Months

It is extremely important that the baby have regular health supervision. Your baby's doctor—whether pediatrician or general practitioner—will check the baby's height and weight on each visit, and make certain he is growing and gaining at a satisfactory rate. Often, the first sign of illness in a baby is a sudden change in his normal height and weight pattern.

Although no two children develop at the same rate, it is possible to make certain generalizations about the normal development of most infants.

By two months a baby often holds his head up when he lies on his stomach or when he is being held up. He recognizes large objects, and he knows his bottle or feeding position. He can probably smile.

Sometime during the second or third month, your physician will start a series of injections against diphtheria, whooping cough, and tetanus (called *DPT*), as well as oral immunizing agents against polio—the *Sabin vaccine.* See the chart on p. 114.

The three-month mark: By three months most babies are eating some solids specially processed for babies—fruits, cereals, vegetables, meats—in addition to having formula. They may, of course, still be entirely on breast milk. Your doctor will also suggest the use of vitamin supplements, in the form of drops, which can be added to the baby's milk or solid food. All babies need vitamins A, C, and D. Occasionally, vitamin B is also prescribed. If fluorides are not present in your drinking water, they are often added to the baby's vitamins to retard tooth decay.

At four months: By four months the baby will look at moving objects. Do not be sur-

formula; its ingredients are likely to be virtually the same. You must switch to a radically different formula, such as one containing no milk at all or no carbohydrates. It is up to your doctor to advise you which modified formula to try.

As to how much formula should be given at each feeding, let the baby decide. If he is satisfied with two-and-a-half ounces, he is probably getting enough. If he wants up to four-and-a-half ounces, give it to him. The amount is not important as long as your doctor feels the baby is in good health.

A final thing to remember about feeding is this: whether you use breast or bottle, you must give your baby the love, warmth, and body contact that he needs. As you feed prised if his eyes cross. This is a normal condition during early infancy, and may even persist for a year.

At about this time, the baby may also learn to turn over from front to back—an important milestone. Some babies may have developed bald or flat places on the back of the head from lying more or less in one position. At about this time the condition should begin to disappear.

Skin rashes: During the first six months, skin rashes are not uncommon. They may be due to overheating or overdressing, or to the use of detergents, powders, perfumes, and oils which cause *contact dermatitis.* In addition, certain foods may make the baby break out in facial rashes. Prolonged contact with wet diapers causes *diaper rash,* from the ammonia produced by urine.

Skin rashes can usually be prevented or controlled by:

• Control of temperature
• Proper clothing
• Avoidance of irritating perfumes, powders, and detergents in laundering diapers
• Avoidance, in certain circumstances, of milk or other foods, as suggested by your physician

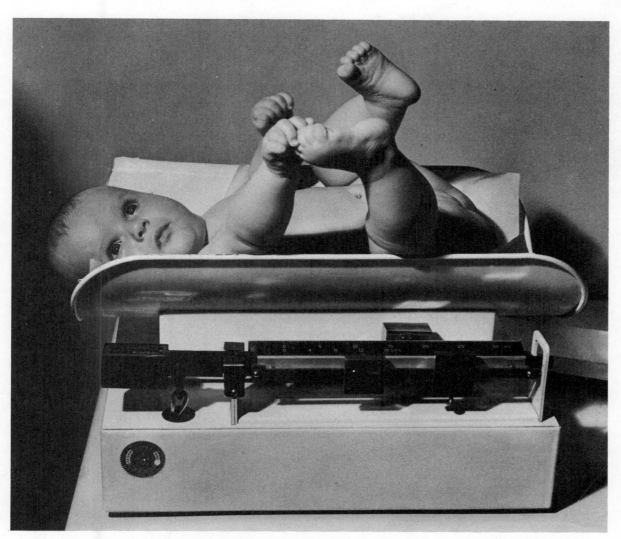

At each checkup, the doctor weighs and measures the baby to make sure he is gaining and growing at a satisfactory rate. A sudden change in the pattern of weight gain may be the first sign of illness.

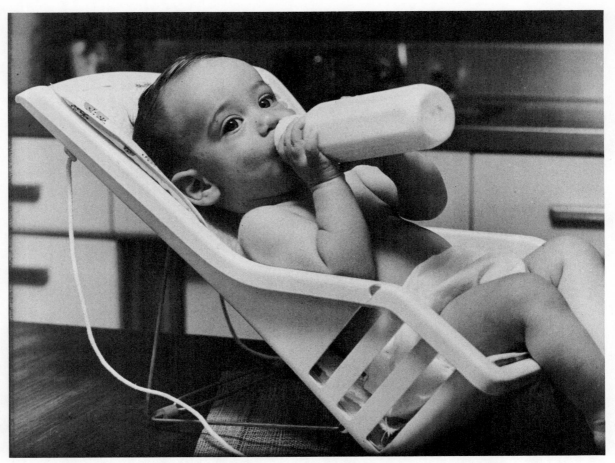

When a baby has developed enough coordination to handle his own bottle, he can be propped up in an infant seat and observe the world around him while he eats.

• Avoidance of rubber pants over diapers
• Applications of ointments to rashy areas.

If a disturbing skin condition persists or gets worse, your physician will check for special infections like impetigo or fungus, and, should they exist, recommend proper treatment.

Cradle cap: This condition is marked by yellowish crusts on the baby's scalp. It is usually harmless, and can be taken care of by regular shampooing. Occasionally, a special soap as well as a very fine comb may be helpful.

Teething: Babies of four to six months drool a great deal and put their fingers in their mouth. These habits, and the telltale small bumps you may detect on the baby's gums, are the signs of teething. But they

don't necessarily mean that the first tooth is about to erupt. That may not happen until he is nearly one year old, although it usually happens earlier.

Teething may or may not be painful. If the baby does fret, medication is available to alleviate the pain. (A little whisky rubbed on the gums is a home remedy that often helps.)

Colic: During the first three or four months, many babies have occasional attacks of *colic,* a general term applied to infantile digestive discomfort. After feeding, the baby may cry out in pain and draw up his arms and legs. His abdomen may feel hard. Apart from making sure the baby is as comfortable as he can be, there's not much that can be done for colic. You must try not to let the baby's crying make you a nervous wreck, for your nervousness will be communicated to the baby, which will only create a vicious circle of increasing tension. Usually colic tapers off at about the third month. If the baby's colic attacks are very frequent or persistent, consult your doctor.

High Fever: As every parent knows, babies can run very high fevers. In itself, a rectal temperature of 103° or 104° is not necessarily cause for alarm. (Normal rectal temperature is about ½° to 1° higher than the oral norm of 98.6°F.) Of course, you should take the immediate step of calling your doctor to find out what's causing the fever. But if a baby's fever climbs over 104°, the baby may experience convulsions. To avoid this possibility, he may be bathed with cool water or with equal parts of water and alcohol. (The alcohol is not necessary.) If convulsions do occur, protect the baby from injuring himself by seeing that his head and body don't strike anything hard. The convulsion, though frightening, is usually brief and ends of its own accord. Get in touch with your doctor without delay.

The Second Six Months

At six months most babies smile when they are brought to the doctor's office. At one year of age a visit to the doctor is more likely to produce tears and screams. The

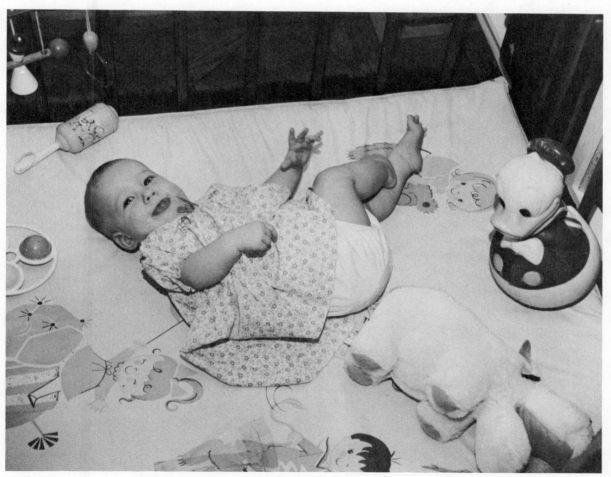

At four months most babies have begun to teethe. They drool a great deal and stick their fingers and other objects into their mouths to relieve the discomfort. Teething may continue for many months.

friendly, sociable attitude of the six-month old gives way to one in which strangers are shunned or mistrusted, and everyone other than mother may qualify as a stranger.

By the sixth month the baby may roll over when placed on his back. He may learn to crawl, sit, pull himself up, and even stand. By a year he may start to walk, although walking unaided does not often occur so soon.

At this stage the baby is full of life and activity. He won't lie still when you change his diaper, and often needs distraction. He cries if you put him down or leave him alone. Unless you are firm and resist running to him at his first whimper, you may set the stage for spoiling him as he gets older. Of course, if he continues to cry for any considerable length of time—not more than half an hour—make sure there is nothing wrong with him besides his displeasure at your not appearing like a genie because he screams and fusses.

Other changes: Other changes occur at this age. Where before he had been a good sleeper, he may now not want to go to sleep or he may awaken at night. Let him know that you are near by, but don't make a habit of playing with him in the middle of the night—not if you value your sleep.

If you should notice, as many parents do at about this time, that your baby seems

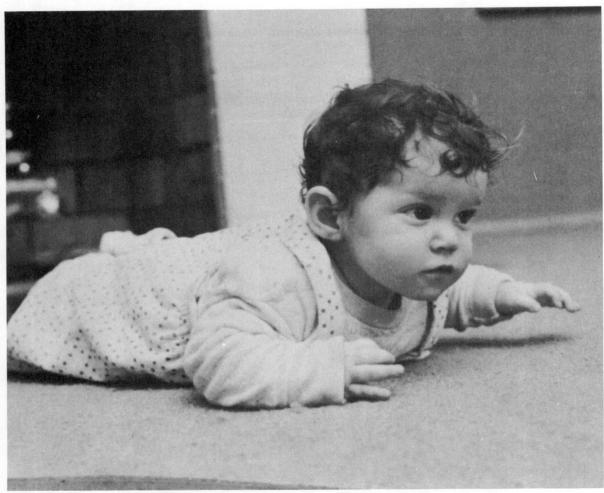

By six months many babies are crawling or making determined wriggles. At first their arms and legs don't coordinate properly, but when they do, crawling becomes an efficient way to get about.

to be left-handed, do not try to make him right-handed. Each of us inherits a preference for one hand or the other, and it is harmful to try to change it. In any case, you are not likely to know for sure which hand your child prefers until the second year of his life.

In this second six-month period, the baby will probably take some of his milk from a cup. Don't be surprised if he takes juices out of a cup but insists on taking milk from a bottle. If he tries to hold the bottle or cup himself, let him. Of course, it may be wise to keep a mop handy at first, but after a few months his skills will improve. In any case, nonbreakable cups are recommended.

Diet and teeth: The baby's diet is soon expanded to include pureed baby foods. You might even want to try the somewhat lumpier junior foods; as more of his teeth erupt, the baby will enjoy the lumpier food more and more. Teething biscuits can be added to the diet, too. By one year he will usually have six teeth (incisors), although, since no two children are alike, he may have none at all. By the end of the first year he will have lost some of his appetite, and his rapid weight gain will cease. This is entirely natural in a period when the outside world is taking on more and more interest.

As he starts to move around he wants to investigate everything. Keep dangerous objects—detergents, poisons, and medicines, especially baby aspirin—out of his reach. Tell him "No" to emphasize the seriousness of certain prohibitions. He should understand what "No" means by the time he is one-year old, and will also probably respond to other simple commands.

It is essential that your baby's health supervision be continued without interruption. During the second six months of his life he will complete his protection against diphtheria, whooping cough, tetanus (DPT), and polio (Sabin), and be tested for exposure to tuberculosis (the tuberculin test).

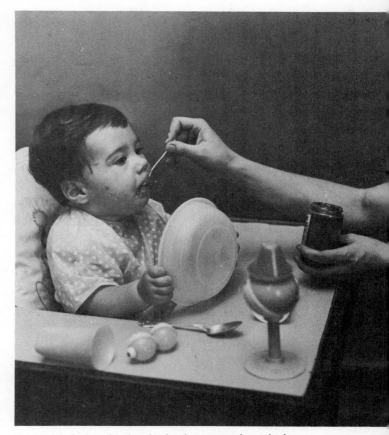

Prepared baby foods—both the pureed and the chunkier junior foods—are gradually added to the baby's diet during his first year. These foods add variety and introduce him to the habit of chewing.

The Toddler Stage

It is in this phase of the child's life that he develops a real relationship with his mother. Mother is the loving, warm, secure comforter in his life, the giver of rewards and disciplinarian of his daily activities, the center of his life. During this period it is imperative that the child's father spend as much time with his son or daughter as he is able to, so that the child begins to recognize the difference between his relationship to his mother and father.

In many homes today the father, because of the demands of business, finds it impossible to spend enough time with his family. This is an unfortunate fact, but one that can be dealt with positively, since it is the quality of the time a father spends with his child, rather than the quantity, that is most important.

Testing Himself and the World Around Him

The toddler is insatiably curious. He wants to explore and investigate everything. Take him outdoors as much as possible. Let him meet children of his own age so that he can play and learn the beginnings of social contact.

Physically, the toddler tries to do many things apart from walking, running, and climbing—including quite a few things that he can't do. He is easily frustrated and may have a short attention span. (Girls are better than boys in this respect.) Don't be impatient with your toddler; don't punish him for his clumsiness. He has a great many experiences ahead of him, and many skills to learn and develop.

You can now expect a negative reaction to your control. Obviously, you must set limits on your child's behavior—on what is acceptable and what is not, while still giving him the freedom to express his emotions and energies in vigorous physical play.

Make the rules easy to understand so that the child will not become confused about what is expected of him. And do not set up impossible standards.

Toilet Training

It is during the toddler stage that you will begin to teach your child how to control his bowel and urinary functions.

A simple question mothers always ask is, "How do I know when my child is ready to be toilet trained?"

A child is ready when he understands what is meant by toilet training and is willing to perform toilet functions without expressing fear of them. This may occur at any age, but is perhaps most apt to start between the ages of 18 and 24 months. With a first child it is usually later than with a second or third child, because the first child has no siblings to emulate. But a first

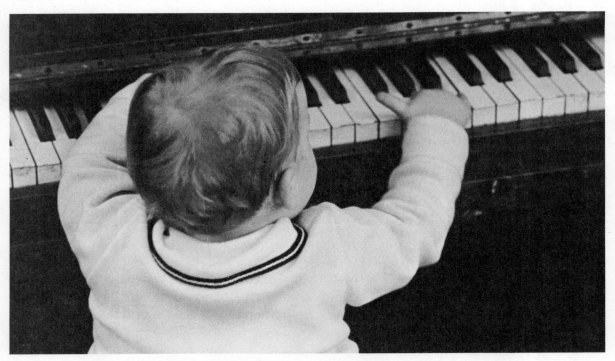

The toddler's insatiable curiosity leads him to explore many things he cannot do. While this frequently results in frustrations, it is through trial and error that he learns and develops.

child should be trained, usually, by the time he is three. Training the child to stay dry through the long night hours may take even longer.

Early toilet training—training that is begun during a child's first year—may work, but as a child develops and asserts his personality and independence, he will resent any insistence on manipulating the control of his bodily functions. He may get even by refusing to empty his bowels when put on the potty. Worse yet, if another baby has entered the scene, the early-trained child may develop constipation, or may revert to wetting and having bowel movements in his training pants.

When you feel the child is ready for training, establish the fact that going to the bathroom is a normal part of daily life. If the child expresses fear, don't struggle with him. Don't fight about it. Take him right off the potty and let him know that you are not concerned or displeased. A genuine complication can arise if the child connects his fear of toilet functions with your displeasure at his failures.

Three to Six Years

The roots of all 20 primary teeth are complete at the child's third year of life. These teeth, which began erupting between 6 and 7 months of age, are called the *central incisors*. The primary teeth, the last of which usually fall out between the eleventh and thirteenth year, are smaller and whiter than the permanent teeth, of which there are 32. The first permanent tooth erupts between 7 and 8 years of age, while the last, the third molars, erupt between the seventeenth and twenty-first year.

This is the age when many children go to school for part of the day and begin learning how to get along with other children in play and in organized activities. They also begin to meet adults other than their parents.

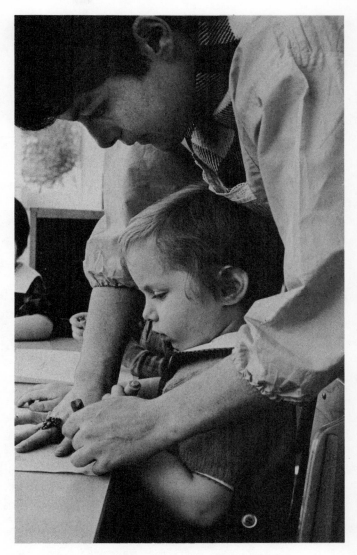

The child's introduction to organized activities is a major step in his social development, for here he has to learn to deal with adults other than his parents.

A child of five grows at a slower rate than in earlier years, but his body is nonetheless changing. The protruding abdomen and knock-knees of the toddler begin to disappear.

Television: Now that television is a part of nearly every family's life, it may absorb a good part of the child's time. Television is an advantage if it does not usurp the time the child would ordinarily spend in vigorous outdoor play or in some quiet indoor activity—working with construction toys, playing house with dolls, playing doctor with a makeshift stethoscope, or just leafing through picture books. A child seldom sticks to television if there is something better going on.

Personal hygiene: Good habits of cleanliness should be established. The child should know that hand-washing before meals is essential even when the hands look clean. He will learn this only if he sees his parents do it. As he gets older he should select his own clean clothing and know that dirty clothing should be washed. A daily routine of washing or bathing should be set up, and the child should be encouraged to observe it.

Six Years to Adolescence

During this period children begin to be more and more individualistic. Some are solitary, others sociable. One likes only other children, another prefers the company of adults. Some children have imaginary fears which disappear with age or when the fears are discussed with an adult who can explain how or why they originated.

Curiosity about sex: The child's earlier curiosity about naked people may change to a concern about being clothed and being with people who are clothed. Questions about sex should be answered simply and truthfully.

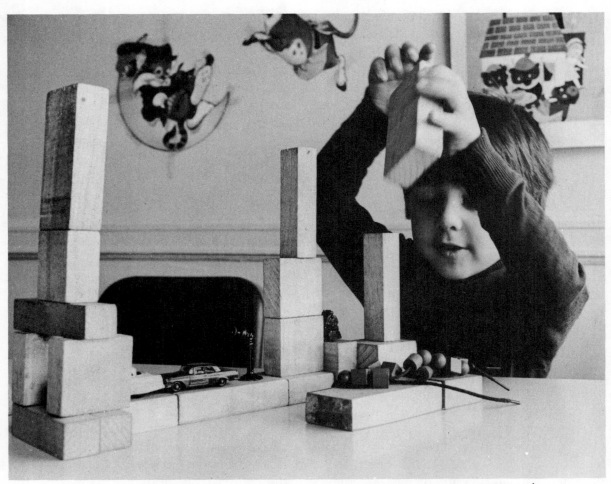

The young child should not watch TV to the exclusion of other important activities, such as vigorous outdoor play and quiet indoor pursuits—role-playing, manipulating building toys, and learning the joys of reading through early exposure to picture books.

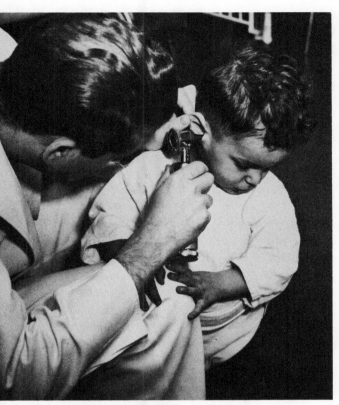

Regular medical examinations—two or three a year for preschoolers—are essential to check normal growth and development and to prevent disorders.

Adolescence: Adolescence arrives anywhere from 9 to 14 years of age. A girl usually enters adolescence at 10, a boy at about 12.

In female children, there is growth of the breasts and nipples; the pelvis matures, and the external genitalia develop. Axillary (underarm), and pubic hair appear. On the average, girls have their first menstrual period around age thirteen, but it can occur between 10 and 16 years of age. Be sure to explain menstruation to your daughter before the beginning of adolescence.

In male children, the penis and testes develop. Facial, axillary, and pubic hair appear. The voice begins to deepen.

In both boys and girls, there is a rapid growth in height and weight which is related to sexual development. In general, the average height of the adolescent is double what it was at age two. See *Puberty and Growth,* p. 122.

Checkups and Immunization

It is no longer true that physicians merely treat disease; they take steps to prevent certain childhood disorders from ever occurring.

During the first year of life, the child is usually seen by his doctor every month. During the toddler stage, there are usually three examinations a year, and during the preschool period, usually two. While in school, children should have an annual preventive checkup; most schools and camps require it. It is best not to wait until June or September, which are likely to be the busiest times for your physician.

DPT injections: DPT stands for diphtheria, pertussis (or whooping cough), and tetanus. DPT injections are usually given in the muscles of the mid-thigh or upper arm, at intervals of one month, sometimes longer. To prevent fever or other severe reactions, the two-to-five-month old baby should receive one grain of baby aspirin within a few hours after the injection. If he nevertheless develops fever or has other severe reactions, your doctor may have to give lower doses, and therefore give more than three injections. Very rarely is a severe reaction reported with smaller doses of the vaccine. If there is such a reaction, no further injections of pertussis vaccine will be given.

Occasionally, redness or a lump appears at the site of the injection. This is a local reaction. It is harmless and will disappear within a few weeks. If it does not, consult your physician.

It is recommended that a booster or recall shot be given at one-and-a-half and at three years of age. Another recall injection of only TD (tetanus-diphtheria toxoid) is given at six years and at twelve years.

Following is a chart listing the recommended schedule for active immunization and tuberculin testing of normal infants and children:

IMMUNIZATION AND TESTING SCHEDULE	
2–3 months	DPT, Sabin Type 3 or Trivalent
3–4 months	DPT, Sabin Type 1 or Trivalent
4–5 months	DPT, Sabin Type 2 or Trivalent
9–11 months	Tuberculin Test
12 months	Measles Vaccine
12–24 months	Mumps Vaccine, Rubella Vaccine
15–18 months	DPT, Trivalent Sabin
2 years	Tuberculin Test
3 years	DPT, Tuberculin Test
4 years	Tuberculin Test
6 years	TD, Tuberculin Test, Trivalent Sabin
8 years	Tuberculin Test, Mumps Vaccine (if not given earlier or if child did not have mumps)
12 years	TD, Tuberculin Test
14 years	Tuberculin Test
16 years	Tuberculin Test

Common Childhood Diseases

Measles: Measles is by far the most dangerous of the common childhood diseases because of its possible complications, such as meningitis, encephalitis, and severe secondary staphylococcus infection. Fortunately, widespread protection is available in the live measles vaccine, which should be given to every child over one year of age.

Measles, a highly contagious disease caused by a virus, has an incubation period of one to two weeks. The most noticeable symptom is the rash which begins on the head and face within a few days after the onset of the disease, and gradually erupts all over the body, blending into big red patches. Other symptoms include fever up to 104° or higher, a severe cough, sore throat, stuffy nose, inflammation of the *conjunctiva* (the mucous membrane on the inner part of the eyelid and extending over the front of the eyeball), sensitivity of the eyes to light, enlarged lymph nodes, and a generalized sick feeling.

Any child who has contracted measles should be seen by a physician and watched carefully for possible complications. Moreover, if he is of school age, the school should be promptly notified. This, of course, is true for any contagious disease.

Measles can be treated only symptomatically. During the incubation period, an injection of gamma globulin will lessen the severity of the disease, or occasionally prevent it. If there are other children at home besides the affected one, they should also receive gamma globulin injections. Antibiotics are of no help unless there is a secondary bacterial infection.

Every parent should make certain that his child is vaccinated against this potentially serious disease.

Rubella (German measles): Rubella once used to be thought of as a benign disease. Then about 20 years ago it was discovered that it could have serious consequences if it were contracted by a woman during the first three months of her pregnancy. The virus that causes rubella is transmitted from the infected woman to her unborn baby, and has been linked to birth defects of the heart, eye, ear, and liver, and to mental retardation.

In addition, a baby who has been exposed to the disease in utero may infect others even though he himself is not affected by it and shows no symptoms. (In fact, most babies are immune to rubella during their first year.) The rubella virus is highly contagious and spreads rapidly.

The incubation period for German measles is two to three weeks. Symptoms include earache, swollen glands behind the

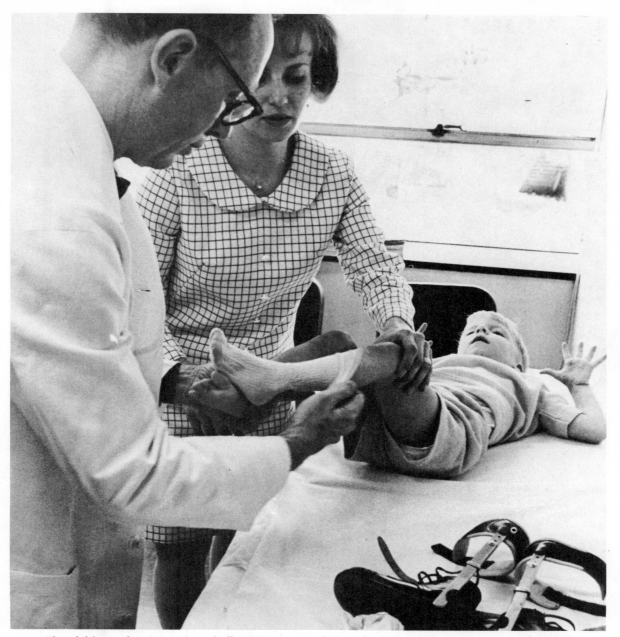

This child was the victim of a rubella (German measles) epidemic in 1964–65. An estimated 30,000 fetal deaths and 20,000 birth abnormalities resulted when mothers contracted the disease during early pregnancy. Such epidemics could be averted if all children over one year were immunized.

ears, a low-grade fever, and a usually mild, blotchy rash which erupts over the body but lasts only a few days.

Most children are only mildly affected by rubella and require little treatment except rest. However, a pregnant woman who comes in contact with the child can contract it. It is, therefore, of great importance that all children over one year of age be immunized with the vaccine that prevents rubella. Any woman of childbearing age who might be pregnant should *not* be given the vaccine, since the effects of the vaccine on an unborn fetus are not known.

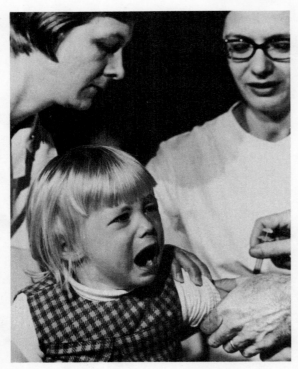

This three-year-old is being vaccinated against mumps, a usually mild disease in young children. In older children it may have serious complications.

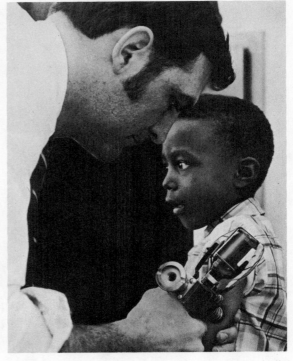

This boy is being immunized with live virus rubella vaccine by a "jet gun," which can give 50 doses of vaccine from a multiple dose vial without reloading.

Mumps: Mumps, a mild disorder in most children, is caused by a virus and has an incubation period of from two to three weeks. The most familiar symptom is swollen glands involving the jaw. The glands usually affected are the *parotid glands*—large salivary glands below and slightly in front of the ear—although other glands may be affected, too. Other symptoms include fever and a generally sick feeling. No rash is present. Mumps lasts about five days; then the swelling disappears, and the child is well.

In an adolescent boy, the disease sometimes causes an inflammation of the testes (called *orchitis*) and may be very painful. In addition, if it involves both testes, there is a possibility—fortunately only a very slight one—that sterility will result.

In older children mumps occasionally produces the complication called *mumps meningoencephalitis*. The signs of this more serious disease are headache, fever, and extreme debilitation. Finally, there may be an inflammation of the pancreas which can cause severe abdominal pain and vomiting.

Since mumps is now preventable, it is important that every boy and girl be given the mumps vaccine. Boys should be given the vaccine before puberty.

Chicken pox: Chicken pox cannot be prevented at this time. It does not usually cause any severe complications in a child, but it can be serious in an adult. It is highly infectious and spreads rapidly.

Chicken pox is caused by a virus. Its incubation period is two to three weeks. Symptoms include those of the common cold, a fever, general malaise, and a rash.

The rash, which may be either mild or severe, is different from that produced by measles or by rubella. The measles rash is red and blotchy. Chicken pox look like bunches of blisters close together.

These blisters are filled with fluid, and there is a reddened area around each lesion. As new blisters appear, the older ones become encrusted. The rash may affect the mouth, nose, ears, vagina, penis, or scrotum. In an older child the symptoms may be more severe than in a younger one, and may be accompanied by headache and vomiting.

The only way to treat chicken pox is symptomatically. The rash is very itchy, and an affected child must be prevented from scratching. Otherwise, he may develop a secondary infection and be left pitted and scarred.

Treatment involves the use of lotions, such as Calomine, which is applied locally to the pox to relieve the itching. If the child is old enough, it's a good idea to let him paint it on himself. Your physician may also prescribe medicine to be taken orally to help the child stop scratching the blisters. In a few days, the rash clears up, the lesions dry, and the crusts fall off.

Scarlet fever: Scarlet fever used to be a disease which everyone dreaded. It is highly contagious, and can result in severe after-effects like rheumatic fever, or the kidney disease known as nephritis.

It is now known that scarlet fever is simply a streptococcal infection—a strain of a specific organism that also causes a diffuse red rash. It can be dealt with quite simply by your physician, the usual treatment being a ten-day course of penicillin, which cures the streptococcal infection and prevents most complications.

Diphtheria: Although diphtheria is a severe infection, it is completely preventable by routine immunization with a specific diphtheria antitoxin, and is now relatively uncommon.

Whooping cough: Whooping cough (also called *pertussis*), like diphtheria a bacterial disease, occurs more frequently than diphtheria because immunity to it wears off, especially in the older child in whom the disease may appear as a severe bronchitis.

Whooping cough can be very serious in young babies because it can cause them to choke and be unable to catch their breath. If your child does contract whooping cough, call your physician immediately. He may give a specific drug against the organism that causes the disease as well as a specific antitoxin against the poison which the bacillus releases.

It is advisable to immunize children against whooping cough as early as possible. The effective triple vaccine known as DPT provides immunization not only against whooping cough, but against diphtheria and tetanus as well.

Tetanus: Tetanus (also called *lockjaw* because it causes spasms of the jaw) can

During the first years of a child's life, frequent check-ups are essential to maintain good health and prevent serious illnesses from developing. This child's ears are being checked for signs of infection.

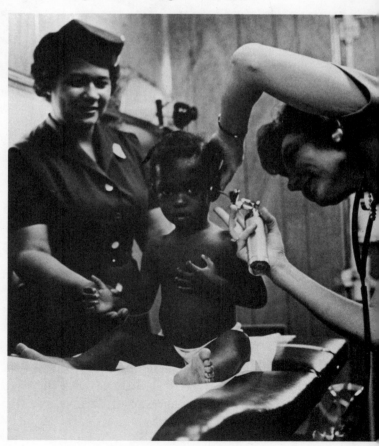

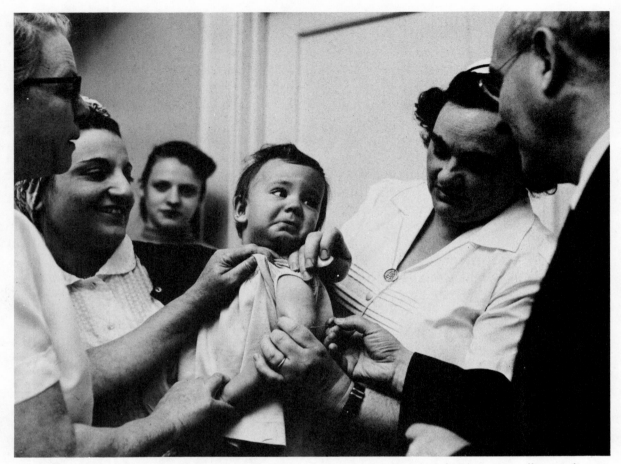

This indignant baby is being vaccinated against smallpox, a disease which has been virtually wiped out in the U.S. Vaccination is now required only for travel to places where smallpox is prevalent.

occur at any age as the result of contamination of a simple wound. The causative organism is usually found in soil, street dust, or feces.

The disease is preventable by immunization. The triple vaccine DPT should be started at two to three months of age. See the chart on p. 114.

When a child suffers a puncture wound, dog bite, or other wound that may be contaminated, ask your doctor to give the child a booster dose of tetanus toxoid if he has not had a shot within one year.

Polio (*infantile paralysis*): Until a few years ago, there was no protection against this disease, which caused paralysis of the extremities and could cause death by paralyzing the muscles used in breathing.

This disorder can now be prevented by giving oral doses of the live virus vaccine (Sabin) which provides immunity without actually causing the symptoms of the disease. Repeated series of booster shots are unnecessary because the immunity persists for years.

It is advisable that a child receive three doses of polio vaccine, six to eight weeks apart, starting at about the age of two months. One method employs *trivalent* vaccine, in which each dose contains three kinds of vaccine—to give protection against three strains of polio. Three separate doses are necessary, however, to insure full protection. The other method employs *monovalent* vaccines, in which each dose insures protection against a different type of polio.

Smallpox: This disease still exists in some countries of the world, but it has been eradicated in the U.S. by the vaccination of babies between the ages of one and two with live calf lymph virus (*cowpox*). Due to the possibility, although slight, of a severe reaction to smallpox vaccination, most authorities now recommend that routine vaccination be discontinued. Instead, the vaccine is administered only to those who are traveling to or from countries where smallpox is still prevalent.

A scratch or multiple needle pressure is used in the vaccination. As there is nearly always some reaction, many people prefer to be vaccinated on the thigh or on another area not readily visible. The scar left from such a reaction, however, is small, and it is advisable to be vaccinated on the outer aspect of the upper arm. No child with eczema should be vaccinated, nor should anyone if another person in the home has eczema.

The typical reaction to a first exposure to the smallpox vaccine is a small red bump that usually appears within three to five days. The skin around the bump is reddish, and the bump soon becomes a blister. In ten to twelve days, a scab forms, darkens in color, and in three to four weeks, drops off. Fever as high as 104° may occur five to ten days after the vaccination. Sometimes there is no reaction at all (a *no take*). In that event, the vaccination is unsuccessful and should be repeated.

If one must be revaccinated—for example, for foreign travel—and still has partial immunity from an earlier vaccination, he will have only a slight reaction.

Abnormalities

Clubfoot: Clubfoot is a bone deformity characterized by an inturning or outturning of the foot. An orthopedist must put the clubfoot and part of the leg into a cast in order to correct the condition. If casting does not cure the abnormality, orthopedic surgery may be necessary.

Occasionally, a benign and easily correctable condition involving a child's legs may have been produced by the position the baby was in while still in the uterus.

The mother can help to correct the condition by daily passive exercises of the baby's feet. She does this by turning the feet correctly for a few minutes every day. To maintain the corrected position, the application of plaster is sometimes necessary. Such a procedure requires the attention of an orthopedic surgeon.

Cleft lip ("harelip"): Early surgical treatment, which leaves only a tiny scar, is by far the best way to treat this condition, for both the child's physical and mental well-being. See p. 403 for a fuller discussion of cleft lip.

Cleft palate: This is a deformity which involves the hard palate. It is much more complex to handle than a cleft lip, although sometimes both deformities appear together. Correction of the condition should take place by the time the baby is a year-and-a-half old.

Since a cleft palate is complicated to repair surgically, it is best to use a team approach, which may involve the services of a pediatrician, surgeon, and dentist. Speech therapy is also recommended following surgery. See also p. 403.

Conditions of the Eyes, Ears, Nose, and Throat

Crossed eyes (strabismus): Do not be alarmed if your baby's eyes do not focus. Crossed eyes are a common condition that usually corrects itself somewhere between the ages of six and twelve months. If crossing of the eyes persists after one year, an ophthalmologist (eye specialist) should evaluate the baby's vision.

If a real problem does develop, one eye —or each eye alternately—may cross, turn

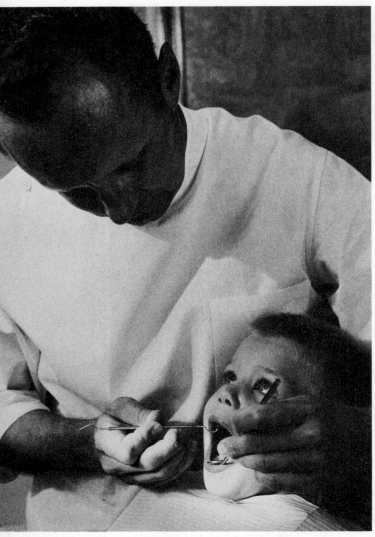

Regular visits to the dentist should start at the age of two or three. The check is important to spot possible orthodontal problems as well as to treat tooth decay.

outward, or focus below or above the other. Frequently the reason for "turning" is that there is a larger refractive error in one eye than in the other. Eyeglasses will often correct this condition.

Occasionally, eye muscle weakness is the cause of crossed eyes. This is most often true of premature children. The weakness of some muscles causes overaction of other muscles.

Eyeglasses will often prevent the need for eye surgery. Sometimes, however, surgery will be necessary to straighten the eyes. Either before or after surgery the eyes may need further attention in the form of eye drops, a patch to cover one eye, or glasses.

Tonsils and adenoids: About thirty years ago every child had to have his tonsils and adenoids out. After that, for a time, very few children had a T and A operation. Now the prevailing opinion lies somewhere in between.

No operation can be guaranteed to be without complications, and a tonsillectomy, however routine as operations go, is still an operation. There is no point, therefore, in performing a T and A unless it really needs to be done. Anesthesia, always necessary in children, is never 100 percent safe.

Frequent throat infections with swollen glands and consequent ear complications, however, are adequate reasons for a T and A. Also, a child who has persistent throat or tonsil abscesses which interfere with his breathing should have the operation.

If it is at all possible, a T and A should not be done before a child is three years of age. Tonsils, which are lymphoid tissue, grow and enlarge until the age of three to five, when they begin to shrink naturally. Sometimes simply waiting avoids the necessity of a T and A procedure.

Dental care: Every human being gets two sets of teeth. While only the baby (or "milk") teeth are visible during the first five years of life, the permanent teeth begin to form in the jaw soon after birth and are nearly completed by the time the child reaches school age.

Regular checkups by a dentist should start at age two or three. When a child enters school, he should be checked not only for cavities but also for cleanliness, gum vitality, alignment of the teeth, and possible orthodontal problems. It is up to parents to stress the necessity of regular brushing of the teeth and gums.

Eyeglasses: Now that infants and youngsters have periodic eye checkups with their physicians, and regular tests are given to all students, more children are wearing glasses than in former years. In addition to *strabismus* (crossed eyes), the three major eye problems encountered in children are *myopia* (nearsightedness), *hyperopia* (farsightedness), and *astigmatism.*

The *myopic* or nearsighted child cannot see distant objects well but can see close objects clearly. A very young child so afflicted may stumble and fall easily. An older child attending school may make errors in copying because he has difficulty in making out the words and figures written on the chalkboard. He may be called a behavior problem or may even be said to be mentally retarded. Most cases of myopia can be helped with glasses.

The *hyperopic* (also called *hypermetropic*) or farsighted eye is shorter from front to rear than the normal eye, and if not corrected will often hinder close work like reading. When a farsighted child reads he often complains of blurring of the printed page, sleepiness, and headache. Farsightedness is often associated with crossed eyes and is usually correctable with glasses.

In *astigmatism* or distorted vision, there is an uneven curvature of the cornea or lens surface of the eye. This condition causes some light rays to focus further back than others and produces a blurred, distorted image on the retina.

Either a farsighted or nearsighted eye can be *astigmatic;* the abnormality can usually be corrected by properly prescribed eyeglasses.

Hearing problems: The doctor begins to suspect a hearing problem when the mother of a young baby tells him that the child does not react to her voice, to noises, or to other auditory stimuli. As the child gets older, he may not speak properly. Since he has never heard speech, he cannot imitate its sound. Sometimes these children, like visually handicapped children, are mistakenly called mentally retarded.

Just as glasses or surgery can help eye problems, simple hearing aids, the surgical removal of excessive lymphoid tissue blocking the Eustachian tube, or special instruction in lip reading can often help a hearing problem and open up a new world for the child afflicted with a hearing disability.

Croup: Croup, a most harassing and terrifying experience for new parents, is a spasm of the windpipe or trachea, especially involving the larynx. When such a spasm occurs, an affected child has great trouble in breathing and produces a cough that sounds like the bark of a dog. In some cases, the child can't breathe at all.

An attack of croup is an emergency. The younger the child, the more dangerous it is. You must get the baby's airway open. The best thing to do is to take the child into the bathroom, shut the door, and turn on the hot water of the shower full force, or of the bathtub and sink if you don't have a shower. The idea is to fill the room with hot steam in order to loosen the mucus plug in the baby's trachea, thus enabling him to cough up the mucus.

Get to your physician as soon as possible so that he can treat the illness. If he finds that the croup is viral in origin, antibiotics may not help; but when the infection is caused by bacteria, your physician will put the child on one of the antimicrobial agents. If your child is subject to croup, it is a good idea to invest in a hot or cold air vaporizer and use it whenever he has congestion due to a cold.

In a really severe emergency, when the windpipe closes completely, a *tracheostomy* must be performed so that the throat can be opened and an airway inserted. A tracheotomy should be performed in a hospital, but if for some reason it is performed elsewhere, the child should be hospitalized as quickly as possible. For a discussion of the emotional development of the child during the first dozen years of life, see *Developing an Awareness of the World,* p. 222.   CHB

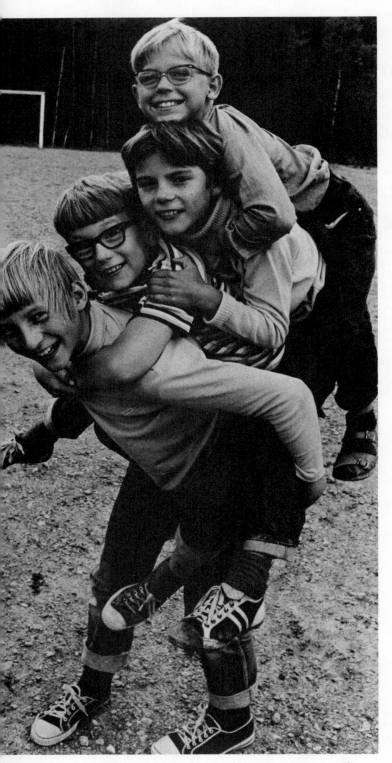

Children need plenty of opportunities to release their energies in rough-and-tumble play. Informal games on the schoolyard or playground also help a child learn to get along socially with others.

PUBERTY AND GROWTH: THE TEENS

The bridge between childhood and adulthood is a period of growth and change called puberty. There seems to be no standard pattern for the physical changes of puberty. Two boys of the same age who have been nearly identical throughout childhood may appear to set off along entirely different paths of physical development as they enter the teen-age years. One may quickly shoot up to a height of 5 feet 8 inches within a couple of years while his companion lags for a while at pre-teen size, then begins growing into a six-footer. One may develop a heavy beard in his early high school years while the other boy will have no use for a razor until he is in college. However, both boys are normal youngsters, and each will eventually attain all of the physical attributes of adulthood.

Similarly, one girl may begin menstruating in her 11th year while a classmate will not experience her first menstruation until she is 16. One girl may need a bra while still in grammar school but her friend will fret about a small bustline for many years. But both girls can look forward to normal motherhood. Each has an individual pattern of development, and if there is any rule of thumb about puberty it is that each youngster has his or her own time schedule for the transformation into a mature man or woman.

Puberty: Changes in Girls

The physical changes that occur in the female body during puberty probably are more dramatic than those associated with a boy progressing into manhood. One definite milestone for the girl is her first *menstruation,* commonly regarded as the first sign of puberty. Actually, the first menstruation, known as the *menarche,* is only one of several signs of puberty, along with the slimming of the waist, gradual broadening of the hips, the development of breasts, the appearance of hair about the genitals and in the armpits, and a change in the rate of growth.

The Menarche

The age at which a girl first experiences menstruation generally varies over a period of 10 years and depends upon the structural development of the youngster, her physical condition, the environment, and hereditary factors. Menarche can occur as early as the age of 7, and most doctors would not be overly concerned if a girl did not begin to menstruate until she was approaching 17. The age range of 9 to 16 usually is considered normal. The median age for the start of menstruation is around 13½ years, which means that 50 percent of all females are younger than 13 years and 6 months when they reach the menarche, and half are on the older side of that age when they first menstruate. In general, the pubertal experiences of a girl follow a pattern like that of her mother and sisters; if the mother began menstruating at an early age, the chances are that her daughters will also.

If the girl has not reached the menarche by the age of 18, she should be examined by a *gynecologist,* a doctor who specializes in problems related to the female reproductive system. A medical examination also should be arranged for any girl who experiences menstruation before she reaches the age of 8 or 9 years.

When menarche occurs on the early side of childhood, the condition is sometimes called *precocious puberty.* The child may suddenly begin menstruating before her mother has told her about the birds and the bees, a situation which can prove embarrassing to both child and parents. It may first be detected by a teacher at school; occasionally, a young girl may be aware of bleeding from the vagina but because of fear or false modesty does not report the event to her mother or teacher. For this reason, parents should be alert for changes associated with early puberty and be prepared to explain the facts of life to their children. Also, in the case of precocious puberty, the mother should arrange for medical consultation to be certain the bleeding actually is the result of first menstruation and not the effects of an injury or tumor.

Growth Spurt Before Menarche

During the year or two preceding the menarche there is a growth spurt of two or three inches. This is because of the hormone changes of puberty. The *hormones* are chemical messengers secreted by glands in various parts of the body and carried rapidly through the bloodstream to organs or other glands where they trigger reactions. The spurt in growth preceding menarche is due to the secretion of a growth hormone which is produced by the pituitary gland, and androgen, a hormone secreted by the adrenal glands. They produce rapid growth of the bones and muscles during puberty. As a result, the girl who is the first among her classmates to menstruate often is larger than those who are of the same age but have not yet reached the menarche.

From numerous research studies of the menarche, it has been learned that poor nutrition and psychological stress sometimes delay the onset of menstruation, that girls reared in cities tend to menstruate earlier, and that climate is a factor, although both tropical and arctic climates seem to be related to early menarche. The first menstrual periods also are likely to occur during the school year, September to June, rather than during the summer vacation.

The First Menstrual Cycles

The first menstrual cycles tend to be very irregular and have been known to be as short as 7 days and as long as 37 weeks.

Even when regularity becomes established, the adolescent menstrual cycle usually is longer than the average for adult women. The typical menstrual cycle of a young girl may be about 33 days, compared to an average of 28 days for an adult woman. About three years elapse before the menstrual cycles become regular. In the meantime, irregular menstrual patterns can be considered as normal for girls during puberty.

The first menstrual cycles also are *anovulatory*. In other words, the young girl's ovaries have not matured sufficiently to produce an *ovum*, or egg cell, or an ovum that can be fertilized by the sperm of a male. There are, of course, the exceptions which make newspaper headlines when a little girl gives birth to a baby. But anovulatory menstruation generally is the rule for the first few months after the menarche.

Delayed Puberty

Delayed puberty probably causes as much anguish as precocious puberty. The last girl in a group of childhood chums to develop breasts and experience the menarche may feel more self-conscious than the first girl in the class to menstruate. If the signs that usually precede menarche have not appeared by the age of 17 or 18, a medical examination should be considered, even though the girl may be a late-late bloomer who is at the other end of the puberty spectrum from the 7- or 8-year-old child who has menstruated.

The absence of menstruation after a girl is 18 can be the result of a wide variety of factors. The cause sometimes can be as simple as an *imperforate hymen,* a membrane that blocks the opening of the vagina. It can be the result of a congenital malformation of the reproductive organs, such as imperfect development of the ovaries. Accidents, exposure to carbon monoxide gas, or diseases like rheumatic fever or encephalitis in earlier years can result in brain damage that would inhibit the start of menstruation. The relationship between emotional upset and delayed menarche was vividly demonstrated during World War II when some girls who suffered psychological traumas also experienced very late signs of puberty.

Preparing Your Daughter for Menstruation

A mother's main responsibility is to convince her daughter at the beginning of puberty that menstruation is a perfectly normal body function. The mother should explain the proper use of sanitary napkins or tampons and encourage her daughter to keep records of her menstrual periods on a calendar.

The mother also should explain that menstruation usually is not a valid reason to stay in bed or avoid school or work. The girl should be advised that bathing and swimming should not be postponed because of menstruation. There are many old wives' tales about menstruation which are not true, including claims that dental work and permanent waves will not last if the girl visits the dentist or the beauty shop while menstruating. But there may be a bit of truth to stories that loss of menstrual blood can be weakening, particularly if the girl's diet does not replace the body stores of iron which may be lowered during menstrual flow. Iron is a key element of the red blood cell, and if iron-rich foods are not included in the meals of women during their years of menstruation they can eventually suffer a form of anemia.

Hormone Activity: Becoming a Woman

Although the sex hormones are the key to what makes little girls grow into women and little boys into men, both sexes appear to receive secretions of male and female sex hormones in approximately equal amounts for about the first ten years of life. But as puberty approaches, the adrenal glands of girls seem to increase production

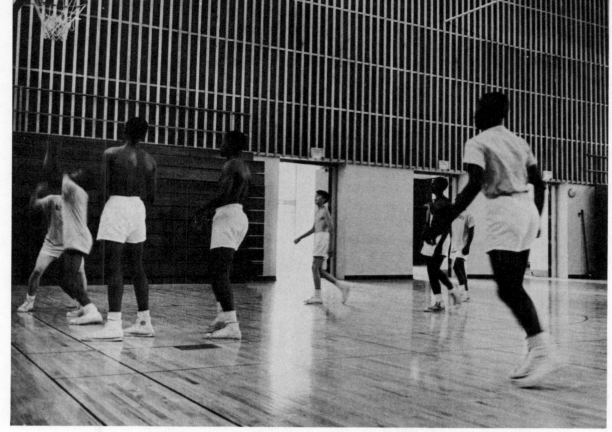

The keen competition of sports is a way for teen-aged boys to experience an outlet for the normal physical and emotional tensions that frequently accompany puberty.

of a female sex hormone, *estrogen*. Meanwhile, a nerve center in the *hypothalamus* area of the brain stimulates the pituitary gland, the master gland of the body, to secrete another kind of hormone, *gonadotropin*. Gonadotropin in turn activates a *follicle-stimulating hormone* which causes a maturation of the ovaries, which are part of the original equipment little girls are born with but which remain dormant until the start of puberty.

During the second decade of life, the hormone activity stimulates the development of body tissues which not only grow in size but give a girl more womanly contours. However, the fully mature contours of a woman usually do not appear until after the ovaries are functioning and still another female sex hormone, *progesterone*, has been introduced in the system. The ovaries, uterus, Fallopian tubes, and vagina gradually mature as the menarche draws near.

Puberty: Changes in Boys

The appearance of male sexual characteristics during puberty is also influenced by hormonal changes. But the manifestation of male puberty is somewhat more subtle. The pituitary gland in a boy also secretes a gonadotropic hormone which stimulates maturation of *gonads*. In the male, the gonads are the *testicles*, the source of *sperm*. But whereas maturation of the ovaries in females leads to the menarche, there is no obvious sign in the boy that *spermatozoa* are being produced.

However, the secondary sexual characteristics, such as the growth of a beard and pubic hair, the spurt of growth of bones and muscles, the increase in size of the sex organs, and the deepening of the voice are all indications of puberty. The changes in a boy's characteristics during puberty are usually spread over a period of two years, beginning with an increase in the size of the penis and testicles and reaching completion with the production of spermatozoa in the testicles. During the two-year period there usually is a noticeable increase in the chest size of the boy, with the broad shoulders of manhood appearing during the peak of bone and muscle growth. Generally, the appearance of pubic and facial hair, as well as hair in the armpits, follows the growth of the shoulder and chest area and precedes the change in voice.

The testicles: The testicles are contained in a walnut-size sac of skin called the *scrotum*. It is held outside the body by a design of nature in order to maintain a temperature for spermatozoa production which is less than internal body temperature. Muscle fibers in the scrotum hold the testicles closer to the body for warmth in cold weather and relax to allow the sperm-producing organ to be farther away from the body when surrounding temperatures are warm.

As the young man passes through puberty, he should be advised that tight clothing which holds the scrotum close to the body can result in sterility because of degeneration of the sperm-developing tubules from body heat. In some cases, the testicles do not descend from the abdomen during development of the male child. The result is the same as that of wearing clothing that holds the scrotum against the body; the boy will be sterile. Other variations are the descent of one testis while the other is retained in the abdomen; or they may descend only as far as the *inguinal* area, at the junction of the thigh and the lower part of the abdomen.

Although undescended testicles usually do not cause any medical problems other than sterility, the danger of malignant change may be sufficient to warrant surgical correction of this disorder. If the testicles become trapped in the inguinal region, they may become inflamed because of the pressure of larger body parts in that area. In many cases, however, the testes descend spontaneously during the second decade of life after being trapped in the abdomen during the early years. Doctors frequently are able to assist the descent by administration of hormones as well as by surgery. At some point during puberty, a medical examination should include the condition of the testicles.

Genital size: Many boys are as sensitive about the size of their genitals as girls are about breast size. In the case of an empty scrotum because of undescended testicles, it is possible to have the scrotum injected with silicone plastic for cosmetic or psychological reasons so the sac appears less flaccid or larger. The size of the penis may become the subject of discussions in the school shower room. If a boy appears sensitive about the subject, he should be assured that there is a wide variation in normal sizes and that like ears, noses, and other body parts the dimensions have little to do with function.

Nocturnal emission: Another cause for concern by adolescent boys is the *nocturnal emission.* The nocturnal emission, sometimes called a *wet dream,* is the automatic expulsion of *semen* through the penis while the young man is asleep. The semen is secreted by the *prostate gland,* the *seminal vesicle,* and other glands which open into the *urethra.* The opalescent white fluid carries spermatozoa during intercourse and if the young male does not engage in sexual intercourse or does not masturbate, the semen simply accumulates until it overflows during a nocturnal emission. It is a harmless, normal occurrence.

Bone Growth

As the growth spurt subsides in the late teens, the *cartilage plates,* or *epiphyses,* in the long bones of the body close. Until the growth plates become filled in with calcium deposits, each long bone is in effect three bones—a central shaft separated from the ends by the cartilage growth plates. The growth plates are not completely replaced by bone until a female is about 20 and a male 23 years old. But the rate of growth begins to taper off as sexual maturity is achieved. After that, young women tend to retain fatty tissue and young men gain in muscle mass. It is a time to begin weight watching so that the hazards of obese adult life can be avoided. But the ravenous appetites developed during the period of rapid body growth and intense physical activity can easily evolve into bad eating habits during the teen years.

Hereditary Influences

Hereditary influences may determine many of the physical and psychological traits that an individual first becomes aware of in the teen years. Because of the various crossovers of the 23 sets of *chromosomes* and the nearly infinite combinations of *genes*, it is not always easy to predict how a child is going to appear as a young adult. But some features, such as hair color and eye color, usually can be identified with one or both parents; other traits may seem to be those of uncles, aunts, or grandparents. Heredity and hormones frequently are involved in the distribution of hair on the body and the oiliness of the skin, both of which can cause concern to teen-agers who are plagued by an overabundance or lack of these cosmetic traits. An example of hereditary influences on hair patterns can be seen in early baldness. A receding hairline is not a trait of the parents but rather an influence of the genetic makeup of a grandparent—the trait skips a generation.

Removal of Excess Hair

While not much can be done about baldness that is hereditary, there are ways of handling the problems of excess hair. If a girl has excess hair on her face, it can be removed by shaving, with wax, by electrolysis, or depilatories. Shaving is the most direct but not always the most satisfactory method of hair removal, since it is intended only as a temporary measure. An alternate shortcut is bleaching with diluted hydrogen peroxide; the hair is still there but it is not as noticeable. Another method involves the use of hot wax spread on the skin and allowed to harden. When it is removed quickly, the hair is pulled away. *Depilatories* are chemicals that destroy the hair at the skin line. Both hot wax and depilatories have longer lasting effects than shaving, but they must be repeated at intervals of several weeks. The only permanent method of removing excess hair is *electrolysis,* which is a time-consuming technique. Each hair root has to be burned out individually with an electric current. Electrolysis is recommended only for small areas and because of the time and expense involved would not be feasible for removing excess hair from regions other than the face.

Acne

There is some evidence that *acne* is partly hereditary. But it is such a common problem among teen-agers—it has been estimated that up to 90 percent of all youngsters endure some degree of acne—that it must have been inherited from a mutual ancestor like Adam or Eve. In fact, one of the deterrents to effective control of the skin disorder is that acne is so common that it is neglected by many youngsters. Waiting to outgrow acne can be a serious mistake, because the pimples, blemishes, blackheads, and boils that make life miserable for so many teen-agers can be eliminated or considerably reduced. They can also cause scarring. A doctor should be consulted in cases of severe or especially persistent acne.

Overactive oil glands: Acne is not a serious threat to the life of a youngster, but it can be seriously disfiguring at a time of life when most young people are sensitive about their appearance. It can occur at any time from puberty into early adulthood, and it is caused by poor adjustment of the skin to secretions of sebaceous glands. The imbalance resulting from hormones in the bloodstream will correct itself eventually. But to prevent permanent scarring, a program of simple skin care must be followed faithfully.

Acne is caused by oil glands in the skin that become overly active at puberty. The glands become clogged, with the result that blackheads or pimples appear. The solution is to wash the skin frequently and thoroughly to remove the oils and to clear the plugged oil glands. The color of blackheads, by the way, is not caused by dirt but rather from a chemical change in the secretions of the oil glands.

Skin care: The face should be washed several times a day with hot water and soap. The skin should be rinsed twice after washing, first with warm water, then with cold. Each time the face should be dried thoroughly with a clean towel. At bedtime, the face should be given a massage with soapsuds and water, rinsed, and patted dry with a clean towel. Any medication prescribed by the doctor should be applied after the final washing of the day. Careless handling of blemishes, such as squeezing blackheads or picking pimples, can result in scarring. Teen-agers also should avoid such habits as supporting the face with the hands or unconsciously rubbing the face.

Other precautions: Young women should not use cold creams or cosmetics unless they have been approved by a physician. Young men who shave must be careful to avoid cutting pimples. The doctor also should be consulted about how diet can help control acne. Although the skin disorder is not a dietary disease, there is some evidence that certain foods tend to aggravate it. However, there is a lack of agreement among doctors as to whether chocolate, carbonated bever-

ages, nuts, sweets, and other specific snack items may be the culprits. And there always is the possibility that since each youngster develops along an individual path, a food item that causes one teen-ager's face to break out with blemishes will not affect a sibling or classmate in the same way.

Diet

A survey by the Food and Nutrition Board of the National Research Council recently showed that 40 percent of boys between 13 and 19 years of age and 60 percent of the girls in the same age group subsisted on diets that were substandard. Generally, the young people surveyed had abandoned the eating routines of their families. They habitually skipped breakfast and failed to make up the nutritional loss during other meals.

Perhaps in rebellion against parental control and to assert their independence, they tended to gather with their friends at candy stores and snack shops. They purchased items that could be held in the hand during informal rap sessions—chocolate bars and cans of soda. The economic standards for the quickie street-corner meals were based on what could be obtained with money from allowances and after-school jobs. The snack habit persisted through the potato chip and carbonated beverage evening routine before a TV set. Their idea of a good meal included a side dish of French fries, a food lacking in almost everything except calories.

Calories and Nutrition

Calories are not all bad. Young people burn hundreds of them daily through dancing, working, athletic competition, and other activities. A typical male teen-ager may burn up to 3,600 calories a day; a teenage girl can easily handle 2,500 calories daily—and calories are easy to come by in snack foods. For example, a chocolate milk shake at 520 calories, two doughnuts, total-

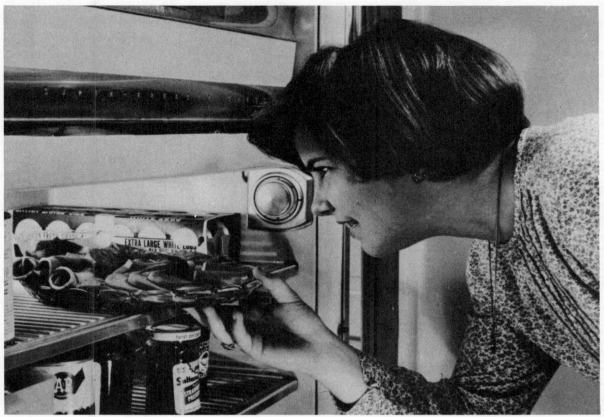

Snacking of this sort is almost synonymous with adolescence; as long as the foods are nutritious—not empty calories—no harm is done and excessive weight gain is unlikely.

ing 270 calories, a chocolate candy bar at 150 calories, a can of soda at 100 calories, and a handful of potato chips at 10 calories each will easily provide half the daily energy requirements for a busy high school girl. Adding French fries, at 15 calories each, and more cans of soda plus other snacks will bring the total up close to the 2,500-calorie level.

However, there is more to nutrition than snacking on calorie-rich foods. An individual obviously can fill up on high-energy goodies but suffer from malnutrition by disregarding the body's normal requirements for proteins, vitamins, and minerals. Also, calories have an insidious way of becoming excess weight. A calorie is a unit of energy, and the human body requires a certain amount of energy each day in order to sustain life and permit the muscle activity of

work or play. To maintain the proper balance between foods consumed and energy used in work and play, the teen-ager, like the adult, must estimate the calories in his meals and check the intake regularly by stepping on the bathroom scale.

People in their teens should develop the habit of weighing themselves at least once a week, recording the weight so it can be compared with previous readings. The weighing in should occur at the same hour each time, and the same scale should be used. Also, the same type of clothing should be worn each time the weight is checked. If an overweight or underweight youngster can find a companion to challenge in a race toward optimum weight, the competition will be an added inducement.

Calcium and phosphorus: Among the important minerals in teen-age diets are cal-

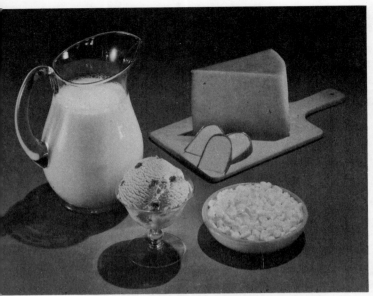

Dairy products are rich and easily-available sources of calcium and phosphorus, essential in teen diets.

cium and phosphorus. Milk is the most easily available source of calcium and phosphorus, which are required for the development of strong bones during the period of life in which the body is still growing. Calcium also is required for the effective contraction of muscle tissues and is vital for normal heart function. The recommended daily intake of milk for teen-agers is four eight-ounce glasses. It can be served as fluid whole milk, as skim milk, buttermilk, evaporated milk, or as nonfat dry milk. Cheese or ice cream can be substituted for part of the fluid milk allowance. One cup of ice cream is equivalent in calcium to one-half cup of milk. A one-inch cube of cheddar cheese is equal to two-thirds of a cup of milk, which also is equivalent in calcium to one cup, or eight ounces, of cottage cheese. Cream cheese can be substituted for milk in a two-to-one ratio; that is, two ounces of cream cheese are equal to one ounce of milk.

Iron: Iron is needed for the formation of *hemoglobin,* the substance that gives red blood cells their red coloration and is responsible for the transport of oxygen and carbon dioxide in the bloodstream. Hemo-globin has such an affinity for oxygen that without it humans would require 60 times as much blood to transport oxygen from the lungs to tissues throughout the body. Studies indicate that girls are five times as likely to need additional supplies of iron in their diets because of blood loss through menstruation. Recommended sources of iron are liver, heart, kidney, liver sausage, meat, shellfish, egg yolk, dark molasses, bread, beans and other legumes. If basic food lists seem drab and boring, the teen-ager might think of the iron sources in terms of a peanut butter sandwich or two hamburgers; either choice would provide the daily iron needs for a girl. Other minerals which are important to a teen-ager's diet include:

• Sulfur is needed by the body for hair, skin, nails, and cartilage, and is available by eating nearly any protein foods.

• Sodium is required for muscle activity and normal body fluid balance, and can be obtained by using ordinary table salt on foods.

• Iodine is needed for normal thyroid control of body metabolism, and is supplied in the form of iodized table salt.

• Potassium is a tonic for the nervous system and the muscles, and is available in adequate amounts in most kinds of meats.

• Magnesium collaborates chemically with calcium and phosphorus for normal muscle and nerve function, and is found in most forms of protein.

Weight Problems

Teens who are seriously overweight or who are contemplating radical weight reduction programs should be examined by a physician. Otherwise unfair comparisons with other persons of the same age and height may lead to wrong conclusions about the need to gain or lose weight. The weight–height standards are based on averages, and there are many youngsters who are above or below the average but quite healthy and normal. Good examples of misinterpretation of weight-height tables can be found among beefy football players who have been rejected by military recruiters because they weighed more than other fellows of the same height.

Another reason for a medical exam is to check the possibility of disease as the cause of the weight problem. The exam will also indicate whether the youngster has some other disorder that could be aggravated by a sudden weight loss.

Achieving optimum weight is only one step toward proper physical conditioning. A youngster who has been able to avoid physical activity by living in an elevator apartment, riding a bus to school, and watching TV after school hours instead of working or playing, could be right on the button as far as weight for his age and height are concerned, but his muscular development and heart and lung capacity could be at the same time at a very low ebb.

Physical Fitness

Good physical conditioning is as important as weight control during the teen years. Everybody cannot be an athletic champion, but almost anyone can improve his heart, lungs, and muscles so that he can cope more effectively with the stresses of young adult life. Physical conditioning can be accomplished with little or no exercise equipment. It can be programmed for city living or country living, in a gymnasium or in an apartment. All that really is required is a little time each day plus a great deal of determination and patience. It is important for young people to understand the major health role of daily exercise. Although many school physical education programs are excellent, some still remain inadequate, and in many cases students are only going through the motions of calisthenic routines and are not really benefiting from the effort.

Bicycling is a healthful, year-round activity that teen-agers can enjoy either alone or in groups. It also provides an economical means of transportation.

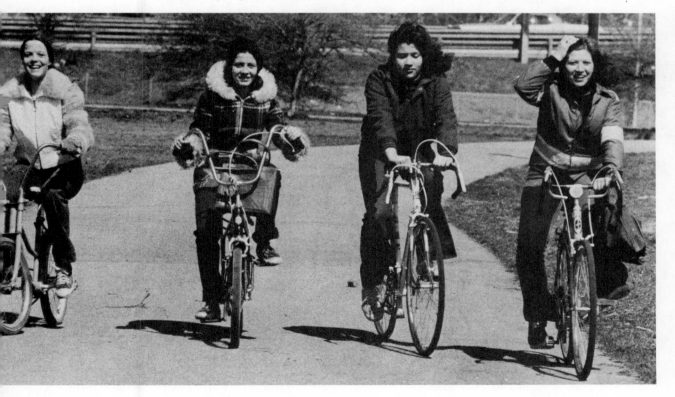

Exercise Goals for Teen-Age Boys

One of the goals of physical conditioning for teen-age boys is muscle development. When muscles are not used they atrophy, or shrink in size. A muscle that has been immobilized because of an injury may shrivel to one-fourth its normal size. Some of the muscle fibers are replaced by non-elastic fibrous tissue. On the other hand, muscles that are exercised regularly and vigorously will grow in size and strength. Exercise causes an increase in the number of individual muscle fibers as well as an increase in the number of blood capillaries supplying the muscle tissue. A fringe benefit

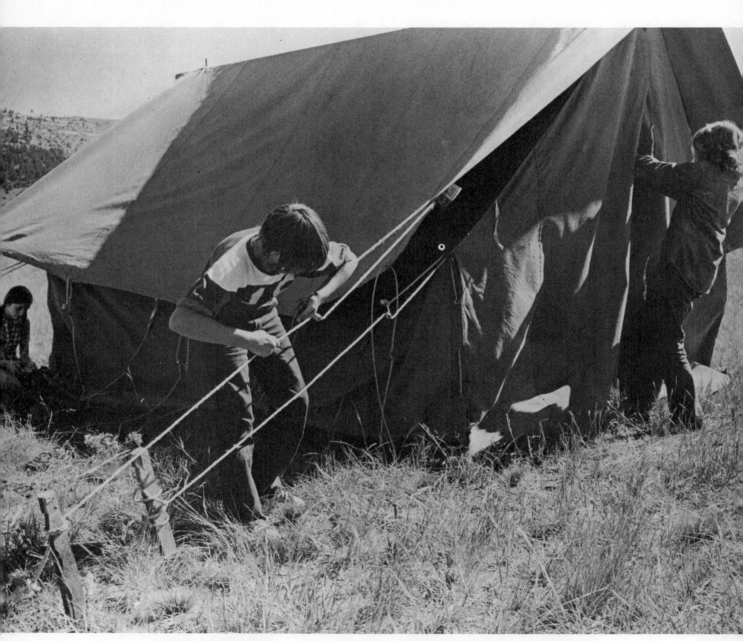

A weekend camping trip gives adolescents a chance to develop self-reliance and learn outdoor skills, such as pitching a tent, while enjoying the beauties of nature.

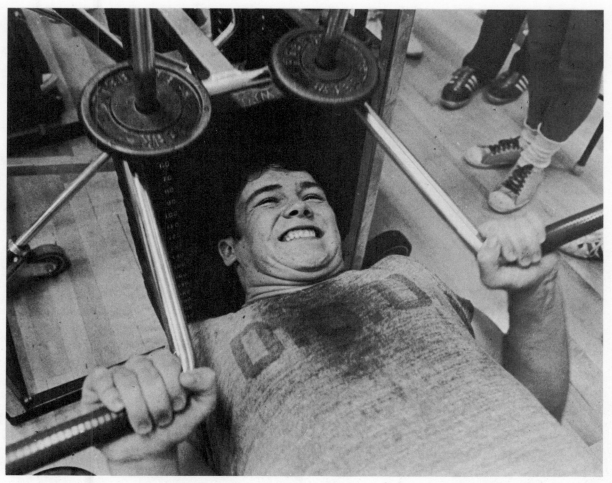

Weight lifting is one of the most efficient means of muscle development, especially of the back and shoulder muscles. Achievement depends on steady practice, gradual improvement, and willpower.

is that muscles become more efficient as they grow in size from exercise. In other words, the muscles can perform more work with less wasted effort.

In addition to muscle development, which every exercise program should provide, physical conditioning should include optimum cardiopulmonary development. This means increased heart activity and greater oxygen consumption and is the basis for the popular aerobics workouts. *Aerobics* means, literally, with oxygen. A goal of aerobics training is to achieve a steady state of exercising in which breathing is heavier than normal. In the steady state, the heart, lungs, and muscles work together as an efficient

machine at an activity level that is more demanding of the body than the resting state. Jogging, running, or rapid walking are examples of aerobic exercises. They can be practiced with no special equipment.

The individual goals for physical fitness should be kept within sensible limits to avoid injury or impaired health. The maximum level of performance can be determined by the appearance of the panting and puffing that occurs when exercise exceeds the normal ability of the lungs to supply oxygen to the muscles. A youngster who is not in good physical condition may huff and puff after walking up a flight of stairs, whereas a classmate in top condition might run a mile without showing signs of excessive breathing.

There are many fine exercise programs which teen-agers can follow, such as those published by the U.S. Air Force and the President's Council on Physical Fitness.

Exercise Goals for Teen-Age Girls

The young girl of today may be as involved in sports and the working world as the male, and the general guidelines for masculine conditioning apply to young women as well. Girls should follow exercise programs which develop muscular strength and the endurance provided by a sound cardiovascular system. Regular exercise causes the heartbeat to grow stronger and steadier and breathing to become deeper. As the flow of blood through the tissues is improved, waste products of the cells are removed more efficiently and complexion problems are reduced. Another benefit is that the body uses energy more efficiently in both physical and mental tasks; coordination is improved. Girls should not worry about developing bulging muscles when they follow a regular, well-balanced exercise routine which includes workouts for the hips and thighs, waist, bustline, calves, and ankles.   KNA

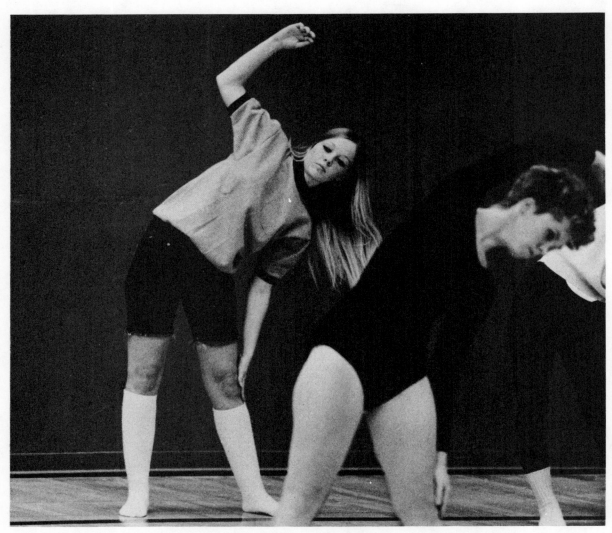

Modern dance, blending body conditioning with aesthetic pleasure, is popular with teen-agers.

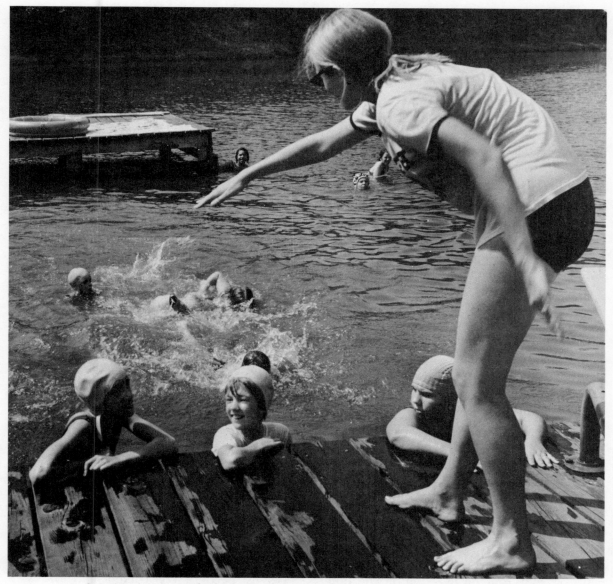

Swimming is among the best of exercises, calling into action most of the muscles of the body. Girls need not postpone the activity simply because of menstruation.

Care of the Teeth

During the teen years, careful supervision by the dentist and cooperation from the teen-ager are especially necessary. The poor eating habits of many teen-agers are reflected in their cavity rate, which is usually higher during adolescence than in later life.

If a young person is conscientious about oral care, he can avoid not only a high cavity rate, but also bad breath and the unpleasant appearance of food particles left on the teeth. These problems are really caused by the same thing—*dental plaque.* For a discussion of plaque removal, see under *Teeth and Gum Care,* p. 93.

Orthodontic Treatment

The development and growth of teeth is completed during the adolescent period.

When oral growth is improper, the adolescent needs treatment by an *orthodontist*, a dental specialist who treats abnormalities of the bite and alignment of teeth and jaws. Correction of such conditions as buck teeth, which mar a person's appearance, is a major reason for orthodontic treatment. But there are also major health reasons for orthodontic care. If teeth, for example, come together improperly, efficient chewing of food is impossible. The digestive system is strained because chunks of improperly chewed food pass through it. Orthodontic treatment will, therefore, result in lifelong better health and appearance.

Need for Frequent Checkups

During the adolescent period, the dentist will often recommend more frequent checkups than in the past. Small cavities are treated before they become deeper and infect the pulp, the inner chamber of the tooth, containing nerves and blood vessels. Should the pulp become infected, the tooth must have special treatment, usually a root canal process, or be extracted.

The dentist also treats tooth decay, or *caries,* more popularly known as cavities, to prevent their spread. While they are not thought to be contagious, cavities begin as a break in the tooth surface, which later enlarges. Food debris can become lodged in the cavity, be attacked by bacteria, and cause a cavity on the next tooth. The only way to avoid such a problem is to have the affected tooth treated immediately.

Front teeth often decay for the first time during this period. They are restored with a silicate or plastic filling close in color to the tooth rather than silver or gold, which would be unattractive. Unfortunately, these materials are not permanent and will need to be replaced in time. As a result, neglect of diet and oral cleanliness by an adolescent may mean that he may need many replacement fillings in the same cavity over his lifetime.   DJC

Stimulants, Drugs, and Alcohol

Initial exposure to caffeine, tobacco, drugs, and alcohol usually occurs during adolescence. Teen-agers should be fully educated regarding their physical effects and potential danger. They should learn how to use them, if at all, sensibly and in moderation and to resist peer-group pressures.

Caffeine

Caffeine, which is naturally present in coffee and tea and is used in many carbonated beverages and medications, stimulates the central nervous system to overcome fatigue and drowsiness. It also affects a part of the nervous system that controls respiration so that more oxygen is pumped through the lungs. In large amounts, caffeine can increase the pulse rate, but there are few long range effects because the substance is broken down by the body tissues within a few hours and excreted. Because of the action of caffeine in stimulating an increased intake of oxygen, it sometimes is used to combat the effects of such nervous system depressants as alcohol.

Nicotine

Nicotine is one of nearly 200 substances in tobacco. It affects the human physiology by stimulating the adrenal glands to increase the flow of *adrenaline.* The blood vessels become constricted and the skin temperature drops, producing effects not unlike exposure to cold temperatures. When comparatively large amounts of nicotine are absorbed by the body, the pulse becomes rapid and the smoker has symptoms of dizziness, faintness, and sometimes nausea and diarrhea. The release of adrenaline, triggered by nicotine, will produce temporary relief from fatigue by increasing the flow of sugar in the blood. But the effect is transient, and the feeling of fatigue will return again after the blood sugar has been expended.

Other properties of tobacco: The nicotine in tobacco can be absorbed simply by contact with the mucous membranes of the mouth; the tobacco does not have to be smoked to get the nicotine effects. Burning tobacco produces a myriad of substances found in the smoke of many plant materials when they are dried and burned. More than 50 different compounds are known to occur in concentrations of one microgram or more in each puff of tobacco smoke. Again, laboratory tests have demonstrated that the substances in burning tobacco do not have to be inhaled; most of the chemical compounds can be absorbed through the mucous membranes while a puff of smoke is held in the mouth for a few seconds. At least ten of the substances in tobacco smoke have been shown to produce cancer in animals. Other chemicals in tobacco tars are known as *co-carcinogens;* although they do not produce cancer themselves, they react with other substances to produce cancers.

Smoking and Disease

The relationship between tobacco smoking and cancer, heart disease, and emphysema-bronchitis are well established, even if some of the cause and effect links are missing. Large-scale studies of the death rates of smokers and nonsmokers have been carried on for the past 20 years. One group, consisting of nearly a quarter-million war veterans, yielded results indicating that smokers are from 10 to 16 times as likely to die of lung cancer as nonsmokers. (The higher ratio is for heavy smokers.) Similar results have been obtained from studies of smokers and nonsmokers with heart disease and lung ailments.

Buerger's disease: One of the possible, although rare, effects of smoking that is particularly insidious is a circulatory disorder known as *Buerger's disease.* As noted above, one of the effects of nicotine is a drop in skin temperatures. Smoking a single cigarette can cause the temperature of the fingers and toes to drop as much as 15 degrees Fahrenheit; the average is a little more than a five degree drop. The temperature change results from constriction of the blood vessels at the extremities. Blood clots may develop in the vessels that have been constricted, cutting off the flow of blood to the tissues of the area. When there is numbness or pain in the extremities. the condition should receive swift medical attention to prevent serious consequences.

Carbon monoxide accumulation: Another little publicized effect of smoking is the accumulation of carbon monoxide in the blood. Carbon monoxide is one of the lethal gases emitted in automobile exhaust. It is also produced by burning plant materials such as tobacco. It is a dangerous gas because of its strong affinity for the hemoglobin of red blood cells. Unlike oxygen and carbon dioxide, which become temporarily attached, then released, from the hemoglobin molecule, carbon monoxide becomes permanently locked into the red blood cell chemistry so that the cells are no longer effective for their normal function of transporting oxygen to the body tissues. With the oxygen-carrying capacity of part of the red blood cells wiped out, brain cells and other tissues suffer a mild oxygen starvation and the results are a form of intoxication.

A strong whiff of carbon monoxide can be fatal. Smokers, of course, do not get that much of the substance into their blood, but they do pick up enough carbon monoxide to render up to eight percent of their red blood cells ineffective. Experiments at Indiana University show that pack-a-day smokers have the same level of carbon monoxide in their blood as subjects who inhale an atmosphere of one-fourth of one percent carbon monoxide. That level of carbon monoxide increases the shortness of breath during exercise by approximately 15 percent, and, the study shows, about three weeks of abstinence from smoking are required to permit the oxygen-carrying capac-

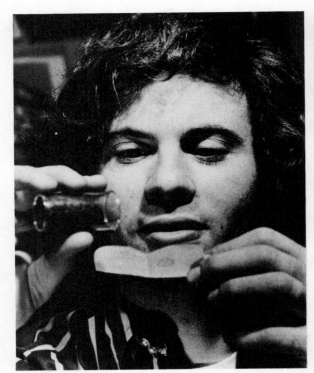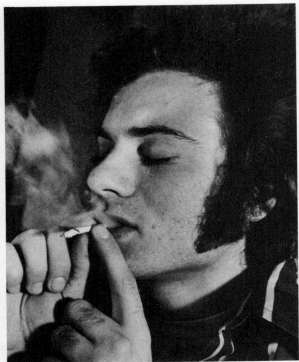

Marihuana is usually used in the form of cigarettes, which produce a mild intoxication. While the drug's effect varies widely, studies indicate possible consequences from frequent smoking, such as deterioration of decision-making ability.

ity of the blood to return to normal. It is the carbon monoxide of burning plant materials that produces most of the "high" associated with the smoking of many substances, including banana peelings.

Drugs

There has in recent years been an alarming increase in drug-use among teen-agers —a problem which is deservedly receiving nationwide attention. Education concerning the hazards and occasional tragedies accompanying drug-use is imperative.

Marihuana

Marihuana affects the central nervous system, including the brain, after it enters the bloodstream. According to some researchers, the substance accumulates in the liver. Some of the effects of marihuana are not unlike those of tobacco. The rate of the heartbeat is increased, body temperature drops, and blood sugar levels are altered. The drug user also feels dehydrated, the appetite is stimulated, coordination of movements becomes difficult, there are feelings of drowsiness or unsteadiness, and the eyes may become reddish. Taken in higher strengths, marihuana can cause hallucinations or distortions of perception.

Varying effects: Scientists are uncertain about the pathways of the drug in the central nervous system and its effects on other body systems. The drug's effects seem to vary widely, not only among individual users but also according to the social setting and the amount and strength of the marihuana used. The effects, which usually begin within 15 minutes after the smoke is inhaled and may continue for several hours, vary from depression to excitement and talkativeness. Some users claim to experience time distortions and errors in distance perception. But others sharing the same marihuana cigarette may experience no effects at all.

Although marihuana is not addictive, in that users do not develop a physical dependence upon the substance and withdrawal of the drug produces no ill effects, there are dangerous results from the use of marihuana. Marihuana users find it hard to make decisions that require clear thinking, some users develop psychotic reactions or an emotional disorder called "acute marihuana panic," and there is some evidence that the active ingredient is transmitted by expectant mothers to their unborn children.

Hallucinogens

Marihuana sometimes is described as a *hallucinogen* because of visual hallucinations, illusions, and delusions reported by users after they have inhaled the smoke from a large number of "joints" or "sticks" of the drug. But marihuana should not be confused with the true hallucinogenic drugs such as *mescaline* and *LSD* (lysergic acid diethylamide) which are known by doctors as *psychomimetic* drugs because they mimic psychoses.

LSD and mescaline: LSD and mescaline have marked effects on perception and thought processes. Teen-agers usually become involved with the use of LSD because they are curious about its effects; they may have heard about its purported "mind-bending" properties and expect to gain great personal insights from its use. Instead of great insight, however, the user finds anxiety, depression, confusion, and frightening hallucinations. The use of LSD is complicated by the reappearance of hallucinations after the individual has quit using the drug; the very possibility of repeated hallucinations causes a sense of terror.

Morphine and Heroin

Besides the hallucinogenic drugs, there are *opium* derivatives, *morphine* and *heroin,* which are literally killers. Morphine is one of the most effective pain relievers known and is one of the most valuable drugs available to the physician. It depresses the body systems to produce drowsiness, sleep, and a reduction in physical activity. It is a true narcotic, and its appeal is in its ability to produce a sense of euphoria by reducing the individual's sensitivity to both psychological and physical stimuli.

Addictive properties: A great danger lies in the ability of the body tissues to develop

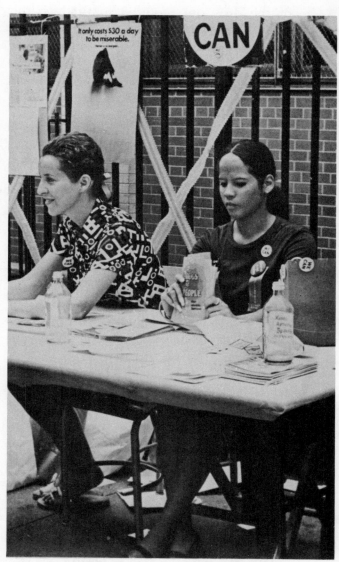

Alarmed at the growing drug problem, communities in both large and small cities have begun educating young people to the hard realities of drug addiction.

a physical dependence on morphine, and its derivative cousin, heroin. The degree to which heroin's "desirable" effects are felt depends in part on how the user takes it. *Sniffing* is the mildest form of abuse, followed by *skin-popping*—subcutaneous injection—and then by *mainlining*—injecting directly into a vein, which is the method used by almost all those dependent on heroin.

The body adjusts to the level of the first doses so that increasingly larger injections of the drug are required to produce the same feelings of euphoria. The ability of the body to adjust to the increasingly larger doses is called *tolerance*. And with tolerance goes *physical dependence,* which means that when heroin or morphine is withdrawn from the user he experiences a violent sickness marked by tremors, sweating and chills, vomiting and diarrhea, and sharp abdominal pains. Another shot of heroin or morphine temporarily ends the withdrawal symptoms. But the user, now dependent upon the drug, must continue regular doses or face another bout of the withdrawal sickness. Heroin has no value as a medicine and is available only through illicit channels at a high price. The heroin addict usually is unable to hold a job because of effects of the drug and must turn to crime in order to finance his daily supply of the narcotic.

Shortened life span: The health of a narcotics addict declines so that his life span is shortened by 15 to 20 years. He usually is in continual trouble with the law because of the severe penalties for illegal possession of narcotics. If he sells narcotics, as many heroin addicts are driven to do to get enough money to support their habit, the punishment is even more severe.

Amphetamines and Barbiturates

Other commonly abused drugs are *amphetamines,* also known as *ups* or *pep pills,* and *barbiturates,* sometimes called *downs* or *goof balls.* Amphetamines are used by doctors to curb the appetite when weight reduction of patients is needed and to relieve mild cases of depression. However, some doctors doubt that amphetamines should be used as a weight-control medication because of the risks involved; other experts have questioned whether the drugs are actually effective for that purpose.

Amphetamines stimulate the heart rate, increase the blood pressure, cause rapid breathing, dilate the pupils of the eyes, and produce other effects such as dryness of the mouth, sweating, headache, and diarrhea. Ordinarily, amphetamines are swallowed as tablets, but a more extreme form of amphetamine abuse involves the injection of the drug, usually Methedrine, directly into the vein.

Dangers of amphetamines: The danger in the use of amphetamines is that they induce a person to do things beyond his physical endurance, cause mental disorders that require hospitalization, and, in large doses, can result in death. Although they do not produce the kind of physical dependence observed in the use of narcotics, amphetamine withdrawal for a heavy user can result in a deep and suicidal depression.

Barbiturates: Barbiturates are sedatives used by doctors to treat high blood pressure, epilepsy, insomnia, and to relax patients being prepared for surgery. They slow the heart rate and breathing, lower blood pressure, and mildly depress the action of nerves and muscles.

Dangers of barbiturates: Barbiturates are highly dangerous when taken without medical advice. They distort perception and slow down reaction and response time, contributing to the chances of accidents. Barbiturates are a leading cause of accidental poison deaths because they make the mind foggy and the user forgets how many pills he has taken, thus leading to overdosage. They also cause physical dependence with withdrawal symptoms that range from cramps and nausea to convulsions and death. See also *Drugs*, p. 649.

Alcohol

Alcohol usually is not considered as a potentially dangerous drug because it is easily available at cocktail lounges, liquor stores, and is served generously at parties. Alcohol has been used by man for thousands of years, at times as a sedative and anesthetic, and when used in moderation has the effect of a mild tranquilizer and appetite stimulant. But when consumed in excess amounts, alcoholic beverages can produce both psychological and physical dependence. It can produce illusions of being a pick-me-up, but studies indicate that this effect is due to a letdown of inhibitions and the weakening of some of the functions of the central nervous system, particularly in the cerebral cortex.

Parents and teachers share an important responsibility to educate young people about the use and misuse of alcohol. Like marihuana, the effects of alcohol on human beings are not thoroughly understood. Some users develop a tissue tolerance for alcohol so that their body tissues require increasing amounts. When alcohol is withdrawn from such users, they develop tremors, convulsions, and even hallucinations. However, there are many varied reactions to the use of alcohol, and an individual may react differently to alcoholic drinks at different times. See also *Alcohol*, p. 626. For a discussion of the emotional development of the teen-ager, see *Social and Sexual Maturation*, p. 235.

KNA

INFERTILITY, PREGNANCY, AND CHILDBIRTH: THE BEGINNING OF A FAMILY

The decision of a young couple to begin a family is usually a happy event, with overtones of great responsibility for the parents-to-be. Although parenthood does bring fulfillment, happiness, and great rewards, it can also involve anxiety and heavy responsibility. Therefore, the decision to have a child should not be made lightly. Before increasing the family unit and thereby complicating it, the husband and wife should have a strong, good marriage, one based on love, understanding, and the ability to compromise and share.

Infertility

Once the decision to have a child has been made, a new set of problems can arise. Though the majority of women are able to conceive within a year, a large number of couples are faced with the problem of infertility. Old census reports and records show that in the early 1800s about one in six marriages was childless—the same proportion as today. However, because of improved medical and surgical techniques, the modern bride has a much better chance of overcoming a condition of infertility. For a description of the female reproductive organs and of the processes of conception and fertilization, see under *Social and Sexual Maturation*, p. 235.

Strain and fatigue: There are many causes of infertility, and an equal number of cures. Nervous strain and mental fatigue can interfere with reproductive capacity, as can

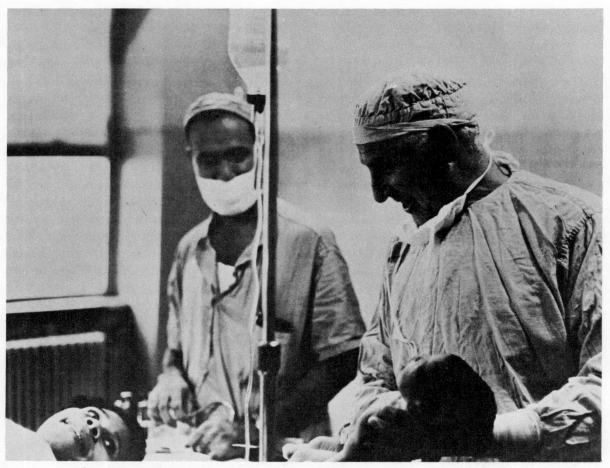

A happy day! Modern birth control methods allow a couple to plan for a child when they are well-prepared both emotionally and financially for the added responsibility.

fatigue from physical work. If a woman has worries or fears about financial security or other matters, she may fail to conceive. It is believed that nervous tension can suppress human ovulation cycles through the relationship of the hypothalamus, a part of the brain, and the pituitary gland, which controls the flow of sex hormones. Recommended treatment for a wife under strain might include a vacation, a temporary interruption in her business or professional goals, or a reorganization of her living pattern to relieve tension.

A similar tension problem can challenge the potential fatherhood of the husband. He may appear to lose his sex drive or suffer from impotency because of stress related to his job. The solution may be a second honeymoon to remove the couple from a stressful environment, or a willingness to accept a lower standard of living until financial security is truly established. Keeping up with the Joneses may put an extra car in the garage, but the penalty might be an empty crib in the nursery.

Timing ovulation: Occasionally, the reason for infertility may be something as basic as timing. Because of misinformation or misapplication of the correct information, husbands and wives may time their intercourse so the husband's sperm does not enter the female reproductive organs during the 24 hours or so of the menstrual cycle in which the ovum is most likely to become fertilized. The wife's menstrual cycles must be watched with extreme care so that the time of ovulation can be judged. Ovulation takes place 14 days before menstruation. In women with a 28-day cycle, ovulation would occur approximately 14 days after the previous period. Women with longer cycles ovulate later in the cycle. For a more accurate method of calculating ovulation, see *Basal Body Temperature*, p. 144.

If the couple is in the habit of having rather frequent intercourse, including at the time of ovulation, they should abstain for a few days before the expected day of ovulation so the sperm count in the husband can build up to a higher level. Then, at the time of ovulation, the couple should have intercourse at least twice with an interval of six to eight hours between. For further assurance of success, the wife should lie on her back with her legs flexed following intercourse so that a pool of sperm will remain near the cervix.

Reproductive incompatibility: Still another factor that can interfere with normal fertility is that of reproductive incompatibility, or an immune reaction, between sperm and ovum. This reaction between the male and female cells is similar to an allergic one, and may happen in one- of two ways. In the more complicated case of reaction between the sperm and the egg cell, the ovum may treat the sperm as a bit of foreign tissue which it will reject. There is at present no foolproof remedy for this problem, but medical scientists are investigating it.

In the second type of situation, there can be an incompatible reaction between the acid environment of the female reproduc-

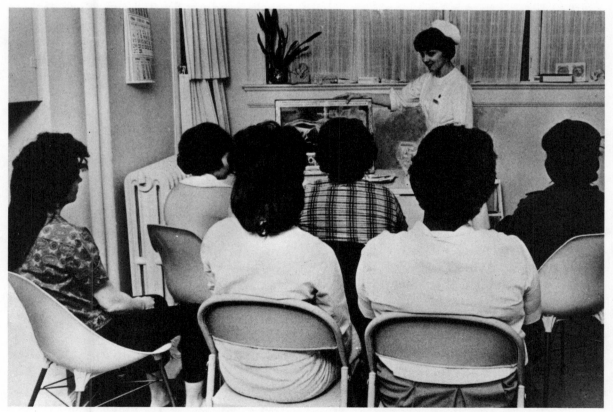

Many hospitals conduct free classes on all aspects of human reproduction, including information on birth control, infertility problems, prenatal and postnatal care.

tive tract and the alkaline male sperm. Although the lining of the vagina usually is acid, it normally becomes alkaline at the time of ovulation to facilitate the survival of the sperm on its way to the cervix. But in some cases, the vagina remains acid enough to kill or immobilize the sperm. In cases of couples unable to have children for this reason, chemicals can be introduced into the vagina to neutralize its acidity.

The Fertility Examination

Although it has been popular for centuries to hold the female partner responsible for childless marriages, the male is just as likely to be the infertile one. But the ego of the man is often such that he may refuse to admit that he is infertile until it has been proved that the wife is indeed capable of bearing children. The easiest way to check out the causes of infertility is to submit to a series of tests by a physician.

The physician giving the tests may be a general practitioner or a specialist. There are two types of specialists who concentrate on the female reproductive system—the *gynecologist* and the *obstetrician*. The gynecologist is a physician who specializes in the care and treatment of women, especially of the reproductive organs; an obstetrician specializes in the birth process. Since the areas of responsibility frequently overlap, the same doctor often handles both specialties and is referred to as an *Ob-Gyn doctor.*

Fertility examinations usually require a series of at least four visits by the wife over a period of about three months, and a similar series of visits by the husband. Both husband and wife usually attend the first meeting, when the doctor explains some of the common causes of infertility and outlines the ground rules for the tests to be performed.

Next, the physician schedules separate conferences with the marital partners so that he can obtain information which hus-

band and wife might be reluctant to discuss in each other's presence. This discussion might touch upon possible venereal diseases of earlier years, previous marital experiences, possible illegitimate pregnancies, and so on. The medical records also will include information about general health, diet, surgery, or diseases such as mumps (which might affect fertility), sex interests and practices, family histories of miscarriages or abnormal children, and contraceptive methods used.

Basal body temperature: The doctor will often suggest that the wife begin the *BBT,* or Basal Body Temperature charts. Using a special thermometer, the BBT is taken each morning at the same hour, before getting out of bed or having a first cigarette, which would alter the results. The BBT record is a remarkably accurate way of determining the day of ovulation, because ovulation causes a sudden rise in temperature. If there is no sudden rise in temperature during the menstrual cycle, it is an indication that no ovum was released by the ovary. If the temperature rises to indicate ovulation and remains elevated for over two weeks, it suggests that a pregnancy has begun. There are factors that can distort the readings, such as a fever or a mistake in reading the thermometer, but in general the BBT charts provide a reliable guide to the fertility cycles of the female partner.

Semen exam: On the second visit to the doctor, the husband is usually asked to bring a sample of semen in a corked bottle. The husband is generally advised to avoid intercourse for at least 48 hours before collecting the semen. The glass container of semen must be protected from both heat and cold, and for this reason should be carried in a paper bag to help insulate it from external temperature variations. A condom should not be used to collect or carry the semen because most rubber prophylactics contain chemicals that are harmful to spermatozoa.

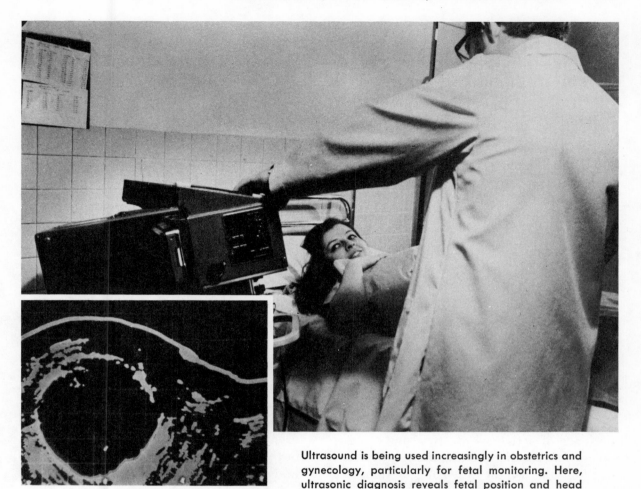

Ultrasound is being used increasingly in obstetrics and gynecology, particularly for fetal monitoring. Here, ultrasonic diagnosis reveals fetal position and head size in diagram (insert) to doctor and expectant mother. Irregularities revealed by ultrasound include multiple pregnancies, breech presentation, tumors, foreign particles in uterine cavity (e.g., coil).

The sperm examination should be made within an hour or so after it is collected so the spermatozoa will be nearly as alive and healthy as they are at the time of intercourse. If for some reason the results are not conclusive, the husband will be asked to bring another sample of semen when he accompanies his wife on her third visit, which will be scheduled about four weeks later.

During the second visit, both husband and wife may be given physical examinations, with emphasis on the pelvic and genital areas. Laboratory tests of blood and urine are made, and the examining physician may decide to make a study of thyroid function.

Tubal insufflation: The doctor generally tries to schedule the third visit to coincide with the 12th day of the wife's menstrual cycle. The examination at that time may include a *tubal insufflation* test. Also known as *Rubin's test,* tubal insufflation involves the injection of carbon dioxide gas, or sometimes ordinary air, into the uterus. Normally, the gas passes up through the uterus and Fallopian tubes and exits into the abdominal cavity. This would be a sign that the tubes are not obstructed. A pressure gauge shows a drop in pressure as the gas passes into the abdominal cavity, and the doctor may listen through a stethoscope for sounds of gas escaping through the tubes. The tubes are very narrow, and even a mild infection or scar tissue from a past infection can block them. Sometimes, forcing gas through the tubes is all that is needed to open them again so that chances of pregnancy will be enhanced.

A fourth visit, scheduled about four weeks after the third, should occur just before normal ovulation time. The couple may be instructed to perform intercourse about six hours before the visit. The tubal insufflation test may be repeated if the results of the earlier test were not satisfactory. In addition, a study of the cervical mucus may be made. In this study, the mucus is stretched into thin fibers or strands, which is possible only at the time of ovulation. During most of the reproductive cycle, the mucus is thick, dense, and jellylike. But the presence of estrogen hormones at the time of ovulation changes the mucus so that it makes a fibrous, fernlike pattern when placed on a glass slide.

The cervical mucus is also studied for the presence of active sperm. By using a high-power microscope, the examining physician can tell whether the cervical secretions are hostile to sperm. This would be the case if an adequate number of sperm are present, but are inactive or dead. The tests can be verified by placing a bit of semen on a microscope slide next to a sample of cervical mucus.

Hysterogram: If the tests up to this point have not revealed the cause of infertility, the doctor (or a recommended radiologist) can inject a special oil into the uterus and tubes and follow its path through the reproductive organs by an X-ray procedure called a *hysterogram.* If there is an obstruction or even a kink in the tubes that might interfere with the movement of an ovum, it should appear in the X-ray photographs, and the doctor can then treat the problem accordingly.

Fibroids: The hysterogram may also reveal the presence of *fibroids,* benign tumors composed of fibrous tissue which usually attach themselves to the walls of the uterus. Fibroids come in varying sizes—from smaller than a pea to larger than a fist—and are present in varying degrees in about 30 percent of all women. Depending on where they occur, they may block conception, in which case they can be removed by surgery.

Other procedures: Depending on what cause of infertility is suspected, the physician may recommend that the wife undergo a *culdoscopy, peritoneoscopy,* or *laparotomy.* The culdoscopy and peritoneoscopy require only a local anesthetic and a brief hospital stay. In these procedures, tubes are used to examine the pelvic organs without making a surgical incision. The laparotomy, requiring a longer hospital stay, involves an incision in the abdominal wall. Depending on the nature of the problem, a laparotomy, and to a lesser extent, the other two procedures allow the gynecologist latitude to make some on-the-spot corrections.

The physician may also decide to do an examination of tissue cells from the vagina or the testicles of the husband in an effort to find out what is causing infertility.

In general, the chances of success in the treatment of infertility vary with the severity of the abnormality and the length of time the disorder has gone untreated. Most minor problems can be treated by surgery, restoring normal hormone balance, proper diet, psychotherapy, or other methods, such as a change in the techniques or frequency of intercourse.

The Expectant Mother

In most marriages there is no problem of infertility. A majority of women between the ages of 20 and 25 become pregnant during the first year of marriage. And that includes a substantial number who have tried to prevent conception with various birth control methods. The fertility prospects usually continue to be satisfactory for newly married women up to the age of 35, but the chances decline if the bride is in her late 30s.

When pregnancy does occur, it should be regarded as a natural process rather than a confining illness. Although some of the bodily functions are altered by approaching motherhood, it should be remembered that women have been bearing children for thousands of years, and the chances for a safe and successful delivery were never better than today.

The expectant mother can look forward to hearing a variety of old wives' tales about the hazards of pregnancy from well-meaning friends. But unless there are complications, there is no reason for anxiety. And many of the complications can be prevented or corrected with good medical care. The woman preparing for motherhood generally can relax and enjoy the state of pregnancy if she follows basic rules of health and hygiene.

Many obstetricians recommend that women refrain from taking any medications, including patent medicines such as cold remedies, during the first three months of pregnancy unless the medicine is essential for the preservation of the mother's health. There are a number of chemical substances in drugs which may or may not affect the development of the embryo. An example of the unfortunate results of drug use during the early months of pregnancy was that of thalidomide, used by a number of women in 1961–1962. The drug was one of the safest sedatives ever developed. But when used by pregnant women, thalidomide caused physically deformed babies.

Eating correctly: Acute dietary deficiencies also can affect the development of an unborn child. As the fetus develops, its growth rate is tremendous—the weight gain is as high as 650 percent per month after the unborn child has passed the third month in its mother's uterus. All of the nutrients needed for fetal growth must be taken from

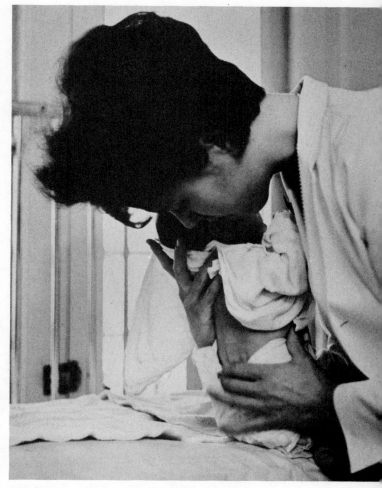

Good prenatal care, with emphasis on proper diet, can prevent many complications of pregnancy and make the delivery of a healthy baby more likely.

the mother's own diet and transmitted through the placenta. If the food eaten by the mother is not sufficient to sustain both mother and child, it is frequently the child who suffers.

This does not mean, however, that an expectant mother should eat double-sized meals because she has to feed two bodies. Obesity can be nearly as great a hazard to normal pregnancy as not eating enough. Overweight women should curb their food intake with such dietary shortcuts as drinking skim milk and eliminating as many fats and carbohydrates as possible. Meals should include a high level of proteins and all the

THE FETAL ENVIRONMENT IN THE UTERUS

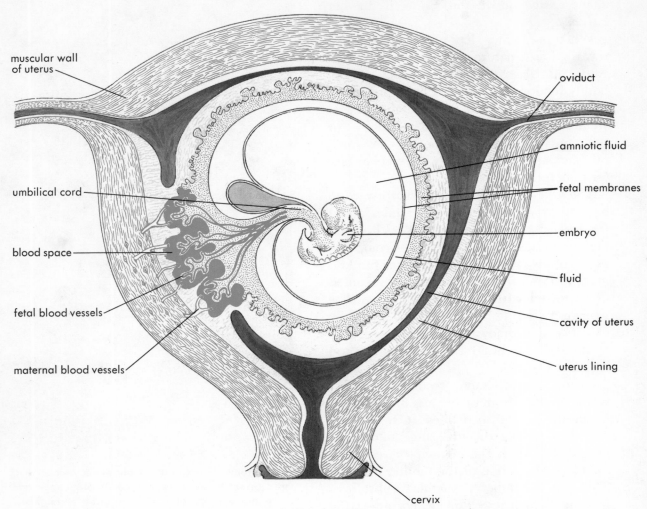

muscular wall of uterus

oviduct

amniotic fluid

fetal membranes

umbilical cord

embryo

blood space

fluid

fetal blood vessels

cavity of uterus

maternal blood vessels

uterus lining

cervix

essential minerals and vitamins. The number of total calories should not be less than 1,800 per day, unless the doctor recommends otherwise.

The rule of thumb on weight gain for a pregnant woman is that she should be about 20 pounds heavier at the end of the nine months than she was before conception. The rate of gain is important. It should be held to around one pound per month during the first three months, and between two and three pounds per month during the last six months.

Throughout the pregnancy, cravings for such foods as strawberries, ice cream, pickles, or whatever, are usually caused by psychological reasons rather than physical ones. However, if the food items craved are nutritious and low in calories, there is nothing wrong with satisfying the whim. Pickles, incidentally, are lower in calories and richer in vitamin C, iron, and other nutrients than most other snack foods.

Heartburn: Many mothers experience heartburn during pregnancy, and investigators have found that the treatment should be related to the length of time the mother has been carrying the unborn child. Heartburn during the first *trimester*, or three-month period, is usually due to anxiety and tension. If the symptoms are severe, the doctor may prescribe antacids or tranquiliz-

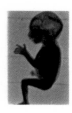

1.
At three months, the fetus is distinctly shaped. The fingers and toes are well outlined, and the eyelids are fully formed.

2.
By four months the fetus has lengthened in size but not otherwise changed markedly in appearance.

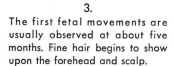

3.
The first fetal movements are usually observed at about five months. Fine hair begins to show upon the forehead and scalp.

DEVELOPMENT
OF THE HUMAN FETUS

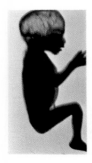

4.
This fetus, also five months old, has been injected with an opaque material to show the delicate network of the arterial circulation.

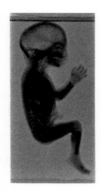

5.
At six months, the fetus has entered its period of most rapid growth. The body is completely covered by fine hair and a protective oily secretion.

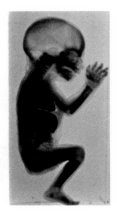

6.
By seven months the fetal skeleton is virtually complete, and the digestive and nervous systems are well advanced.

FOOD AND NUTRITION

The human body needs energy to carry on its many physical and mental activities. It also requires material from which to build new tissues and replace old "worn out" tissues. Food supplies the source of both energy and building material. The basic foodstuffs are proteins, carbohydrates, fats, minerals, vitamins and water. The proteins and minerals are the principal building materials, carbohydrates and fats yield most of the energy units, the vitamins regulate certain important bodily functions, and water serves as a vehicle for the other foods.

All bodily activities (even building of tissue cells from proteins) require energy. The body derives this needed energy by burning (oxidizing) the food it consumes at a low temperature (about 99° F). Different types of food components yield varying amounts of energy units or calories. Thus, fats are a more concentrated source of calories than proteins.

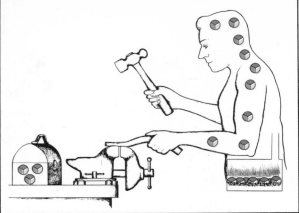

Daily caloric requirements are not the same for everyone, but due to many factors, such as the type of work done, vary from one person to another. By determining these requirements for a great many persons, it has been possible to calculate the average caloric output for the average person during various types of activity. These are shown in the section below.

The amount of food consumed in 24 hours should yield the same number of calories as the body requires for that period. If this is true and the diet is well balanced with the main food components, then good nutrition will result.

At the left is a diagrammatic representation of a working man using the food he eats (in lunch box) for energy and building material. The red-blue-yellow circles represent proteins, carbohydrates, and fats. His body is burning these food components as he works, and they are also being used to replace his tissue cells or placed in storage.

Rates of Metabolism — Caloric Output — In 24 Hours

RESTING	LIGHT WORK	MODERATE WORK	HEAVY WORK
1500 Calories	2500 Calories	3500 Calories	6000 Calories

The Main Components of Food

PROTEINS

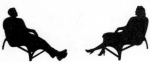

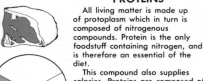

All living matter is made up of protoplasm which in turn is composed of nitrogenous compounds. Protein is the only foodstuff containing nitrogen, and is therefore an essential of the diet.

This compound also supplies calories. Proteins are composed of amino acids, which are needed to build and replace tissue cells. It is in the form of amino acids that proteins are absorbed through the intestinal wall into the blood.

CARBOHYDRATES

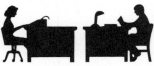

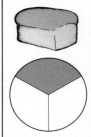

Carbohydrates include the large chemical group of sugars and starches. These substances are all reduced to simple sugars before being absorbed into the blood. From the blood they are used by the tissue cells for energy or are carried to the liver and muscles where they are stored as glycogen for future use. If the tissue cells deplete this store of glycogen, then the fat reserves are used for energy.

FATS

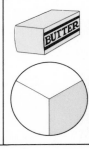

Fats are the richest source of energy. Weight for weight, they yield more than twice as many energy units as either carbohydrates or proteins. Fats are utilized by the body in metabolism either as such or as fatty acids of which all fats are composed. Stored fats serve as a reserve supply of energy and to a certain extent as insulation in the body. They are also an integral part of certain tissue cells.

VITAMINS

Vitamins are chemical substances manufactured in plants and found deposited in animal tissues. They are essential to life and good health. In extremely small amounts, they govern and regulate many important functions of the body such as metabolism. They may be supplied from natural sources such as illustrated below. Some are also available as synthetically prepared compounds.

A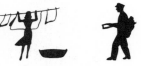

Fish liver oils (cod, halibut and shark), yellow vegetables (like carrots), butter, and egg yolk contain vitamin A.

B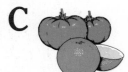

The B vitamins, including thiamine, riboflavin, niacin and others, may be obtained from whole-grain cereals, yeast, and liver.

C

Oranges and other citrus fruits are the best natural sources of vitamin C. It is also found in tomatoes and raw cabbage.

D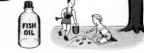

Vitamin D is produced in the skin during exposure to direct sunlight or an ultraviolet lamp. Fish liver oils are another source.

MINERALS

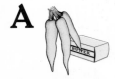

For building and repairing tissues the organism needs minerals such as calcium, phosphorus, iron, iodine, sodium, potassium, manganese, fluorine, chlorine, and magnesium.

ROUGHAGE

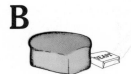

Certain foods contain indigestible fibers and other material which aid in digestion. They give bulk to the intestinal contents and promote the movement of waste through the intestinal tract.

SEASONING

Appetizing substances in our food also help digestion by stimulating directly and indirectly the secretion of digestive juices.

WATER

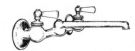

Water transports food, serves as a part of living matter, regulates temperature, and aids in eliminating waste products.

Edited by Ervin, Gordon and Neyman

THE CIRCULATORY SYSTEM

The circulatory system distributes blood to the body, bringing nourishment and oxygen to the body cells and removing their wastes. During one cycle, dark blood (represented by the color blue in the illustration) with much waste carbon dioxide and little oxygen is pumped by the right side of the heart to the lungs. There carbon dioxide escapes, and oxygen enters the blood, turning it bright red. It then flows into the left side of the heart. Next, the left side of the heart pumps the blood (represented as red in the illustration) via main arteries to organs and tissues throughout the body. Nutrients of the blood are absorbed through capillaries, and the blood is returned through veins to the right side of the heart, completing the circuit.

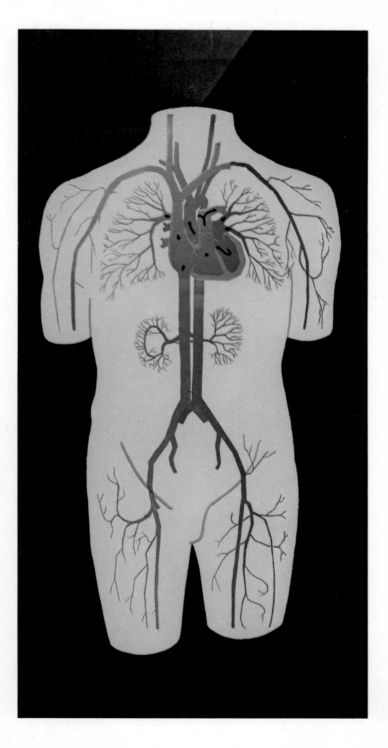

SKIN AND OUTER MUSCLES OF FACE, NECK, CHEST AND ABDOMEN

In this model the skin on one side has been removed to show the important outer muscles of the face, neck, chest, and abdomen. Symmetrical muscles of the face open and close the eyes and mouth, and also express emotion. Muscles of the neck aid in movements of the head. The large, fan-shaped muscle of the chest gives strength to the arm and shoulder, and a pair of long, flat abdominal muscles compress the abdomen and help bend the body.

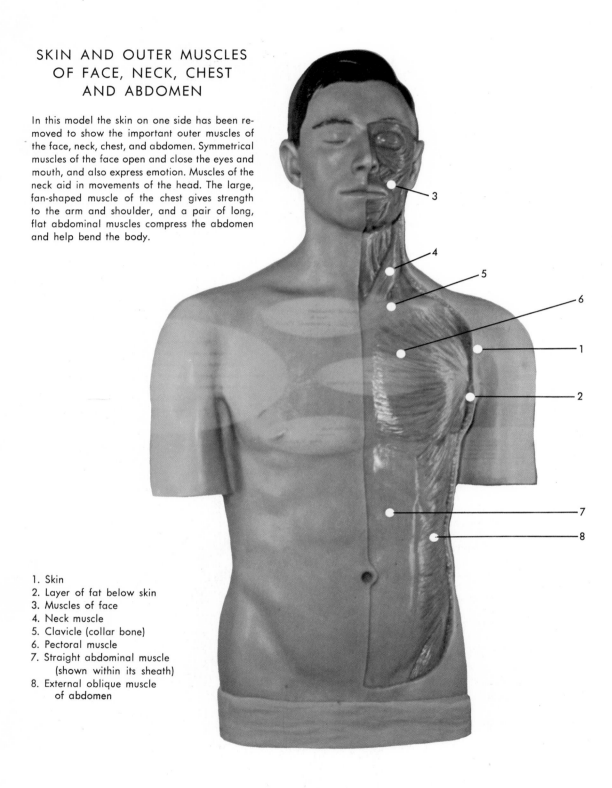

1. Skin
2. Layer of fat below skin
3. Muscles of face
4. Neck muscle
5. Clavicle (collar bone)
6. Pectoral muscle
7. Straight abdominal muscle (shown within its sheath)
8. External oblique muscle of abdomen

LEFT LUNG
AND RIGHT RIBS;
AND MUSCLES
OF THE ABDOMEN

In this model most of the outer muscles and the ribs on the left side have been cut away to show the lung on the left side and the ribs on the right side. The location of the heart is indicated, and the various layers of the muscles that make up the abdominal wall are shown in the lower part of the model.

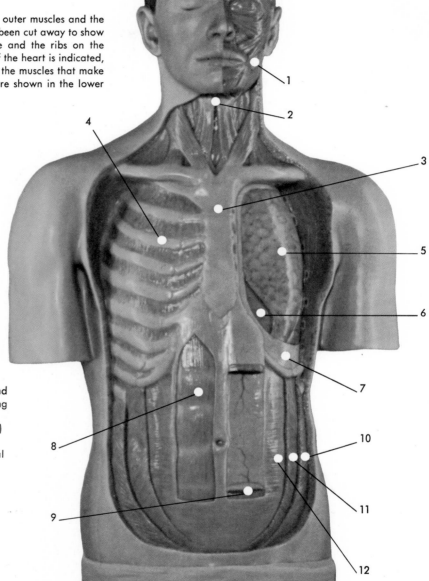

1. Parotid (salivary) gland
2. Hyoid bone (supporting the tongue)
3. Sternum (breast bone)
4. Ribs of right side
5. Left lung in its pleural sac
6. Apex of heart behind pleural sac
7. Lower part of pleural sac
8. Straight abdominal muscle
9. Straight abdominal muscle in section
10. External oblique muscle
11. Internal oblique muscle
12. Transverse muscle

LARYNX, THYROID GLAND, LUNGS, HEART, STOMACH AND INTESTINES

Here the muscles of the face, neck, and ribs, and the covering of the heart have been removed. The model shows the larynx and the trachea, the thyroid gland, the jugular veins and carotid arteries, the heart, the lungs, and part of the diaphragm. Abdominal muscles have been removed to show the edge of the liver, the end of the gallbladder, part of the stomach, and the intestines.

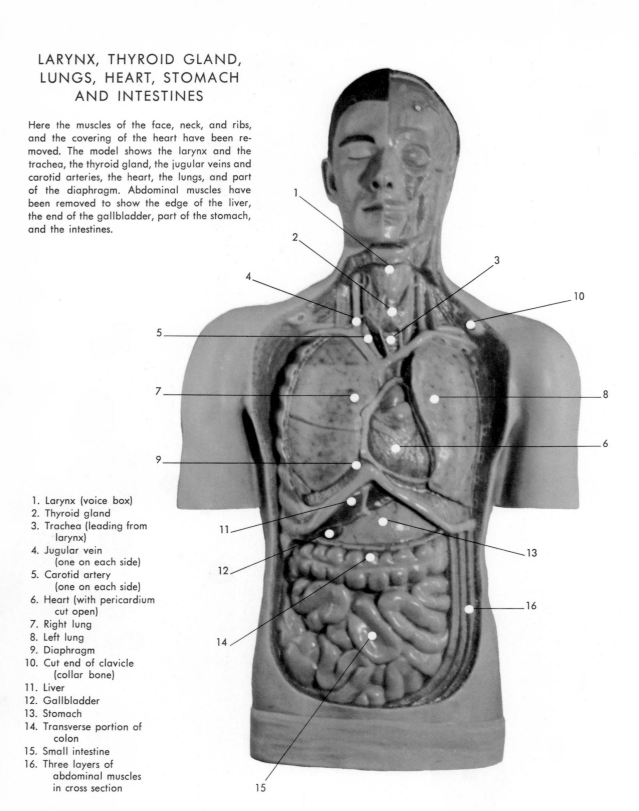

1. Larynx (voice box)
2. Thyroid gland
3. Trachea (leading from larynx)
4. Jugular vein (one on each side)
5. Carotid artery (one on each side)
6. Heart (with pericardium cut open)
7. Right lung
8. Left lung
9. Diaphragm
10. Cut end of clavicle (collar bone)
11. Liver
12. Gallbladder
13. Stomach
14. Transverse portion of colon
15. Small intestine
16. Three layers of abdominal muscles in cross section

SECTIONAL VIEWS OF LUNGS AND HEART; STOMACH, LIVER, DUODENUM AND COLON

Still deeper cuts have been made in this model to show the inner covering of the brain, the inside of the larynx and trachea, sectional views of the lungs, and the heart with its four chambers.

The liver below the diaphragm has been lifted up to show the gallbladder, pancreas, and duodenum. The transverse colon and the small intestine have been partially removed to show the remainder of the colon as well as the bladder.

1. Inner covering of the brain
2. Roots of upper teeth
3. Upper end of esophagus
4. Larynx in section
5. Superior vena cava
6. Right atrium
7. Right ventricle
8. Pulmonary artery
9. Left atrium
10. Left ventricle
11. Aorta and its branches
12. Cut surface of lung, showing branching of pulmonary artery, pulmonary veins, and the bronchi
13. Diaphragm
14. Liver (lifted up)
15. Gallbladder
16. Stomach
17. Pancreas
18. Duodenum
19. Cut end of small intestine
20. Cecum (beginning of colon)
21. Appendix
22. Ascending colon
23. Cut end of transverse colon
24. Descending colon
25. Sigmoid colon
26. Top of urinary bladder

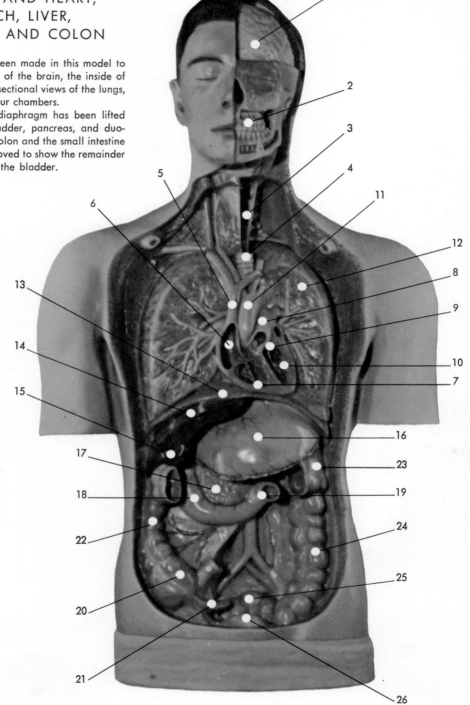

BRAIN; AORTA, TRACHEA AND ESOPHAGUS; KIDNEYS, URETERS AND BLADDER

In this model, the cerebral and cerebellar portions of the brain have been exposed. The lungs and heart have been removed from the chest cavity to reveal the aorta, the trachea, and the esophagus. The aorta and the esophagus pass through the diaphragm to enter the abdomen. Below the diaphragm are the spleen, the kidneys and the ureters leading from the kidneys into the bladder.

1. Brain with coverings removed
2. Cerebellar portion of brain
3. Inside of esophagus
4. Inside of larynx
5. Vocal Cord
6. Trachea
7. Right bronchial tube
8. Left bronchial tube
9. Aorta
10. Esophagus
11. Diaphragm
12. End of esophagus
13. Spleen
14. Inferior vena cava
15. Abdominal aorta
16. Right kidney
17. Adrenal glands
18. Left kidney
    (cut section to show its relation to ureter)
19. Left ureter
20. Right ureter
21. Urinary bladder
22. Beginning of rectum
23. Peritoneal lining of abdominal cavity

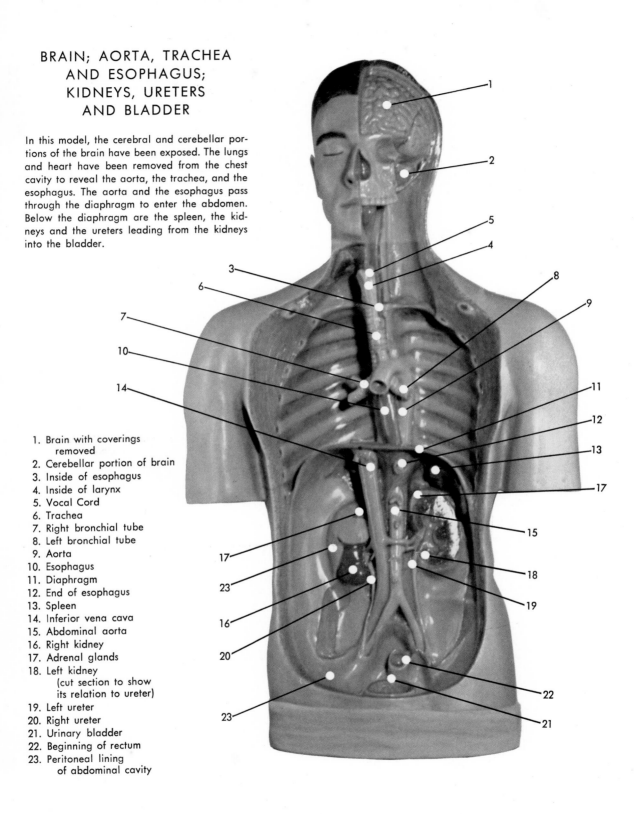

ers. Heartburn during the last six months is usually due to the crowding of the enlarged uterus within the abdomen, which lessens stomach capacity. The solution in such cases is to eat a number of smaller meals during the day rather than three large ones. Expectant mothers with heartburn should also use additional pillows so they sleep with the head and shoulders higher than the rest of the body, avoid tight clothing that squeezes the abdominal area, and not stoop or bend over after eating.

Smoking: Should an expectant mother smoke? A study of more than 16,000 pregnancies shows that mothers who smoke cigarettes are more likely to have stillborn babies, premature babies, and babies who are below average in weight than nonsmoking mothers. Other researchers have found that cigarette smoking stimulates contractions of the uterus, which could lead to premature birth. Mothers who smoke are also more likely to have spontaneous abortions or miscarriages.

Morning sickness: Morning sickness, characterized by nausea and vomiting, is one of the most common complaints of mothers-to-be. Although it is unpleasant, morning sickness rarely becomes so serious that special medical treatment is needed. While friends and relatives may try to convince the expectant mother that the sick feeling is all in her mind—and she certainly may feel some anxiety about her pregnancy—there is good evidence that there is also a physical cause. The level of gastric acid in the pregnant woman's stomach declines during the first trimester of pregnancy. Also, stomach activity during that period is at low ebb, and digestion is one to two hours slower after a meal than before pregnancy.

In most cases of morning sickness, the mother is unable to hold down her breakfast. The feeling of nausea usually subsides by lunch time, and does not appear again until the following morning. For the majority of women, the feeling fades away en-

tirely by the 12th week. If it continues into the last two trimesters, the condition may not be related to the pregnancy.

Food for periods of morning sickness should include crackers and dry toast, lemonade or soft drinks served at cold temperatures, and hot soup, tea, or coffee. Items to be avoided are greasy foods and liquids that are only lukewarm.

Toxemia of pregnancy: The expectant mother should visit her doctor as frequently as he suggests and follow his instructions carefully. She should report to her doctor any signs of puffiness of the hands and face, headaches, or visual disturbances that she experiences. Such signs and symptoms, especially in the last trimester of pregnancy, suggest *toxemia*. It is one of the most serious complications of pregnancy, and it affects about five percent of all expectant mothers.

Toxemia of pregnancy is a catch-all term that covers *hypertension,* or abnormally high blood pressure, and *edema,* or swelling of tissues due to fluid accumulation. Other symptoms are weight gain, *proteinuria,* or excretion of protein, and, in severe cases—when the disorder is sometimes called *eclampsia*—convulsions and loss of consciousness. Toxemia in late pregnancy is sometimes called *preeclampsia.*

Weight gain can amount to over two pounds a week and may be due almost entirely to fluid retention. Proteinuria usually does not appear until after high blood pressure and weight gain have appeared. But even these clinical signs may develop before the mother-to-be knows that she has toxemia, As the problem progresses, she may have visual disturbances, puffy eyelids, headaches, and abdominal pains. When the latter symptoms occur the disease is rather well established.

The cause of toxemia is believed to be a failure of the mother's body to adjust to the metabolic and physiological stresses of pregnancy. With careful management, toxemia can be controlled with the help of drugs, regulation of weight gain and fluid intake, bed rest, and in some cases by early delivery of the baby. The fact that delivery of the child seems to resolve the problem of toxemia reinforces the theory of metabolic–physiologic relationships in the stresses of pregnancy in some women.

During pregnancy a number of complex changes take place in the mother's body— a different pattern of hormone activity, alterations in the glands secreting hormones, increased blood supply with greater demands on the heart, and a rapidly growing parasitic human in the uterus, which also grows and presses against other organs within the body. Each woman reacts somewhat differently to these changes, and toxemia is one of the reactions.

Backaches and other disorders: Some expectant mothers are concerned about whether the baby should be carried high or low. There is a belief among some women that a baby carried high will be a boy. The truth is that no single pregnancy is either high or low for the entire nine months. Some babies seem to be carried higher at certain stages of pregnancy while at other times they seem to be carried low. The position has nothing to do with the sex of the future offspring.

Where the baby is carried also has nothing to do with a common complaint associated with pregnancy—backache. Backache in pregnant woman is usually caused by changes in posture, and only rarely by abnormality of the organs within the pelvis. Usually it is due to bending, lifting, or walking without properly compensating for the added strain of the weight of the child, especially in the later stages of pregnancy. Generally, backache responds to rest, heat, and drugs, which relax the muscles—although the drugs should be used only on a doctor's recommendation. The physician also may recommend that a lightweight maternity girdle be worn to help minimize the strain.

Improper posture in the final weeks may also be responsible for numbness and tingling or crawling sensations in the hands and arms. The hand-and-arm complaints frequently are related to what is called the *lordotic posture*, where shoulders are slumped, the spine curved forward, and the neck bent forward. The tingling sensations usually vanish when the posture is corrected. Exercises are used to help change the lordotic positioning of the spine and shoulders.

The mother-to-be must be careful about the use of seat belts when traveling by automobile or airplane. In the final months of pregnancy the belt should be fitted snugly around the lower third of the abdomen to protect the uterus from the steering wheel or dashboard in the event of an accident or sudden stop.

Occasionally, a doctor will want to have X rays made of the pelvis of the mother to determine whether it is adequate to permit an uncomplicated childbirth. There is little hazard in a brief diagnostic X ray if modern equipment is used. Nevertheless, the mother should avoid exposure to unnecessary X rays, particularly during the first three months of pregnancy. Embryonic tissue is highly sensitive to radiation because the cells have not reached the degree of differentiation found in the fetus in the later months of pregnancy. In other words, the embryo tissues are much more likely to be adversely affected by radiation.

Urinary tract disturbances are not unusual during pregnancy, and may be recurrent in women who were treated for kidney or bladder infections before pregnancy. It is not unusual for women to void as frequently as once an hour or oftener, and half a dozen times during the night. The disorder may be accompanied by fever and a burning sensation while voiding the urine. But most cases respond to medications and special hygiene instructions prescribed by the doctor.

Leg cramps and varicose veins: Leg cramps and varicose veins affect a significant number of pregnant women. Leg cramps are the most common problem, and probably 85 percent of expectant mothers experience an occasional spasm of the calf muscles while carrying a child. The leg cramps may occur suddenly and be quite painful; at other times, the cramp may feel more like a simple kink in the muscles. The cramps occur more frequently in the last three months of pregnancy and are more likely to be experienced during a second or third pregnancy than during the first. Sluggish blood circulation and a dietary deficiency of calcium are thought to be the causes of leg cramps. The treatment consists of applying heat to the legs, massaging them, and sitting or lying down with the legs elevated. Drinking fortified milk will add calcium and vitamin D to the diet. In severe cases, muscle-relaxing drugs may be prescribed.

Varicose veins are more likely to appear during the second or third pregnancy, and tend to disappear after the birth of the baby. They are caused by a pooling of blood in the veins of the legs. Normally, the contraction of the leg muscles during walking has the effect of pumping blood from the legs back up toward the heart. But just the strain of standing can produce varicose veins even in normally active people who are on their feet for long periods. The strain of pregnancy also can upset the normal return flow of blood in the legs, so the veins become dilated. As with leg cramps, some relief can be had by sitting or lying with the feet raised. Additional relief can be obtained by wearing elastic stockings. If the varicosities remain after pregnancy, they can be treated by drugs or surgery.

Immunization: There are certain facts about immunization that a woman should know if she contemplates pregnancy. One is that the vaccinia of smallpox vaccine can be transmitted through the placenta to the

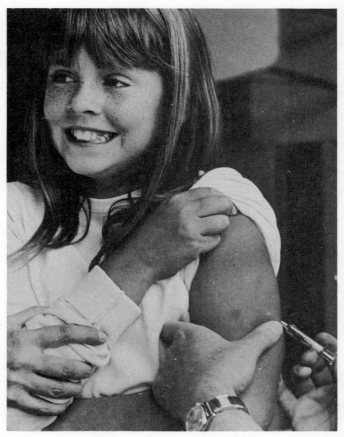

Rubella vaccine will protect this girl from contracting the disease in later child-bearing years and will prevent her spreading the disease to pregnant women.

fetus. The disease can be fatal to an unborn child. But if the mother must travel to an area where there is a chance of smallpox infection, she should take the risk of vaccination.

If she plans to be pregnant during the winter months, she should arrange to receive a series of influenza shots beginning in September and ending by mid-December. If she has been immunized against influenza within the past two years, a booster shot should be sufficient.

German measles, or rubella, can be a serious threat to the normal development of a baby if contracted during the first 12 weeks of pregnancy. The rubella vaccine normally given to children should be given to women of child-bearing age only with caution.

Some medical scientists believe that the virus can be transmitted by the vaccine to the fetus if conception occurs within two months after the vaccine is given. If the virus infects the unborn child, particularly during the first trimester, the child may be afflicted with cataracts, deafness, or damage to the heart and nervous system.

Immunizations should also be obtained for diphtheria, malaria (if in an area where this is common), and mumps. If these diseases occur during pregnancy they result in spontaneous abortion in about one-third of the cases.

Tetanus is regarded as one of the most serious complications of pregnancy. The period of incubation for tetanus is shorter in pregnant than in nonpregnant women. It is particularly hazardous during the period immediately after abortion or childbirth. But the threat can be avoided by receiving proper tetanus immunization before pregnancy.

The Rh Factor

Blood incompatibilities between the mother and father can be another complication of pregnancy. The condition is caused by a blood protein known as the *Rh factor*. A person whose blood contains the protein is called *Rh-positive; Rh-negative* people lack the blood factor. Approximately 85 percent of the population is Rh-positive. The term *Rh* is derived from the first two letters of the name of the Rhesus monkey, a laboratory animal which was used for much of the basic research on the blood incompatibility problem.

About ten percent of all marriages in the United States involve an Rh conflict. If both husband and wife are either Rh-positive or Rh-negative, there is no problem. But if the wife has Rh-negative blood and her husband Rh-positive, the child of such a union may be threatened by death or mental retardation, particularly after the first pregnancy.

The Rh-factor is inherited, and if the unborn offspring inherits the Rh-positive factor from its father while the mother has Rh-negative blood, the mother's blood may develop antibodies that destroy the baby's blood. The threat to the unborn child can be modified by a blood transfusion to the newborn infant or to the fetus before birth. The mother also can in effect be immunized against the development of antibodies by the injection of a gamma globulin blood fraction rich in passive Rh antibodies.

Usually, the first child is not affected by Rh blood conflicts. The red blood cells of the fetus can cross the placenta and trigger the reaction in the mother's blood system. But they do not reach their peak of entry into the mother's blood supply until the time of delivery. Thus, to prevent sensitization of the mother, doctors must eliminate the fetal red cells around the time of delivery—before the buildup of antibodies can begin. Once the antibodies have developed in the mother's blood, all future Rh-positive babies will be threatened unless preventive steps are taken.

If the husband has Rh-negative blood, or if he carries genes for both Rh-negative and Rh-positive, the baby will probably inherit the Rh-negative factor, and there will be no blood conflict. In nearly every case of Rh conflict today the baby can be saved and the production of antibodies suppressed in the mother. But the blood of both parents should be checked at the start of pregnancy plans, and arrangements made to protect the fetus if there is a threat of blood incompatibility.

Other genetic factors: The genetic background of each marital partner has an influence on the fetus, since hereditary factors have a tendency to show up in the offspring. In addition to desirable hereditary traits, over 1,200 congenital defects have been catalogued. However, genetic factors do not always appear in a new generation, and environmental influences do not always affect mothers in the same manner. During the thalidomide episode of the 1960s, for example, only 20 percent of the pregnant women who used the drug had deformed babies; the other 80 percent had normal offspring.

While the expectant mother should take all normal precautions and follow her doctor's orders faithfully with regard to diet, hygiene, and exercise, if she and her husband have normal family histories she should not be concerned with congenital birth defects. However, there are cases where there is cause for legitimate worry about the chances of an inherited disorder. If there are cases of *cystic fibrosis, phenylketonuria (PKU), sickle-cell anemia,* or other genetic diseases in the background of either prospective parent; if the prospective mother is over 40 (at which age there is an increased chance of giving birth to a child afflicted with *Down's syndrome* or *Mongolism*), or if the parents or others in the family have previously given birth to a mentally retarded child, then it is recommended that the couple seek the advice of a *genetic counselor.*

Genetic counseling is available through a network of genetic counseling and treatment centers which were set up to help couples who are planning a family but are troubled by the possibility that their children may be born with a genetic disorder. When the wife gets pregnant a prenatal diagnosis is made. This procedure, known as *amniocentesis,* involves obtaining a small sample of the amniotic fluid that surrounds the fetus by inserting a hypodermic needle through the abdominal wall. The sex of the fetus can also be determined by this method, and since many inherited disorders are sex-linked (for example, transmitted only from mother to son), this information can be critically important. If the fetus is found to be affected with the suspected disorder a therapeutic abortion is performed, if so desired by the parents. Those interested in consulting a genetic counselor should write

to the National Genetics Foundation, Inc., 250 West Fifty-Seventh Street, New York, New York 10019.

Miscarriage

About ten percent of all pregnancies end in a *miscarriage,* often called a *spontaneous abortion.* A miscarriage can occur for a variety of reasons, many of which are related. Some of the reasons may be hormone malfunction or deficiency; a faulty sperm or ovum, which would, in the vast majority of cases, result in a cruelly malformed child or one incapable of staying alive if the pregnancy were carried to term; a poor *endometrium,* or lining of the uterus, in which the ovum is implanted; changes in the mother's body chemistry; or other factors that interfere with normal development of the child within the uterus.

Hormone deficiency: Hormone malfunction is responsible for many spontaneous abortions. Once the placenta is established on the inner wall of the uterus, it ordinarily produces sufficient hormones to maintain the pregnancy. But the condition of the endometrium at the time the embryo becomes implanted in the uterine wall affects the later development of the placenta. That situation, in turn, may affect the secretion of the hormones needed to continue the pregnancy. The level of one hormone, called the human chorionic gonadotropic hormone, is frequently used as a barometer of the condition of the uterus. When the amount of that hormone excreted in the urine suddenly decreases, it is a warning signal that spontaneous abortion may be imminent.

Other physiological barometers are thyroid function and the rate of excretion of a substance known as sodium pregnanediol. Normally, there is a rise in thyroid activity when a woman becomes pregnant. The level remains elevated as long as the pregnancy continues, declining when the pregnancy is terminated either by delivery of a child or abortion. The expectant mother who has an underactive or overactive thyroid gland needs special medical attention because the hormone secreted by the gland seems to influence both the ovaries and the pituitary gland. Thyroid dysfunction is associated with infertility and the tendency toward spontaneous abortions.

Hormone deficiencies can contribute to the failure of the ovaries to produce thriving ova. In younger girls, the ovaries may be too immature to yield ova that are capable of continuing life after they are fertilized. In older women, the egg cells may be faulty because of approaching menopause. Even if the egg cell is perfect, defective sperm from the husband may be responsible for failure of the egg cell to develop into a healthy embryo after fertilization.

Still another cause of spontaneous abortion related to unfavorable hormone levels is the infantile or underdeveloped uterus, which may not have the capacity to maintain the fetus as it grows toward normal size for delivery. The undersized uterus can be treated with a hormone, estrin, to make it large enough to sustain a full-term pregnancy.

Fibroid tumors or polyps in the uterus can interfere with both conception and pregnancy. Congenital malformations, such as a divided uterus, may also result in miscarriage. These problems can usually be corrected by surgery. A retroverted, malpositioned or tipped uterus can also be corrected to make carrying to term possible if this situation has caused a spontaneous abortion. An abnormality of the uterus called incompetent cervix used to be the cause of many spontaneous abortions in the last half of pregnancy, but in recent years a simple operation has been devised to correct the defect.

Bleeding and cramps: Spontaneous abortions usually are classified as threatened or inevitable. Generally, an abortion is considered to be of the threatened type when there is bleeding or cramps or both. Even when bleeding and cramps seem to be severe, it is possible that they will stop, or can be stopped, and the pregnancy will continue. If the bleeding and cramps become progressive and there is dilation of the cervix with the passage of tissue, the abortion is considered inevitable. Doctors sometimes can estimate the length of time that a spontaneous abortion has been progressing by examining the blood. If the blood is dark brown rather than bright red, it suggests that bleeding may have started at some time in the past. The longer the bleeding continues, the less chance there is that the fetus will survive.

Ectopic pregnancy: Bleeding and cramping are not always signs of spontaneous abortion. Bleeding may be caused by a polyp or a malignant growth on the cervix. Cramps or bleeding can also occur if there is an *ectopic pregnancy*, a pregnancy outside the uterus. For example, the fertilized egg may become implanted in a Fallopian tube or even in the abdominal cavity instead of in the uterus. Many cases of ectopic pregnancy go undiagnosed because the symptoms are quite similar to those of a threatened abortion. Most ectopic pregnancies end in miscarriage when the pressure of the growing fetus causes the tube to rupture. In rare cases, the fetus may lodge in the abdominal cavity after rupture and continue to grow and develop. Such a fetus can be delivered by Caesarian techniques, but is thought to be extremely dangerous for the mother. Most physicians prefer to perform a therapeutic abortion if this situation occurs.

Habitual abortion: Among some women, spontaneous abortion occurs repeatedly and is known as habitual abortion. Habitual abortion usually threatens at the same stage of each pregnancy, and the measures needed to prevent a repetition of the miscarriage should be started as soon as the expectant mother knows she is pregnant. The usual prenatal care should be followed conscientiously, including the rules about nutrition and exercise. Cigarette smoking should be curtailed or eliminated because, among other reasons, tobacco use seems to affect the carbohydrate metabolism of smokers, and pregnant women are particularly sensitive to changes in carbohydrate balance. The cells which form the placenta and fetal membranes require large amounts of carbohydrates that can be assimilated easily. Even before the fertilized egg cell becomes implanted in the lining of the uterus, the cells of the endometrium demand unusually large quantities of glycogen, or body starch, that has been converted to simple sugar molecules. Other nutrients are also needed, of course, but the demand for them is not as critical as that of carbohydrates.

Induced Abortion

Not all abortions are involuntary. The induced abortion is a deliberate interruption of the development of an embryo or fetus because of therapeutic or nonmedical reasons. Although there are minor variations in the procedure, an induced abortion usually consists of simply removing the embryonic tissue from the lining of the uterus. Such an abortion, usually performed in a hospital or clinic, requires antiseptic conditions. Local anesthetics are used if needed. In the procedure called *dilation and curettage,* or *D and C,* the doctor simply enlarges the opening of the womb to permit entry of the surgical tools used to scrape the lining of the uterus. The tissue is removed from the lining with a pair of tweezers. Some doctors employ a device which pulls the embryonic tissue from inside the uterus by suction. If the abortion is delayed beyond the first three months, more complicated surgery may be required. An alternative method called *salting out* involves the injection of a saline solution into the amniotic fluid. The salt water induces labor, and the fetus is delivered, thus terminating the pregnancy.

If an induced abortion is performed by a doctor in a hospital or clinic equipped with facilities to cope with possible complications—standard procedure in states where induced abortion is legal—the experience should be completely safe and harmless. The notion that women are rendered sterile or more likely to have spontaneous abortions or premature deliveries of wanted children in later years can be true; but this is almost always so only in those cases where women went to illegal abortion mills and had the procedure performed under unsanitary conditions or by someone who was medically incompetent.

Some women do experience psychological upsets or feelings of guilt after having an induced abortion, but these feelings can perhaps be more easily overcome than the problem of bearing an unwanted child.

Approaching Delivery

When all is going well with a pregnancy —and it does in the vast majority of cases— a favorite guessing game becomes the prediction of delivery day. There are several ways in which to estimate the approximate birth date of the new addition to the family. One is to calculate 267 days from the date of conception. Another approach is to count 280 days from the first day of the last menstrual period. This method is easier, since women are more likely to know about the last menstrual period than the last time they ovulated. Still another method commonly used is to count back three months from the first day of the last menstrual period and add seven days. No matter what method is used it will probably be wrong, since surveys show that fewer than five percent of all babies arrive on the day they were expected. However, the majority of babies make the scene within five days of the anticipated date.

As delivery day approaches, the doctor usually wants to make some last-minute studies of the position of the child and its

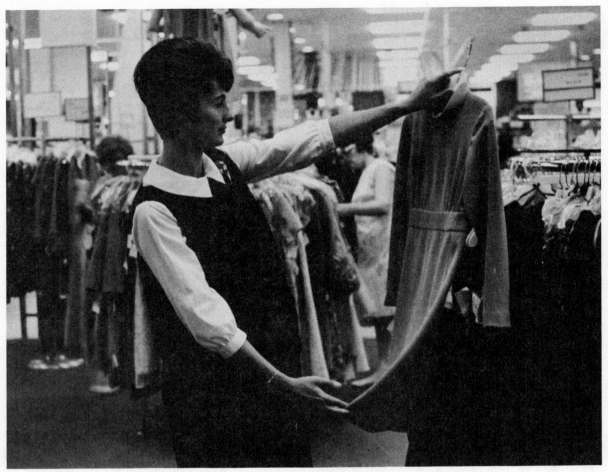

There are many methods used to calculate an approximate delivery date. Perhaps the simplest is to count 280 days from the first day of the last menstrual period.

general condition. He may also want to check the size of the bony areas of the mother's pelvis in an effort to determine in advance whether there will be any complications in delivery. During the examination, the doctor usually looks for varicose veins around the vulva and vagina; they are a common occurrence among pregnant women, and some women claim they can tell when they are pregnant—even before a period is missed—by the appearance of these varicose veins.

By pressing the abdomen with the palms of his hands and his fingers, the doctor can determine the position of the unborn child in the uterus. He also can get a fair idea of the size of the fetus and can tell how low

it is in the pelvic region. The doctor listens to the heartbeat of the fetus and, if labor is near, he may mark the position of the fetus on the skin of the mother's abdomen so that he can tell later if it has moved and in which direction.

In about half of all pregnant women, reddish streaks appear on the skin of the stretched abdomen. The streaks sometimes have the appearance of broken skin fibers due to stretching, but most doctors agree that the streaks are the result of hormone activity. It is another sign of a successful pregnancy.

In the final days before delivery, the doctor usually makes an estimate of the space through which the baby must move to reach the outside world. He also must make a rough guess about the weight of the baby at birth. If the baby weighs less than five pounds at birth it is *premature* by definition and may require special care which the doctor would want to schedule.

Lightening: The phenomenon of *lightening* is a sign that pregnancy is approaching an end and that birth can be expected within about three weeks. When lightening occurs, the mother feels less pressure on the upper part of the abdomen and more dis-

comfort in the pelvic region as the head of the fetus descends toward the birth canal. Lightening may be accompanied by strong contractions of the uterus, which may be mistaken for labor pains. If lightening does not occur during the final weeks, the doctor may conduct further examinations to learn if the delay is due to a large fetus, twins (though a possible multiple birth is usually discovered earlier in the pregnancy), or another reason such as an unfavorable fetal position. When lightening does occur

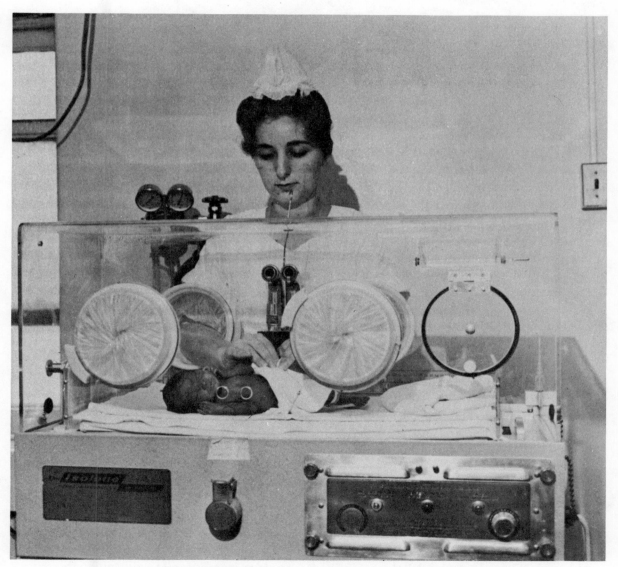

Infants weighing less than five pounds at birth are considered premature and require a specially controlled environment within an incubator to regulate oxygen and reduce the risk of infection.

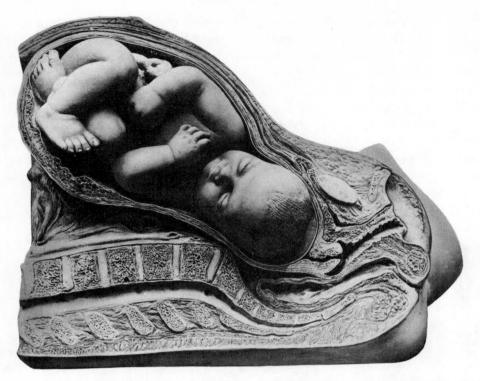

Before the onset of labor, 95 percent of all babies are in the head-downward position. The widest part of the uterus accommodates the baby's feet and bottom; the narrower portion fits its head.

on schedule, the doctor usually assumes that the head of the fetus is low in the pelvic region and can pass through the birth canal without difficulty, since it has already completed the first part of the obstacle course to the outside world.

Fetal position: With X rays and fetal electrocardiograms, it can be determined whether the unborn baby is upside down or in some other position in the uterus. A fetal electrocardiogram is made by placing electrodes on the mother's abdomen while she is lying on an examination table. The electrical impulses of the fetal heart muscle will produce a pattern revealing the direction of the heart which, in turn, tells which way the head is positioned. If the pattern indicates the head is toward the top of the abdomen rather than the bottom, a *breech presentation* can be expected in the delivery room.

Although 95 percent of all babies are in the head-downward position when labor begins, about three percent are in the more difficult breech presentation. Some doctors believe that a breech presentation is more likely if the fetus is delivered before term, since nearly 40 percent of the fetuses are in the breech presentation at the 20th week of pregnancy. However, this percentage declines as delivery day approaches, because the growing fetus finds it more comfortable to move its feet and bottom into the widest part of the pear-shaped uterus while the head fits into the narrow part.

Labor

The contractions of labor pains are something of a mystery. They are independent of the will of the mother. Women who are paralyzed or who feel no labor pains because of severed nerves can have a normal delivery. The uterus may even continue contractions automatically after the uterus has been removed from the body.

The first stage of labor is characterized by regular pains which may occur at intervals of 5 to 15 minutes. During this stage the cervix becomes dilated and forms a passageway into the vagina. There is a rest period between the labor pains which lasts at least a minute and gives the mother a brief respite while permitting the flow of oxygen to the fetus by way of the placenta. (If the uterine contractions were continuous they would cut off the baby's oxygen supply.) During uterine contractions, the uterus rises in the abdomen; the change in shape can be observed at the start and end of each labor pain.

The so-called *bag of waters*, which actually is the *amniotic fluid* within the membrane, may be discharged at almost any time during labor. Sometimes the bag of waters ruptures before the labor pains begin, but this usually occurs during one of the strong contractions. The fluid generally comes out with a gush, but it may also be discharged in small amounts with each contraction. The term dry labor is used to describe contractions that begin after the bag of waters has ruptured. Ordinarily, the contractions become stronger and more frequent and the cervix dilates more rapidly after the amniotic fluid has been discharged.

Occasionally, the baby is delivered with the amniotic membrane still intact about its head. The membrane in such a case is known as a *caul*. At one time, a caul was regarded as a symbol of great superstitious value; midwives sold cauls to sailors who carried them for good luck on voyages.

Labor—Stage Two

Rupture of the bag of waters frequently climaxes the first stage of labor, which may last over 12 hours if it is the first pregnancy. The second stage of labor is considerably shorter and can be expected to last around 2 hours in a first pregnancy, 30 minutes for a woman who had children previously. The second stage may begin with rupture of the bag of waters if the amniotic fluid was not released earlier. The contractions are more intense and frequent, occurring at intervals of 2 to 3 minutes rather than the 5- to 15-minute intervals of the first stage. There also

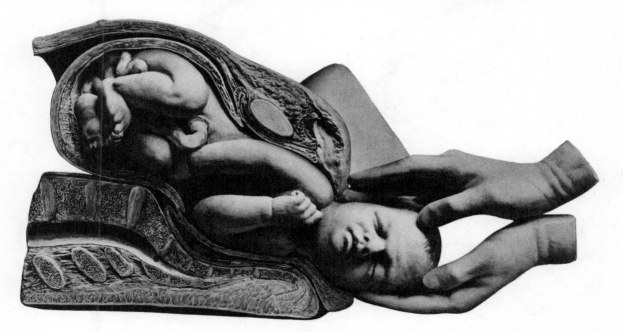

In a normal delivery, the baby's head is turned sideways and is often slightly elongated for easier passage through the birth canal. The right shoulder and upper torso rotate to take up less room.

is a consciousness on the part of the mother to help expel the fetus. She may feel additional pains, pressures, or irritations because of the presence of the fetus in the lower pelvic area.

During this series of labor pains the baby gradually makes its appearance outside the mother's womb. At first a bit of the scalp shows, then recedes as the labor pain subsides. With the next labor pain more of the head appears. Finally, the entire head is outside the mother's body, followed by the shoulders, trunk, and lower extremities.

Anesthetics and Drugs

Although it is standard practice to refer to the uterine contractions as labor pains, the amount of actual pain varies, and there are numerous methods for reducing the pain. True painless labor is rare, and when it occurs it is sometimes attributed to an abnormality of the nervous system.

The doctor is as concerned about the welfare of the mother and baby as the mother herself, and this concern is reflected in the approach taken to provide relief from labor pains. The drug or anesthetic the doctor chooses to use will be one that gives optimum relief to the mother without creating an environment in the womb that would threaten the life of the baby. A number of rather common drugs that could be used to relieve pain without harm to the mother could very easily be fatal to the infant, who would share through the placenta substances injected into the mother's bloodstream.

The type of anesthetic or drug administered to the mother is usually one that affects only the part of the nervous system associated with pain. If the substance also affected the motor nerves, the delivery would become stalemated. On the other hand, it would be very simple to handle the

BABY SQUEEZING THROUGH BIRTH CANAL

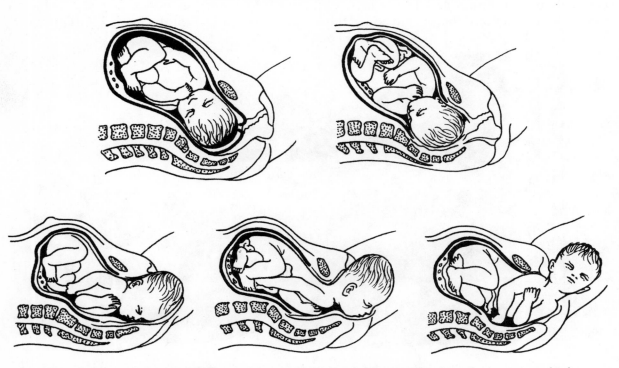

This sequence of drawings illustrates how a baby's head must squeeze through the narrow birth canal. Usually there is little danger of deformity, for the skull has not yet calcified, i.e., it is still soft.

childbirth in a satisfactory manner as far as the baby is concerned if the mother were given no relief from pain.

Drugs used as aids in childbirth include analgesics, tranquilizers, barbiturates, and the type of drugs used in so-called twilight sleep—scopolamine and morphine. They can be given orally or by injection. In nearly all cases the drugs are used with caution, and they are frequently administered in combination with a gas anesthetic.

The gases frequently used during delivery are nitrous oxide, which provides intermittent relief from pain during the second stage of labor, and cyclopropane, which may be administered for Caesarian section or cases of delivery in which there are complications requiring unconsciousness or deep analgesia (incapacity to feel pain). Nitrous oxide sometimes is provided during labor pains on signal from the mother. When she wants relief for a few moments or when she feels a pain starting, the mother signals the anesthetist, who places the mask over her face so she can take a few deep whiffs. The procedure is repeated when the next labor pain begins. Nitrous oxide may also be used in conjunction with ether or one of the other standard anesthetic gases. When properly administered, ether is safe and reliable for producing deep anesthesia or relaxation.

Still another anesthetic commonly used during delivery is a drug injected either for local anesthesia or for putting the mother to sleep for the period of delivery. Sodium pentothal is injected intravenously in many cases, particularly when forceps are used to assist in delivery. However, the doctor has to work fast in these cases, because this is one of the drugs that can be transmitted through the placenta in a short time.

A caudal anesthetic can be used to block pain in the entire pelvic area. In this case, a drug is injected into the area at the bottom of the spinal column. Most women who have had caudal anesthesia like it as a

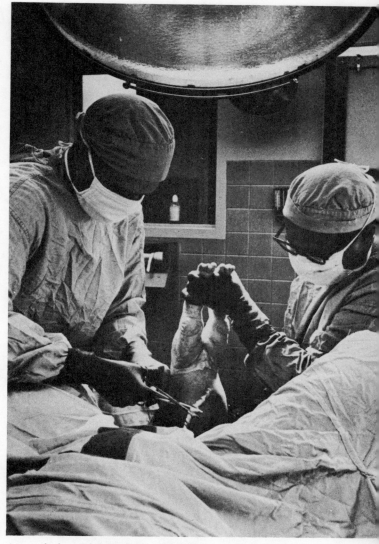

A new baby girl enters the world and is held upside-down as the attending surgeon cuts the umbilical cord.

means of obtaining relief from labor pains, but it requires the presence of specially trained personnel.

When delivery can be timed rather precisely, a spinal anesthetic, sometimes called a *saddle block,* is injected into the spinal cord in the lumbar area while the mother is in a sitting position. After the injection, the mother lies on her back and, in most cases, is free of pain for the remainder of labor and delivery.

Natural childbirth: Natural childbirth methods are preferred by some women who

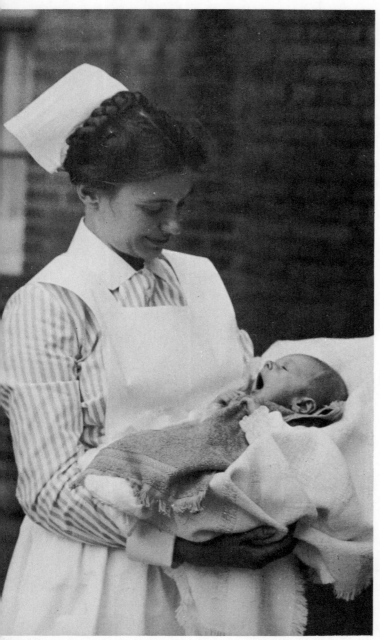

Babies who are picked up at regular intervals appear to develop faster than babies who are undisturbed.

episiotomy incision, to make the vaginal area large enough for passage of the baby, drugs to relieve tension when requested, and *oxytocin*. Oxytocin is a hormone naturally secreted by the pituitary gland to help the muscles of the uterus contract normally.

A woman who chooses the natural childbirth technique developed by Dr. Ferdinand Lamaze conditions herself for labor pains by substituting a different response. Instead of crying out, for example, her response is a pattern of rapid, shallow breathing which she begins at the first sign of a uterine contraction. The conditioning exercises take about 30 minutes a day and should be started two months before the expected delivery date. Although some women who start natural childbirth training lessons are not able to complete the course for various reasons, most agree that they were better prepared for labor because of what they learned about the control of muscles and breathing.

Hypnosis sometimes is used instead of drugs or anesthetics for childbirth. But only a minority of women are able to accept the long period of training for the effective deep trance required, some applicants are not susceptible to hypnosis, and few obstetricians are adequately trained to control the hypnotic situation during delivery. Many doctors feel that the type of woman who would be a good subject for child delivery while hynotized would get along just as well with the natural childbirth method.

Caesarian section: A Caesarian section may be performed in cases of diabetic mothers with rapidly growing fetuses, when delivery is complicated by breech or shoulder presentation, if the uterus is weak due to previous surgery or other reasons, or when the mother has a history of losing the child after carrying it to the time of delivery. There are several variations in Caesarian techniques, some requiring a general anesthetic and others using local anesthetics and other medications. But all ap-

want to participate as consciously as possible in the act of bringing a child into the world. Others, by contrast, want to go into the delivery room completely anesthetized —to enter a pregnant woman and awaken as a mother. In natural childbirth, most women receive a local anesthetic for the proaches are directed toward the same goal of saving the lives of both mother and baby. In nearly all instances, the uterus is closed after the baby and placental material are removed. Only in extremely rare cases is it necessary to remove the uterus. Most mothers who have Caesarians can have more children in the future if they so desire.

Labor—Stage Three

After the baby is delivered through the normal birth canal, the placenta is expelled by the same route. This is called the third, or placental, stage of labor. The placenta, also known as the *afterbirth,* is connected to the baby by the umbilical cord. The cord is not cut until the blood has drained from the placenta into the baby's body; to help the flow the placenta is held above the level of the baby to get an assist from gravity.

Before the infant leaves the delivery room, it is examined for a normal heart beat, possible abdominal distention or evidence of fluid in the abdominal region, possible abnormalities of the ears, and possible deformities of the mouth area, such as cleft palate or lip. The health of newborn babies is scored by the *Apgar system* when the baby is 60 seconds old. Five items of physical condition are noted and scored on a scale of 0 to 2. They are heart rate, muscle tone, respiration, nerve reflexes, and skin color. Babies that score 8 to 10 points are considered in excellent condition and are given routine postnatal care. If they score 7 points or less, additional measures are taken to get the infants off to a normal start in life. Since the system was started, nearly three-fourths of all newborn babies tested have passed with 8 points or more.

Breast and Bottle Feeding

Whether the infant is to be breast fed or bottle fed is usually a personal matter to be decided by the new mother. For the average healthy baby, there are no obstacles to breast feeding if the mother desires it and is able to produce and deliver milk. A few women are unable to produce a sufficient supply of milk and must supplement their output with bottle feedings. In a few cases, babies are allergic to mother's milk, but in such instances the allergen can be identified and removed from the mother's diet.

Feeding problems are sometimes fewer and less serious among breast-fed babies. The mother's milk contains most of the necessary nutrients and is available when needed at the proper temperature. It also is more likely to be fresh and free of infectious bacteria than bottled milk.

The mother's milk during the first few days after birth is yellowish in color and

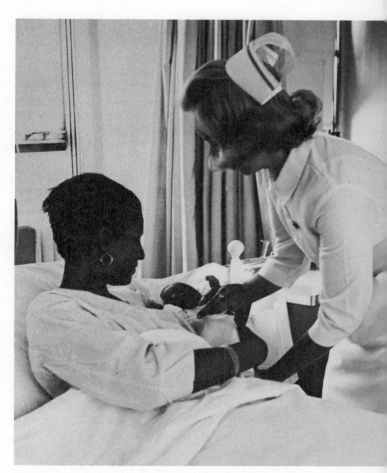

Few satisfactions equal that of a mother with her newborn. The long wait and ordeal of labor are over, and at last she can turn her attention to the baby.

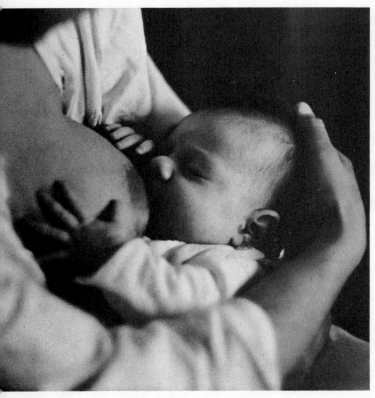

During the first few days after delivery, mother's milk (called at this stage colostrum) is yellowish in color and very rich in proteins and minerals. It is gradually changed into regular milk in the first four weeks.

rich in proteins and minerals. It is called *colostrum,* and is replaced gradually by regular human milk by the fourth week. Mother's milk is low in iron and may lack vitamins C and D. However, the baby arrives in the world with enough stores of iron in its tissues to last through the first few months of life. Compared to cow's milk, human milk is richer in carbohydrates, but cow's milk has a greater proportion of proteins and minerals. The vitamin content of both mother's milk and cow's milk varies with the vitamin intake of each.

Mother's milk generally is more easily digestible in the baby's stomach than cow's milk, since the curd of mother's milk is fine and more rapidly metabolized. On the other hand, mothers who breast-feed sometimes suffer from fissuring or cracking of the nipples, *mastitis* (breast inflammation), or diseases which require temporary or permanent discontinuance of breast feeding.

Surveys indicate that more than three-fourths of babies today are bottle fed. Many mothers avoid breast feeding because they feel it is socially unacceptable, that it interferes with employment or social life, that it will affect their physical attractiveness, or because of fear of failure. For mothers who select bottle feeding over breast feeding, the procedure is much simpler today than in previous years. Many of the differences in nutritional values of mother's milk and cow's milk have been reduced or eliminated by improved formula development. Equipment for preparing the bottled meals is superior to that used in previous generations. And there is less danger today of bacterial infection from cow's milk because of improved dairy sanitation methods. New mothers who choose not to breast-feed are usually given hormones, along with ice packs and analgesics, to relieve any breast discomfort that may appear during the first few days.

If the mother wants to breast-feed the baby, plans should be made in advance of delivery. The first feeding can be started as soon after delivery as is feasible for both mother and child, usually within hours after birth. Although the first breast feeding can be delayed for several days, because of the stimulation of milk secretion immediately after delivery, the first ten days to two weeks are crucial in the establishment of a breast feeding program. The sucking reflex of the baby at the mother's breast triggers release of the hormone oxytocin, which in turn influences the release of another substance of the pituitary gland, prolactin, needed for the production of milk in the mother's breast. See also *Birth, Infancy, and Maturation,* especially pp. 102–104. For a discussion of the emotional aspects of the beginning of a family, see *Marriage and Parenthood,* p. 246.   KNA

KEEPING FIT:
THE MIDDLE YEARS

Physical Changes

Physically, middle age should be a pleasant plateau—a time to look back on a vigorous youth, enjoy an active present, and prepare for a ripe old age.

Middle age should not be measured by chronological age but by biological age, the condition of various parts of the body. You might say that the middle-aged body is like a car that has been driven a certain number of miles. It should be well broken in and running smoothly, but with plenty of reserve power for emergencies, and lots of mileage left.

Biological age should be measured by the state of the heart, arteries and other essential organs, the length of life and comparative health of parents and grandparents, temperament and outlook on life, and outward appearance. The way you have fed or treated yourself is important. Eating the

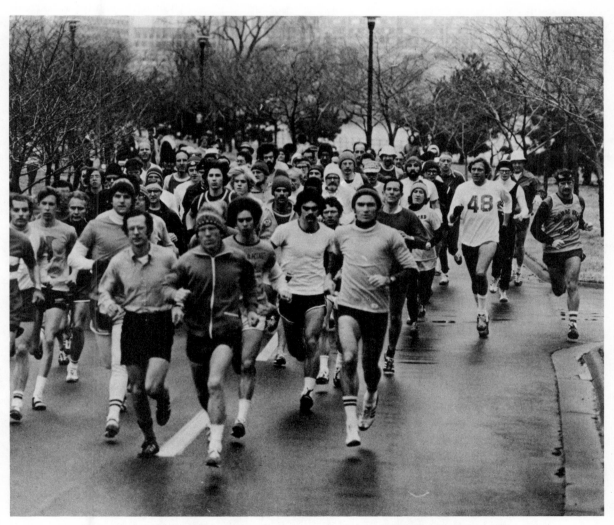

Many people in recent years have discovered the health benefits of running and jogging, sports that can be enjoyed from youth through the later years.

wrong kinds of food, being overweight, smoking too much, or worrying too much can add years to biological age.

However, no one should be surprised if he is not in quite the shape he was when he was 25 to 30 years old. At age 40 to 50 it is perfectly normal to have only 80 percent of the maximum breathing capacity, 85 percent of the resting cardiac output, 95 percent of the total body water, and 96 percent of the basal metabolic rate. These factors, however, should not slow anyone down very much.

There is one difference though, that can be anticipated in middle age. Reaction time and decision-making processes may be a bit slower. This is because the nervous system is one of the most vulnerable to aging. The cells of the central nervous system begin to die early in life and are not replaced, while other organs are still growing and producing new cells. Specific response to input is delayed because it takes a greater length of time for an impulse to travel across the connections linking nerve fibers.

Thus, though you may function as usual under normal conditions, you may find it a little harder to respond to physical or emotional stress. However, if you have followed a sound health maintenance program, including good nutrition, enough mental and physical exercise and rest, and moderate living habits, you should respond to unusual physiological or emotional stress quite adequately.

The Importance of Checkups

Physical disabilities associated with chronic disease increase sharply with age, starting with the middle years. While more than half (54 percent) of the 86 million persons who have one or more chronic conditions are under age 45, the prevalence of disability from illness is greatest in the 45 and older age group. Of those under 45 who have chronic conditions, only 14 percent are limited in activity as compared with almost 30 percent of the 45 to 64 age group. And only 1 percent of those under 45 with chronic illness are completely disabled, as compared with 4 percent in the 45 to 64 age group.

These figures suggest that it is wise to have an annual checkup so that any disease process or condition can be nipped in the bud. Further evidence of the value of medical checkups comes from the Aetna Life Insurance Company, which compared two groups of policyholders over a five-year period. Those who did not have checkups and health counseling had a death rate 44 percent higher than the group who did. Regular checkups will not only help prolong life, they will also help you to live it more comfortably.

Here are some other good reasons for having a physical checkup:

• If an organ has been attacked by serious disease in youth, it may deteriorate at an early adult age.

• Heredity may play an important role in determining the speed at which various organs age. If your parents and grandparents had arteriosclerosis, there is a chance you might develop this condition in your middle years.

• Your environment (smog, poor climate, etc.) might affect the rate at which your body ages, particularly the skin.

• Individual stresses and strains, or abuses or overuse (of alcohol, for example) may create a health problem in middle age.

• The endocrine glands (pituitary, thyroid, parathyroids, adrenals, ovaries, testicles) play important roles in aging. Serious disease of one or more of these glands may lead to premature aging of an organ dependent upon its secretions.

• At middle age you are more likely to be beset by emotional strains at work or at home that could make you an early candidate for heart disease, arteriosclerosis, and other degenerative disorders.

• The earlier a chronic disease is detected, the better the chance that it can be arrested before permanent damage is done. This is especially true in the case of glaucoma, diabetes, heart disease, lung cancer and other cancers—all of which could have their onset in middle age.

To help detect disease and other debilitating conditions, many physicians utilize automated medical screening, which combines medical history with selected physiological measurements and laboratory tests to give the doctor a complete health profile of the patient. This profile should indicate the probability of any chronic condition, which the physician could then pinpoint with more thorough tests.

Also, annual checkups enable the doctor to observe changes taking place over a period of time. For example, he is able to observe gradually changing blood chemistry levels or a progressive increase in eye pressure that could signal the onset of disease.

Don't Try To Be Your Own Doctor

A panel of medical specialists from the University of California at Los Angeles recently found that many men of 40 years and older were dosing themselves with unnecessary pills and "conserving" their energy by increasing bed rest to the point that it actually became enervating.

These doctors point out that increasing dependence on pills can be harmful as well as expensive. Laxatives are a good example of a popular commercial medicine taken unnecessarily by large numbers of people. Perhaps only one person in 100,000 may have an actual motor disability of the bowels, and most constipation can be easily corrected through proper foods and exercise, without resorting to laxatives. Also, taking vitamin pills or avoiding high-cholesterol foods is unnecessary—unless recommended by a physician.

But, most important, "conserving" energy through prolonged bed rest or avoiding ex-

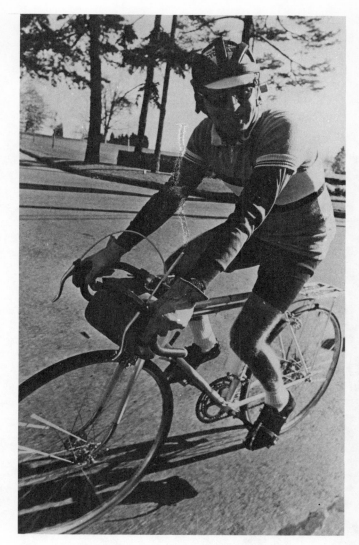

Regular exercise over age 40 can improve chances of survival while preserving a youthful, fit appearance.

ercise can be fatal. The panel members pointed out that before age 40, a man exercises to improve his performance, but that after age 40 he exercises to improve his chance of survival.

Physical Fitness and Exercise

In middle age most of us drop exercise that we must do, and do only those forms of exercise we enjoy doing. In other words, we find it easier to bend an elbow than lift weights. This is unfortunate, because in

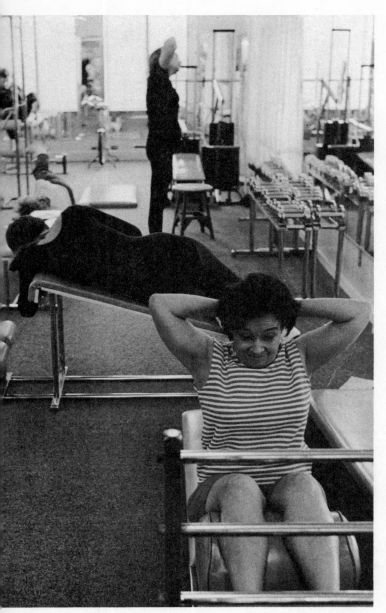

It's not easy, but this kind of continued effort will in time improve the function of the body's systems.

required to move blood to active regions of the body through exercise or movement, the more efficient they become. Protracted exercise also improves the work of the lungs by increasing their ability to expand more fully, take in more air, and utilize a greater proportion of the oxygen in the inhaled air.

While exercise alone cannot eliminate obesity, it can help prevent it by improving digestion and bowel movements and by burning up excess calories. Exercise can also make you feel, look, and think better. Some traditional formal exercises, however, like touching the toes while keeping your knees stiff, or doing deep knee bends, are potentially harmful in middle age; they put too much stress on weak parts of the back and legs.

Despite protests about not having enough time, everyone has time to exercise, particularly if it is worked into the daily routine—for example, walking instead of riding to the train, office, store, or bus stop. You might find you'll get there faster, especially in traffic-clogged metropolitan areas, and you'll save money as well. More important, those minutes of "stolen" exercise accrue over the years in the form of improved health.

Sports and Games

If you don't like formal exercise, you can get exercise informally—through a favorite sport, whether it be golf, tennis, swimming, jogging, skiing, cycling, or whatever. Many sports and games are stop and go activities that do not provide helpful, rhythmic exercise, but here's how you can make them more beneficial.

Golf: Instead of riding in a golf cart between shots, walk—in fact, stride vigorously, lifting your head and chest. And don't make golf a cut-throat competition or business pursuit. Relax and enjoy it—count your blessings rather than your bogeys.

Tennis: Like golf, tennis can be a cut-throat competitive sport or a pleasant pursuit. If it's played with muscles tied in knots

middle age most of us need regular exercise to maintain both mental and physical fitness and to increase endurance, strength, and agility.

As noted earlier, in middle age there is some decrease in breathing capacity, cardiac output, and metabolic rate; yet exercise can improve these functions. The more often the normal heart and circulatory system are

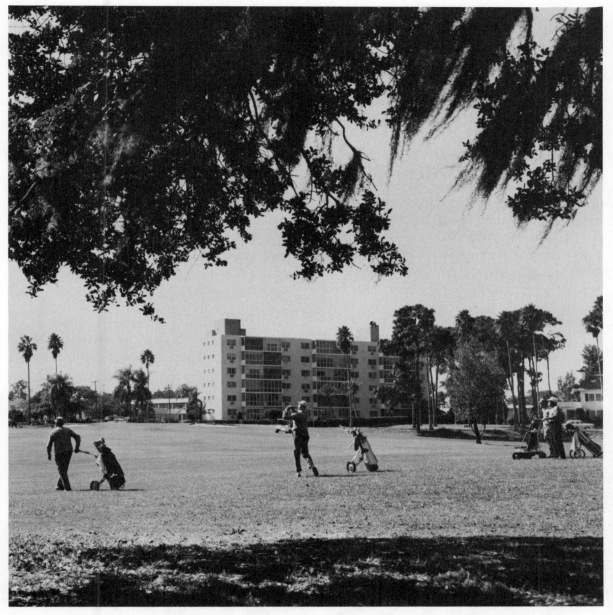

Although the stop and go nature of golf does not provide the kind of rhythmic activity that is most desirable in exercise, the game can be made more beneficial by striding vigorously between shots.

from nervous tension, it will not provide any fun or healthful exercise. Also, players over 30 are well-advised to play more doubles than singles, and to avoid exhausting themselves in the heat of competition.

Swimming: Along with fast walking and jogging, swimming is one of the best all-around exercises. When swimming, most of the muscles are exercised and lung capacity and cardiac output are improved. The exercise potential can be increased by doing pull-ups with the diving board or ladder and by bobbing up and down in the water.

Jogging: This popular sport can be combined with walking, done in a group or alone, either outdoors or indoors, and alternated with other exercises. Moreover, it doesn't require any special equipment and has been recognized by fitness experts as one of the best exercises for the heart and circulation. However, it is wise to get your doctor's advice and approval before embarking on a jogging program.

Skiing: Skiing is healthful as well as fun. You can get in shape for skiing and improve your ability by jogging and by practicing some of the techniques needed in skiing—such as the rhythmic left-right-left-right twist of foot, knee, and leg in short turns. To do this exercise, stand up straight with your feet quite close together and flex your knees forward so that the weight goes onto the balls of the feet. Now, arms apart for balance, twist your feet and knees to the left without twisting your upper body. As you do this, try the modified half-bends of the traversing position that all ski schools teach. Then reverse the position to the right, and keep repeating.

Other sports: Other worthwhile sports for healthful exercise include badminton, bicycling, canoeing, rowing, table tennis, skating, and squash. However, they should be sustained for at least 30 minutes at a time, and ideally four times a week, and should be combined with supplemental exercises.

A word of warning: Everyone should beware of becoming a weekend athlete and punishing himself with an overdose of exercise or sports only on weekends. It makes as much sense as stuffing yourself on weekends and starving the rest of the week. It's far more sensible—and healthful—to engage in sports activities for an hour or so at a time on a daily basis.

Exercises

Participating in sports activities is not the only way to keep fit. Special exercises can

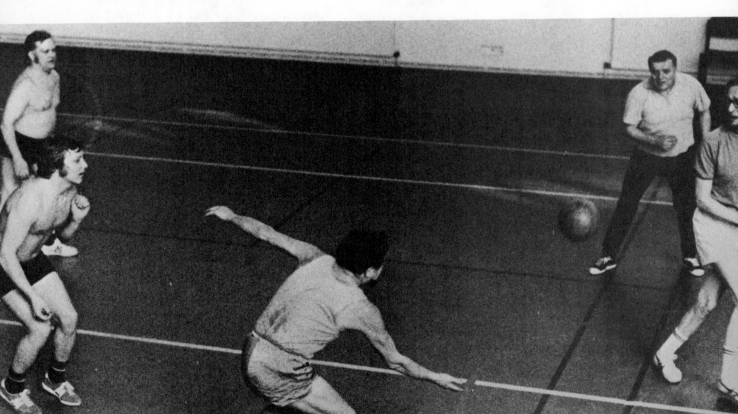

A brisk game of volleyball can help dispel the tensions that accumulate during the working day.

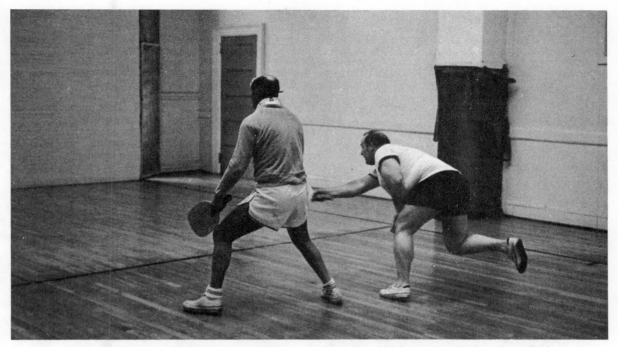

Paddle ball is just one of many sports that can provide healthful exercise if played regularly.

help reduce tension and build muscles. For instance, one way to relax is to do rhythmic exercises, particularly for the trunk, that help to improve circulation. You can also try exercises that will relieve tense muscles and improve breathing. The exercises described below were developed by Dr. Josephine L. Rathbone of Columbia University.

Breathing to relax: Lie on your back on the floor with knees bent and feet resting on the floor. Take a deep breath, letting both the abdominal wall and chest rise. Hold the air for a few seconds, then expel it through your mouth with a gasp. Repeat four or five times at regular intervals.

For tense arms: Standing erectly, swing both arms forward, then to the side, letting them drop during the swings so that your hands brush your thighs with each motion. Keep your shoulders low. Repeat a few times. Then, sit on the edge of a chair and clench one hand tightly. Swing your arm vigorously in large circles, keeping your hand clenched. Then repeat with other arm.

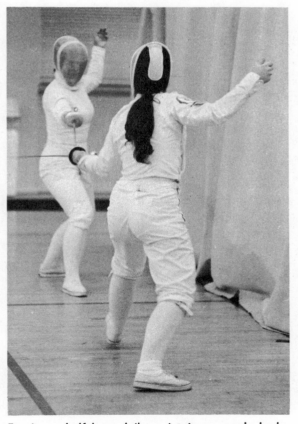

Fencing a half hour daily maintains a supple body.

For tense legs: Sit on the edge of a table with lower legs hanging free. Then, alternately, swing them backward and forward. Try to keep your legs moving in rhythm.

For stomach tension: Kneel with your feet under your hips and swing your trunk down to one side and around, sweeping your arms in a wide circle, coming up again on the opposite side. Or stand with your hips supported against the wall, feet apart and a few inches from the wall. Bend your body forward, arms drooping, and let your body sway from side to side, with your arms and head loose.

Relaxing at work or home: Relieve tension while sitting by holding the spine erect, shoulders low. Turn your head so that the chin touches first one collarbone, then the other. Move slowly and rhythmically.

Yoga: You can also relax and become revitalized through various Yoga exercises. Courses are taught at many recreational centers. Some of the exercises require only a minimum of time, and can be done not only before and after the workday but in the office during the lunch hour.

Isometrics: Isometric exercises—pitting one muscle against another without moving —can also be practiced at odd moments. These exercises should, however, be done only by healthy persons, and not by anyone with a cardiac problem. To strengthen arm

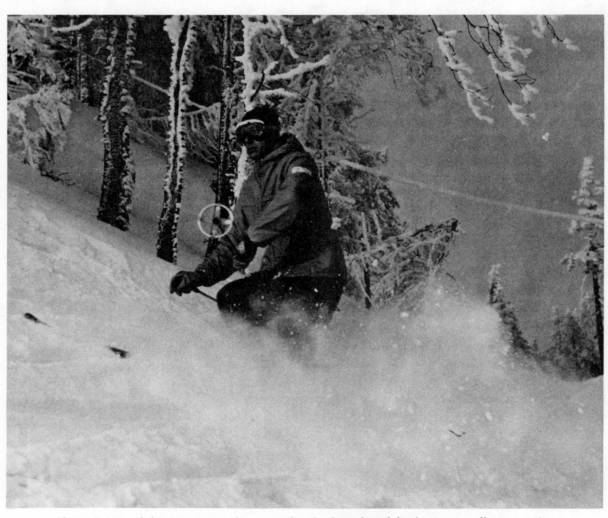

Skiing is an exhilarating sport that provides the benefits of fresh air as well as exercise.

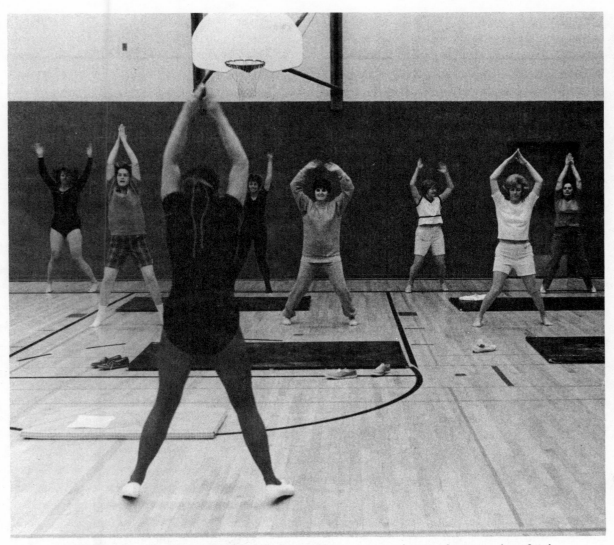

Calisthenics may lack the competitive challenge of group sports, but can be just as beneficial. A good leader who knows how to pace the class is important—so is regular attendance.

and shoulder muscles through isometrics, put the fist of one hand against the palm of the other and push without moving. Or push up with your arms from a chair or the edge of a table. Strengthen arm and neck muscles by grasping the back of the neck with laced fingers and pulling forward—again, without movement.

All of the above exercises and sports can put you on the road to physical fitness. Just remember, whatever form of exercise or sport you choose, make it fun and do not strain yourself unduly.

Care of the Feet

"My feet are killing me!" is a complaint heard more frequently in middle age, especially from women. The devil in this case usually takes the shape of fashionable shoes, where the foot is frequently squeezed into shapes and positions it was never designed to tolerate. Particularly unhealthy for the foot was the formerly fashionable spike heel and pointed toe.

Any heel two inches or higher will force the full weight of the body onto the smaller

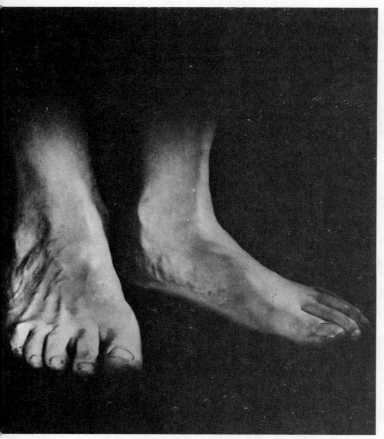

Weak arches are the source of much pain and discomfort in the foot. Orthopedic shoes with arch supports can provide considerable relief.

give the muscles in the back of the legs a chance to return to their normal position. It's highly desirable to wear different shoes each day, or at least alternate two pairs. This gives the shoes a chance to dry out completely. Dust shoes with a mild powder when removed.

Shoes should not be bought in the morning. They should be tried on near the end of the day, when the feet have broadened from standing and walking and tightness or rubbing can be more easily detected.

As to hosiery, socks and stockings should extend a half-inch beyond the longest toe. Stretch socks are fine in many cases, but plain wool or cotton socks help if your feet perspire a lot.

Foot Exercises

Exercise your feet by trying these simple steps recommended by leading podiatrists:

• Extend the toes and flex rapidly for a minute or two. Rotate the feet in circles at the ankles. Try picking up a marble or pencil with your toes; this will give them agility and strength.

• Stand on a book with your toes extended over the edge. Then curl your toes down as far as possible, grasping the cover.

• After an unusually active day, refresh the feet with an alcohol rub. Follow this with a foot massage, squeezing the feet between your hands. When you are tired, rest with your feet up. Try lying down for about a half-hour with your feet higher than your head, using pillows to prop up your legs.

• Walk barefoot on uneven sandy beaches and thick grass. This limbers up the feet and makes the toes work. Walking anywhere is one of the best exercises for the feet if you learn to walk properly and cultivate good posture. Keep toes pointed ahead, and lift rather than push the foot, letting it come down flat on the ground, placing little weight on the heel. Your toes will come alive, and your feet will become more active.

bones in the front of the foot and squeeze the toes into the forepart of the shoe. This hurts the arch, causes calluses on the sole of the foot, and can lead to various bone deformities.

The major solution to this problem is to buy good shoes that really fit. The shoes should be moderately broad across the instep, have a straight inner border, and a moderately low heel. To fit properly, shoes should extend one-half inch to three-fourths inch beyond the longest toe.

Avoid wearing shoes that have no support; also, avoid wearing high heels for long periods of time. Extremely high heels worn constantly force the foot forward and upset body balance. Changing heel height several times a day will rest the feet and

Foot Ailments

Doing foot exercises is particularly important in middle age, because the foot is especially vulnerable to the following problems:

Bunions: A bunion is a thickening and swelling of the big joint of the big toe, forcing it toward the other toes. There is also a protuberance on the inner side of the foot. Unless treated, this condition usually gets progressively worse. Surgery is not always necessary or successful. Often, special shoes to fit the deformed foot must be worn.

Stiff Toe: People suffering from this problem find that the big joint of the big toe becomes painful and stiff, possibly due to a major accident or repeated minor trauma. This condition usually corrects itself if the joint is protected for a few weeks, usually by a small steel plate within the sole of the shoe.

Hammer toe: This clawlike deformity is usually caused by cramping the toes with too small shoes. The pressure can be eased with padding and, in some cases, the deformity can be corrected by surgery.

Ingrown toenail: Cutting the nail short and wearing shoes that are too tight are major causes of ingrown toenails; the edge of the nail of the toe—usually the big toe—is forced into the soft outer tissues. In some cases the tissues can be peeled back after soaking the foot in hot water, and the offending part of the nail can be removed. To prevent ingrown toenails, the nails should be kept carefully trimmed and cut straight across the nail rather than trimmed into curves at the corners. For severe or chronic cases of ingrown toenails it is best to seek professional treatment.   PAD

Care of the Teeth

Neglect of oral hygiene and the forgoing of dental checkups are commonplace in the middle years. An often-heard excuse is that the eventual loss of teeth is inevitable. Years ago, loss of teeth really was unavoidable. Today, however, thanks to modern dental practices, it is possible for nearly everyone to enjoy the benefits of natural teeth for a lifetime.

Restorations and Fillings

Although *periodontal* (gum) disease and cavities continue to threaten oral health, two other problems may assume prominence in the middle years—replacing worn-out restorations, or fillings, and replacing missing teeth.

No filling material will last forever. The whitish restorations in front teeth eventually wear away. Silver restorations tend to crack and chip with age because they contract and expand slightly when cold or hot foods and drinks come into contact with them. Even cast gold restorations, the most permanent kind, are subject to new decay around the edges which may spread underneath.

If a needed restoration is not made or a worn-out restoration is not replaced, a deep cavity may result. When the decay—properly called *caries*—reaches the inner layer of the tooth, the *dentin*, temporary warning

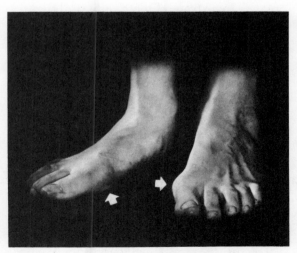

Bunions, caused by tight-fitting shoes, arthritis, or imbalance in foot muscles, are difficult to relieve and painful. Sometimes special shoes can be helpful.

twinges of pain may occur. If the tooth still is not restored, the decay will spread into the *pulp*, the tissue that fills the inner canal of the tooth. A toothache results because the pus and gas formed by the decaying pulp produce pressure against the rigid walls of the tooth socket. Although the pain may subside, the pulp dies, or is no longer vital, and an abscess forms at its root.

Root canal treatment: An abscessed tooth does not always require extraction; it can often be saved by root canal treatment. The dead pulp is removed and the canal is filled with special materials. Since the dentist or *endodontist* (a specialist in root canal treatment) must take elaborate precautions to remove all bacteria from the canal prior to filling it, a number of appointments are generally required. However, saving a tooth this way is less costly than having it extracted and replaced.

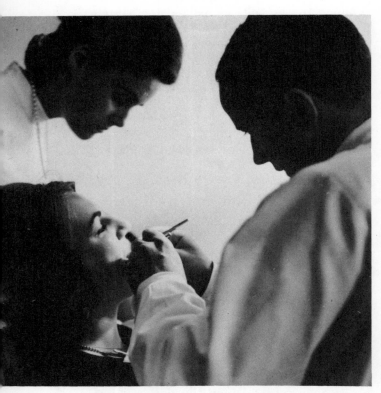

The best way to preserve natural teeth is to follow a program of regular checkups combined with careful oral hygiene and a sensible, varied, nutritious diet.

Replacement Teeth and Dentures

Lost teeth, even one lost tooth, should be replaced. Most people want missing front teeth replaced, but many are unconcerned about replacing lost back teeth if they do not show. Appearance, though a major reason why teeth are replaced, is not the most important reason.

Each tooth functions to hold the ones next to it and opposite to it in place. If a tooth is lost, the others shift because there is no counterforce to keep them in place. Food then packs in the improper spaces created by shifting teeth, plaque forms, and irritation of the gums results. If the irritation is not removed, periodontal disease causes the loss of more teeth. The loss of additional teeth may take years if the teeth move slowly, but can happen within a few years if they tilt and shift rapidly into the empty space.

Bridges and partial dentures: Several different types of dental appliances are constructed to fill empty spaces. A bridge, usually gold, is used to replace teeth if there is a sound tooth on each side of the space. The bridge is cemented into place and is brushed like a natural tooth.

If there are no teeth behind the space created by extracted teeth, a partial denture is used to replace the missing teeth. This appliance fastens by a clasp onto the last tooth on each side of the mouth, and often has a bar on the inside of the front teeth for stability. The partial denture is removed for cleaning with a special brush, usually cone-shaped to fit into the clasp and its little prongs. It should be cleaned whenever natural teeth are brushed. In addition, the dentist should periodically check it to see whether the clasp is loose. A loose clasp may rock the teeth to which it is attached, causing their loss.

The bridge and partial denture prevent further deterioration of the mouth if they are kept clean and in good condition. DJC

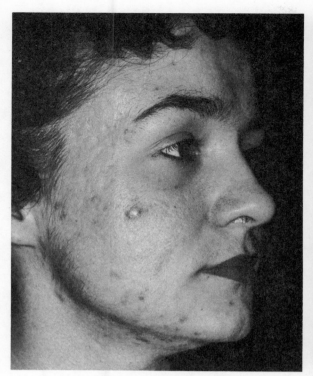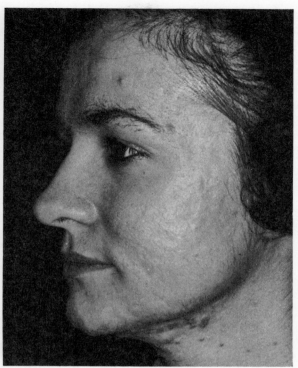

Before and after treatment by dermabrasion, or skin planing, used here to improve appearance of an acne patient; the technique can be helpful in minimizing middle-age wrinkles.

Problems of Aging

When the human body reaches middle age, a number of problems and conditions which are the result of advancing years begin to make themselves felt. These include wrinkling of the skin, baldness, varicose veins, menopause and the male climacteric, and the body's decreased ability to deal with nicotine, caffeine, alcohol, and excess calories.

Skin

The skin usually starts to show its age in the mid to late 30s. At that time it starts to lose its elasticity and flexibility, and becomes somewhat thinner. Little lines—not yet wrinkles—start to show up, usually crow's feet around the eyes.

Wrinkling takes place at different times with different people, and sometimes in different areas of the skin. Heredity may play a part. For instance, one family may have the trait of wrinkling around the mouth rather than the eyes. In another family, wrinkling or crow's feet may start early and then stop.

Treatment for wrinkles: While wrinkles do not hurt, many people want to do something about them. Experienced physicians and dermatologists have a number of techniques for removing or minimizing wrinkles. One accepted method is *dermabrasion,* or planing of the skin. The doctor sprays on a local anesthetic, then scrapes the skin with a motor-driven wire brush or some other abrasive tool. The treatment usually takes one session, and no hospital stay is required. There will be some swelling and scab formation, but this should clear up in a week to ten days.

Another method is called *cryotherapy,* in which the doctor freezes the skin with carbon dioxide. This induces peeling, which improves the appearance of flat acne scars and shallow wrinkles.

Still another procedure involves the application of chemicals, which are neutralized when they have obtained the desired action.

Skin texture change: Besides wrinkling, the skin has a tendency in some people to become thinner, leathery, and darkened as they move towards the 40s and 50s. This effect can be minimized if the skin is toned up with cold cream and other emollients that provide the moisture and oil the skin needs. Also, overexposure to the sun—one of the prime agers of the skin—should be avoided.

In fact, most doctors feel that the sun is a lethal agent, and that exposing the face to too much sun is like putting it in a hot oven. Many say that the sun destroys some inherent good qualities of facial skin, and ruins any chance of improving the appearance through cosmetic surgery.

Cosmetic Surgery

Cosmetic surgery for both men and women is becoming increasingly popular and sophisticated. Cosmetic surgery procedures include *rhinoplasty* (nose); *facial plasty* or *rhytidoplasty* (face lift); *blepharoplasty* (upper eyelids and bags under the eyes); breast augmentation and reduction; as well as the dermabrasion and other methods mentioned earlier. See *Plastic and Cosmetic Surgery*, p. 402.

Baldness

While cosmetic surgery for men is relatively new, the problem of baldness has its roots in ancient history. Men were worried about baldness 4,000 years ago—and they were just about as successful as we are today in finding a cure. Dr. Eugene Van Scott, head of the Dermatology Service of the National Cancer Institute, expressed the opinion of most authorities when he said: "Baldness is caused by three factors: sex, age, and heredity. And we can't do a thing about any of these."

Other causes of baldness include infections, systemic diseases, drugs which have a toxic effect, mechanical stress, friction, and radiation.

Diet does not usually affect baldness, but chronic starvation or vitamin deficiencies can contribute to dryness, lack of luster, and hair loss. Also, excessive intake of vitamin A can cause hair loss.

In women, loss of hair is quite common toward the end of pregnancy, after delivery, and during menopause. In these cases, most hair eventually grows back.

There are two common types of baldness in men: *male pattern baldness* and *patchy baldness.*

Male pattern baldness: Male pattern baldness (*alopecia*) usually begins in the late twenties or early thirties. Hair falls out from the crown until a fringe of hair remains at the sides and along the back of the head from ear to ear. At the onset, a bald spot may appear on the crown of the head, and balding spots in other areas may merge to form the fringe pattern. There is little one can do to prevent or restore hair lost through typical male pattern baldness.

Patchy baldness: In patchy baldness (*alopecia areata*) hair might fall out suddenly in patches. In this case, hair eventually returns after going through three growth periods. The new hair may be thinner than the original hair. Although patchy baldness is self-limiting and usually self-curing, therapy is indicated in some patients. This usually consists of injections of insoluble steroid suspensions directly into the scalp. Regrowth generally begins in three to four weeks, but remains localized at the site of injection.

Treatment for other types of scalp disorders varies. Dermatologists can usually diagnose a disorder caused by a toxic agent, and they can usually clear up scalp infections with antibiotics. But there is no effective cure, treatment, or drug for male pattern baldness.

In some cases, *hair transplantation* can help. Using a skin biopsy punch and a local anesthetic, a doctor can remove small grafts from the sides and back of the scalp and transplant them to bald areas. As many as 20 transplants can be made in one hour. However, this procedure works only if the baldness is not extensive.

Wigs: Some men who wish to hide their baldness find it easier and less expensive to buy a wig. Not surprisingly, wigs shops exclusively for men are opening throughout the country. Men can buy synthetic stretch wigs in many natural colors for as little as $25 or less. They are made with tapered back and sideburns, and it's reported that they can even be worn when swimming.

Of course, wigs for women are even more prevalent and fashionable. Some women own a wardrobe of wigs in a variety of colors and styles to match their moods, clothes, and the climate.

Excess hair: For some middle-aged women, the problem is too much hair in the wrong place, instead of too little. Excess hair can grow on the face, chest, arms, and legs. In some instances, unwanted hair may be a sign of an endocrine disorder that can be detected by a doctor. In other cases, it can be caused by chronic irritation, such as prolonged use of a cast, bandage, or hot-water bottle; it can also be due to excess exposure to the sun, iodine or mercury irritation, or localized rubbing.

Excess hair can be bleached, shaved, tweezed, waxed, or removed by chemical depilatories and electrolysis. Only electrolysis is permanent. See *Hair Removal*, p. 387.

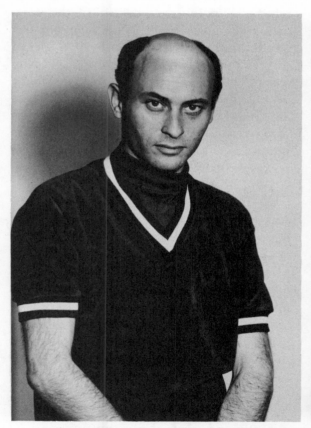 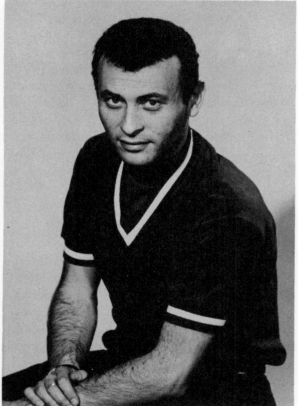

The tendency to lose hair is determined largely by heredity, age, and sex. Male pattern baldness (*left*) often starts in late twenties. Although there is no cure for baldness, today's wigs (*right*) are so well made and styled that it is often impossible to tell when one is being worn.

Varicose Veins

Another complaint of middle-aged women is *varicose veins*. About half the women over 50 years of age have these enlarged veins with damaged valves in their thighs and calves.

Varicose veins are usually caused by years of downward pressure on the veins, causing the valves to break down. This often happens to people who must stand for many hours at a time. The large, bluish irregularities are plainly visible beneath the skin of the thighs and calves, and they cause a heavy dragging sensation in the legs and a general feeling of tiredness and lack of energy.

Treatment: In most instances, the best treatment involves surgery to tie off the main veins and remove all superficial veins that lend themselves to this procedure (called *stripping*). In other cases, varicose veins can be relieved by wearing elastic stockings or compression bandages.

Varicose veins that remain untreated can cause *varicose ulcers,* which usually form on the inner side of the leg above the ankle. Treatment calls for prolonged bed rest, warm applications, and surgical ligation and stripping of the varicose veins responsible for the ulcers. Thus, it is wise to consult a doctor if varicose veins appear.

Menopause

At some point during middle age, women go through what is often called the *change of life*, when the capacity to bear children comes to an end. The start of the menopause usually comes between ages 40 and 50. However, about 12 percent of women reach the menopause between ages 36 and 40; 15 percent between ages 51 and 55; and another 6 percent earlier or later. As a general rule, it may be said that the later in a girl's life menstruation begins, the sooner menopause starts.

While menopause is sometimes abrupt, the onset is usually gradual, and the process normally lasts several years. The ovaries gradually reduce their ovulation and hormone secretion. Menstruation becomes irregular and finally ceases.

The periods between, during, and after the menopause are called premenopausal, menopausal, and postmenopausal. Premenopausal symptoms include skipped menstrual periods and scanty or lessened menstrual flow. During the menopausal period, menstruation ceases, and there are sometimes various systemic disturbances. The postmenopausal period is characterized by the return of bodily equilibrium and a renewed feeling of good health.

Symptoms of menopause: Physical symptoms of the menopause are believed to be caused by an estrogen deficiency which upsets the hypothalamic control of the autonomic nervous system. While many women go through menopause with little or no distress, about one out of five may feel hot flashes and chills, nervousness, insomnia, heart palpitation, dizzy spells, or increased or diminished appetite. Generally, most women suffer from only a few of these symptoms, sudden hot flashes and dizziness being the most common.

Surgical menopause: Many women develop benign uterine tumors called fibroids, and these tumors may cause irregular bleeding, prolonged menstrual periods, massive hemorrhages, or pain and discomfort due to pressure on other organs. In these cases a *hysterectomy,* or surgical removal of the uterus, may be performed. In cases where the cervix is also removed, the procedure is called total hysterectomy. It is only when the complete removal of the ovaries and tubes, called radical hysterectomy, is also necessary, that the production of ova and the normal menstrual cycle are stopped abruptly and surgical menopause occurs.

Though more abrupt and severe than menopause that occurs naturally, surgical menopause is treated in much the same manner as natural menopause. Tranquilizers or sedatives may be prescribed. In some cases, the doctor may prescribe hormone replacement therapy to supplement the body's reduced supply of estrogen. This can be especially beneficial in the relief of hot flashes.

Emotional Aspects of Menopause

In addition to physical symptoms, a woman often has a pronounced psychological reaction to menopause. Though there is no medical basis for believing that menopause adversely affects her sex life or appearance, a woman may feel this is true. Common emotional problems may include the following: the feeling that she has lost her beauty, sex appeal, or sexual desire; a fear of cancer; the idea that the onset of menopause means the loss of her husband's love; fears that her job may be lost because of illness, bad nerves, or general debility; or a feeling the menopause means that she has lost youthful energy and spirit and is becoming old.

Most of these fears are groundless and can be avoided or cured by maintaining an active, healthy life and placing mind over matter.

Advice to the husband: A husband can help his wife through this difficult period if he makes an effort to be especially considerate. For example, he can take special care to show her that she is appreciated and still physically attractive. He can pamper her and show his interest by remembering anniversaries and birthdays and by taking her out more often. Instead of crouching behind a newspaper or watching television in the evening, he can talk to his wife and show an interest in what she is doing.

When one's wife is in a bad humor or moody and depressed, sympathize with her moods and remain tolerant. Invite her out for an evening's entertainment or plan a trip to take together.

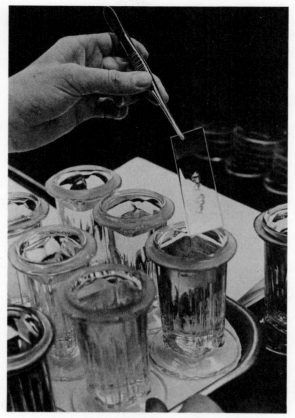

A sample of vaginal fluid is prepared for microscopic study. The procedure, known as the Pap test, enables early, simple, painless detection of uterine cancer.

By taking a realistic view of menopause as a natural process of life, and with the aid of an understanding husband, friends, and family, most women can get through the menopause without frequent visits to a family doctor. However, if a woman experiences any unusual symptoms—abnormal vaginal discharge, spotting between periods, excessive or too frequent periods, periods that last too long, or unusual irritation of the genitals—she should by all means see a doctor.

Pap test: Cancer may be a major fear during the menopause, especially cancer of the cervix. Such fears can easily be allayed by having a simple diagnostic test called the *Papanicolaou* (or *Pap*) *smear.* This is a painless process in which the cervix is exposed by an instrument which dilates the cavity to make it more visible. The doctor can then take samples of the cells, which are examined for the possible presence of cancer. All women should have a pelvic examination and Pap test at least once a year.

A number of other forms of cancer, including cancer of the lining of the uterus, cancer of the ovaries, cancer of the breast, and cancer of the vulva and other sexual organs, appear more frequently in women over 50. However, these conditions can be detected before they do much, if any, damage by having regular examinations during and after the menopause. If such cancers are caught in an early stage, they are much easier to treat and cure.

Male Climacteric

Many men go through a psychological equivalent of the menopause, which may be called the "foolish forties," the "frenzied fifties," or the *male climacteric*.

According to Dr. Charles Wahl, a psychiatrist at the University of California (Los Angeles), some men tend to blame all sorts of symptoms—forgetfulness, self-doubt, worry, depression, and a declining sexual interest—on this mythical male menopause. "These symptoms are of psychic origin," says Dr. Wahl, "when found in a middle-aged man who is not afflicted by a specific disease. The body undergoes no organic or functional changes that might account for such complaints."

This may be of small comfort to the man who—for whatever emotional reasons—goes through this period of psychological upset. But there is some help in this remark from Dr. John F. Briggs, Associate Professor of Clinical Medicine at the University of Minnesota: "The best way to steer a successful course through the hazards of the frenzied fifties is to assay your assets and liabilities dispassionately, and adapt to the circumstances and changes they dictate."

Advice to the wife: Just as a husband can help his wife through her menopause, so can a wife help her husband. The thoughtful wife can bolster her husband's ego by being aware of what deflates him and what builds him up. Concentrate on building up his self-confidence and avoid nagging criticisms and arguments. Show your husband how much you need him and depend on him; sustain his sense of self-importance. Be affectionate and give him tender loving care, especially if you feel that he is worried or tense. He may want more company than usual, or he may prefer not to go out socially. Whatever the case, give in to him. He will assume his normal pace after a while.

There can be a physical reason for the male change of life, called primary *testicular failure*. In such cases, the testes fade out earlier in life than might be expected. Since it is an illness, like diabetes or kidney trouble, testicular failure can happen at any age. When it does occur, the physical discomforts may be surprisingly similar to a woman's symptoms in menopause.

Any man who suspects he may be really ill should see a doctor who can make a thorough examination. This is necessary because any treatment with hormones (androgen) could hurt as much as it could help if the case is not a true testicular failure. Androgen could also be harmful in the case of prostate trouble, which becomes more prevalent after the age of 40. See under *Aging and What to Do About It,* p. 188, for a fuller discussion of prostate trouble.

Other than testicular failure, which is rare, there is no physical reason why a man should be impotent in middle age. As the late Dr. Kinsey reported: "Only a slight portion of the male population ever becomes impotent before death."

If a man thinks that he needs "one last fling" before his virility is curtailed by glandular deterioration, he will not find support for this idea from Dr. Josiah Brown, an endocrinologist with the University of California (Los Angeles). Says Dr. Brown: "There is no significant change in the endocrine function between the ages of 40 and 55."

Also, if a man looks for a sex stimulator for flagging interests, he need look no further than this statement by the late Dr. Kinsey: ". . . good health, sufficient exercise, and plenty of sleep still remain the most effective of the aphrodisiacs known to man."

Nicotine

Used in moderation, nicotine is not harmful, and according to some researchers may be helpful, improving memory and learning ability, perhaps by stimulating the flow of adrenaline. Nicotine also stimulates the adrenal glands, causing blood vessels to constrict and skin temperatures to drop.

Interestingly enough, nicotine is thought to get into the system through the membranes of the mouth and related areas. Thus, a person who holds an unlighted cigar in his mouth may absorb nicotine.

While a little nicotine is not harmful, most steady smokers absorb too much nicotine for their own good. Lung cancer kills over 50,-000 persons a year, about 80 percent of whom are cigarette smokers. Also, cigarette smoking is believed to be a primary cause of *emphysema* (a disease that decreases efficiency of the lungs) which kills over 15,000 persons a year. Approximately 100,-000 cigarette smokers die from heart attacks each year.

In their book *Vigor for Men Over 30*, the authors, Drs. Warren R. Guild, Stuart Cowan and Samm Baker suggest these tips on giving up smoking:

Try a program of enjoyable physical activity: They suggest that if the urge to smoke becomes overpowering, the smoker should take a brisk walk, do a set of invigorating exercises at home or in the office, or engage in an enjoyable sport.

Don't use antismoking drugs or other nostrums without a doctor's advice: Such devices may do more harm than good. Your doctor is the one who can advise you on the best way to cut down on smoking, and he can help you cope with any withdrawal symptoms such as nervousness, dizziness, or insomnia.

Don't try to cut down on too many things at the same time: Concentrate on cutting down on your smoking, and relax about cutting down on diet and drinking, too. One reduction at a time is best.

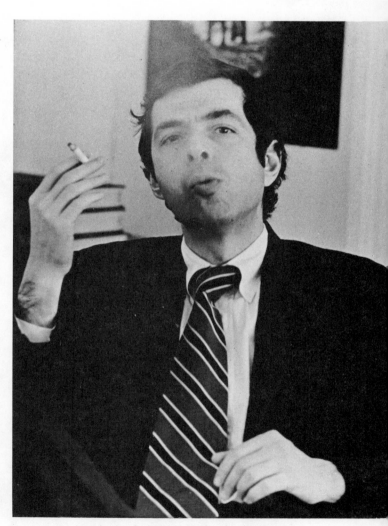

Reasons to break the habit: the risk of developing lung cancer is greater for smokers, and scientists have found that smoking contributes to other kinds of cancer, heart disease, bronchitis, and emphysema.

You've got to quit completely: Like the alcoholic, you've got to say, "This is my *last* cigarette"—and mean it.

Quit when there's a major break in your routine: The recovery from an operation or illness is a good time to stop. After you have established the habit of *not* smoking, make that habit a part of your daily life.

Try something different to throw desire off the track: Take a shower—you can't light a match under water. Also, you can't hold a cigarette if you're playing table tennis or practicing your golf swing.

Caffeine

Like nicotine, *caffeine* can be a pleasant stimulant if used in moderation. Laboratory studies show that caffeine appears to work on the central nervous system: fatigue and drowsiness fade while mental activities quicken. But too much caffeine can produce headaches, irritability, and confusion.

Although tea leaves contain almost twice as much caffeine as an equal weight of coffee, smaller amounts of tea are used to make a cup of tea, thus lessening the per-cup intake rate. Cola and chocolate also contain caffeine. Although these drinks are not addictive, they do create a physical dependence similar to a narcotic. Caffeine drinkers who "withdraw" from their accustomed cups of coffee may have headaches for a short time.

Ordinarily, drinking a few cups of coffee or other caffeine beverage is not harmful—unless your doctor tells you to cut down for some reason. But if you find that you need a caffeine beverage to keep going, you might be better off taking a rest instead.

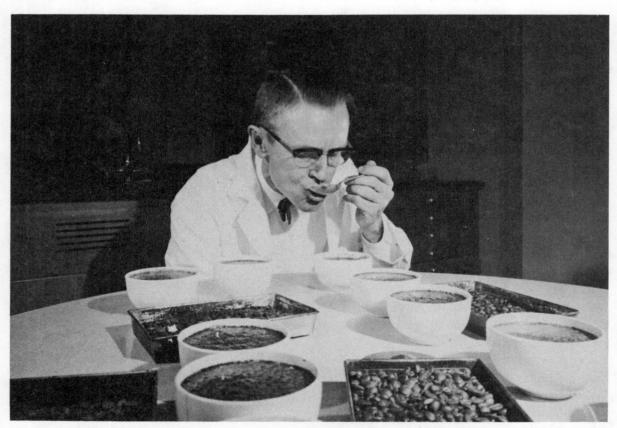

Coffee beans are tested by the U.S. Dept. of Agriculture. Coffee contains caffeine, which stimulates mental and physical energy. Ordinarily harmless, it should be used in moderation.

Alcohol

Many doctors feel that a person's capacity to handle liquor diminishes after age 40, and that alcohol intake should be cut down after this age. Also, some people seem to develop a reaction to alcohol that is almost like an allergy—an allergy that can be fatal. One doctor described the extra dry martini as "the quick blow to the back of the neck."

Drinking too much and too fast can jar the whole system. It tends to make the drinker nervous and on edge instead of providing calming relief from tensions. The hard-pressed executive is especially vulnerable to the quick, fast drink he takes to provide instant relaxation when he is fatigued.

"The key to the real value of alcohol is intelligent drinking," says Dr. Harry J. Johnson, of the Life Extension Institute. Dr. Johnson says that he sometimes recommends a drink or two before dinner, which he says is the best time to indulge. However, Dr. Johnson suggests a tall, well-diluted, highball taken in a peaceful, quiet setting.

How to Avoid Drinking

If you find that drinking is a problem at business luncheons, conventions, and cocktail parties, Dr. Warren R. Guild recommends the following commonsense tips to pass up drinks:

• Say "no thanks" if you do not like the taste or effect of alcohol. Order a juice or nonalcoholic beverage just to have something to sip. Actually, many more jobs and clients have been lost through drinking too much than by not drinking at all.

• Wait for others to order drinks. If someone else refuses a drink, you can decline too. Or, you could say, "I'm not having one but you go ahead." This usually sets the pace for drinking.

• Instead of a powerhouse martini, try vermouth on the rocks, beer, wine, or a well-diluted highball.

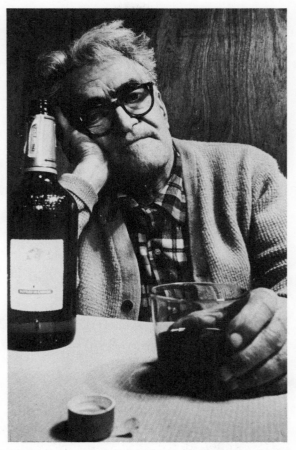

Alcoholism, one of the most prevalent diseases in the United States, is a major health problem. Five out of six alcoholics are men between 30–55 years old, but the percentage of women drinkers is on the way up.

• Use dieting as a reason to cut down or out on drinking. You have a good excuse—a drink has 100 or more calories.

• Make arrangements with your favorite restaurant or bar to serve you "your usual." You could make this a nonalcoholic drink.

Remember that alcohol definitely decreases your ability to concentrate, absorb, or produce thoughts or ideas. After drinking you will not be as efficient at writing, drawing, handling objects, or driving. If the level of alcohol in your blood exceeds 0.05 percent—which, depending on weight, is approximately the equivalent of two ounces of hard liquor or two bottles of beer at one session—*you are not a safe driver.*

Treating a Hangover

What if you do drink too much and have a hangover? Is there anything you can do about it? Dr. Harold T. Hyman, formerly of the Columbia University College of Physicians and Surgeons, recommends calling a physician if the case is particularly bad. He will probably prescribe a large dose of paraldehyde or a tranquilizer such as Librium or Thorazine, and put the patient to bed.

Less acute sufferers should, on awakening after a binge, take warmed fluids (tea, consommé, clam broth). As soon as your stomach feels in shape, eat warm, soft foods at frequent intervals—poached egg, milk toast, pureed soup, mashed potatoes. Despite your craving for cold, carbonated fluids, avoid them; they may cause stomach cramps.

To prevent a hangover as you drink, Dr. Guild recommends taking *fructose*. Fructose, or *levulose*, is a crystalline sugar, the sweetest of the sugars. It increases the rate at which the body metabolizes and eliminates alcohol. It seems to work best when the alcohol is combined with something naturally high in fructose, as the tomato juice in a Bloody Mary, for example. Or, you could just sip tomato juice between drinks.

Looking for quick panaceas in the medicine cabinet to cure a hangover or any other condition seems to become increasingly popular after age 40. Panaceas are all right up to a point, but indiscriminate self-treatment can do a great deal of harm, since it may mask a more serious illness or may prevent a condition from clearing up if left alone. In drinking, as in eating, the key is moderation.

Weight and Health

Overweight is one of the biggest deterrents to successful middle age, and is also one of the greatest threats to health and longevity.

As one doctor said, "Consider how few really obese persons you see over 60 years of age." Unfortunately, in middle age most of us maintain the eating habits of our youth while we cut down on our exercise. The result: added weight that acts as an anchor to our physical well-being.

The overweight person is more likely to develop arthritis, cancer, diabetes, heart disease, high blood pressure, kidney trouble, and many other disabling or fatal disorders. As the American Heart Association said recently: "Pity the fat man; the statisticians number his days."

As reported in *Nation's Business*, "If you are overweight by 10 percent, your chances of surviving the next 20 years are 15 percent less than if you had ideal weight; if you are 20 percent overweight, your chances are 25 percent less; if you are 30 percent overweight, 45 percent less." In other words, the odds are against the overweight.

If you do not know what your ideal weight should be, a doctor can tell you. To check yourself, try the "pinch" test. Take a pinch of skin on your upper arm just below the shoulder. If more than a half-inch separates your fingers, you are too fat. Try the same test on your stomach when you're standing erect. And, of course, your mirror can reveal the tell-tale signs of middle-age fat—the double chin, sagging belly, flabby arms and legs.

Good Eating Habits

Is there any magic way to reduce? The only sure way is to *eat less*, and to continue this practice all the time. It will not help if you go on a crash diet and then resume your normal eating habits. And while exercise will help control weight and burn up excess calories, probably the best exercise is to push yourself away from the table before you've overeaten.

Calories do count, and usually the caloric intake of a person in the 40 to 55 year age bracket should be about one-third less than that of a person between ages 25 and 40. Again, your doctor or a good calorie-counter can help you determine what to eat and how much.

Here are some additional tips from nutritionists to help you lose weight:

Cut down on quantity: Eat just enough to satisfy your appetite—not as much as you can. Even low-calorie foods will add weight if you eat enough of them.

Eat less more often: Spread your food intake over several meals or snacks. Some hospitals have been experimenting with five meals a day, spreading the recommended total food intake over two full meals a day (brunch and dinner) and three snacks (continental breakfast, afternoon snack, and night cap). They find that the stomach handles small amounts of food better, that metabolism keeps working at a good pace all day, and that blood sugar levels (your energy reserve) do not drop between meals. Also, the process of digestion burns up calories.

Avoid high-calorie foods: Cut out breads, rolls, butter, jellies, hams, sauces, gravies, dressings, creams, and rich desserts. These are the villains that add calories and are not as rich in nutrients.

Look for natural flavors: Cultivate an interest in the natural flavor of what you eat. Try vegetables without butter, coffee and tea without cream and sugar. You might want to substitute a pinch of salt or a squeeze of lemon on your vegetables or noncaloric sweeteners in your beverages, but chances are you will find the natural flavors new and interesting.

Serve only just enough: Keep portions small and put serving dishes with leftovers out of sight. Taking seconds is often just a habit. Cultivate the idea of just one serving, and you will find it satisfies the appetite. Another idea: serve meals on smaller plates. The portion will look big if only in relationship to the size of the plate.

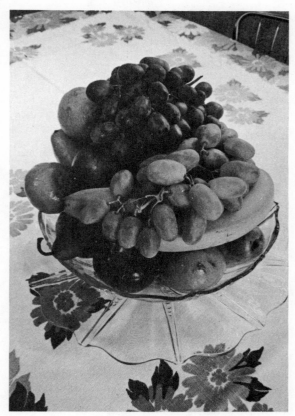

Fresh fruits, rich in vitamins and low in calories, are among the preferred foods for many weight watchers.

In order to maintain a healthy body and a youthful appearance while dieting, you must make sure you eat the necessary proteins and nutrients. This can be done by selecting foods from the four basic food groups. See *Basic Nutritional Requirements,* p. 295.

As a panel of experts on middle age said in a recent interview: "Two factors are vital to successful middle age: physical activity and a variety of interests. Move around but don't rush around. Keep an open mind and a closed refrigerator. Remember that variety is more than the spice of life—it's the wellspring of life. The person who pursues a variety of activities will usually stay fit long after middle age." For a discussion of emotional problems encountered during the middle years, see *Living Life to the Fullest,* p. 261.   PAD

AGING AND WHAT TO DO ABOUT IT: THE LATER YEARS

Growing older could mean growing healthier. In many ways you are as old as you think and feel. Consider these points:

• No disease results just from the passage of years.

• We age piecemeal—each organ separately rather than uniformly.

• In retirement you have less daily stress and strain, and you have more time to take better care of yourself.

What, then, makes a person think and feel old?

The Aging Process

Physically, we mature at about age 25 to 30, when the body reaches maximum size and strength. Then, body tissues and cells are constantly being rebuilt and renewed. Nutrition, rest, exercise, and stress influence the length of time a person's body can maintain a balance between the wearing down and rebuilding of body tissues. When more cells die than can be reproduced, they are replaced by a fibrous, inert substance called *collagen*. The living process slows down to compensate, and we begin aging; strength and ability start to decline.

But this happens at various intervals. For instance, vision is sharpest at age 25; the eye loses its ability to make rapid adjustments in focus after age 40. Hearing is sharpest at about age 10, then diminishes as you grow older. Sensitivity to taste and smell lessens after age 60.

The decline in strength and muscle ability is long and gradual; there are even gratifying plateaus. At age 50, a man still has about four-fifths of the muscle strength he had when he was 25.

Although physical abilities may decline, mental abilities may actually improve dur-

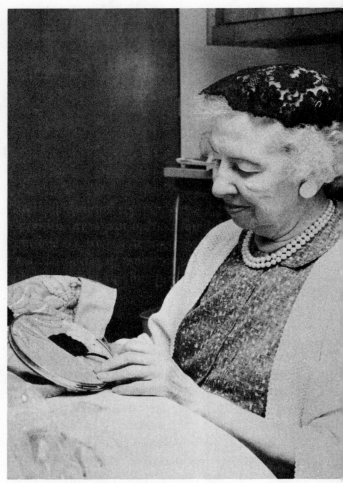

The dignity of purposeful activity is reflected in this woman's face as she concentrates on her embroidery.

ing the middle years, and memory and the ability to learn can remain keen. Dr. Alfred Schwartz, dean of education at Drake University, was asked: "Can a 70-year-old man in reasonably good health learn as rapidly as a 17-year-old boy?" Dr. Schwartz answered:

Indeed he can—provided he's in the habit of learning. The fact that some older people today are not active intellectually is no reflection on their ability to learn. There is ample proof that learning ability does not automatically decline with age.

Regardless of what you may have heard, organic brain damage affects less than one percent of those over age 65.

But in thinking about physical change, remember that this is just one aspect of aging. Age is determined by emotional and intellectual maturity as well as by chronological years.

Can a person do anything to retard aging?

Most *gerontologists* feel that the reason more people don't live longer is that they are not willing to follow a regimen of diet, exercise, rest, recreation—coupled with the exclusion of various excesses. And while there isn't anything you can do to set back the clock, you can keep in good health by making sure to have regular physical examinations, sufficient exercise, adequate rest, nutritious food, and a positive mental attitude.

A Positive Mental Attitude

Mark Twain once said: "Whatever a man's age he can reduce it several years by putting a bright-colored flower in his buttonhole." A lively, fresh outlook is essential for enjoyable living at any age. Most doctors believe there is a direct connection between one's state of mind and physical health. This is especially true when you are faced with the challenges of retirement. Plato said: "He who is of a calm and happy nature will hardly feel the pressure of age, but to him who is of an opposite disposition, youth and age are equally a burden."

Experts in the field of aging have found that most older people can relieve transitory depression by a deliberate shift of thought or by physical activity. If you look upon retirement as an opportunity to take better care of yourself and to pursue old and new interests, you'll go a long way toward better health.

The Annual Checkup

For peace of mind and to maintain and improve your health, make it a habit to see your doctor at least once a year. To remind themselves, many people make an appointment on their birthday. An annual checkup

is especially important in later years and should not be put off or neglected.

During a routine checkup, the doctor pays special attention to enlarged lymph nodes of the neck, armpits, and groin, and the front of the neck. He also checks the condition of veins and arteries and looks at your knees and arches—which are of particular importance to older people.

He makes tests for arteriosclerosis, high blood pressure, diabetes, brain tumors, and other diseases. He can feel and tap your body to check your lungs, liver, and spleen, and he can take *electrocardiographs* to detect changes in your heart. Simple tests can note bladder and kidney conditions.

In addition, the doctor usually asks about personal habits—smoking, drinking, eating. He also wants to know about any unusual symptoms you might have. Be completely frank with your doctor, answer his questions as directly as possible, and give all information that might be helpful.

When explaining the nature of your ailment or symptom, tell him what part of the body is involved, what changes are associated with the symptoms, and whether symptoms occurred after a change of diet or medicine. Tell him about any previous experiences with this condition and what treatments you might have had.

It is extremely important to tell your doctor about any pills you are taking—including aspirin, tranquilizers, and sleeping tablets. Even the most common drug can affect the potency of medication he might prescribe.

After he has taken your case history and after he has all the reports from your tests, the doctor will want to talk with you, explain his findings, and perhaps make some recommendations. Take his advice; don't try to be your own doctor.

If you have questions, don't be afraid to ask them. Have him explain the nature of your ailment, how long it may take for relief or cure, how the therapy or medication is

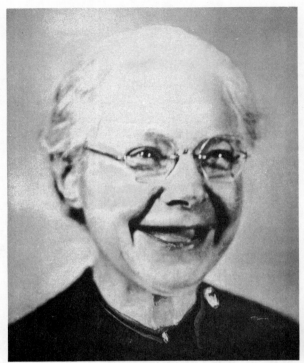 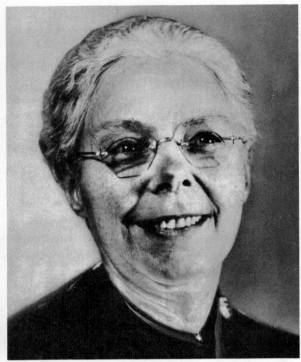

Although the chief value of dentures may be practical, their contribution to a handsome appearance is also of real importance, as these illustrations show.

expected to work, and the possible impact on your everyday activities.

Hopefully, by following his advice you'll stay healthy and well. However, if you are at home and feel ill, call your doctor if:

• Your symptoms are so severe you can't endure them.

• Apparent minor symptoms persist without explainable cause.

• You are in doubt.

Oral Health

It is especially important in later years to have regular dental checkups. After age 50, over half of the American people have some form of *periodontal disease,* and at age 65 nearly all persons have this disease.

Periodontal disease begins when a sticky film called *dental plaque* forms on the teeth. Soft at first, this deposit soon hardens into a cement-like crust (*calculus*) that becomes a breeding place for most bacteria. If not removed, the bacteria-laden crust irritates the gums, which become red and swollen and bleed when the teeth are brushed.

Should the inflammation (*gingivitis*) not be treated, it spreads along the roots. The gums separate from the teeth to form pockets which fill up with more food particles and bacteria. As the disease progresses, the bone support for the teeth is weakened. The affected teeth begin to loosen and drift from their normal position. Finally—unless the disease is treated in time—the teeth must be removed. For illustrations of this process, see p. 95.

Brushing teeth and gums regularly is a defense against periodontal disease. Use dental floss to remove all food particles and plaque from areas between the teeth, especially after each meal.   PAD

Dentures

If you do lose some teeth, they should be replaced with bridges or partial or full *dentures,* because the cheeks and lips will otherwise sag and wrinkle and make you look older than you really are. Chewing ability and the clarity of speech are also impaired if missing teeth are not replaced.

Fitting of dentures: Modern techniques and materials of construction and the skill of modern dentists assure well-fitting, natural-looking dentures. The dentist selects the tooth shade and shape that is best for your face, size, and coloring. People sometimes want perfectly white straight teeth. No one, however, has perfectly arranged, perfectly white natural teeth. Tooth color is inherited and complements a person's particular complexion, and teeth darken as one grows older. The dentist considers all of these factors in designing dentures.

Although dentures do not change with age, the mouth does. It is still necessary, therefore, for the denture-wearer to have dental checkups. At the checkup, the dentist checks denture fit, measuring present oral conditions and examining the oral tissues for irritation. Continuous irritation may cause infection or more serious complications. The dentist seeks to correct any irritations and polishes the denture, making it smooth and easier to brush and keep clean. If correction is not possible, a replacement may be recommended.

Dentists are now working to develop implant dentures, in which artificial teeth will be fastened to the jawbone.

Care of dentures: The use of adhesives and powders are temporary solutions to ill-fitting dentures. In time, the dentist may recommend *relining* the denture to fit the present conformation of one's mouth. Relining is the rebuilding of the inner (gum) side of the denture. If the mouth tissue changes greatly, it may be necessary to be fitted with a new denture. Never attempt to do relining yourself; you may be so accustomed to the fit of your dentures that you don't notice

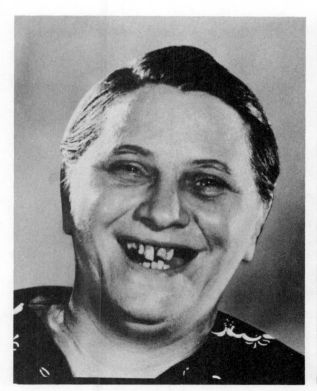
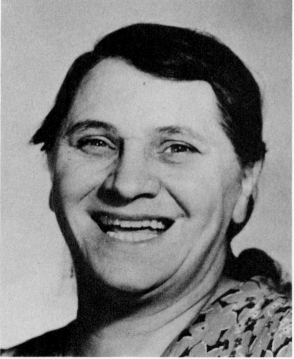

When selecting dentures, the dentist selects the tooth shade and shape that best suit the patient's face and complexion. Dentures are made to look slightly irregular to appear natural.

an irritated area that may nevertheless do great harm to the mouth.

Ethical technicians work only from a dentist's order, because only a qualified dentist has the necessary background to make a thorough examination of the mouth, determine its condition, and design the proper denture.

In the past, you might have had to wait a long time after an extraction before getting a denture. Today, no such delay is necessary. Back teeth are removed, and as soon as these areas have healed, the front teeth are removed; dentures are inserted the same day. Immediate dentures do require relining or replacing, usually within a year, because of the expected tissue change. Although there are some people for whom immediate dentures are not advised, most people are capable of wearing them.

Cleaning of dentures: Dentures should be cleaned daily with a denture brush and toothpaste; once a week they should be soaked for seven or eight hours in a denture cleaner. To avoid breaking them during the brushing process, fill the wash basin with a little water. If they are dropped while cleaning, the water will cushion the fall. A harsh abrasive such as a cleanser should not be used because it scratches the surface of the dentures. Scratches allow stains to penetrate the surface of the denture, creating permanent discoloration.

The rules of dental health are the same in later years as in any other period of life. Keep the teeth clean at home and visit the dentist regularly.   DJC

Diet and Health

Just what are your food requirements as you grow older? Basically you need the same essential nutrients that you have always needed, except that you face special problems. You need to:

• Select food more carefully to eat adequate proteins, vitamins, and minerals—while cutting down on calories.

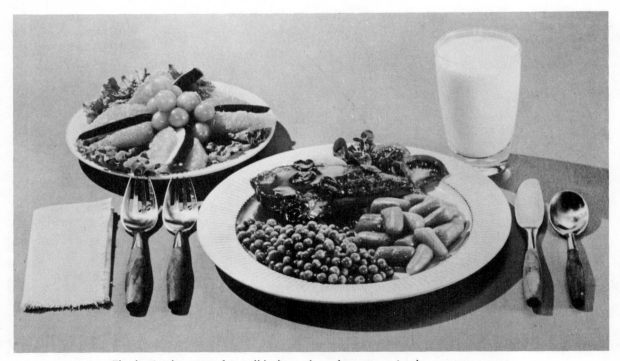

The basic elements of a well-balanced meal are very simple: meat, a green and yellow vegetable, green salad, fruit, and a beverage such as milk.

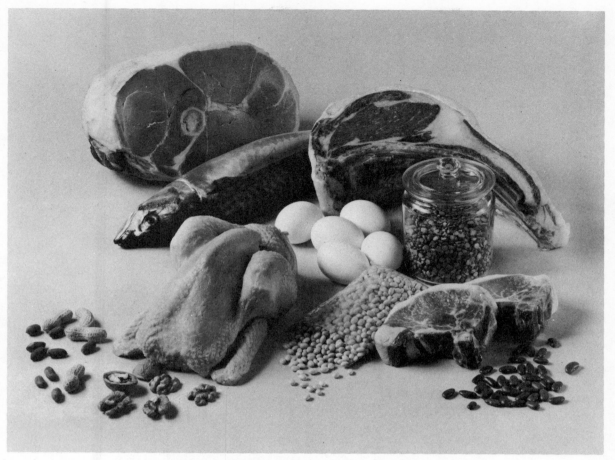

The meat group—one of the four basic food groups—includes fish, poultry, eggs, dry beans or peas, nuts, and eggs, as well as the various kinds of meat. All of these foods are especially rich in protein.

• Get the most nutritious food for the least money and make the most of what you buy.

• Avoid bad eating habits—make mealtime a pleasure rather than a chore.

• Learn new techniques to stretch meals, use leftovers, and substitute lower-priced items with the same nutritional value for higher-price foods. In other words, learn how to shop well.

Basic Requirements

How can you get the essential nutrients every day? A good rule is first to eat recommended servings from the Basic Four Food Groups (see below) established by the National Research Council. Then, eat other foods that you like, as long as they do not go over the recommended daily caloric intake. The average man in the 55 to 75 year age group should consume 2,200 calories a day; the average woman in the same age group, 1,600 calories a day. This is a drop of between 500 and 600 calories a day from what was needed at age 25. As you grow older, your physical activity decreases and your metabolism slows, causing body fats to build up at a much higher rate, and making you more prone to hardening of the arteries and certain heart conditions.

Here are the Basic Four Food Groups:

Meat group: Two or more servings from this group of foods are recommended daily. A serving is 2 to 3 oz. of cooked meat, fish,

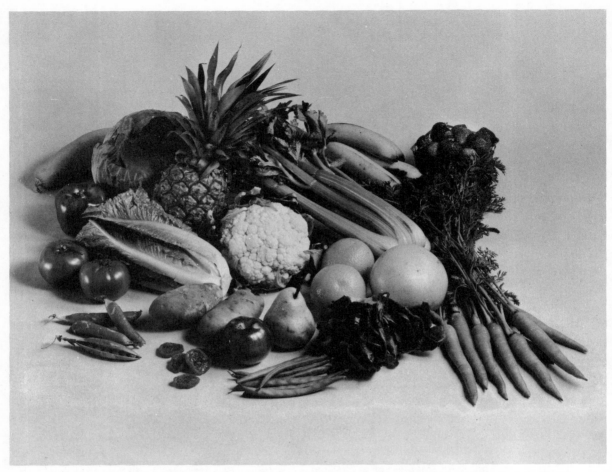

The vegetable and fruit group is a rich source of vitamins, minerals, and carbohydrates. Green and yellow vegetables should be eaten daily, preferably at both noonday and evening meals.

or poultry; 2 eggs; occasionally 1 cup of cooked dry beans or peas; ½ cup peanut butter; or 1 cup cottage cheese.

Dairy foods: Dairy food requirements may be satisfied by two cups of milk or its equivalent in cheese, ice cream, etc. A 1⅓ oz. slice of cheddar-type cheese or one scant pint of ice cream is equivalent to 1 cup of milk. Imitation ice cream or ice milk where vegetable fat has been substituted for butterfat has just as much protein.

Vegetables and fruit: The daily vegetable and fruit requirement consists of four or more servings. A serving is one-half cup. Include one serving of citrus fruit each day and dark greens or deep yellow vegetables every other day.

Bread and cereal group: Each day have four or more servings of whole grain, enriched, or restored products such as breads, cereals, rice, hominy grits, noodles, or macaroni. One serving is a slice of bread; one-half to three-fourths cup cooked cereal, pasta, or rice; one medium potato.

Use other foods such as sweets, baked goods, desserts to complete meals and treat the sweet tooth. But remember to count calories. Nutritionists have found that skinny animals live longer than fat ones, and this seems to be true of people, too.

Beware of food fads and so-called health foods unless these are recommended by your doctor. Also, do not buy vitamins and mineral tablets unless prescribed. When you obtain vitamins from food, your body uses the amount necessary to maintain proper health, appetite, and resistance to infection. Your body promptly eliminates excesses of vitamin C and the B complex, and stores an excess of vitamins A and D in your liver and other body organs. It may take up to seven years of practically complete deprivation for a previously healthy adult to show signs of a vitamin deficiency.

Some older people may go on low-fat diets because of the cholesterol fear caused by talk and advertisements for unsaturated fats. Get a doctor's recommendation before curtailing your fat intake—too little fat and dairy products can be as harmful as too much.

Also, unless prescribed, do not take iron tonics or pills. Usually, you'll get adequate iron intake if you eat meat, eggs, vegetables, and enriched cereals regularly. Adding more iron to a normal diet may even be harmful.

Eating Habits

If you find that mealtime is a chore rather than a pleasure, try these tips to enhance your meals:

• Try a two-meal-a-day schedule. Have a late breakfast and early dinner when you

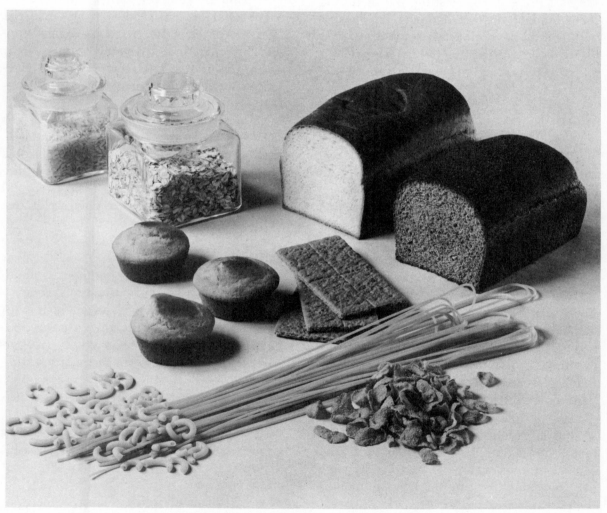

The bread and cereal group is particularly rich in carbohydrates, the primary source of calories. Unless overweight, children should have several daily servings of bread or a cereal product.

are really hungry. But be sure to get your Basic Four requirements in these two meals.

• Drink a glass of water as soon as you wake up to promote good digestion, weight control, and bowel movements.

• Try a walk or light exercise to stimulate appetite and to regulate body processes. Moderate exercise also will help regulate weight since it burns up calories.

• You might sip a glass of wine before dinner. Recent research shows wine is very useful to older people in improving appetite and digestion. Port, a light sherry, and vermouth with a dash of soda are good appetite stimulators.

• Make meals interesting by including some food of distinctive flavor to contrast with a mild-flavored food; something crisp for contrast with softer foods, even if it is only a pickle or a lettuce leaf; some brightly colored food for eye appeal.

• Pep up your food with a judicious use of herbs and spices or flavor-enhancers like wine, bottled sauces, fruit juices, and peels.

• If some food causes you distress, eliminate it and substitute something else of equal nutritive value. Green salad may include too much roughage for the intestinal tract; ham or bacon may be supplying your body with too much salt, which increases water retention. Or you may be drinking too much coffee, tea, or soft drinks.

• Be realistic about your chewing ability. Food swallowed whole may be causing digestive problems. If your teeth are not as good as they were or if you are wearing dentures, try cubing, chopping, or grinding foods that are difficult to chew. Let your knife or meat grinder do part of the work.

• Try a different atmosphere or different setting for your meals. Use candlelight, music, and your best linen on occasion. Move outdoors when the weather is good; eat your lunch in the park and dinner on the patio.

• Occasionally invite a friend or relative to dine with you. It's surprising what stimu-lating conversation and an exchange of ideas can do to boost your mood and appetite.

• Try a new recipe or a new food. Thanks to modern transportation, foods are available in larger cities from many areas and other countries. Eat eggplant or okra, avocado or artichoke, gooseberry jam, or garbanzo beans in a salad. And why not have a papaya with lemon juice for breakfast?

Cooking Hints

Try these ideas for preparing food more easily; they are especially useful if you have only a single gas or electric burner:

• Combine your vegetables and meat—or some other protein food—into a single pot or pan. You can cook many hot, nourishing meals of this kind: Irish stew, braised liver or pot roast with vegetables, ham-and-vegetable chowder or fish chowder, a New England boiled dinner.

• Combine leftovers to make a one-dish meal. Leftover meat combines beautifully with vegetables, macaroni, or rice. Add a cheese or tomato sauce or a simple white sauce and heat in a baking dish. Chopped tomatoes or green onions or chives will give extra flavor and color to the dish.

• Round out one-dish meals with a crisp salad topped with cut strips of leftover cooked meat or poultry or another raw food, bread, a beverage, and perhaps a dessert.

• Mix leftover cooked vegetables with raw fresh ones, such as chopped celery, cucumber slices, tomatoes, green pepper, shredded cabbage, to make an interesting salad.

• Cream vegetables, meat, fish, or chicken. Or serve them with a tasty sauce. Use canned tomato or mushroom soup for a quick and easy sauce. If the dish is a bit skimpy, a hard-boiled egg may stretch it to serving size.

• Add a bit of relish, snappy cheese, or diced cucumber to a cooked dressing for meat or vegetable salad.

• If you cook a potato, an ear of corn, or some other vegetable in the bottom of a double boiler, you can use the top to warm rolls, heat leftover meat in gravy, or heat such foods as creamed eggs or fish.

The Value of Exercise

As you grow older, exercise can help you look, feel, and work better. Various organs and systems of the body, particularly the digestive process, are stimulated through activity, and, as a result, work more effectively.

You can improve your posture through exercise that tones supporting muscles. This not only improves appearance but can decrease the frequency of lower-back pain and disability.

Here are some other benefits of exercise: it can increase your ability to relax and tolerate fatigue; it improves muscle tone; reduces fat deposits; increases working capacity of the lungs; improves kidney and liver function; increases volume of blood, hemoglobin, and red blood cells, leading to improved utilization of oxygen and iron.

Also, physically active people are less likely to experience a heart attack or other forms of cardiovascular disease than sedentary people. Moreover, an active person who does suffer a coronary attack will probably

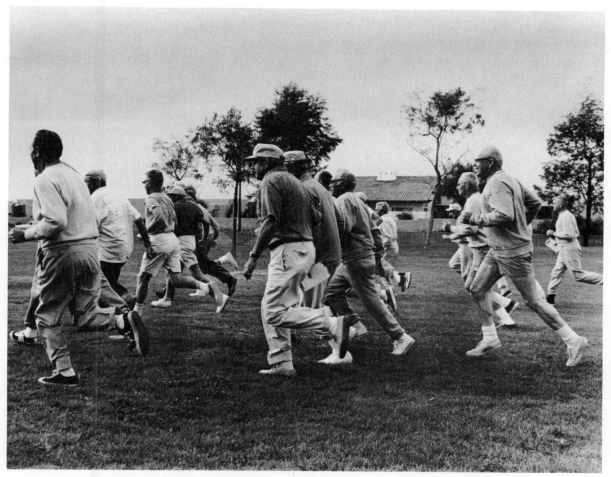

Jogging is an especially valuable exercise because it stimulates the heart muscle and blood circulation. Although there are joggers of all ages—including some in their 80s—no one of or beyond middle age should take up jogging without first consulting his physician.

have a less severe form. The Public Health Service studied 5,000 adults in Framingham, Mass., for more than a decade. When any member of the group suffered a heart attack, his physical activity was reviewed. It was found that more inactive people suffered more fatal heart attacks than active members.

Walking for Exercise

Exercise need not be something you *must* do but rather something you *enjoy* doing. One of the most practical and enjoyable exercises is walking. Charles Dickens said:

> Walk and be happy, walk and be healthy. The best of all ways to lengthen our days is to walk, steadily and with a purpose. The wandering man knows of certain ancients, far gone in years, who have staved off infirmities and dissolution by earnest walking —hale fellows close upon eighty and ninety, but brisk as boys.

The benefits of walking were revealed in a recent Health Insurance Plan study of 110,000 people in New York City. Those who had heart attacks were divided into two groups—walkers and nonwalkers. The first four weeks of illness were reviewed for both groups. At the end of that time 41 percent of the nonwalkers were dead, while only 23 percent of the walkers were. When all physical activity was considered, 57 percent of the inactive had died compared to only 16 percent of those who had some form of exercise.

Walking is as natural to the human body as breathing. It is a muscular symphony; all the foot, leg, and hip muscles and much of the back musculature are involved. The abdominal muscles tend to contract and support their share of the weight, and the diaphragm and rib muscles increase their action. There is automatic action of the arm and shoulder muscles; the shoulder and neck muscles get play as the head is held erect; the eye muscles are exercised as you look about you.

Other Types of Exercise

Swimming and bicycling exercise most of the muscles, and gardening is highly recommended. The fresh air, the bending, squatting, and countless other movements exercise most parts of the body.

Surprisingly, most games do not provide good exercise. According to a physical fitness research laboratory at the University of Illinois, the trouble with most games is that the action is intermittent—starting and stopping—a burst of energy and then a wait. The bowler swings a ball for 2.5 seconds and gets about one minute of actual muscular work per game. Golf is a succession of pause, swing, walk—or, more often, a ride to the next pause, swing, and so on. Also, you spend a lot of time standing and waiting for the party ahead and for your partners. Tennis gives one more exercise but it too involves a great deal of starting and stopping, as does handball. No game has the essential, tension-releasing pattern of continuous, vigorous, rhythmic motion found in such activities as walking, running, or jogging.

For formal exercises, you could join a gym, but you might find your enthusiasm waning after a few weeks. You could also exercise at home; there are many excellent books on exercise that provide programs for you to follow at home on a daily basis.

But everyone's exercise capacity varies. It is best to discuss any new exercise program with your doctor, especially if you have some illness or are out of practice. Then select an exercise which is pleasant for you and suitable to your condition.

It is most important always to warm up before any strenuous exercise. The U.S. Administration on Aging's booklet, *The Fitness Challenge in the Later Years*, states:

> The enthusiast who tackles a keep-fit program too fast and too strenuously soon gives up in discomfort, if not in injury. A warm-up period should be performed by starting lightly

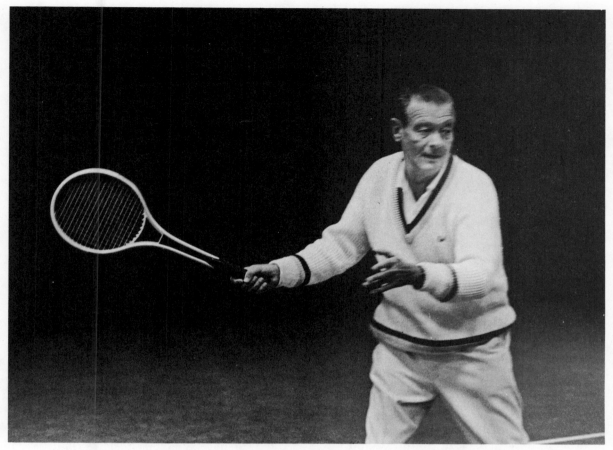

Many healthy, older people, like this 67-year-old, keep up their participation in active sports. The trick is knowing how to adjust your game to a slower and more comfortable pace.

with a continuous rhythmical activity such as walking and gradually increasing the intensity until your pulse rate, breathing, and body temperature are elevated. It's also desirable to do some easy stretching, pulling, and rotating exercises during the warm-up period.

The booklet outlines an excellent program —*red* (easiest), *white* (next), and *blue* (the most sustained and difficult). Each program is "designed to give a balanced workout utilizing all major muscle groups." For a copy of this booklet, send 30 cents to the Superintendent of Documents, U.S. Government Printing Office, Washington, D.C. 20402.

A word of caution: You may be exercising too strenuously if the following happens:

• Your heart does not stop pounding within ten minutes after the exercise.
• You cannot catch your breath ten minutes after the exercise.
• You are shaky for more than thirty minutes afterwards.
• You can't sleep well afterwards.
• Your fatigue (not muscle soreness) continues into the next day.

Sensible, moderate exercise geared to your own physical capacity can help to give you a sense of all-around well-being. As Dr. Ernest Simonson, associate professor of physiological hygiene at the University of Minnesota Medical School, has said:

Those who exercise regularly never fail to mention that it makes them feel better in every way. It's common logic if one feels better, his attitude towards others will be more congenial. When one is in a cordial, happy frame of mind, he will likely make wiser decisions, and his world in general will look better.

Skin Problems

As a person grows older, his skin begins to wrinkle; oil and sweat glands slow down, causing the skin to become dry. Also, the skin may lack the elasticity and tone of normal skin, and this might cause changes in facial contours.

However, the skin, like other parts of the body, tends to age according to various factors. Among prime agers of the skin are exposure to sunlight and weather; the sailor and chronic sunbather may have older looking skin than their years. Also, hereditary and racial factors influence skin age.

Itching: The skin often itches as one grows older. Itching usually stems from external irritations or internal diseases. External irritations may be more severe in winter because of lack of humidity and because the skin oil does not spread properly. Too many baths or wearing wool garments could also cause itching. You can correct this by cutting down on bathing, maintaining correct temperature and humidity, and applying skin creams.

If itching does not clear up in about two weeks, the trouble may be due to any of a number of internal diseases, some of them serious. Thus, it is wise to see your doctor if itching persists.

Skin cancer: Skin cancer can be easily diagnosed and treated. The two most common types are *basal cell* and *squamous cell*.

The basal cell type begins with a small fleshy *nodule*, usually on the face. It may take several months to reach one-half to one-inch in diameter. In about a year it begins to ulcerate and bleed. Then it forms a crust which it sheds at intervals, leaving another ulcer. If you notice anything like this, see your doctor. He can usually remove the ulcer by a local operation.

Squamous cell cancer is often aided by smoking and exposure to the sun. The lesions may appear on the lips, mouth, and genitalia, and they tend to spread and increase in size. Horny growths in exposed areas—face, ears, neck, and scalp—may be forerunners of squamous cell cancer. Again, your doctor can treat or operate effectively.

Vitiligo: Vitiligo, loss of pigment, is not caused by a disease, but it could be a hereditary problem. The affected area of skin has patches of whiteness throughout, but these can be masked by cosmetics.

Senile purpura: Sometimes the skin develops *senile purpura* as one grows older. The characteristic hemorrhages of this condition usually appear on the extremities, and the purple color gradually fades and leaves mottled areas of yellow-brown. Generally, the skin is thin, fragile, and transparent in appearance.

Stasis dermatitis: Sometimes in association with such conditions as varicose veins, the skin may develop *stasis dermatitis*, an acute, chronic condition of the leg, associated with swelling, scaling of the skin, and in some cases, ulcer formation. It may exist for years with or without ulceration.

If any of the above conditions develop, it is wise to consult your doctor rather than try to treat yourself.

Other skin conditions: Other skin conditions that may develop in the later years may include an increase in coarse hairs on exposed places such as the upper lip or chin. The downy hairs in the ears and nose become thicker and more apparent, and the eyebrows may become bushy. Graying hair is popularly associated with aging, but its onset often depends upon genetic factors and varies so much that it cannot be used as a reliable measure of age.

The ear lobes may elongate as you grow older and the nails may become coarse and thickened or thinner and brittle.

Relieving skin conditions: As mentioned earlier, you can use some creams to relieve dryness and scaliness in older skin. The best of such creams are the water-in-oil emulsions (cold creams) such as Petrolatum Rose Water Ointment USP XVI, or oil-in-water emulsions such as Hydrophilic Ointment USP XVI. Wrinkle creams will not help much, but some conditions may be masked by regular cosmetic items such as powder, rouge, mascara, hair dyes, etc.

Sunscreens may aid in preventing acute and chronic overexposure to the sun's rays.

Various types of surgery may be performed to correct older skin conditions, but they won't work for everyone. Among some of the more common types of surgery are *plastic surgery, dermabrasion* (skin planing), *chemosurgery* (chemical cautery), *cryosurgery* (freezing of the skin), and *electrosurgery* (employing electricity). See *Plastic and Cosmetic Surgery,* p. 402.

Hearing Loss

About three out of ten persons over age 65 have some hearing loss; at age 70 to 80 this percentage increases greatly.

Causes

While some hearing loss can be blamed on bad listening habits (tuning out people and conversation a person does not want to hear), the two major causes are *conduction loss* and *nerve defects.* A person with conduction loss hears high-pitched sounds best; a person with nerve impairment hears low sounds best. A combination of the two is called *mixed deafness.*

Conduction loss can be caused by wax, diseases of the ear, disturbances of the eardrum, or abnormalities inside the ear. It can also be caused by *otosclerosis,* a bony growth over the window to the inner ear. Most of these conditions can be treated by an ear doctor (*otologist*). He can remove wax from the ear, repair or replace eardrums, remove bony growths, and loosen or remove fixed ear bones.

Nerve defects may be another story. They are caused by wear and tear on the ear, disease, certain drugs, and blows and skull fractures, and usually cause permanent damage that cannot be helped by surgery or medical treatment.

Some persons complain about ringing in the ears (*tinnitus*) that may start without warning and vary in intensity and quality. What causes tinnitus in one person may not cause it in another, but often it is caused by wax in the ear, middle ear infection, arteriosclerosis, or certain drugs.

Hearing Aids

In some cases, a hearing loss may be helped by a hearing aid, but be sure your doctor refers you to a hearing clinic. A recent National Health survey showed that most persons over 65 bought their aids directly from a hearing aid dealer rather than from a physician or a hearing aid clinic. Many of these older people discontinued using their hearing aids after buying them.

Be sure your doctor thinks a hearing aid will help you and directs you to a nonprofit hearing aid clinic. You can get addresses from your community health organizations or by writing to the National Association of Hearing and Speech Agencies, 919 Eighteenth St., N.W., Washington, D.C. 20006, or to the American Speech and Hearing Association, 9030 Old Georgetown Rd., Bethesda, Md. 20014.

At a hearing aid clinic, trained *audiologists* will scientifically measure your hearing and will assist you in trying on several kinds of hearing aids. These audiologists do not sell aids, but will give you an idea of what kind is the best for you.

Basically, there are four kinds of aids:

• Body types operate by a cord running to the receiver mold in the ear from a miniature microphone carried in a pocket, pinned to the clothing, or worn in a special carrier.

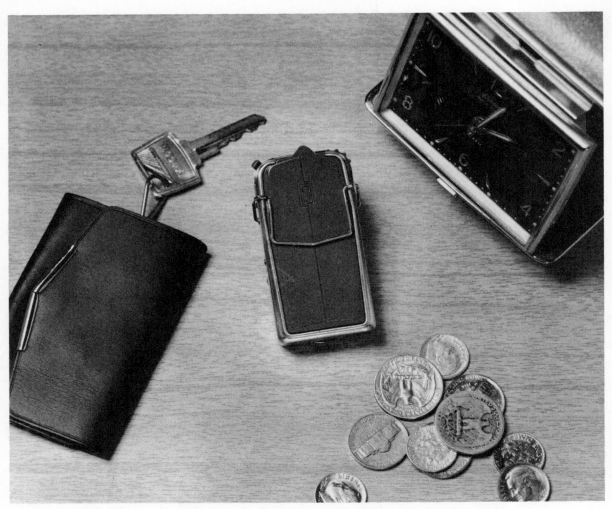

Shown here with other articles to indicate its size, this microphone is carried in a pocket or special case. It is equipped with a cord that runs to a receiver in one ear.

They are about 1 to 1½-inches long and weigh about 2 ounces.

• Behind-the-ear types weigh only about ½ ounce and fit behind the ear. A plastic tube leads from the microphone to the receiver which fits in the ear.

• In-the-ear types are almost invisible. But they are not as powerful as other aids, and they may be affected by dirt, wax, or perspiration.

• Eyeglass models are built into the temple piece of spectacles. The bigger the temple piece the more powerful the aid.

The Veterans Administration, which annually tests aids, points out that there is no

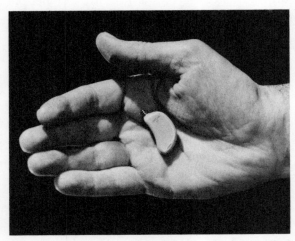

This aid tucks behind the ear and conveys amplified sounds by means of a thin tube to the ear opening.

best hearing aid for all individuals. "Aids that test well for one person may not test well for someone else."

Buying a hearing aid: One good way to test an aid is to have a friend or relative along when you are being fitted. A familiar voice provides a yardstick to help you judge which aid is best.

It takes time to get used to a hearing aid. An aid amplifies all sounds—wanted and unwanted. Voices may sound unnatural or tinny. Normal sounds may be harsh and brutal—mainly because the patient is not used to them and cannot tune them out. However, the maximum power outlet of a hearing aid is below the threshold of pain, and will not amplify sounds over a certain level. Also, special circuiting in some aids limits the sound level reaching the eardrum. Nevertheless, every person who wears an aid must go through some adjustment process.

If a person does not want to wear an aid or cannot adjust to one, he can try lip reading or speech reading. This involves watching the lips and vocal cords to determine what the person is saying. While you may not catch every word that is spoken, you will be able to understand enough.

Talking to the hard-of-hearing: If you are talking to someone who has some hearing difficulty, he'll understand you better if you speak slowly and distinctly and use the lower range of your voice. Face him when you speak; let him see the movements of your lips. It also helps to point to visible objects.

Above all, don't shout. In fact, raising your voice sometimes pitches it into a higher frequency which a hard-of-hearing person may find difficult to understand.

Other Health Problems

The following health problems might also confront an older person. (Many of these conditions are discussed at greater length elsewhere in the book; in such cases, cross-references are supplied for your convenience at the end of the section.)

Heart Disease

The heart is the strongest, toughest muscle in the body. It is like an engine that

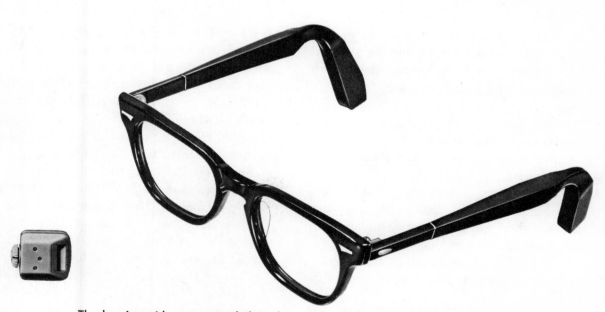

The hearing aids are concealed in the temple pieces of the eyeglasses. The small aid at the left is worn in the ear with no cords, wires, or tubes required.

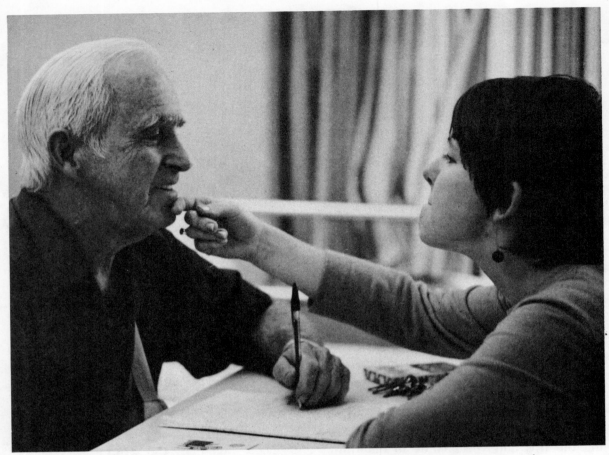

Impairment of mobility caused by stroke can often be corrected to some extent—and sometimes wholly—by therapy. This stroke patient is being given speech therapy.

could run 70 years or more without an overhaul. The heart has a complete maintenance and repair system, enabling many heart disease victims to continue long and useful lives.

While heart disease is not necessarily a product of aging, some heart and blood vessel problems become more acute as one grows older.

The following symptoms do not necessarily indicate heart disease, but it is wise to see a physician if you notice any of them:

• Shortness of breath
• A feeling of tightness in the chest or pain directly related to exertion or excitement
• Swelling of the feet and ankles
• Unusual fatigue.

There is much that doctors can do to prevent heart conditions or to relieve them once present. But there is much that you can do to help yourself. You should watch:

Weight: Extra pounds of fat mean more work for the heart.

Diet: The rules of sound nutrition apply to proper heart care.

Smoking: Heavy cigarette smokers suffer three times as many heart attacks as do pipe or cigar smokers. Nonsmokers are safest.

Exercise: Exercise improves the pumping action of the heart as well as circulation, digestion, and general health.

Worry: Worry increases tension and elevates blood pressure. Try to cultivate a philosophical approach to the daily ups and downs. See *Heart Disease,* p. 500.

Strokes

Strokes are not hopeless; even severely paralyzed patients may make remarkable progress. A *stroke* occurs when the blood supply to a part of the brain tissue is cut off and, as a result, the nerve cells in that part of the brain can't function. When this happens, the part of the body controlled by these nerve cells can't function either.

Whenever the blood supply is cut off from an area, small neighboring arteries get larger and take over part of the work of the damaged artery. In this way nerve cells that have been temporarily put out of order may recover, and that part of the body affected by the stroke may eventually improve or even return to normal.

Once a stroke has occurred, a sound rehabilitation program can help the patient resume as many normal activities as possible. This program can be worked out in cooperation with the doctor, patient, family, and local organizations. See under *Diseases of the Circulatory System*, p. 484.

Arthritis

There are two main types of arthritis: *rheumatoid arthritis* and *osteoarthritis*.

Rheumatoid arthritis—which can cause pain and swelling in joints, nerves, muscles, tendons, blood vessels, and connective tissue in the whole body—can strike at any age, but it occurs mainly in the 25 to 40 year age group.

The exact cause of rheumatoid arthritis is unknown, but it is believed to be a type of reaction similar to an allergy, caused by a bacterial infection.

Osteoarthritis is a degenerative joint disease that affects almost everyone who lives long enough; it is a product of normal wear and tear on the joints over the years. Poor posture and obesity are contributing causes, as are heredity and trauma.

Osteoarthritis is usually mild, and it seldom cripples. Pain is generally moderate.

Unlike rheumatoid arthritis, which is inflammatory, spreads from joint to joint, and affects the whole body, osteoarthritis confines its attack locally to individual joints. Rarely is inflammation a problem.

Osteoarthritis is likely to develop in any joint which has been required to take a lot of punishment or abuse: the knee or hip joints of someone who is overweight; joints injured in an accident; joints injured or overused in sports; joints subjected to unusual stresses and strains in work or play; joints with hidden defects that were present at birth.

There is no specific cure for arthritis, but the pain and swelling can be controlled. In other than acute cases, common aspirin has proved the safest and most popular medication.

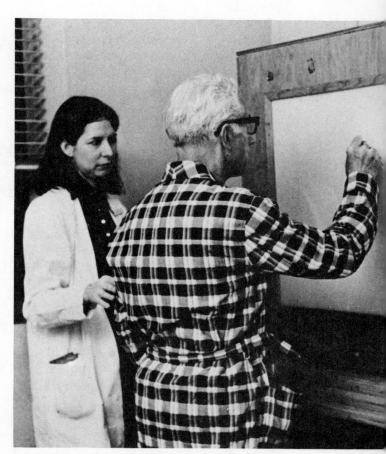

Having suffered a stroke that affected his right arm, this patient is practicing better hand coordination.

Adequate rest for both the body and the affected joint is a fundamental treatment. Heat, controlled exercise, hydrotherapy, and massage are all effective if done under a doctor's supervision. See under *Diseases of the Skeletal System*, p. 448.

Cancer

Cancer strikes at any age, but it does strike more frequently in the later years. Many factors are believed to contribute to cancer: frictional and chemical irritations like cigarette smoking, irritation of the skin and mouth (such as poor dentures), exposure to the sun, X rays, or radioactive elements. Common sites are the lips, mouth, stomach, intestines, rectum, liver, lungs, breast, kidney, bladder, skin, uterus, and prostate.

Early detection and prompt treatment are the best protection against cancer. If any of the following seven danger signals lasts longer than two weeks, be sure to get a checkup:
- Unusual bleeding or discharge
- A lump or thickening in the breast or elsewhere
- A sore that does not heal
- Change in bowel or bladder habits
- Hoarseness or cough
- Indigestion or difficulty in swallowing
- Change in wart or mole.

Great strides have been made in treating cancer through surgery, *radiotherapy*, and *chemotherapy*. See *Cancer*, p. 609.

The Eyes

The eye does age. After age 40, failing vision is usually caused by natural hardening of the lens, making it difficult to see close objects. However, failing vision may also be the first symptom of a serious bodily disorder, or of glaucoma or of a cataract, which requires a physician's immediate attention.

Both glaucoma and cataract can be treated effectively. About 90 percent of

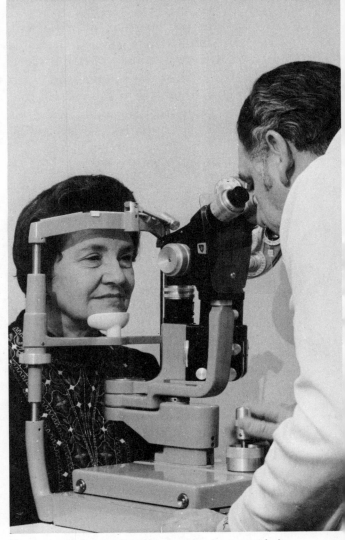

The patient is being given an eye examination with the aid of a biomicroscope, or slit lamp, which provides highly concentrated illumination and magnification.

glaucoma cases can be checked with eye drops and about 95 percent of cataracts can be removed by a painless operation.

Other diseases that may develop in later years affect the blood vessels of the eye. A common condition is *senile macula degeneration* which causes a blind spot to appear when the victim looks directly at something. The exact cause of senile macula degeneration is not known. See under *Diseases of the Eye and Ear*, p. 584.

Diabetes

Most likely candidates for diabetes are overweight persons past 40, particularly those who have a hereditary history of diabetes, and especially older women.

The exact cause of diabetes is not known, but it is a functional disorder in which the body cannot handle certain foods—mainly sugars and starches. Symptoms include increased thirst, constant hunger, frequent urination, loss of weight, itching, easy tiring, changes in vision, and slow healing of cuts and scratches.

Treatment and control consist of planned diet, exercise, and, in many cases, insulin shots or oral medication. Well-controlled diabetics can lead active lives. See *Diabetes Mellitus*, p. 573.

Constipation

There is no truth in the notion that a daily bowel movement is necessary for good health. A movement every day or twice a day may be all right for one person; for another every three or four days may be enough.

The two most common causes of chronic constipation are physical inactivity and poor food and water habits. Ironically, constipation may be caused by swallowing a *cathartic* nightly to induce a bowel movement. The habit eventually leads to chronic constipation because normal bowel movement ceases and bowel evacuation depends on using a cathartic.

To maintain proper bowel movement, try the following:

• Drink eight to ten glasses of water a day. Take two glasses of water on an empty stomach as soon as you get up.

• Drink more fruit juices and eat more dried and fresh fruits.

• Get at least one-half hour of moderate exercise daily. Walking, for example, is excellent, particularly if you relax while you walk.

• Give yourself enough time for normal bowel movement and set up a regular time for evacuation.

• If you are constipated, consult your doctor to make sure it is simple and functional. See under *Aches, Pains, Nuisances, Worries*, p. 430.

Back Problems

As we grow older, the back muscles—weakened by inactivity, poor posture, and almost unavoidable wear and tear—start to complain.

Other causes of back problems are muscle and joint strain, changes in the spine, psychological tension, and internal diseases. Here are some tips to help avoid backache:

• Learn to lift correctly. Use your leg muscles, which are stronger than back muscles, by placing your feet closer to the base of the object, bending your knees outward, and pushing up with your legs.

• Avoid subjecting your back to any sudden, erratic motion.

• Try to improve your posture when sitting and walking.

• Sleep on a firm bed; a bed board may be helpful.

• Get regular exercise of a type that stimulates all your muscles rather than just a few.

• If you have to sit for a long period, get up and stretch occasionally.

• Beware of excess weight. Extra weight on the abdomen pulls on the vertebrae at the small of the back, increasing the spine's normal curve and causing pain.

• Try never to become overfatigued or exhausted, either physically or mentally. Emotional pressure, from work or personal problems, causes muscle tension. See *Backaches*, p. 415.

The Feet

Since the feet are farthest away from the heart's blood supply, they are often the first areas affected by circulatory diseases. Also,

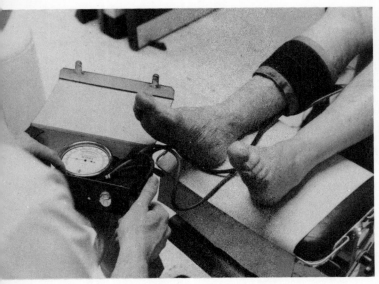

Measuring blood circulation to the feet can be valuable in the diagnosis of some circulatory disorders.

arthritis and diabetes might first show up in the feet.

Warning signs include continued cramping of the calf muscles, pain in the arch and toes, and unusually cold feet—especially if accompanied by a bluish skin. Brittle or thickened toe nails or burning, tingling, and numbness may also signal a circulatory disease.

Foot ulcers may be one of the first signs of diabetes. Some *bunions*—swollen, tender, red joints—are caused by arthritis. Swelling around the foot and ankles suggests a possible kidney disorder.

If you have any of these symptoms, go to a *podiatrist* (a foot doctor) or to your own doctor. They are trained to recognize these symptoms.

Most older people, however, suffer from minor aches and pains in the feet that are caused by poor foot care or abuse. See *The Vulnerable Extremities*, p. 421.

Care of the Feet

To prevent these problems, treat yourself to daily foot care.

Dry your feet thoroughly and gently after bathing and inspect the skin for abrasions, rough spots, or cracks. Dry carefully between the toes. If the skin is dry or scaly, lubricate it with lanolin or olive oil. Next, apply a medicated foot powder recommended by your doctor over the entire foot, especially between the toes, as a preventive measure against athlete's foot.

When you cut your nails, do it with a strong light and be careful to cut straight across the nail to prevent ingrown toe nails. Avoid the use of strong medications containing salicylate and strong antiseptics like iodine, carbolic acid, lysol, or bleach. Harsh chemicals that attack toughened skin can irritate normal tissue and cause infection. Avoid using hot water bottles, electric pads, or any form of extreme heat or cold. Diabetics should visit a podiatrist regularly.

The Prostate

Men over 50 may have an enlarged *prostate*—but this is *not* caused by sexual excesses or venereal disease. The exact cause is not known, but it's estimated that some type of enlarged prostate is present in about 10 percent of 40-year-olds and 80 percent of 80-year-olds.

The prostate is a rubbery mass of glands and muscle tissue about the size and shape of a horse chestnut. It is wrapped around the urethra and base of the bladder at the point where they join. The prostate functions as part of a man's sexual apparatus, providing a fluid that transports and nourishes the spermatozoa.

Symptoms of an enlarged prostate include difficulty in urination. There might be an initial blocking of the urine, or the stream may lack force. You may feel that you can't empty the bladder, and you may have urgent needs to urinate. You may have pain or blood in the urine from straining.

If you have any of these symptoms, your doctor can easily check for enlarged prostate by a simple rectal examination. If he discovers an enlargement, he can usually treat it in early stages with simple massage.

But if it has progressed too far, he may have to operate.

An operation is usually performed through the urethra or by an incision in the lower abdomen. The choice depends upon the individual problems of the patient and the judgment of the surgeon. In either case, the patient usually recovers completely in a short time.

A rectal examination can also discover early stages of cancer of the prostate, which is not uncommon in men over 40. Some 20 percent of men over 60 have this condition, and it is most common in men over 70.

Unfortunately, this disease does not manifest itself early, so it is most important that older men have the diagnostic rectal examination. If the disease is detected early and treated—usually by surgery, hormonal therapy, and possibly radiation—the cure rate is very high. If found late, the cure rate is low.

When treatment is by surgery, the entire prostate and upper urethra may be removed. In some cases, the disease may be retarded or relieved by treatment with female hormones. (The male hormone is known to hasten prostate cancer.)

In both enlargement and cancer of the prostate, early detection is vital to a successful cure. That is why it is important to have a rectal examination.

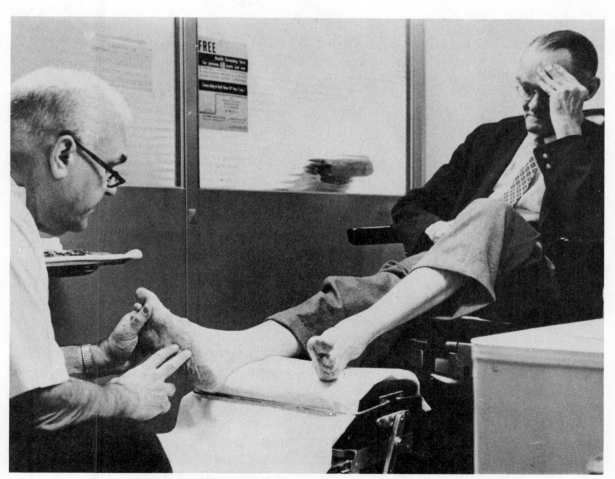

Although many older people experience minor aches and pains in their feet due only to poor foot care, unusual or very uncomfortable symptoms may be warning signs that require the attention of a podiatrist.

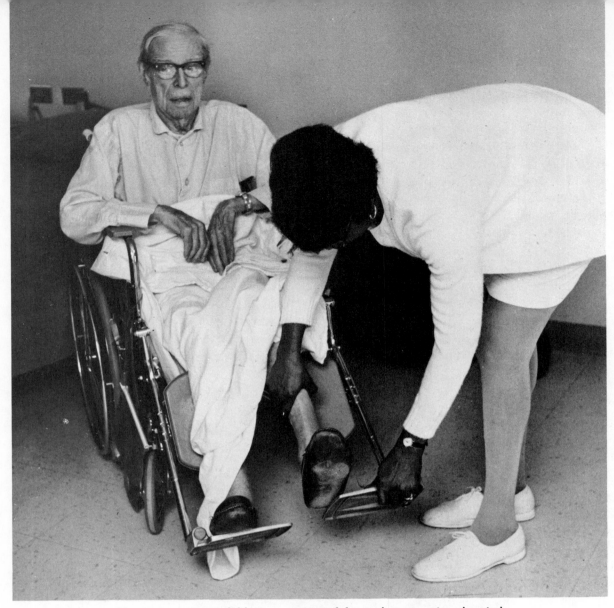

Nursing care is available in a variety of forms: home nursing, hospital care, and nursing homes. Medicare can help pay for some of these costs.

Financing Medical Care

Older people have recourse to many community facilities and programs, all aimed at easing the financial burden of medical care.

There are over 2,000 hospitals, visiting nurse associations, and similar agencies eligible to provide benefits to persons over 65 under Medicare. Those under 65 may also receive aid, although arrangements for payments will differ.

All such agencies provide skilled home-visiting nursing service and one or more additional services, such as physical therapy, occupational therapy, medical-social services, or homemaker-home health aide services.

The Visiting Nurse Service provides a full slate of nursing services: bed baths, injections, physical therapy, diet and nutrition guidance, and related professional nursing services. Costs, averaging around $18–$20 per visit, are adjusted to the patient's ability to pay; fees may be covered by public welfare funds or health insurance benefits.

There are more than 800 agencies in all providing Homemaker-Home Health Aide service in forty-nine states and Puerto Rico. This service offers specially trained women who handle any marketing, cooking, serving, and cleaning requirements of the client.

Many major cities provide a Home Delivered Meals program often sponsored by the women's auxiliaries of county medical associations. This is a catering service for the ill and handicapped confined to their homes. Wholesome, balanced meals are delivered to the homes of the handicapped persons whose finances are slim; those receiving this service pay a minimum fee for the food.

The American Dental Association has entered the home-care program by developing portable equipment for home dental service and dental school programs to train undergraduates in the care of elderly, home-bound patients, and by setting up central-service headquarters and supply departments—usually at a hospital, dental clinic, or state health department.

For those who are able to pay moderate dental costs but can't stand a heavy financial strain, the dental profession has set up prepaid dental care by establishing non-profit dental service corporations similar to the programs sponsored by Blue Shield and Blue Cross.

Your family doctor should be aware of these community programs. In many cases, your doctor must request the service. He receives regular, periodic reports on your condition.

Also, practically every metropolitan area in the United States and Canada has an Information and Referral Service, usually staffed by the United Crusade or Welfare Department. This service answers many questions, such as how to locate a nursing home or borrow a wheelchair, where to find a doctor or a hospital to meet a specific need, and other inquiries of that nature. To find the number of your Information and Referral Service, consult your local telephone directory.

Medicare and Health Insurance

Medicare offers free hospital benefits to persons 65 and older and optional medical benefits for $7.20 a month (as of July 1, 1976).

As of January 1, 1976, the hospital insurance program pays the cost of covered services for the following hospital and post-hospital care:

• The first 60 days in a hospital (except for the first $104), and all but $26 per day for an additional 30 days for each spell of illness

• A lifetime reserve of 60 additional hospital days if you need more than 90 days hospital care in the same benefit period and all but $52 a day

• Up to 20 days in an extended care facility and all but $13 per day for an additional 80 days for each spell of illness—services provided only after a hospital stay of at least 3 days

• Up to 100 home-health visits by nurses or other health workers in the 365 days following your release from a hospital or extended-care facility.

If you sign up for optional medical benefits under Medicare, you agree to pay a premium of $7.20 monthly. The medical insurance will pay 80 percent of the *reasonable* charges for the following services after the first $60 in each calendar year:

• Physicians' and surgeons' services

• Home-health services even if you have not been in a hospital—up to 100 visits a year

• A number of medical and health services, such as diagnostic tests or treatment and certain services by podiatrists.

Benefits have been steadily expanded—some new provisions include coverage for medical equipment needed in your home, provisions for doctors' unpaid but itemized bills to be sent directly to Medicare for payment.

When you reach 65, you are automatically qualified for free hospital benefits.

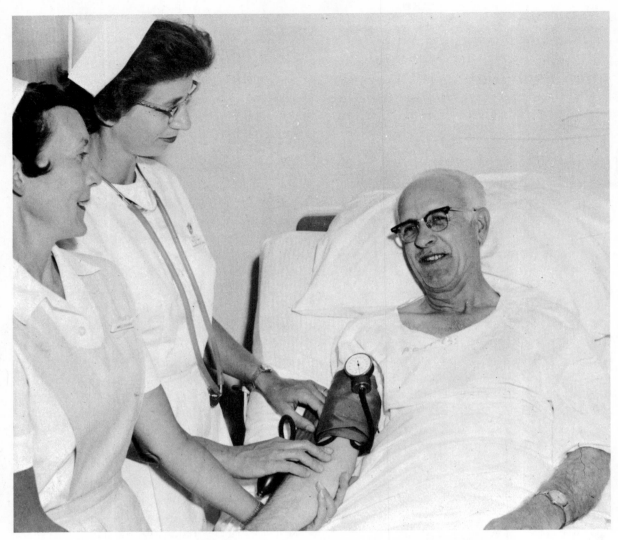

Free hospital benefits through Medicare are available to all persons 65 years and over. Optional medical benefits are also included at a small monthly charge.

You may sign up for the optional medical benefits during the first three months of any calendar year (January to December) after your 65th birthday. To sign up for these benefits, or for further information, contact your nearest social security office.

Private insurance companies offer policies to fill some of the gaps in Medicare coverage and to supplement provisions. Check with your local insurance agent or write to Health Insurance Institute, 277 Park Avenue, New York, N.Y. 10017 for further information.

Nursing Homes

While Medicare pays most of the cost of 100 days in an extended-care facility, you must be referred after a 3-day hospital stay. If your condition—or that of a friend or relative—requires a longer stay in a nursing home, you are faced with different circumstances.

First, there is a confusion of terms. "Nursing home" can mean almost any type of facility that provides some sort of health or custodial care short of that offered by a regular hospital. Thus, convalescent homes, homes for the aged, rest homes, geriatric hospitals, senior care homes, and many other euphemisms all may be loosely classified as nursing homes.

The services they offer vary from skilled nursing and medical attention to strictly personal service. The confusion in terminology has become so great that responsible professionals in the field of health care have recommended that the term "nursing home" be erased from our vocabulary. Others feel that eliminating it might cause even more confusion.

Choosing a Home

Thus, picking the right home for the patient is not easy. The first step would be to have your physician recommend a place suited to the patient's condition. If you are in doubt or if you do not have a family physician, try your local health and welfare or community service agency. Sometimes, these agencies have a referral service that can direct you to a nursing home.

You could also try the Family Service Association or your county medical society. Another source of information is your state affiliate of the American Nursing Home Association, 1101 17th St. N.W., Washington, D.C. 20036.

The next step would be to visit the home, if possible. Try to find out as much as you can about the qualifications, staff, and services they offer. The American Nursing Home Association suggests you ask these questions:

• Is the facility licensed by the state or local government? Avoid an unlicensed home.

• What level of nursing care is provided? It should have a Registered Nurse or Licensed Practical Nurse on hand for both day and night shifts.

• Is there a staff physician who spends some time at the nursing home? Can a patient have his own physician? Does the

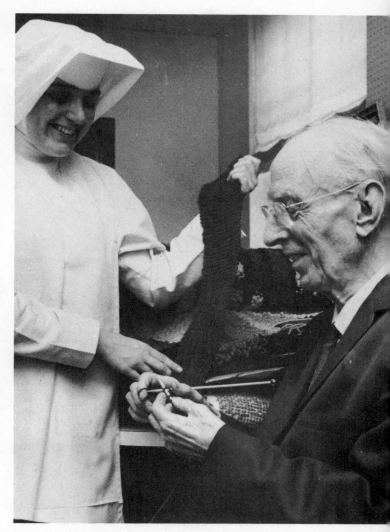

Factors to consider in selecting a nursing home include cost, quality of medical and nursing care, state or local licensing, expenses, and religious affiliation.

home make a special effort to keep physicians advised of their patients' conditions?

• Does the home have an organized program of diversional activities? What does it include? Are arrangements made for the religious life of the patient?

• What provisions does the home make for visiting patients?

• What facilities are there for rehabilitation and physical therapy?

• Are nursing personnel and other staff members trained in motivation and rehabilitation techniques?

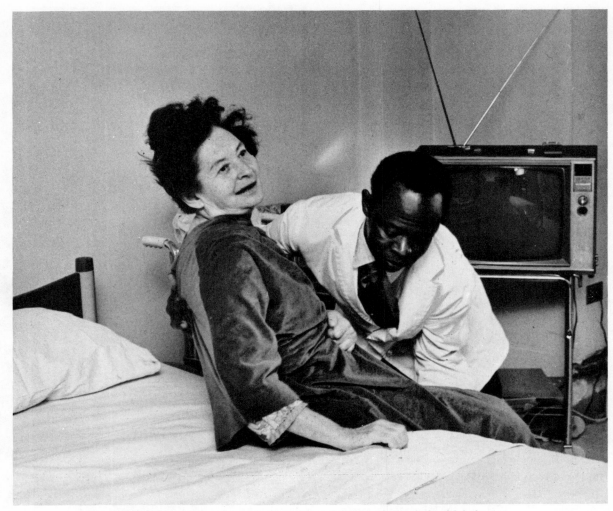

A visit to a nursing home before the patient is admitted should help answer questions about the quality and standards of nursing care. Some homes offer excellent personal service but little in the way of nursing care.

• Does the home have arrangements with a nearby hospital for easy transfer of patients? Is emergency transportation readily available?

• Does the home maintain a planned menu at least a week or two in advance? Are there arrangements for handling patients who require special diets?

• Is the place basically safe? It should have an automatic sprinkler system, be fire resistant, or have an automatic alarm system. It should have escape routes in case of emergencies, and it should have grab bars and rails in hallways and bathrooms.

Also, ask about the food service and dental care. The place should have a general homelike atmosphere rather than a cold, institutional look.

Costs

Most important: *find out about all costs!* Generally, expect to pay about $7,000 to $12,000 a year for a good place ($600 to $1,000 a month) for room, board, and nursing care. You may be charged extra for doctor calls ($10 to $30 a month); drugs ($10 to $50 a month). Also, extra charges may be made for special diets, extra nursing care, personal services (shampoos, haircuts, and shaving).

What about tips? Strange as it seems, tipping is a fact of life in many nursing homes. Wages are low, and many staff personnel rely on tips to provide good service. Have a frank talk with the administrator about tipping—it could make a big difference in the service you receive.

In some cases, you might get financial aid to pay part of the cost. As noted above, Medicare could pay part of the tab if the patient was referred to the home from a hospital. Second, check with your local welfare or public assistance office to determine whether you are eligible for assistance under the Medical Assistance for the Aged program or the Medicaid program. It's *not* always necessary for an individual to be drawing public assistance payments to be eligible for one of these medical assistance programs.

Finally, check with any fraternal organizations you might belong to—they may have their own facilities—and if you are a veteran, check with the Veterans Administration office, or call one of your local veterans organizations for addresses and phone numbers.

Frauds and Quacks

It is estimated that older people spend over $2 billion a year on unnecessary health supplements—worthless electronic devices, skin lotions and cosmetics, and other false products purported to aid health.

Tragically, many claims of quacks and their worthless remedies—particularly in respect to cancer—are death warrants for people who might have been saved had they gone to reliable sources soon enough.

The American Medical Association provides a list to help in spotting quacks. A practitioner may be a quack if he:

• Uses a special or secret machine or formula

• Guarantees a quick cure

• Advertises or uses case histories and testimonials

• Clamors for medical investigation and recognition

• Claims medical men are persecuting him

• Tells you that surgery, X rays, or drugs will do you more harm than good.

For a discussion of emotional problems of the later years, see *Meeting the Challenge of Leisure*, p. 274.   PAD

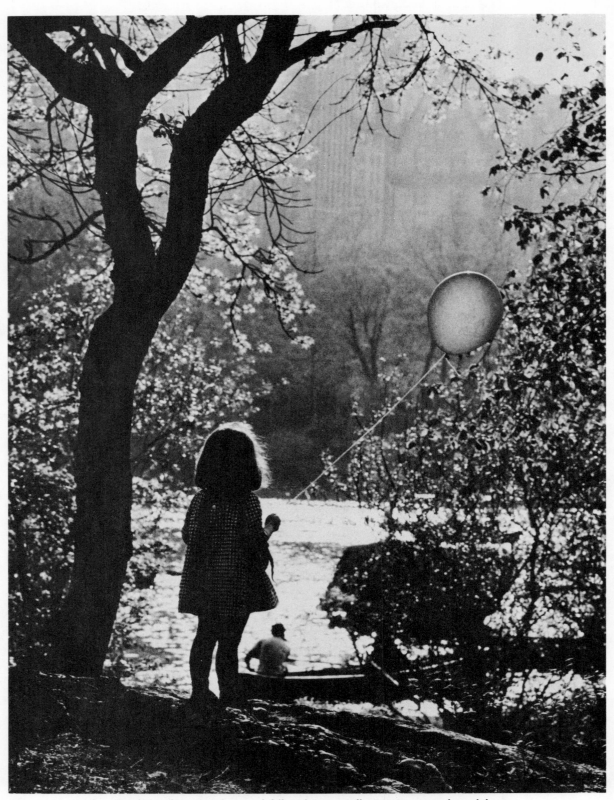

Emotional development during childhood is crucially important to the adult years.

CHAPTER 3

Feeling Good: Maintaining Emotional Health Through the Years

The ability to adapt is central to being emotionally fit, healthy, and mature. An emotionally fit person is one who can adapt to changing circumstances with constructive reactions and who can enjoy living, loving others, and working productively. In everyone's life there are bound to be experiences that are anxious or deeply disturbing, such as the sadness of losing a loved one or the disappointment of failure. The emotionally fit person is stable enough not to be overwhelmed by the anxiety, grief, or guilt that such experiences frequently produce. His sense of his own worth is not lost easily by a setback in life; rather, he can learn from his own mistakes.

This chapter deals with emotional and intellectual development at various ages. See Chapter 2 for a discussion of physical development at these age levels.

Communication and Tolerance

Even the most unpleasant experiences can add to one's understanding of life. Emerg-

ing from a crisis with new wisdom can give a sense of pride and mastery. The emotionally fit person can listen attentively to the opinions of others, yet if his decision differs from that being urged by friends and relatives, he will abide by it and can stand alone if necessary, without guilt and anger at those who disagree.

Communicating well with others is an important part of emotional fitness. Sharing experiences, both good and bad, is one of the joys of living. Although the capacity to enjoy is often increased by such sharing, independence is also essential, for one man's pleasure may leave others indifferent. It is just as important to appreciate and respect the individuality of others as it is to value our own individual preferences, as long as these are reasonable and do not give pain to others.

Ways of Expressing Disagreement

Communication should be kept open at all times. Anger toward those who disagree may be an immediate response, but it should not lead to cutting off communication, as it so frequently does, particularly between husbands and wives, parents and children.

Emotional maturity enables us to disagree with what another says, feels, or does, yet make the distinction between that person and how we feel about his thoughts and actions. To tell someone, "I don't like what you are doing," is more likely to keep the lines of communication open than telling him "I don't like you." This is particularly important between parents and children.

It is unfortunately common for parents to launch personal attacks when children do something that displeases them. The child, or any person to whom this is done, then feels unworthy or rejected, which often makes him angry and defiant. Revenge becomes uppermost, and communication is lost; each party feels misunderstood and lonely, perhaps even wounded, and is not likely to want to reopen communication. The joy in a human relationship is gone, and one's pleasure in living is by that much diminished.

The Function of Guilt

The same principles used in dealing with others can be applied to ourselves. Everyone makes mistakes, has angry or even murderous thoughts that can produce excessive guilt. Sometimes there is a realistic reason for feeling guilty, which should be a spur to take corrective action. Differentiate clearly between thoughts, feelings, and actions. Only actions need cause guilt. In the privacy of one's own mind, anything may be thought as long as it is not acted out; an emotionally fit person can accept this difference.

The Role of the Subconscious

Emotional disorders are similar to other medical diseases and can be treated by doctors or other professionals just as any other disease can be treated. Fortunately, this truth is widely accepted today, but as re-

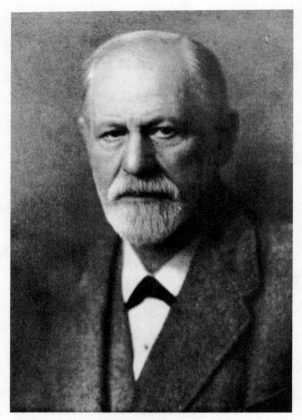

Sigmund Freud (1856–1939) taught that memories stored in the subconscious mind influence the individual's mental life and can cause mental illness. Freud's method of treatment is called psychoanalysis.

cently as 200 years ago it was believed that the emotionally ill were evil, possessed by the devil. Their illness was punished rather than treated. The strange and sometimes bizarre actions of the mentally ill were feared and misunderstood.

Freud and Psychoanalysis

Although we have penetrated many of the mysteries of the mind, much remains to be discovered. Significant steps toward understanding mental functioning came about through the work of Sigmund Freud. Building upon the work of others before him and making his own detailed observations, Freud demonstrated that there is a subconscious part of the mind which functions without our awareness.

He taught that mental illness resulting from subconscious memories could be cured by *psychoanalysis,* which brings the memories out into consciousness. He believed that dreams are a major key to the subconscious mind and that thoughts, dreams, fantasies, and abnormal fears follow the rules of cause and effect and are not random. This is called *psychic determinism,* meaning that emotional disorders can be understood by exploring the subconscious. *Psychiatrists* help the patient understand how his mind works and why it works that way—often the first step toward a cure.

Does psychic determinism rule out will power as a function of the mind? No, because the subconscious is only one part of the mind. Although it has an important influence, there are other forces influencing behavior and thought: the *id,* or instinctive force, the *superego,* or conscience, and the *ego,* or decision-maker. The more we know about how our minds work, what underlies our wishes and thoughts, the more control we can exercise in choosing how to behave in order to achieve our goals.

Role of Sexuality

Freud discovered that young children and even babies are aware of the sensations, pleasurable and painful, that can be experienced from all parts of the body. The sexual organs have a rich supply of nerves; the baby receives pleasure when these organs are touched, for example, during a bath or a diaper change. The child learns that when he touches these organs he obtains a pleasant feeling; therefore he repeatedly touches and rubs them (*infantile masturbation*).

This concept, that the child derives pleasure from his body and sex organs, is called *infantile sexuality.* It does not mean that the baby has adult sexual ideas or wishes. These do not develop until puberty. It *does* mean that parents have the responsibility to see to it that children learn early that sex is associated with tenderness and love between man and woman. Even young children are aware of what their parents do and how they treat each other.

Treating Emotional Problems

When should help be sought for an emotional problem? Sometimes individuals themselves realize that they need help and seek it without urging. They may have symptoms such as anxiety, depression, or troublesome thoughts that they cannot put out of their mind. But many others who need help do not know it or do not want to know that they need it. They usually have symptoms that disturb others rather than themselves, such as irritability, impulsive behavior, or excessive use of drugs or alcohol that interferes with their family relationships and work responsibilities.

Other people in need of psychological guidance are those who have a physical disease that is based on psychological factors. They react to stress internally rather than externally. Instead of displaying anger, they feel it inside. We are all familiar with headaches or heartburn caused by tension; more serious diseases clearly associated with emotional factors are asthma, certain skin disorders, ulcerative colitis, essential hypertension, hyperthyroidism, and peptic ulcer. Other physical symptoms that may be related to psychological factors are some types of paralysis, blindness, and loss of memory.

In all these situations the patient's enjoyment of life is curtailed. He has no feeling of control over what he does and little or no tolerance for himself and others. Such an existence is unnecessary today, with the many agencies and specialists capable of treating these problems.

Who can help those with emotional problems? Confusion about the different professions in the mental health field is understandable. To add to the muddle, self-appointed counselors without professional

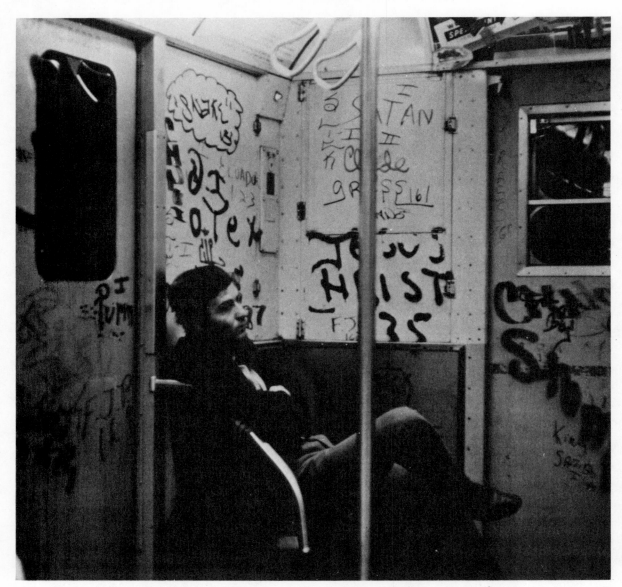

Life in the big city, with its noise, dirt, and impersonality, can contribute to mental depression. Fortunately, many kinds of help and therapy are available.

training and experience have set themselves up in this field, so it is necessary to know whom to consult to obtain the best help possible.

Psychiatrists

Psychiatrists are medical doctors; that is, they have graduated from a medical school, served internships and afterwards residencies specializing in emotional disorders. They are specialists in the same way that a surgeon or an eye doctor is a specialist. Most are members of the American Psychiatric Association. They are experienced in treating medical illnesses, having done so for many years before being certified as specialists in emotional disorders. Generally they can be relied upon to adhere to the ethical and professional standards of the medical field.

The American Psychiatric Association, 1700 18th Street, N.W., Washington, D. C.

20009, can supply the names of members. The American Board of Psychiatry and Neurology, 1603 Orrington Avenue, Evanston, Illinois 60201, examines and certifies psychiatrists who pass its tests, so that the term "board certified" means that the psychiatrist has passed its tests. If a family doctor is consulted about an emotional problem, he will often refer the patient to a psychiatrist, just as he would to any other specialist.

Psychologists

Psychologists have gone to college, majored in psychology, and sometimes have advanced degrees, for example, a doctorate in psychology. They are not medical doctors and may get a degree in psychology without ever working with a human being, e.g., by working in animal behavior, experimental psychology, or other fields. They may or may not have clinical training, but many acquire this training and experience with human beings. There is no guarantee that a psychologist has this background without looking into the qualifications of each individual.

Psychotherapy

Psychotherapy is the general term for any treatment that tries to effect a cure by psychological rather than physical means. A psychotherapist may be as highly trained as a psychiatrist, or he may be a psychologist, or may even have no training at all. Anyone can set up an office and call himself a psychotherapist, psychoanalyst, marriage counselor, family therapist, or anything else he desires. It is up to the patient to check on the training and background of a therapist. Any reputable therapist should be pleased to tell patients his credentials and qualifications for helping them. A psychoanalyst, for example, may by a psychiatrist with several years of additional training in psychoanalysis, or may be someone such as a social worker with a few college psychology courses.

Social Workers

Social workers are another group of trained persons who may also counsel those with emotional problems. They may work either with individuals, families, or groups after meeting the educational requirements for the profession, which include a bachelor's degree and two years of professional training leading to a master's degree in social work.

Professionals should be associated with recognized groups of their peers, or perhaps with a medical center or hospital. Generally a person with emotional problems should consult a psychiatrist first, who will then either treat the problem or be in a good position to advise what is necessary and who can best be available for treatment.

Treatment

There are many types of treatment available, from tranquilizers, to psychotherapy, psychoanalysis or counseling, group therapy, and so on. The psychiatrist is best able to decide what is needed.

What can be expected from treatment? Does a person who has been through treatment emerge bland, uncaring about others, with absolutely no problems, and without guilt for his misdeeds? Absolutely not. What treatment can do, said Freud, is to change neurotic misery into common unhappiness. There will always be things in life that are disappointing or otherwise upsetting. No treatment can eliminate such problems. After successful treatment, however, one should be better able to handle these stresses with flexible and constructive responses and to see his own difficulties in relation to the problems of others.

To feel emotionally fit is to have a capacity for enjoyment of life, working well, and loving others. Fears, shame, and guilt about undergoing needed treatment should not prevent anyone from reaching that potential.

JJC, RWC

DEVELOPING AN AWARENESS
OF THE WORLD:
THE FIRST DOZEN YEARS

Until about the beginning of the twentieth century, little attention was paid to emotional development in infants and children. The years of childhood were felt by most to be a time of peaceful, idyllic innocence, with the main tasks considered to be those of learning to be an adult. Children were felt to be miniature adults without special needs, feelings, or impulses; they were supposed to be seen and not heard.

The last half century of research on children has clearly shown the crucial importance of emotional development in childhood and has shown further that much of an adult's emotional makeup is accounted for by his emotional development as a child. This work has also revealed that children have special needs, feelings, and impulses that are sometimes similar to, sometimes quite different from those of adults. These

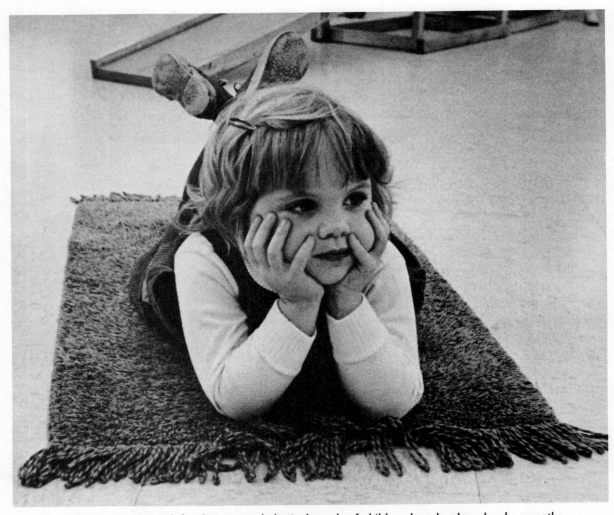

An understanding of the distinct psychological needs of children has developed only recently.

needs, feelings, and impulses also differ at various stages and ages during a child's development.

Infancy

During a child's first year he needs a warm and loving emotional environment in the home. It is during this time that a child establishes what psychiatrists and psychologists call basic trust. That is, he learns to be a trusting individual who feels that his important needs—those of being cared for, fed, and comforted—will be met by other human beings, initially by his mother.

Emotional needs: Such activities as holding and cuddling the infant, talking to him, and playing with him in an affectionate, relaxed way are important for his emotional growth. Experiments with animals have shown that if the infant animal does not get sufficient cuddling and physical contact from its mother during its early development, it is unable to perform adequately as an adult later in life. It has also been shown that infants growing up in an environment lacking warm, loving, close physical and emotional contact with a mother or a mother-substitute often fail to thrive and may even die.

Fondling and Sucking

During the first year, most of an infant's satisfactions and gratifications are through his skin's perception of being touched—through physical contact with his mother and other caring adults—and through the mouth, especially sucking. Infants have a great need to suck even when they are not hungry, and this sucking should be both allowed and encouraged.

Mothers frequently worry that if they respond to a baby's crying by picking him up they will spoil him, and the baby will cry often in order to get attention. In general, it could be said that during its first year an infant cannot be spoiled. When an in-

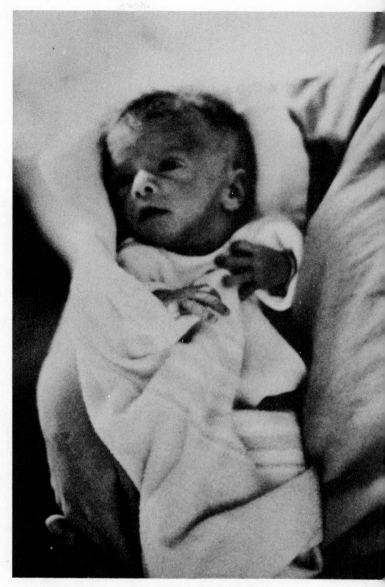

Cuddling and close, frequent, physical contact are as vital as food itself if the infant is to thrive and develop the basic trust that his needs will always be met.

fant cries he usually does so because he is uncomfortable, hungry, sick, or needs some physical attention.

Social Responses

As he matures one of a child's tasks is to begin to see himself as separate from the world around him. During early infancy, the infant does not see himself as an individual who is separate from his mother, from other adults, and from the rest of the world. But, gradually, sometime within the first year of life, this feeling of separateness and individuality begins to emerge in the developing infant.

One of the important and gratifying events in the early months of a child's life is the smiling responses. For the first time the infant can respond in a social way to other human beings. It is often at this time that the infant's mother and father begin to think of him as a real person and an individual. Thus the smile could be considered one of the infant's first social communications.

Suspicion of Strangers

Somewhere around the age of eight months, an infant who has in the past without complaint allowed anyone to pick him up begins to distinguish his mother from other individuals. When picked up by another the infant usually cries, acts frightened, and, in general, looks unhappy. This response indicates that he can now tell his mother and other individuals apart—an important and normal step in an infant's development.

Fear of separation: Sometime later, usually around the age of one year, the infant begins to become fearful upon separation from his mother. When his mother walks out of the room or leaves the baby with a sitter, the child may respond with crying, fear, and anger. This again indicates that the infant can now tell his mother from strangers and does not like being separated from her. Although the response is normal and usually subsides within three to four months, parents should learn to leave the child in the hands of a competent sitter, and walk out without guilt or anger. The child must learn that separations are temporary and that parents do return.

The Second Year

It is during the second year of a child's life that he begins to develop independence and separateness from his mother. Beginning with his growing ability to walk, usually sometime early in the second year (age

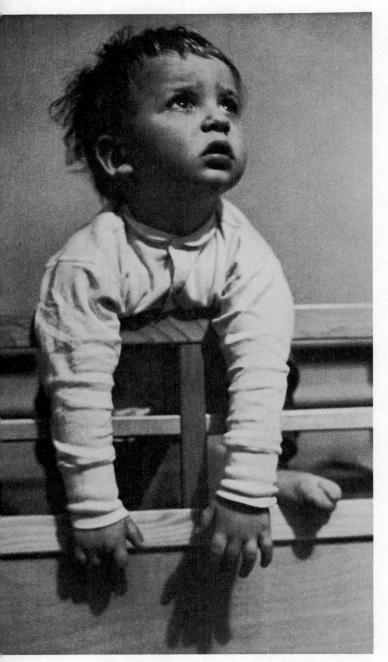

Fear of strangers and of separation from parents is common toward the end of the first year. The child will gradually realize that separations are temporary.

12–16 months), an infant starts to explore the world around him more actively. He experiments with greater and greater distances and increasing independence from his mother.

Towards the end of the second year, children frequently become quite independent, trying to do many things for themselves, and resenting their mothers or other well-meaning adults doing things for them. Even if the child is not yet capable of performing the tasks he attempts, he should be encouraged in these early moves toward independence. It is also during the second year that speech begins to develop, with the first words usually being "ma ma," "da da," "milk" and that ever-present word, "no."

The Third Year

The third year is extremely important. Children are usually toilet trained, show marked growth in their language abilities, and demonstrate a continuing and growing independence.

Toilet Training

Toilet training is an important step in the life of an infant. Generally, children do not have muscular control over their bowel movements and urination until about the age of two, so attempting to toilet-train a child much before this is usually wasted effort. If it is accomplished, the result is usually a training of the mother rather than of the infant. Toilet training should usually take place sometime between the age of two and three and one-half.

Training can usually be facilitated by praise from the parents for putting the bowel movement and the urine in the proper place, rather than by punishment. Excessive punishment or the threat of it usually results in anger on the child's part and increasing stubbornness and resistance to toilet training. Praise immediately following

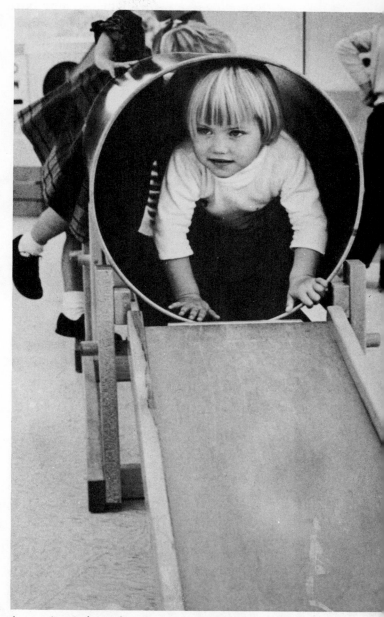

A growing independence and interest in the world around him marks the three-year-old child, who is usually ready for a play-group or nursery school.

the proper performance of the act is far more effective in encouraging compliance with the parents' goals.

Negativism

From two to about three and perhaps beyond, a child is extremely negative. When asked to do anything or when asked about anything, he often responds by saying, "No, no, no, no, no." This saying of the word "no" on the slightest provocation indicates a child's wish to become separate and independent from parents, to do what he wants to do when he wants to do it, and to be free from the control of others.

The child's desire for independence can be respected and encouraged by parents within limits, but this does not mean that a parent must give in to a child on every issue. A parent should try to determine what is really important and not make an issue over petty matters that can best be handled with relaxed good humor.

Language Development and Play

A rapid spurt in language development takes place at this time. A child may increase his vocabulary from about 50 words at the beginning of the third year to an almost countless vocabulary at the end of the third year. It is during this year, too, that children first show marked interest in imaginative play activities. Play, including making up stories, using toy trucks and cars, blocks, dolls, and toy furniture, is vital activity for children and should be encouraged by parents. It is through play that children express their feelings, often feelings that cannot be expressed in ordinary ways. The child also experiences what it feels like to be an adult by playing the role of doctor, fireman, policeman, teacher, mother or father. In addition, during play children discharge tensions and learn to use their muscles and bodies.

Exploring the Body

From very early infancy, all children show a strong interest in their own and in other's bodies. During infancy this takes the form of playing with his own and his mother's body. A baby puts his fingers in his own mouth, in his mother's mouth, ears, eyes, and pats her on the tummy or on the breast. An infant also explores and touches his own body, including the genital region. This interest is normal and need not be discouraged.

The Preschooler: The First Separation From Mother

During the ages of three and four, the preschooler develops increasing interest in the world around him, in children his own age, and in himself. One of the key problems

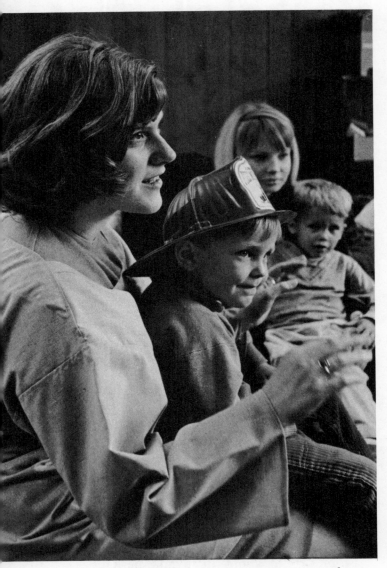

Let's-pretend games are an important part of growing up, permitting a child to experience what it might be like to be a fireman, teacher, or mother.

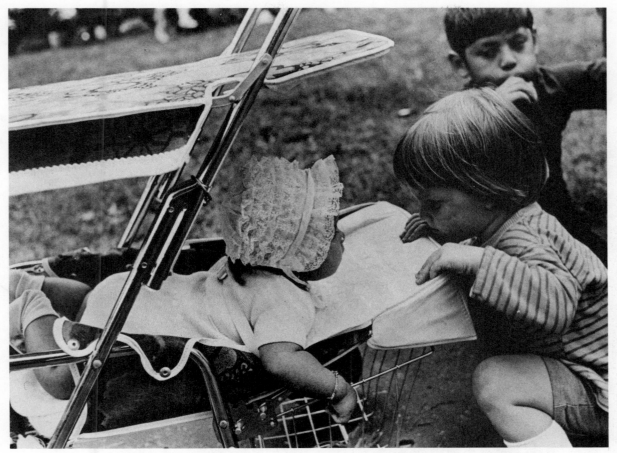

Young children are naturally curious about each other and the world around them. A stroll in the park provides a fine opportunity to strike up a new friendship.

that the preschooler has to deal with is his impending separation from his mother when he becomes old enough to go to school. This can often be made less painful by arranging for the child to spend at first short and then increasingly longer periods of time away from his mother. By using baby-sitters both in the evening and during the day, by later having the child spend three or more half-days a week at a pre-school, and lastly by enrolling him in kindergarten for either all day or half a day, five days a week, the mother can ease the child's adjustment to the world outside the home.

Although his first nearly full-time separation from mother is difficult for the child, it may be difficult for the mother as well.

Mothers often feel that this initial separation from their child will eventually lead to their child's growing up and leaving home. Parents are often nostalgic and somewhat regretful about their children's first going off full time to school. The child's fearful anticipation of a strange situation can be eased by a mother's anticipating school with the child, talking with him about it and reassuring him regarding his fears of abandonment or separation.

A word might be mentioned here concerning differences between boys and girls. At the age of five most girls are ready to attend kindergarten; they can sit in their seats for long periods of time, pay attention to a teacher, and be interested in a task. Boys, because of their somewhat slower rate

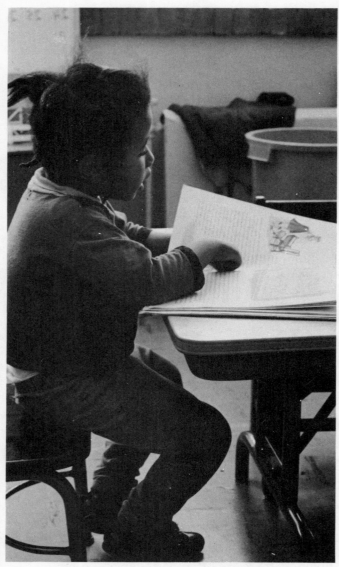

Girls usually mature more rapidly than boys, making it easier for them to sit still and concentrate when they are ready to enter kindergarten at the age of five.

of maturity, are often less ready than girls for coping with a classroom situation at the age of five.

School-Age Children: Parent-Child Relationships

Beginning around the age of four, boys show a decided preference for their mothers. A boy may, for example, tell his mother that when he grows up he would like to marry her and kick father out of the house. At times he may even suggest that he would work to support her and that life would be much nicer if daddy were not around.

This interest in his mother is often expressed in what may be thought of as sexual ways. That is, the child of this age enjoys his mother's affection, including kissing, hugging, and close bodily contact. This wish to have mother all to himself and to have father out of the picture is called by psychiatrists and psychologists the *Oedipal complex,* after the ancient Greek tragedy, *Oedipus Rex,* in which Oedipus kills his father and marries a woman whom he later discovers to be his mother.

At about this same age, similar emotional developments take place in a girl. She will likely be somewhat seductive, coy, and coquettish with her father, and may talk about marrying father (or a man like father) and having mother out of the picture. This phase of emotional attachment between a girl and her father is called the *Electra complex* after the Greek play, *Electra.*

At these times, both the girl and the boy have a strong, although not always conscious, wish to displace the parent of the same sex and have the opposite-sexed parent all to themselves. Strong conflicts disturb children in this phase of development, for they also realize that they love and need the same-sexed parent to instruct them, to guide them, to provide for them, and to love them.

Identification

Both males and females eventually resolve these conflicts by abandoning their so-called sexual attachment to the opposite-sexed parent, forming a closer attachment to the same-sexed parent and trying to be like that parent. This is not a conscious decision, but one that a child makes without realizing it. This process of *identification* with the parent of the same sex starts very early, perhaps as early as the second year, and continues through adolescence, but it is especially noticeable from five to ten.

Much of the energy that had previously been utilized in loving the parent of the opposite sex is now spent in loving the parent of the same sex. The boy follows father around, wants to do whatever he does, and holds as his greatest ambition to be exactly like father when he grows up— even to marry a woman like the one father did.

The girl during this same period spends the energy that was once expended in love for her father in an attempt to learn to be

like mother and perhaps eventually to marry a man resembling in some way her father. This, however, does not mean that children do not continue to love the opposite-sexed parent; it means only that their primary attachment during these years is to the same-sexed parent. It is this process of identification with the same-sexed parent that facilitates the chief task of the school-age child from 5 to 11: the task of learning.

The years from 5 to 11 have generally been regarded as quiet years as far as emotional development is concerned. Many of the tasks of earlier childhood have been completed, and the relatively stormy years of

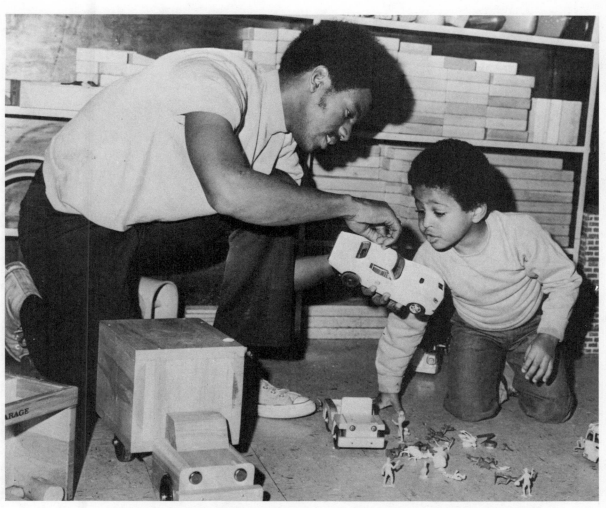

Between the ages of five and ten the identification that children feel for the parent of the same sex becomes especially obvious; this emulation helps the child's emerging self-image.

adolescence have not yet begun. A child's interests begin to turn more and more away from his family and to other children his own age, usually children of the same sex. At this stage, a child's interest in learning is broad and intense.

Discipline

There are no easy answers or sure guides to the discipline of children; but there are some basic principles that, if followed, can make life together more enjoyable and tolerable for parents and children alike. All children, whether they be normal, retarded, geniuses, sick or well, need and want discipline in their daily lives, even though they will say, when asked, that they would rather do as they please. From time to time almost every parent has been jolted to realize that his only interactions with his children seem to be when he is nagging them to do something or reprimanding them for doing something wrong.

The Effect of Praise

One of the most important principles of discipline is that praise is more effective than punishment. As has been noted by many students of human behavior, children crave attention from their parents. In order to gain this attention, they will behave in

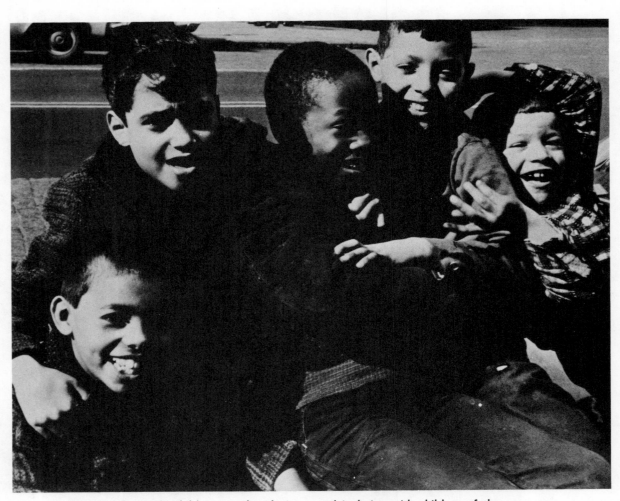

The "middle-aged" child is most keenly interested in being with children of the same age and sex. This is an emotionally stable age, but rivalry between the sexes can cause tensions.

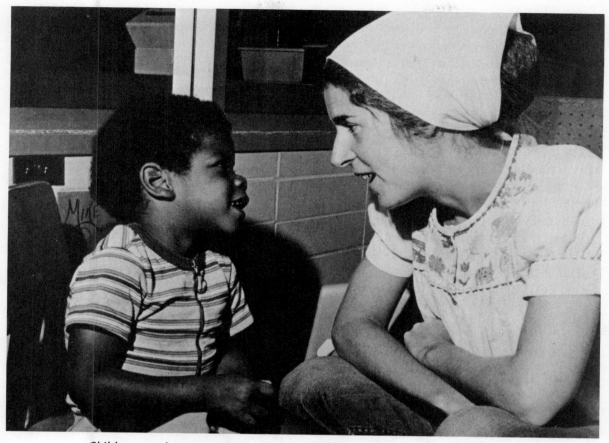

Children need a sympathetic adult listener to share their joys and sorrows.
If both parents have to work, a teacher or day-care worker can help fill the role.

any way necessary; if misbehavior is the only action that receives attention, the child misbehaves. Parents should make a point of being attentive to their children when they are behaving properly and should reinforce good behavior with praise. The result will usually be an increase in good behavior and a decrease in misbehavior.

Basic Principles

In order for discipline to be effective, a number of other principles should be remembered.

Consistency: Consistent discipline is important. Children should know what is expected of them and should know what the consequences of their misbehavior will be. Once a promise or threat is made, it should be carried out. Failure to carry out a

threat encourages a repetition of the undesirable behavior. Failure to carry out a promise may cause the child to lose faith in the parent.

Physical punishment: Severe physical punishment should be avoided. Ideally, punishment should be carried out because it has an instructional value for the child rather than because it helps a parent relieve his or her feelings of anger or frustration. Severe physical punishments—for example, the use of sticks, belts, or hard blows to the body—are extremely frightening and may even be permanently injurious to the child. Frequently, this kind of discipline can evoke even further anger on the part of the child and lead to further misbehavior.

Duration: Punishments should not be long and drawn out, but should be as immediate as possible and last only a reasonable length of time. For example, withdrawal of television privileges for a month for a seven-year-old's misbehavior would be excessively long, because at the end of the month it would be difficult for him to remember what he had done that was wrong. Excessively long punishments are also difficult to enforce. If possible, a punishment should be related to the misbehavior for which the child is receiving the punishment.

Immediacy: Punishment "when father gets home" or a day later frequently has little meaning for the child and is unlikely to help him stop misbehaving. Rewards for good behavior should also be immediate; affection and approval for most children are often more powerful rewards than candy and money.

Thoughts vs. Deeds

Children often feel as guilty about bad thoughts as they do about bad deeds. After being angry, a child may feel as badly about having had a fleeting wish to hurt his mother as he would have felt had he actually hurt her. A child should be helped to understand that his thoughts are his own, that his thoughts cannot harm anybody, and that he will not be punished for his thoughts. He should understand that it is only actions of certain kinds that cannot be

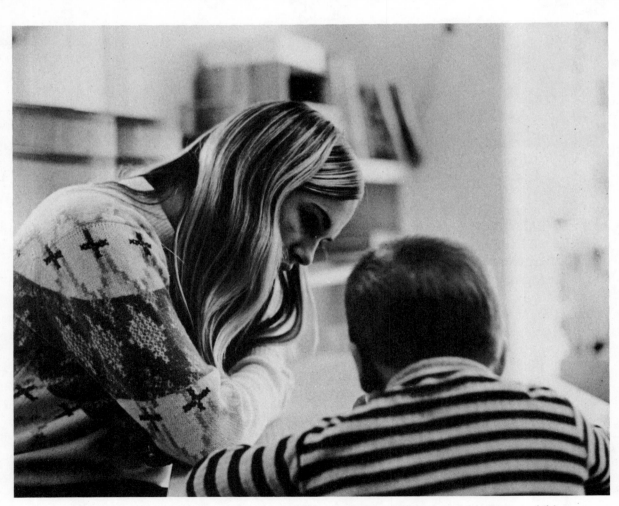

Parents and children should understand the differences between thoughts and actions. A child should not be made to feel guilty for wishing harm; he is responsible only for his deeds.

allowed and that will result in a reprimand or punishment. In other words, a child should not be made to feel guilty for angry or aggressive thoughts toward other members of his family, but only for angry and aggressive acts.

A parent might say to a child, "I understand that you really disliked your brother when you hit him, in fact, even hated him and would have liked to hurt him. It's okay for you to be angry with him, but I am not going to let you hurt him." This could be called the principle of accepting the feelings that the child has but not accepting his actions.

Especially Stressful Situations for Children

There are a number of occasions which may subject a child to unusual stress. One of the most difficult of these is hospitalization.

Hospitalization

Most children at some time in their first 15 years of life require at least one hospitalization, ranging in time from a few days to many months. This is a frightening experience and may leave permanent emotional scars on a child. Parents can do many things to make the experience less harmful.

Hospitalization for an operation or an illness affects children at different stages of their development in different ways. Very young children are particularly worried about the separation from their mother. Parents can help with this fear by assuring a child that he will not be separated permanently from his mother.

If at all possible, it should be arranged so that the child's mother or another member of the family is with the child much of the time he is in the hospital. Of course, during an extended hospitalization this becomes very difficult. Barring accidents, children should always be forewarned of a hospitalization, for if they are not, they feel

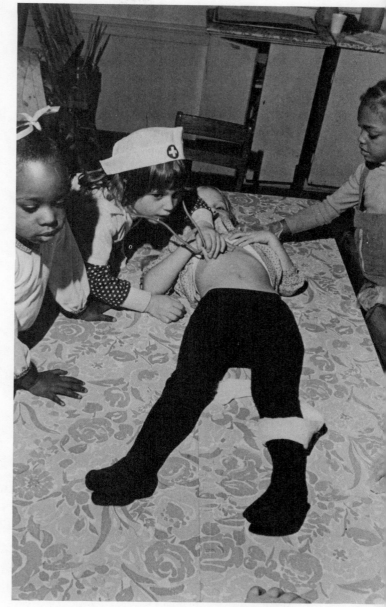

Young children's fears of doctors and hospitals can be minimized by letting them act out the roles of doctor, nurse and patients in a play situation.

that they have been deceived by their parents and lose trust in them.

Children of about 4 to 10 or 11 are more worried about possible damage or mutilation to their body than they are about separation from their family. They often have unrealistic fears that a part of their body is going to be cut out or in some way permanently harmed. They often feel that when they come back from the hospital they will not be the same as they were when they went in. Matter-of-fact reassurance by parents can be helpful in alleviating these fears.

Older children, ages 10, 11, and 12, often fear the anesthetic that goes along with an operation. Again, reassurances by the parents and the providing of opportunities for the child to talk of his fears can prevent anxieties from getting out of hand.

Other Upsetting Situations

In general, children, as do adults, prefer stability and constancy in their home environment. Emotional upsets often occur around changes in the regular routine. Some of the changes that especially bother children are: separations from parents; divorce and consequent separation from one of the parents; illnesses or deaths in the family; transition points in a child's life—for example, starting school; moves from city to city; changes in schools; the birth of a new sibling.

Although these kinds of changes are difficult for children to manage, they are part of life and children will cope with them if they are discussed openly. Children should be given an opportunity to express their feelings about them without punishment or disapproval.

Sex Education

Children need and deserve to have access to correct information about sexual functioning. If there is a natural openness in a family about questions of all types, children first start asking questions about sex when they are three or four; it is then that parents can begin describing sexual functioning to their children.

The first questions about sex usually have to do with the functioning of body parts. For example, children want to know where urine comes from, what happens to food when they eat it, where feces come from, and where babies come from. Explanations should be given in a straightforward, unembarrassed manner. Children should not be overloaded with information that they do not understand, but parents should be willing to answer questions to the best of their ability.

With older children, particularly 11- and 12-year-olds, it is often helpful for sexual questions to be answered by the parent of the same sex. Reading a book on sexual development together with the child can be a good experience for both parent and child. Parents frequently wonder if sex education may not lead children to engage in experimentation. Most of the evidence on this question indicates that children are more likely to experiment sexually when they are ignorant than when their questions about sex are reasonably and accurately answered.

The Retarded Child

In recent years scientists have begun to understand more about mental retardation, its causes, and its treatment. Evidence of severe retardation usually is seen in a child's first year, often taking the form of delayed developmental landmarks—for example, late sitting, late standing, late walking, and delayed talking. If retardation is suspected by parents, medical advice should be sought immediately and a thorough evaluation of the child conducted. Some types of retardation can be greatly benefited by medical and educational treatment. It should be emphasized that all retarded children can learn and that many can be helped to the extent that they can become productive citizens.

For a description of the physical development of the child during the first dozen years of life, see *Birth, Infancy, and Maturation*, p. 99.
                                                    GKF

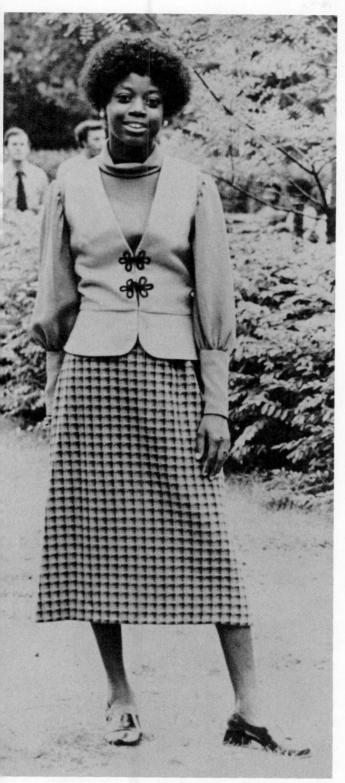

Seemingly poised and confident on the outside, adolescents are frequently troubled by conflicts that can seem to them to be both overwhelming and unique.

SOCIAL AND SEXUAL MATURATION: THE TEENS

The Prospect of Adulthood

As a youngster passes from childhood into adolescence, it is the psychological adjustments rather than the physical changes that are most likely to produce difficulties. The emotional problems, of course, are related to the hormonal activity of the developing body. However, the conflicts which frequently are upsetting to both the adolescent and other members of his family are the result of adjustments which must be made between the young person and the society in which he must live.

In certain primitive cultures, for example, the boy becomes an "instant adult" by undergoing puberty rites. There may be no restrictions on sex play between boys and girls; the girl does not have to be concerned about dating procedures because her parents select her husband. There is no question about economic independence; the young couple becomes a part of the economic unit of the parents.

In our own culture, the teen-ager must continually adjust to a complex set of rules and regulations. He frequently may feel that he must accept the responsibilities of adulthood before he is entitled to the privileges of being treated as an adult. Childhood is only a step behind, but he has learned to suppress or ignore childhood relationships. He can easily forget the point of view of children and even resent the ability of his parents to recall the "cute" incidents of his earlier years. At the same time, he may be startled by the suggestion that within a few short years he and his teen-age friends will face the selection of a career, marriage, establishment of a home, and a lifetime of responsibilities he may feel ill-prepared to assume.

Future Outlook for Girls

For a girl, the future is somewhat more complex than it was for her mother at the same stage of life. In her mother's day, a teen-age girl might look forward to a brief period of work as a secretary, store clerk, or factory hand between the day of her high school graduation and her wedding day. After the wedding, there followed a couple of decades or more of being a housewife and mother. Today's teen-age girl can still follow the pattern of her mother's life. Or she can plan a lifetime professional career as a doctor, lawyer, or scientist. She can compete with men as a business executive, writer, or aquanaut, and she can schedule marriage and motherhood to complement rather than compete with career goals.

Future Outlook for Boys

The adolescent boy also has a wider choice of goals. He may or may not follow in his father's footsteps. If he decides to join a family business venture, the chances are that he will go to college and contribute a working knowledge of computer techniques or tax laws to the accumulated experience and business contacts his father acquired by starting as an apprentice and working for many years.

Advanced Education

The educational requirements for the jobs of tomorrow place an added strain on the pace of growing into adulthood. Although going steady may begin at an earlier age for both sexes, marriage may have to be postponed until the boy and girl have completed college, which may include the time needed for an advanced degree. An alternative is marriage and the start of a family while the boy and girl are still in college and dependent economically upon their parents. Also complicating the relationship is the matter of the boy's military obligation. The couple must decide whether to get

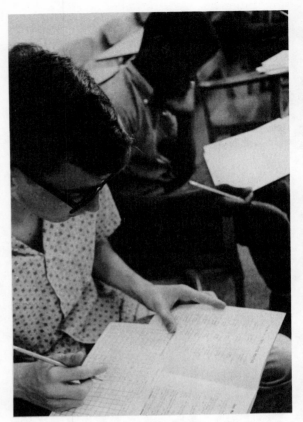

Tomorrow's careers require educational preparation that frequently results in postponement of marriage.

married before the boy's induction into military life or postpone the wedding until he has been discharged. Either choice can mean a long period of physical separation at a stage of life in which the natural wish is to live together and start a family.

Need for Independence

Just as natural as the boy-girl relationships of the teen years are the needs for independence and privacy. Sometimes a youngster feels it necessary to demonstrate a mind of his own by taking independent action, although such action could be considered as rebellion against parental authority. A recent survey showed that a girl may go steady with a boy, not because she really likes the boy that much but to prove she is capable of handling a relationship which her parents have criticized. Carried to a sometimes tragic extreme is the compulsion of a boy or girl to marry a person the parents dislike in order to demonstrate so-called independence. The wise parent will avoid efforts to force a young person into a position in which the alternatives are a surrender to the will of the parents or an action such as a premature marriage that might have unfortunate consequences.

Conflicts Between Parent and Teen-Ager

Some conflicts between the generations are avoidable. The parents may be protective and slow to cut the apron strings because they love their children and want to prevent them from becoming involved in unhappy situations. The teen-ager resents the overprotective actions of the parents, regarding them as evidence that they do not trust their own children.

What parents should try to make clear to their children is that they are offering their years of experience as guidelines. Teen-agers should value the counsel of more experienced members of the family; they should cooperate by listening to the adult viewpoint. If, after serious consideration of the parents' point of view the youngster still wants to make his own decision in the matter, it should be understood that he may have to accept the responsibility for the consequences. A keystone in the training for adulthood is the concept that being an adult consists not only of privileges and the authority to make decisions; along with decision-making goes a responsibility to the family and society for the consequences of one's decisions.

Few parents, of course, would refuse to bail out a teen-age son or daughter in real trouble. And even when a youngster is rebellious enough to leave home, he should know that the door will always be open to him when he decides to return. Again, limiting the options available to a teen-ager can lead to a snowballing of bad decisions and resulting complications.

In many cases, the conflicts between parents and teen-agers derive from the illusion that a younger child has more freedom of choice. A small child may actually seem to have a freer choice of friends he can bring into his home and the games he can play with them. But there are always limitations to a child's choices, and parents are more understanding of the bad choices by attributing mistakes to the fact that "he's only a child."

Older youngsters become involved in situations in which the decisions are more important. A boy and girl at the age of five can "play house" together in an atmosphere of innocence. However, the same boy and girl could hardly suggest to their parents that they intended to play house at the age of 15. If the boy and girl, although next-door neighbors, are of different social or ethnic backgrounds, they may become aware of parental prejudices in addition to new rules of propriety as they grow into their teen-age years.

Decisions of the teen years can involve the use of tobacco, alcohol, owning an automobile, handling of money, overnight trips with friends, association with friends who use drugs illegally, and relationships with members of the opposite sex. The consequences of all alternatives should be outlined for the adolescent.

Search for Identity

Part of the youngster's struggle for independence will involve what sometimes is described as a search for identity. A child accepts without much questioning that he is a member of a certain family and lives in a certain neighborhood. But as he grows older, he becomes aware of his status in the family as well as the status of his family in society. A seven-year-old could not care less about the background of his family or that of his second-grade friends. As he becomes a teen-ager he learns that such subjects may be matters of concern to parents and their circle of friends. He may imitate the attitudes of his family or disregard them, perhaps inviting criticism that he is rebellious.

More important to the youngster, however, is a growing concern about his position and role in life and where it may lead. He is still in the so-called formative years and is sensitive to countless influences in the world about him. Teen-agers become concerned with approaching education and career decisions. It is natural for them to identify with older members in the family, teachers, and celebrities.

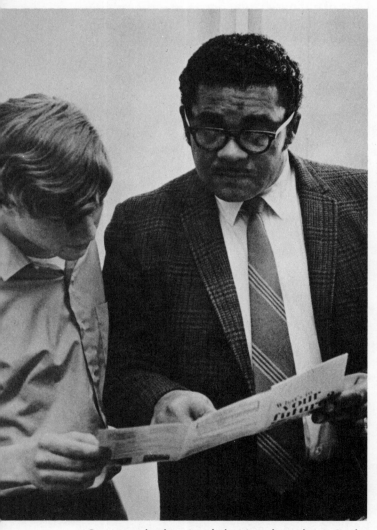

Career and educational decisions loom large in the lives of teen-agers; the advice of respected adults or professional counselors can often provide insight.

Need for Privacy

For the teen-age girl, party invitations, dances, and diaries are important and an increasing amount of privacy is required. Even if she must share a room with a sister, there should be a part of the room which is her territory. She should have personal belongings which are not shared by a parent or sibling. If she has her own room, everything in the room probably will be regarded as her property. Even her mother should respect her privacy by knocking on the door and getting permission to enter her private world.

Although somewhat less sensitive about such matters, boys also are likely to insist on a certain amount of privacy as they grow older. They may share a room with a brother but they need trunks or other containers with locks in which they can keep personal possessions. Proof that such desire for privacy is not a passing fad for young men is found in their adult compulsion for private offices and a den or workshop area at home.

Contacts With Older Friends

Young teen-agers, through part-time jobs as baby-sitters or errand boys, usually come in contact with young adults outside the family circle for the first time. The young adults may accept the teen-agers as peers, which is flattering to the youngsters, who may in turn admire and imitate the young adults. If the teen-ager has been able to identify closely with his family's sense of propriety, the contacts can be a good social experience. But if the youngster has not been able to identify effectively with his parents and family members, he may be vulnerable to misguiding influences. Because of the urge for adult status, the teen-ager may find a premature outlet for testing his abilities to live the adult life in the company of young adults. He (or she) can absorb a lot of information—and misinforma-

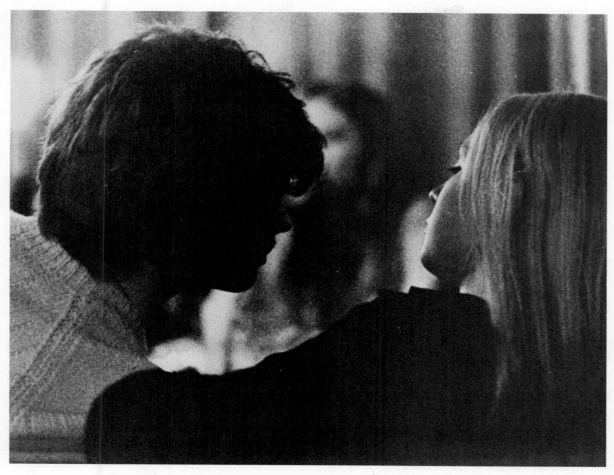

During the teen years, young people begin to develop an interest in the opposite sex. Boy-girl parties and group outings are usually followed by a growing attachment to one person and, often, steady dating.

tion—about sex, alcohol, drugs, and other subjects.

Teen-agers certainly should not be cautioned against contacts with all young adults, but they should have a reliable older person aside from their own parents with whom they can discuss matters they would not discuss with a mother or father. The alternate adult might be a clergyman, the family doctor, a teacher, or even a favorite aunt or uncle. Such an arrangement provides the youngster with a means of learning a bit more about life in an independent manner and from a different point of view than could be obtained within his own immediate family circle.

Relationships With the Opposite Sex

First teen-age contacts with the opposite sex tend to be awkward and sometimes embarrassing despite the best efforts and intentions of parents. The meetings may be at school dances or movie dates, perhaps in the presence of a chaperon who is a teacher or parent.

Overcoming insecurity: Some youngsters will feel more secure than others in social gatherings; those who feel insecure may not participate at all when such opportunities first arise. As the youngsters grow older, however, they find that more and more of their friends are dating or going to dances or parties to meet members of the opposite sex.

Some boys or girls who feel insecure may find that they are more gregarious or less ill-at-ease if they fortify themselves with a couple of drinks of an alcoholic beverage, or with drugs, before they join their friends. Youngsters who feel the need for stimulants or depressants in order to enjoy parties usually can be helped with psychological counseling to overcome their fears of inadequacy.

Young people should be assured that getting together at parties of mixed sexes is a natural thing to do. It has been going on for generations and although an individual youngster may feel ill-at-ease at his first few dances or parties, he probably will survive. As the boy or girl attends more parties the chances increase that he or she will meet a person of the opposite sex who is particularly attractive. If the feeling is mutual, the acquaintanceship may develop into more or less steady dating.

Going steady: Steady dating, which leads to a formal engagement and marriage in many cases, should not be encouraged at an early age or before a young person has had an opportunity to date a number of prospective partners. At the same time, it should not be discouraged to the point of producing a rebellious reaction. As was pointed out earlier, some girls admit going steady with a boy for no other reason than to demonstrate their independence of judgment.

Controlling the Sexual Impulse

Teen-agers who spend a lot of time together at parties, in their homes, or at recreational meetings such as beach outings, are likely to be physically attracted to each other. It may begin with kissing, dancing, holding hands, or simply a natural urge to neck or pet. In more primitive societies, the couple might simply indulge in sexual intercourse without any concern for the possible consequences. But in our own society,

young people are expected to control their natural urges.

Influence of the mass media: Complicating sincere efforts of a teen-ager to make the right decisions in relations with the opposite sex is the constant exposure of youngsters to movies, magazine articles, books, and other media suggesting that sexual relations between unmarried couples is not only acceptable but a common practice. Compared to the image of young love as displayed in movie promotion advertising, a teen-age boy and girl may believe that a few ardent hugs and kisses in a secluded spot may be as innocent as making a plate of fudge together in the girl's kitchen.

Some girls, but not all, are as easily aroused as boys by close bodily contact with the opposite sex. Physical contact for most boys arouses sexual desire, partly because of the physiological makeup of the male. The male impulses are related to the accumulation of sperm in the sex gland region.

The sex drive in boys: Males are so constituted that during periods of abstinence from female contact, their sperm builds up to a level beyond which it is automatically discharged during sleep. The event is called a *nocturnal emission*—in the vernacular, a *wet dream*—and is a normal periodic occurrence among unmarried males. During periods of sperm buildup, the male sex drive is stronger than immediately after the expulsion of sperm-laden semen. There are no standards or averages for the male sex drive; instead there is a wide variety of sexual appetites and abilities.

A girl who cuddles too closely to a boy may trigger a response she did not expect and may not want. Depending upon the boy and the status of his sex drive at that time, he might accept the girl's approaches as a suggestion that she were willing to have intercourse or were at least interested in petting. If the girl is simply being friendly, the results can be embarrassing to one or both of the youngsters. If the boy is the type who likes to discuss the details of his dates with friends, the girl may discover a sudden change in attitude by other boys of the group.

Walking hand-in-hand, or with an arm around the waist, and kissing which is not too passionate usually are acceptable ways for young teen-agers to display affection. And there are activities such as hiking or bicycle riding which afford a boy and girl a chance to be together and apart from the rest of the world. There also are picnics, ball games, movies, and concerts which permit togetherness without setting the stage for hard-to-control sexual impulses.

Masturbation

Another manifestation of the natural sex drives of young persons is masturbation. Prohibited by the rules and regulations of modern society from fulfilling sex urges in the same manner as married couples, teen-agers discover they can find sexual satisfaction in masturbation. Despite the old wives' tales that warn of physical or mental decay for youngsters who masturbate, there is no evidence that the practice is harmful unless the parents make an issue of it.

If there are dangers in masturbation, they are likely to be the isolation and loneliness associated with the practice and the confusion and anxiety which can result if the youngster feels guilty, or is punished or criticized for masturbating. Masturbation is such a natural reaction that most youngsters discover it by themselves even if the subject is never discussed by friends or family members. And like many other matters that seem important during the teen-age years, masturbation usually diminishes as a matter of concern as adulthood is reached.

Sex Education

Since boys and girls in their teens may be capable of producing children and are known to have strong sexual urges, they

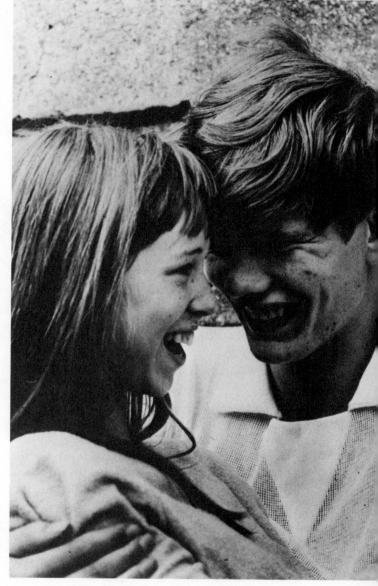

The high spirits of adolescence are reflected in these two teen-agers as they share a moment of laughter.

should be provided with authoritative information about human reproduction and birth control. It is up to the parents to make decisions regarding the proper sources of such information, how much information should be given, and at what age.

One of the reasons for the popularity of sex education in the schools is that teachers can get the parents off the hook by explaining the facts of life to youngsters. However, by forfeiting their prerogative to explain sex and human reproduction to their own children, parents must depend upon the teacher to make an acceptable presentation to the youngsters. The likely alternative is that youngsters will obtain a considerable amount of misinformation from friends and acquaintances at street-corner seminars or by experimentation.

In the days when the majority of the population lived on farms or near rural areas, children learned a few things about sex and reproduction simply by working with farm animals. They learned that cats begat kittens, dogs begat puppies, cows begat calves, and so on. This on-the-job type of sex education also provided farm youngsters with a smattering of genetics, because cross-breeding strains of animals frequently had economic consequences. And it was not too difficult for the rural youngsters to relate their barnyard education to human experience.

Children enrolled in sex education classes in the urban areas of America today receive similar information—dogs have puppies, cats have kittens, etc.—by watching movies and reading books. However, the lessons may be superficial or incomplete, depending upon the teacher and the prescribed curriculum. For example, the children in one eastern school were taught that the baby develops in the mother's abdomen, which led some youngsters to believe the baby lived in the mother's stomach until born. "Why isn't the baby digested by the stomach acid?" asked one confused girl. And when asked how the baby gets out when it's time to be born, the teacher told the students that such questions should be answered by their parents. The point here is that parents should establish some rapport with their children to be sure they are learning a practical set of facts about adult love, sex, and reproduction, including the possible emotional and physical consequences of premarital sexual intercourse.

Although parents may find it difficult or embarrassing to explain the facts of life to their own children, it is one of the most important contributions that can be made to a maturing youngster. At the present time, at least one out of six teen-age girls in the United States can expect to marry a boy-friend so that she will not become an unwed mother. Obviously, thousands of parents and teachers are not providing adequate instruction in sex education subjects.

The Male Reproductive System

Any instruction in the facts of life should begin by use of the proper names for the body parts involved. In the male, the external sex organs are the *penis* and the *testicles,* or *testes.* The penis contains a tiny tube, the *urethra,* through which urine is eliminated. Much of the fleshy part of the penis is composed of spongy tissue. When the penis is stimulated sexually, the spongy areas become filled with blood which makes the penis larger and firm, a condition called an *erection.* The testicles contain male *sperm cells,* also called *spermatozoa.*

THE MALE REPRODUCTIVE SYSTEM

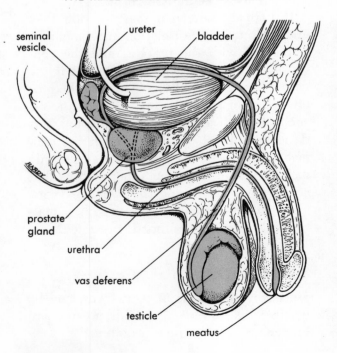

THE FEMALE REPRODUCTIVE SYSTEM

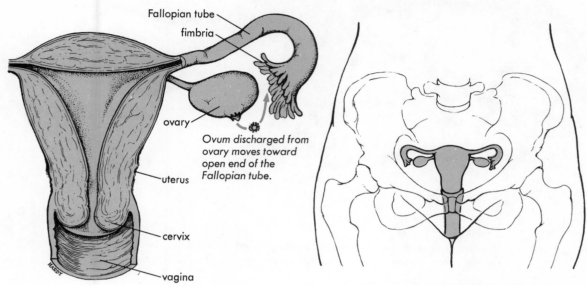

Fallopian tube
fimbria
ovary

Ovum discharged from ovary moves toward open end of the Fallopian tube.

uterus

cervix

vagina

Location of the Reproductive Organs

The sperm travel up tubules inside the abdomen to a storage organ, or reservoir, the *seminal vesicle.* The sperm storage area also contains a thick white fluid called *semen* which is secreted by glands which open into the urethra. One of the glands, the *prostate,* serves partly as a control valve to prevent urine from mixing with the semen, since both are discharged through the urethra. The semen, containing millions of sperm, empties periodically in a more or less automatic action, being squeezed out of the seminal vesicle by pulsating contractions. The contractions and ejection of semen is called *ejaculation.* During the sex act, or *intercourse,* with a female, the semen is ejaculated into the woman's vagina.

The Female Reproductive System

The *vagina* is the proper name for the tubular female sex organ. At the end of the vagina is an opening, called the *cervix,* which leads into the *uterus.* The uterus, or *womb,* is shaped somewhat like an upside-down pear. When a baby develops within the mother's abdomen, it grows inside the uterus. The uterus also is the source of the bloody discharge which occurs periodically during the fertile years of women. When the blood is discharged it is called *menstruation,* or the menstrual period. The menstrual blood passes out through the vagina, which stretches to become the *birth canal* when a baby is being born. The urethra of a female empties outside the vagina.

The menstrual cycle and conception: Unlike the male reproductive organs, which produce perhaps millions of spermatozoa each day, the female reproductive system ordinarily releases only one germ cell, called an *ovum* or egg, at a time. An ovum is released at an average frequency of once every 28 days. It should always be remembered that the 28-day figure is only an average; the actual time may vary considerably for reasons that are only partly known. The cycles are more likely to be irregular for teen-age girls than for mature women. An ovum is released from one of the two *ovaries,* or sex glands, comparable in function to the male testicles, located on either side of the uterus. The ovum or egg is transported from the ovary to the uterus through a *Fallopian tube.*

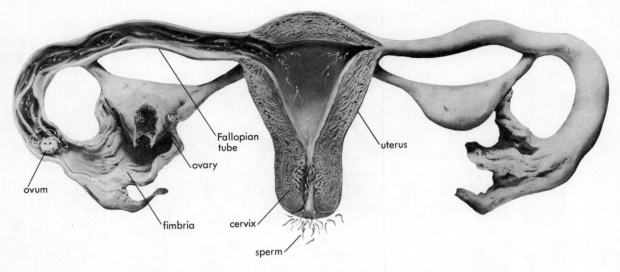

If ovum, released here from left ovary (shown in cross section), meets sperms during passage through Fallopian tube to uterus, fertilization is likely.

If the ovum encounters male sperm during its passage from the ovary to the uterus, there is a good chance that fertilization, or *conception*, will occur through a union of a spermatozoon and the egg. The fertilized ovum, called a *zygote*, soon divides into a cluster of human tissue cells which become the embryo of a baby. For further information about pregnancy, see under *Infertility, Pregnancy, and Childbirth*, p. 141.

During the time that the egg is maturing in the ovary and passing into the uterus after its release, the membrane lining of the uterus becomes thicker because it accumulates blood and nutrients. If the ovum is fertilized, it finds a spot in the membrane where it becomes attached and develops rapidly into an embryo, gaining its nourishment from the blood and nutrient-enriched lining of the uterus. If the ovum is not fertilized, it passes through the uterus, and the blood-rich membrane sloughs off. The blood and some of the cells of the membrane become the discharged material of menstruation. The unfertilized ovum could pass through undetected since it is nearly microscopic.

After menstruation has begun, the female reproductive cycle starts over again. The lining of the uterus once more builds up its supply of blood and nutrients to support a fertilized ovum. Ordinarily, the next ovum will be released about 14 days after a menstrual period begins. If a female does not have intercourse, or avoids intercourse during the time the ovum is released, or in some other manner is able to prevent sperm from reaching an ovum, she will not become pregnant but will experience a menstrual period at intervals which average around 28 days.

When fertilization of an ovum occurs, menstruation ceases and no further egg cells are released until the outcome of the pregnancy has been determined. In other words, the cycles of ovulation and menstruation start anew after the baby is born or the pregnancy has been terminated by abortion or miscarriage.

Contraception

The first rule of birth control is that no method is guaranteed to be 100 percent effective. Sexual intercourse nearly always is accompanied by some risk of pregnancy, and the teen-agers who try to beat the odds should be willing to take the responsibility for the results. Teen-agers should be provided with the basics of birth control as early in life as they are told the facts of life about the human reproductive processes. But the emphasis should be on the relative unreliability of the techniques which do not require a visit to a physician's office. There are many birth control devices and substances that can be purchased without a doctor's prescription. But if young men and women were aware of their chances of effecting a pregnancy while using such methods, they probably would have second thoughts about taking the risk. See under *Marriage and Parenthood*, p. 246, for a full discussion of birth control methods.

Venereal Disease

Equally important in the education of teen-agers is a knowledge of the hazards of venereal disease. A poster prepared for a New York campaign against venereal disease carried the words, "If your son is old enough to shave, he's old enough to get syphilis." The American Social Health Association estimates that 300,000 teen-agers each year become infected with one or more forms of venereal disease. Most insidious has been the recent increase in gonorrhea, partly because girls who carry the infection may show no symptoms. A girl may have a slight but seemingly unimportant vaginal discharge. She may not be aware that she has gonorrhea until she is contacted by health officials after her boyfriend has reported to a doctor for treatment.

Two reasons for the rising incidence of gonorrhea after it was once thought to be virtually eliminated by antibiotics are that condoms, once used as a mechanical barrier by males, have become less popular since teen-age girls have obtained the use of oral contraceptives, and new strains of the bacteria are resistant to the antibiotics. Some boys delay treatment when they realize they are infected with VD; they believe it makes them appear "tough" to be able to go without medical treatment even when

it endangers their health. Because of rebelliousness, youngsters may have a venereal disease and either refuse to tell their parents or boast about it, depending upon which approach they think will make them appear independent.

It is a bitter irony for many parents to realize that their children might carry the spirit of independence and privacy into areas which could endanger their health, for untreated syphilis can result in blindness, insanity, and heart disease. Such grave consequences can be avoided in most cases by establishing effective channels of communication between parents and teen-agers, or between teen-agers and another responsible adult.

The Generation Gap

Despite the attention devoted in recent years to the so-called generation gap, the gap is nothing new to the process of evolving from childhood to adulthood. Every generation has had its generation gap—a period in which the fledgling adult tests his ability to make his own way in the world. In previous eras youngsters were considered old enough to take on an adult role when they were big enough physically. A boy left home to become a farm hand or a factory apprentice. A girl would leave home to become a live-in maid with another family. Sometimes the generation gap was masked by great social upheavals such as a war or a wave of emigration. The fictional hero of many romantic stories is a young man who leaves home to make his own way in the world, discovering in the process a girl who wants to be rescued from her environment. With a few jet-age variations the adolescent boys and girls of today experience the same emotional struggles as nature develops their minds and bodies toward becoming another generation of adults. For a description of the physical development of the child beginning with the onset of puberty, see *Puberty and Growth*, p. 122.   KNA

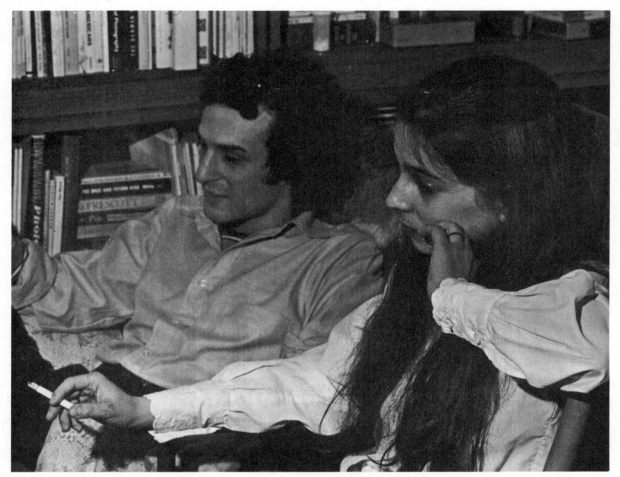

Today's young couples frequently marry before finishing school. While they are physically ready for parenthood, they may not be ready for the added responsibility of raising children.

MARRIAGE AND PARENTHOOD: THE BEGINNING OF A FAMILY

Early Marriage

The average age of young men and women who marry today is nearly five years lower than it was a generation ago. Boys and girls begin going steady and becoming engaged at an earlier age. It is not uncommon for couples to be married and begin having children while they are still in college. In some high schools, sex education programs now include maternity training for girls who may become mothers before they graduate.

Although the young newlyweds are ready physically for marriage, and can prove it by having babies, they are not always ready for the responsibilities of marriage. Often, the parents of the newlyweds have to contribute to the support of the family in one way or another. If the older generation can afford it, they may help the young couple to purchase a home or help them finance an apartment that would not otherwise be available to them. Sometimes the newlyweds will move into the home of the parents of the bride or the groom.

In the view of some experts, a number of teen-agers enter marriage as a kind of initiation into adulthood. These young couples marry not for sexual reasons but to satisfy a desire to have the status of adulthood. About 40 percent of today's brides are no more than 18 years old; half are married before they are 21. The average age of bridegrooms is 23. But 50 percent of these marriages end in divorce within five years. The couples find that marriage and adult status do not offer the magic they had expected, and the bride and groom find themselves locked into a life which can be quite mundane and dull.

When the wife realizes that instead of a life of magic she faces a life of pots and pans and diapers, and the husband discovers that two cannot live as cheaply as one, arguments may evolve. Not all marriages of young couples are destined for failure, of course, and millions of unions that are threatened by divorce survive the rocky first years to develop into well-adjusted and realistic lifetime partnerships.

Marriage Counseling

At some point in the early years of marriage, the couple may decide to consult with someone outside their inner circle of friends and family when personal problems arise which defy an amicable solution. An outside point of view can be more objec-

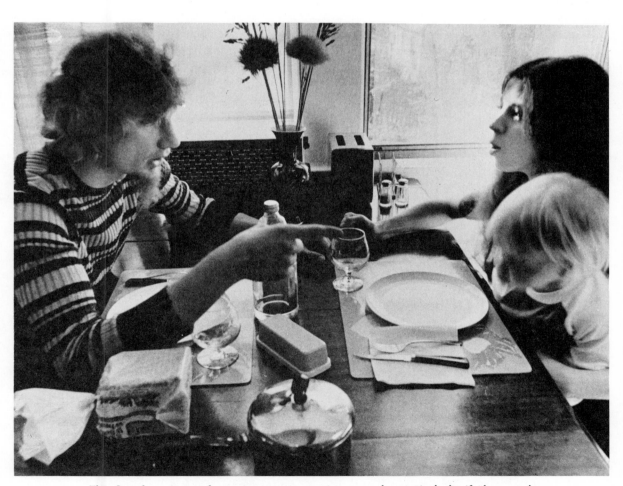

The first few years of marriage are sometimes rough, particularly if the couple has a totally romantic, unrealistic view of what marriage and raising a family entail.

tive, and the conflict may involve matters the couple would not want to discuss with family, friends, or a clergyman.

Rather than face separation or divorce, they can take their problems to someone professionally trained, such as a psychiatrist, psychologist, or a marriage counselor. However, they should be forewarned that solutions are not quick and easy. Several sessions, at least, may be needed. If the problems are serious enough to warrant professional help, the couple can expect that it will take time for a stranger to separate facts from emotions and develop a future course acceptable to both parties.

Selecting the right counselor can be a problem in itself, since not all counselors are equally qualified. A family doctor or a psychiatrist may be asked to give direct help or to make a referral. A counselor who uses systems or formulas, such as astrology charts or computer analysis, or who communicates by mail or telephone, should be avoided. Marital problems require a personal approach; it is unlikely that a marriage counselor could have simple solutions that might be applied to any couple who come to him with questions ranging from sexual incompatibility to the handling of family finances. The couple should also be suspicious of a counselor who offers a contract for his services or who suggests that a certain set number of sessions will be required.

Sexual Compatibility

The normal young American housewife, according to a study made by the American Psychiatric Association, is not the mate-swapping, cocktail circuit, jet-set female portrayed in some movies and television dramas. She is emotionally well adjusted, average or above-average in physical attractiveness, content with her lot in life, and realistic about her social aspirations. She tends to idealize her husband and is confident of his fidelity. She does not try to dominate her husband; if she has children, they tend to be emotionally healthy.

Their husbands are well-adjusted, normal males whose responses to social and psychological tests are so similar to their own that psychiatrists are convinced that "like marries like." The couples experience deep, meaningful pleasures in stable relationships with each other and in raising their children.

Most of the wives, according to the study, married with full parental consent; more than 80 percent had a religious ceremony. The wives had reached approximately the same level of education as their husbands, tended to be of the same religious faith, and usually were of the same age or slightly younger than their husbands.

The Honeymoon

During the first weeks or months of marriage, the husband and wife have an opportunity to become better acquainted on an intimate basis. The honeymoon period usually provides ideal settings for intimate living, away from the daily pressures of earning a living and the social pressures of well-meaning friends and relatives. Even so honeymoons frequently are disappointing, perhaps because of the disproportionate emotional investment in them. This does not, by any means, indicate that the marriage is doomed to fail.

Fatigue

After the honeymoon, both partners may suffer a bit from mental and physical fatigue in the evenings, particularly if both are employed; sexual intimacies might be fewer and less frequent than the couple had anticipated. The wife may be in the mood for sex play but the husband might be tired or distracted by financial worries. Or the husband may be in the mood, but the wife may be too tired physically or emotionally upset. However, if fatigue serves as a frequent excuse for not having sexual relations, it may be a rationalization, and the attitudes of both partners toward sex should be examined. One of the best ways to get the marriage off to a pleasant beginning is to make sure that the husband and wife can retire in the evening and leave the cares of the day for tomorrow.

Importance of Foreplay

Despite the seemingly open attitude toward sex among today's young people, many marital partners can be rather inept in the bedroom. If the sex act were a complicated procedure, the human race would not be around today. However, the many superstitions, fears, and restrictions superimposed upon a normal function almost from the time of birth until marriage can lead to emotional conflicts and frustrations when the young man and woman are face to face in a double bed.

If the husband does not take into account the importance of sexual foreplay and timing, the wife may not respond in the manner he expected, and he may reject her as frigid. Or the husband may experience premature ejaculation in his sexual excitement and complete the sex act before the wife has had time to respond. Premature ejaculation is one form of impotence. In another form, because of shyness or other psychological reasons, the man may not be able to sustain an erection.

The wife may not experience a true orgasm until after several months of marriage, and it may take the same amount of time for the husband to develop his techniques to the point that the wife is satisfied. The idea that practice makes perfect in *coitus,* or the sex act, may seem facetious, but it is nevertheless true. Patience and consideration for each other's preferences should result in a mutually pleasurable sexual adjustment.

Frigidity and Impotency

Only a small percentage of women fail to achieve orgasm eventually, and probably a

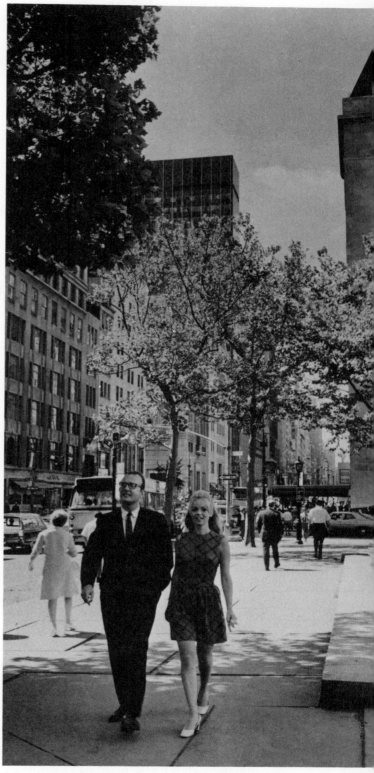

A honeymoon can provide a bride and groom with the privacy to begin exploring their new relationship without the distractions of relatives and friends.

smaller percentage of men remain impotent for an extended period of time. The most frequent cause of frigidity and impotency is psychological. For those who do feel frustrated in the sex act after many weeks or months of serious effort, advice should be sought from a psychotherapist, or the family doctor may make a referral to a doctor who specializes in this area of medicine. In some cases, impotence can be treated with drugs or medication. On the other hand, the wrong kinds of drugs or alcohol may interfere with normal sex functions.

Birth Control

Female frigidity can be caused by nothing more serious than fear of an unwanted pregnancy. If the couple has agreed to postpone starting a family or adding to it, the wife might feel insecure about her birth control method, especially if she depends upon a technique known to be less effective than the oral contraceptive.

Oral Contraceptives

Although "the pill," or *oral contraceptive,* has received a bad press in recent years, it probably ranks second only to sterilization as a birth control method. Oral contraceptives are composed of synthetic sex hormones; they are manufactured by pharmaceutical companies from substances found in plant materials such as Mexican yams. The hormones are chemical cousins of the hormones naturally secreted in the female body during a normal reproductive cycle. They work by "fooling" the woman's reproductive system with a simulated pregnancy.

How "the pill" works: Normally, an ovum is released from the ovaries once during each menstrual cycle. If the ovum becomes fertilized by male sperm and implanted in the uterus, the hormones send back chemical signals that tell the ovaries to suppress ovulation until further notice. If this natural defense did not occur, a woman could find herself carrying several embryos and fetuses of different ages at the same time.

In other words, when an ovum is fertilized, the mother's reproductive machinery is mobilized to protect and encourage the development of the newly created life, and the monthly release of ova is halted until the birth of the baby. The synthetic hormones in the pill are of the type that signal the body that a pregnancy has been started, even though it is not true. Ovulation is suppressed and menstruation is delayed as long as the pills are taken.

At the end of a series of approximately 20 pills, one per day, a normal menstruation is allowed to occur. Then the series of pills is resumed for another menstrual cycle, but the hormones again suppress ovulation with a false pregnancy message. Since no ovum is released, there is very little chance that pregnancy will result from intercourse while the pills are used. Oral contraceptives are

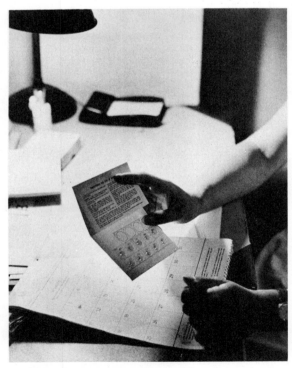

Synthetic hormones in "the pill" act to simulate pregnancy, effectively suppressing ovulation and delaying menstruation for as long as the pills are taken.

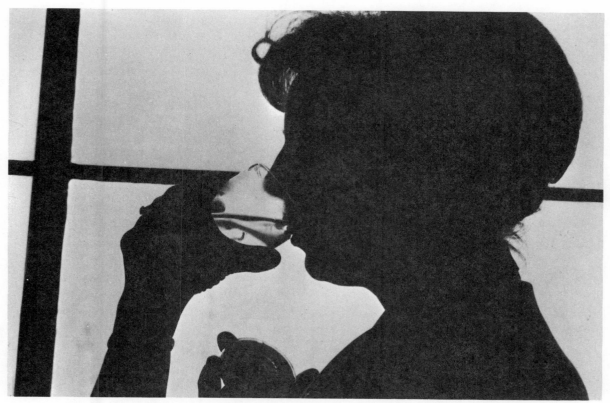

Although oral contraceptives are almost 100 percent effective, pregnancies have occurred as a result of human error, when the female has forgotten to take one of the series of twenty pills.

almost 100 percent effective, but errors occur from time to time, usually human errors in which the wife forgets to take a pill each day.

Side effects: Some women who use the pill have experienced undesirable side effects, which may range from break-through bleeding or cramps to hypertension, neurologic disorders, or *thromboembolism* (the blocking of a vein or artery by a blood clot). However, the most unpleasant side effects, such as blood clots and hypertension, usually occur when the woman taking the pill has high blood pressure. Therefore, women with this condition should not take the pill unless under strict medical supervision.

Although there is a danger of circulatory disorders and other side effects from the use of oral contraceptives, many doctors agree that the hazards of pregnancy are a greater threat to possibly millions of women.

However, it is advisable for women using the pill to have periodic checkups.

The IUD

Next in popularity after the pill is the IUD, or *intrauterine contraceptive device*, a plastic or metal coil inserted in the uterus. A plastic coil can be produced at a cost of about 10 cents and inserted easily by a doctor with a syringelike device. However, the costs usually run much higher for the patient because of follow-up examinations and related care.

IUD's come in a variety of shapes and sizes. One is a plastic spiral, another has a double-S loop, still another looks like a tiny hour-glass. Each is about an inch and a half in length, and most have a tail that extends through the cervix.

How it works: Once the IUD is inserted, the woman can make her own examination,

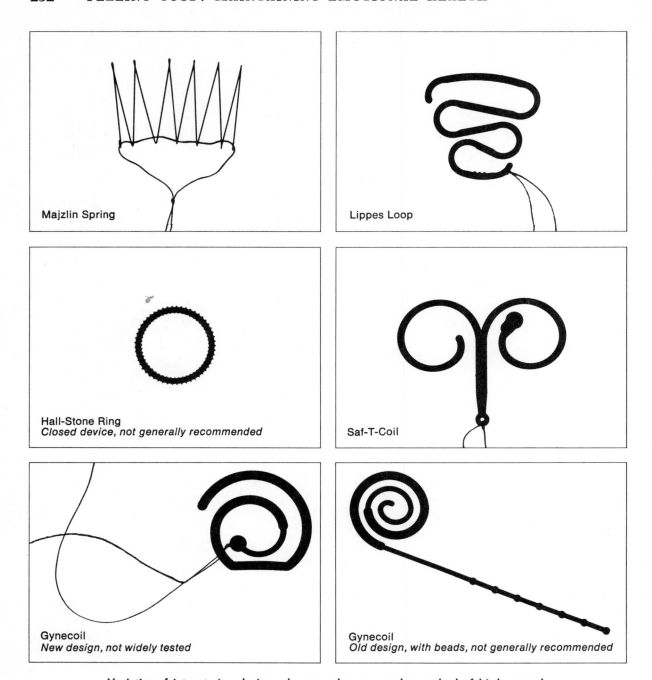

Majzlin Spring

Lippes Loop

Hall-Stone Ring
Closed device, not generally recommended

Saf-T-Coil

Gynecoil
New design, not widely tested

Gynecoil
Old design, with beads, not generally recommended

Varieties of intrauterine devices, the second most popular method of birth control.

usually once a week, to determine whether it is still in place. If, by feeling the tail of the IUD, the woman suspects it has slipped out of place, she notifies her physician immediately. Otherwise, if there are no side effects, the IUD remains in place indefinitely, to be removed only when the woman wants to become pregnant. The IUD apparently functions by interfering with the natural implantation of a fertilized ovum in the wall of the uterus.

Side effects: Side effects might include pelvic pain, irregular bleeding, occasional perforation of the uterus, or pelvic infection.

Some doctors feel that IUD's are better suited for the woman who has already had one or more children because of minor problems in fitting the device through the cervix.

Diaphragms and Cervical Caps

The oral contraceptive, the intrauterine contraceptive device, and two kinds of mechanical sperm barriers, the *cervical cap* and *diaphragm,* require a visit to the doctor's office. The diaphragm or cervical cap must be fitted to the size and shape of the female reproductive organs at the opening of the uterus.

How they work: The main difference between the diaphragm and the cervical cap is that the diaphragm is placed at the back of the vagina in such a way that it serves as a barrier against spermatozoa that would be ejaculated during intercourse. The cervical cap, as the name suggests, is a cap that fits over the cervix to prevent the passage of spermatozoa.

The diaphragm must be coated on both surfaces as well as along the rim with a contraceptive jelly or cream. The soft rubber cup is placed at the back of the vagina before intercourse and should be left in place for at least 6 hours but not more than 16 hours after coitus. When removed, it should be cleaned according to directions and not used again for a period of 6 to 8 hours. Because of changes in weight and other factors, the diaphragm should be refitted at least once every two years. It should be replaced periodically, regardless of changes in size, because, being made of rubber, it does deteriorate with use, and the flaws are not always obvious to the naked eye.

A cervical cap may be made of rubber, plastic, or metal. It is carefully fitted over the cervix by a physician. During use, it is filled with contraceptive cream or jelly. The metal variety can be left in place from the end of one menstrual period to the beginning of the next, but other types should not remain in place for more than 24 hours. The cervical cap should be checked from time to time, since it can slip out of position during intercourse.

Condoms

Among birth control devices that do not require a visit to the doctor is the *condom,* usually made of soft rubber and shaped to fit as a sheath over the penis. They are inexpensive and are the preferred method of contraception for many couples, since they require the least advance preparation of all the methods except the oral contraceptive and the IUD.

Although condoms manufactured in the United States for the past 35 years have been subjected to quality control tests and are checked by federal inspectors, they are not immune to failure. For this reason, many women insert a spermicidal jelly or cream in the vagina when the man uses a condom.

The condom frequently is used by newlyweds as a birth control device while the wife waits to be fitted with a diaphragm after the first weeks of marriage. It also permits intercourse when one of the partners has an infectious disease affecting the genitals.

Because the condom dulls the sensation of intercourse somewhat, it is recommended for men who experience premature ejaculation. On the other hand, some men object to the lessened coital sensation associated with the wearing of a condom.

The Rhythm Method

At about the same level of effectiveness as the diaphragm, cervical cap, or condom is the *rhythm method*—if used in conjunction with basal body temperature readings. In the rhythm method, the couple schedules intercourse before or after ovulation. In order for this method to be effective, a woman must keep extremely accurate charts of her basal temperature with a basal body thermometer in order to determine exactly when she ovulates. One problem with the rhythm method is that few women, especially newly marrieds, have had experience keeping careful records of this kind and often misinterpret the results without a doctor's counsel. About one in five women simply does not have regular menstrual cycles, which is the key to avoiding days of peak fertility.

Spermicides

Spermicides in the form of jellies, creams, foaming tablets, gels, aerosol foams, and suppositories are available in nearly any drug store and can be obtained without a prescription. The chemical substances are inserted with special applicators and form a film over the vaginal lining. The tablets and suppositories melt inside the vagina to spread a film over the lining.

The main objection to the use of chemical contraceptives is that coitus must take place within an hour after the substances are applied. When tablets are used, up to 15 minutes must elapse before coitus can begin. Generally, the chemicals should remain in the vagina for at least six hours after intercourse. If coitus is repeated during that period, another dose of chemicals must be inserted in advance.

Coitus Interruptus and Douching

Two of the least reliable birth control methods are *coitus interruptus* and *douching*. Coitus interruptus requires that the husband withdraw his penis from the vagina before ejaculation. If carried out to its ideal conclusion, the technique requires a lot of self-control and split-second timing. Ejaculation is triggered by an automatic nerve reflex after the seminal vesicles are filled with semen; once the message gets through the nervous system, there is little the man can do to prevent ejaculation. Needless to say, the coitus interruptus technique has a high rate of failure. Beyond that it is

psychologically bad because it places undue anxiety on both partners during coitus.

Douching with water or special solutions works on occasion, but it is rated only as better than no birth control method at all. The douching, or flushing, of the vagina seems to have some effect in that it reduces the number of spermatozoa in the female reproductive system. Water alone is sufficient to kill sperm, although special preparations are available. The important factor with a douche is timing. The douche must be used immediately after intercourse, since spermatozoa can be moving through the cervix within a couple of minutes after ejaculation and are able to reach the Fallopian tubes within 45 minutes.

Sterilization

About ten percent of the couples in the United States have chosen to have one of the partners sterilized as a permanent form of contraception; most are parents who have acquired all the children they feel they can support or who fear the mother's life would be endangered by pregnancy. A rather quick and simple operation called a *vasectomy* may be performed on the male to remove a portion of the *vas deferens,* or sperm ducts, thus preventing semen from reaching the seminal vesicles, where it would ordinarily be discharged during intercourse. A vasectomy can be performed in a doctor's office with no more than a day or two lost from work.

The operation to sterilize a female is more involved; the abdomen is opened and the Fallopian tubes are cut or tied. A general anesthetic is employed and the operation is performed in a hospital. It is a safe and almost bloodless operation requiring hospitalization for only a few days.

The problem with sterilization is that it is generally not reversible. It does not interfere with sex activity once the patient has recovered, but if the couple decides later to have more children, or if the sterilized part-

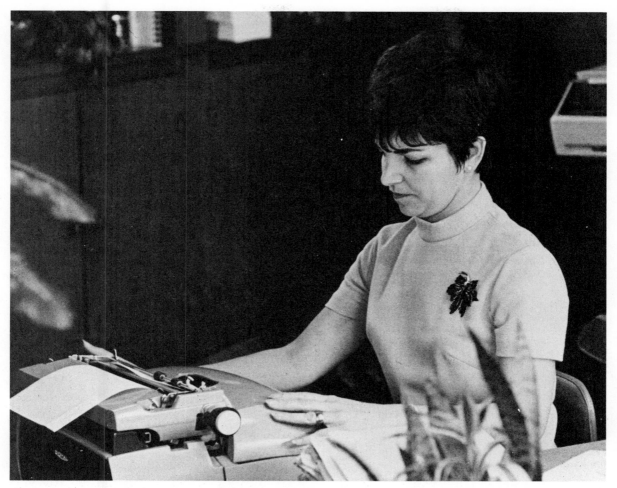

Wives and mothers are becoming an increasingly vital part of the work force. Some women work because their salary is necessary to family support, others because it makes them feel fulfilled.

ner remarries and wants to have children, the odds are against success in patching together the Fallopian tubes or the sperm ducts so that normal reproductive function can be restored.

Research on Other Methods

There are other birth control methods in the research and testing stage, such as oral contraceptives for men, morning-after contraceptives, and once-a-month shots. Eventually, some scientists speculate, foods in the supermarket will be treated with harmless substances that prevent conception. They will be similar to the iodine in iodized salt or the vitamin D added to

homogenized milk. When the wife wants a baby, she merely changes the menu for a few days to exclude birth-control foods or switches to the foods in a special dietetic grocery store.

The Working Mother

A woman's place is in the home—and in the office, laboratory, factory, classroom, or any other place where she is qualified to fill a position that will pay her for her talents and help her fulfill her own needs and achieve professional goals. Since World War II, when women took over the assembly lines and women in uniform released military men from office tasks, the role of the working mother has been generally accepted as an integral part of the modern social scene.

And just as a wife does not mind the amount of time a husband must devote to his job as long as he does not neglect his family, psychologists have found that men are happy and content with working wives and mothers, as long as they do not neglect their husbands or the needs of their children.

Agreement on Priorities

Managing a home and a job and trying to raise a family at the same time can be a frenzied routine beset with tension and emotional strain. The strain is frequently related to the priorities a working wife and mother assigns to her various responsibilities. If the family really cannot subsist adequately on the husband's income, most women can devote a considerable amount of time to an outside job without feeling they are somehow neglecting other duties. Also, mothers who pursue a career for the sake of self-fulfillment have probably calculated the assorted risks and feel little or no anguish about the goals they have chosen.

The women most likely to suffer are the ones who believe that total, full-time devotion to home and family is necessary. These women may have intense guilt feelings if they take an outside job in order to improve the standard of living in the home.

The decision of a mother to take on a full- or part-time job should be based on mutual understanding and a thorough discussion between husband and wife. It is most important that both husband and wife realize each other's feelings and the changes a job can bring about. For example, the husband should realize that if his wife agrees to remain at home despite her desire to get a job, her frustrations will undoubtedly be transmitted to her children. He must also realize that if the couple cannot afford the services of a maid to help with the housework, he himself must help with the housework or care of the children.

On the other hand, the wife must realize that her husband's position may require him to work occasional evenings—at which time he cannot also help her with housework—and that she may have to entertain clients or other people for him, even on days when she has worked a full day and is tired. The important thing is to weigh all aspects of the problem and base the decision on whatever brings the most satisfaction to everyone concerned. When both husband and wife are satisfied with the home-and-job decision, the children will be in a more secure position, regardless of which choice was made.

Age of Children

The age of the children should also be considered. Although many experts feel that mothers should postpone working outside the home if possible until the children are about six years of age, others maintain that this is not necessary if the children are well cared for in her absence and are given ample love and attention by both parents. A child of six or younger is particularly vulnerable, and his emotional needs must be served just as completely as are his physical needs.

Parents' Division of Labor

The roles of both parents are often subjected to revisions and modifications in a family where both parents work. The father usually assumes more responsibility for the care of a child at the end of a workday, when the working mother must get dinner ready. This may actually enable father and child to know one another more intimately and may also result in the father's feeling more sympathy and understanding toward the problems involved in child care.

Limitations on the mother's time: One recent study revealed that working mothers spend an average of 34 hours a week at housework, compared to about 56 hours a week for mothers who stay at home. Since the 34 hours are in addition to the time spent on her job plus commuting time, the working mother obviously has little time for recreation or community activities.

However, many women drive themselves to exhaustion by trying to prove they can hold a job and be perfect housekeepers and community leaders. The working mother must be able to accept limitations and decide what is most important; otherwise, she may feel guilty and insecure as well as continually tired. At some point the couple might consider alternatives; perhaps the mother should give up all extracurricular activities in favor of a career, or she might drop out of the work force for a few years, resume community activities, and return to work when the children are old enough to be more self-sufficient.

She also might consider a part-time job until the children are older. Even when the children are in the early years of grammar school, the mother may want to find employment that allows her to be at home when they are dismissed from class in the afternoon.

Economics and Others Factors

If economic factors are the prime motive for the mother's outside job, her take-home pay should be considerably greater than the costs of a baby-sitter, maid, or house-

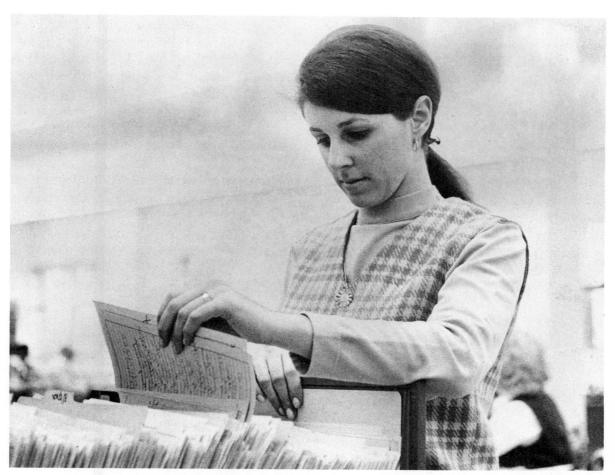

For some mothers, a part-time job that enables them to be home in the afternoon when their children are dismissed from school is the best solution until the children are more self-sufficient.

keeper, nursery school or day care center, clothing needed for the job, transportation, lunches, and so on. The economics of the situation may be complex. For example, the couple may decide that even though the wife's earnings are not that sizable to begin with, she will be a far better wage earner in the long run if she continues working now rather than tries to return to a career at some later date when her skills will be rusty or completely outdated. Besides, economic considerations are not the only criteria; the woman's emotional needs to be productive or challenged intellectually must also be considered.

Care of the Child

The baby-sitter must be a person responsible enough to assume the role of the parents in their absence, although the sitter does not have the authority to treat the child as she might her own. Because of the many gray areas, such as whether the sitter is authorized to punish the child, some firm ground rules should be established by the parents before the sitter begins work. Even if the sitter is a close relative, such as a grandmother or aunt of the child, there should be an understanding about what the child can and cannot do in the absence of the parents and what the sitter can and cannot do.

Teen-age sitters: If the sitter is a teen-ager, she should be instructed as to whether she can let her friends visit her at the home where she is baby-sitting, whether she can chat with her friends on the telephone while she is sitting, and so on. She should have the telephone numbers where the parents can be reached if a problem arises, as well as the telephone numbers of doctors, friends, and neighbors who could assist in an emergency.

Usually, the main job of the baby-sitter is the safety and welfare of the child. But when a sitter is expected to spend as much as a full working day with a child, five days

a week, parents should try to find a sitter who is emotionally compatible with the child and can provide warmth and companionship, particularly for the preschool-aged child.

If the sitter is a close relative, she probably will know all about changing diapers, bottle feeding, minor first aid for bumps and bruises, and so on. A teen-ager, however, may not be experienced in these areas. Just because she has never changed a diaper doesn't mean the girl is unqualified for the job of sitter. But the parents should learn in advance how experienced the sitter is. She may need only a brief lesson in formula preparation or diaper changing to make the grade.

Nursery Schools

There are good nursery schools and not-so-good nursery schools, as well as children who do and those who do not benefit from a nursery-school experience. The facilities should supplement rather than substitute for home care of a child. Although the child may at first be reluctant to leave his home, he should be mature enough to spend part of each day away from home. The staff, physical setting, and equipment should be appropriate for the needs of the individual child.

Many states have strict licensing requirements for nursery schools, while others do not, so it is up to the parents to investigate thoroughly. Under no circumstances should a child be parked for the day in any facility in order to solve emotional conflicts of the child or the parents.

Nursery school can be a rewarding and enriching experience for the preschool youngster. Perhaps the most important purpose of nursery school is the opportunity it provides for children to experience peer relationships. This is particularly necessary if children lack frequent opportunities to play with other children. For most preschoolers, nursery school is the first time

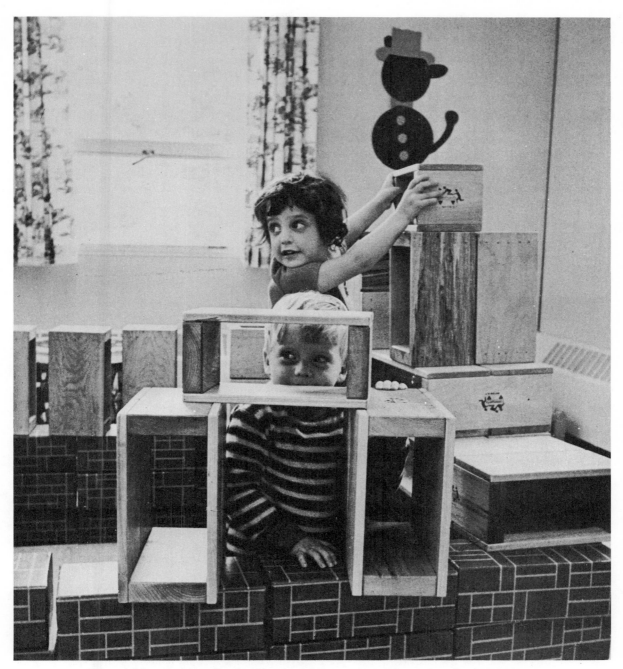

Some children are initially shy, but most thrive on a good nursery-school experience.

they experience a group situation, and what they learn in nursery school in terms of cooperation with others prepares them for the dynamics of the more formal learning situations to come.

The programs for nursery school children may include excursions, exposure to music, story books, creative work with clay and paints, and organized games. It is wise to investigate several schools in terms of staff, facilities, and professional standards before making a decision. Under no circumstances should a school be chosen simply because it is cheaper.

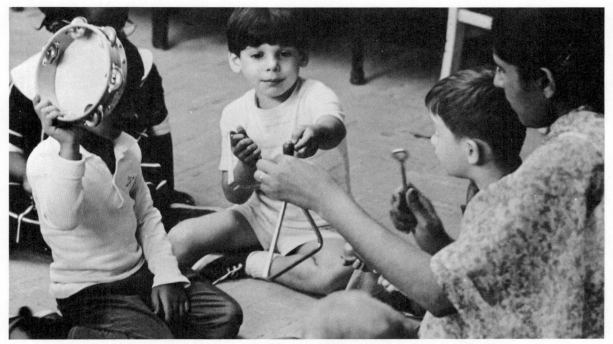

The staff, program, and facilities should be considered before a nursery school is chosen.

Parental Responsibilities

Parents who are separated from their children because of the demands of their jobs should not abdicate their responsibilities as mother and father either to baby-sitters or nursery school staff members.

Need for Strong Father

The father, particularly, must not avoid his responsibilities in the child raising department. Too often today's father makes himself unavailable for guidance by telling a child to "ask your mother," when what the youngster wanted was a decision from the father. Families need a male authority who can command the respect of the children, but the father cannot expect to have a voice in family discipline when he passes the responsibility to the mother.

Agreement on Discipline

Many children learn at an early age that they can play the parents against each other to gain their objectives. If the father con-

tinually tells a child to ask his mother for a decision, the youngster may learn to work the game into a "yes" from the mother whenever he wants his own way. This should not be interpreted to mean that the father should be harsh or stern, but rather that he be actively concerned and involved in all phases of his child's growth, particularly in guiding his behavior.

If parents cannot agree on a course of discipline, the effect on a child can be as bad as no direction at all. In such a home the growing child has difficulty in learning to discipline himself because of uncertainty as to whom to model himself after. Although the female influence in child raising may seem more immediate because it is the mother who nurtures the baby during his first few months, growing children need two loving and attentive parents to give them support and provide them with behavioral models.

For a description of physical problems relating to childbirth, see *Infertility, Pregnancy, and Childbirth*, p. 141.   KNA

LIVING LIFE TO THE FULLEST: THE MIDDLE YEARS

No wise man ever wished to be younger.
—JONATHAN SWIFT

Staying young is looked on by most of the rest of the world as a peculiarly American obsession. This obsession is certainly fostered and exploited by the advertising industry, but its causes have to be looked for elsewhere.

In many countries, it is the old who are venerated for their wisdom and authority. This point of view is likely to prevail in societies that stay the same or that enjoyed their greatest glories in the past.

America is another matter. Because of its history, it is literally a young country. It is also a nation built on the idea of progress and hope in the future. And to whom does the future belong if not to youth?

Keeping up with change is unfortunately identified by too many people with how they look rather than how they think or feel. To be young in heart and spirit has very little to do with wearing the latest style in clothes—no matter how unbecom-

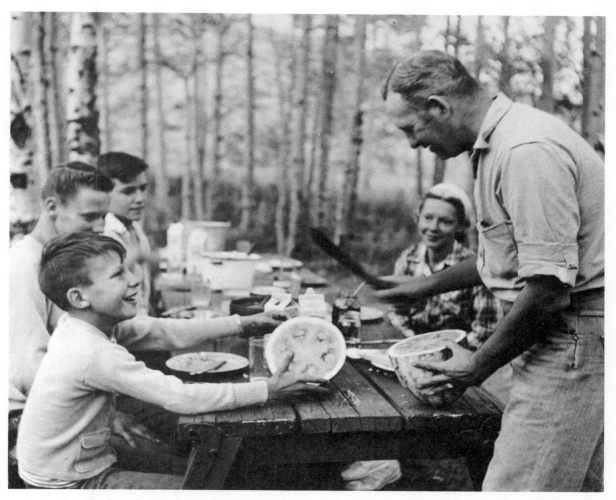

As inner knowledge increases during the middle years, so can the capacity for enjoying life.

ing—or learning the latest dances. Maintaining an open mind receptive to new ideas, keeping the capacity for pleasure in the details of daily living, refusing to be overwhelmed by essentially unimportant irritations can make the middle years more joyful for any family.

A Critical Time

Nowadays, the average American can expect to reach the age of 70. Thus, for most people, the middle years begin during the late thirties. Ideally, these are the years of personal fulfillment accompanied by a feeling of pride in accomplishment, a deeper knowledge of one's strengths and limitations, and a growing understanding and tolerance of other people's ideas and behavior.

Emotional Pressures: In many families, however, the pleasures of maturity often go hand in hand with increased pressures. It's no simple matter for the typical husband and wife in their forties to maintain emotional health while handling worries about money, aging parents, anxiety about willful teen-agers, tensions caused by marital friction, and feelings of depression about getting older. To some people, the problems of the middle years are so burdensome that instead of dealing with them realistically—by eliminating some, by compromising in the solution of others—they escape into excessive drinking or into sexual infidelity. It doesn't take much thought to realize that those escapes do nothing except introduce new problems.

Physical symptoms of emotional problems: For others, deep-seated conflicts that come to a head during the middle years may be expressed in chronic physical symptoms. Many physicians in the past intuitively understood the relationship between emotional and physical health, but it is only in recent years that medical science has proved that feelings of tension, anxiety, suppressed anger, and frustration are often the direct cause of ulcers, sexual impotence, high blood pressure, and heart attacks, not to mention sleeplessness and headaches.

Of course, there are no magic formulas that guarantee the achievement of emotional well-being at any time of life. Nor does any sensible person expect to find a perfect solution to any human problem. However, it is possible to come to grips with specific difficulties and deal with them in ways that can reduce stress and safeguard emotional health.

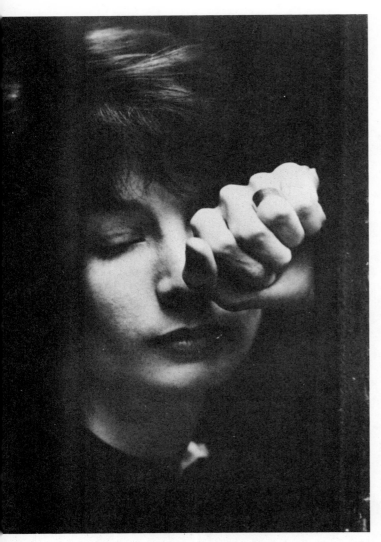

Emotional conflicts that come to a head during the middle years may express themselves in chronic physical symptoms, including ulcers and heart trouble.

Sexuality During the Middle Years

In spite of the so-called sexual revolution and all its accompanying publicity, it is still very difficult for most people to sort out their attitudes towards sexual activity. It is a subject that continues to be clouded by feelings of guilt and anxiety, surrounded by taboos, and saddled with misinformation. For each individual, the subject is additionally complicated by personal concepts of love and morality.

Many people were shocked when the Kinsey reports on male and female sexual behavior appeared. More recently, militant efforts have been made in various communities to prevent the schools from including sex education in their courses of study. Yet marriage counselors, family doctors, ministers, and all other specialists in human relations can attest to the amount of human misery caused by ignorance about sex—all the way from the ignorance that results in a 15-year-old's unwanted pregnancy to the ignorance of a 50-year-old man about his wife's sexual needs.

Pioneering Work in Sexual Response

According to the research of Dr. William H. Masters and Mrs. Virginia E. Johnson, directors of the Reproductive Biology Research Foundation in St. Louis and authors of *Human Sexual Response* and *Human Sexual Inadequacy*, 50 percent of all married couples can be considered sexually inadequate. These authorities define sexual inadequacy as the inability to achieve sexual communication in marriage or insecurity about whatever sexual communication does exist.

In the intensive sexual therapy they offer to married couples professionally referred to the Foundation, Dr. Masters and Mrs. Johnson concentrate on the relationship between husband and wife. They stress the concept of sexual activity as communication between two human beings, each with unique needs and desires that must be fulfilled by the other. The basic attitude they hope to instill in those who come to them for help is that pleasure in sex is natural and can be achieved through an understanding of giving and receiving it.

Emotional Causes of Sexual Inadequacy

It is not unusual for a couple whose marriage begins with a satisfactory sexual adjustment to find the relationship deteriorating as they approach their forties. From the point of view of how the body itself functions during the middle years, there is rarely a physical reason for a decline in the ability to perform sexually. Almost always, male impotence or lack of female responsiveness is caused by psychological factors, some deeply buried, others superficial.

The Impotent Husband

Because of particular circumstances and differing personalities, many middle-aged men spend their days in a state of impotent anger. They may have suppressed feelings of hostility against an unreasonable boss; they may feel put down by a successful neighbor; they may be unable to deal effectively with a rebellious son. With such men, a chain of cause and effect sometimes develops that cannot be broken without professional help.

The tensions generated by impotent anger may result in impotence during the sex act. Since the underlying causes for sexual impotence are probably unknown to him, a middle-aged husband may develop deep anxieties about his waning sexuality. These anxieties in turn cause the sexual incompetence to continue.

There is also the husband who unconsciously builds up resentments against his wife because he thinks she is paying too much attention to the house and the children and too little to him. Their surface

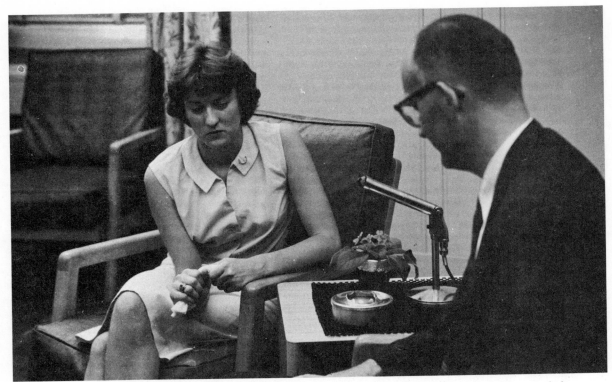

Mounting worries may cause either partner to become sexually unresponsive; counseling can help.

relationship may not be affected, but his body will express his feelings by withholding itself from her as a form of punishment.

Another typical cause of temporary impotence is a feeling of guilt about an adventure in sexual infidelity. Impotence with the marital partner under these circumstances is usually the husband's way of punishing himself for behavior that he considers sinful.

The Unresponsive Wife

Many men complain about their wives' waning interest in sex during the middle years. It is true that women often give or withhold themselves from their husbands as a reward or a punishment, but more commonly, wives who are unresponsive are likely to be expressing resentment about the fact that the only time they get any attention is in bed, and even there, the attention is apt to be perfunctory rather than personally gratifying and meaningful.

When this is the case, the breach in a marriage is likely to widen unless there is a willingness on the part of both partners to confront the problem openly, if necessary with a marriage counselor, minister, or doctor, so that a satisfactory solution can be found. Otherwise, the wife's resentment of neglect expressed in sexual coldness may lead her husband to look elsewhere for gratification.

Sometimes a woman seems unresponsive only because she feels she is being used as a sex object instead of having her needs satisfied. This unconscious feeling may express itself in the lack of responsiveness that is mistakenly called frigidity. As a result of their experience in helping many couples achieve good sexual relationships, Dr. Masters and Mrs. Johnson assert that the word *frigidity* has little meaning. There are very few women incapable of being physically aroused and satisfied by an understanding sexual partner.

Being Honest

In most cases of sexual inadequacy, insight and honesty about feelings are usually a more effective treatment than hormones, sex manuals, and so-called aphrodisiacs.

Any married couple whose sexual problems have become acute during the middle years should look for the causes in their own emotions about themselves and each other. They should also examine any persistent feelings of tension and anxiety that might be the result of practical matters in their daily lives, such as worry about money or children.

Emotional Problems and the Menopause

The physical aspects of the menopause are in many cases the cause of emotional disturbances that can be alleviated with estrogen therapy. (See under *Keeping Fit,* p. 165, for a discussion of the physical aspects of menopause.) However, these disturbances are by no means inevitable. Many women have superstitious notions about the natural bodily changes that occur during the middle years.

It is only normal to feel sad occasionally about growing older, but there is no need to identify the menopause with loss of attractiveness, an end to sexual desire, or a so-called nervous breakdown. For anyone who is emotionally unstable, this transition may be especially hard to weather, but for such a personality, any time of change—such as marriage or motherhood—might also be accompanied by emotional turbulence.

Probably those women who see their total identity in terms of motherhood are the ones hardest hit when faced with the loss of their child-bearing functions. A woman who has a more complete sense of herself can accept the menopause with equanimity and can also face the tapering off of her child-rearing activities without feeling useless and discarded.

The most satisfying way to continue to express a strong maternal instinct after the menopause is in the role of grandmother, and if there are no grandchildren, in the role of occasional baby-sitter. Volunteer work in the children's ward of a local hospital or as a helper in a day-care nursery has also brought satisfaction to women who miss mothering as their own children leave them.

A Healthy Attitude Toward Change

The old-fashioned term "change of life" that used to describe the menopause really isn't accurate, since change is a rule of life at all times. It is the ability to adjust to different circumstances and to find contentment in new outlets that marks the happy woman of any age.

Instead of feeling frustrated, or wallowing in self-pity, or hunting for sexual adventures, a woman whose emotions are disturbed during the menopause should find better ways of coping with them.

If depression and anxiety are deep enough to result in a loss of interest in daily affairs, the wisest thing to do is to have an honest conversation with the family doctor or gynecologist. He may be able to alleviate these symptoms with such medicines as hormones or tranquilizers. Or he may feel that a few sessions with a psychiatrist would be helpful. It is no sign of personal failure or weakness of will to need professional guidance, and no woman should feel guilty if she seeks it out. See under *Keeping Fit,* p. 165, for a discussion of the male climacteric, which is the male counterpart to menopause.

Beyond Motherhood: New Goals

There are many women casting about to find ways of spending their newly found spare time, women who are bored by bridge

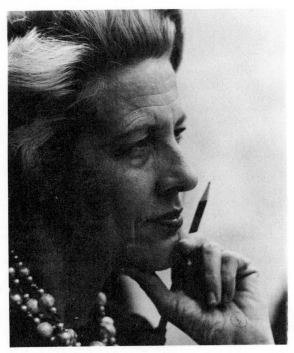

Some colleges offer special courses for women who want to resume their education after a long absence.

to hire them—on a part-time basis if necessary—because they are usually serious, competent, and reliable. Colleges make special provisions for women who want to complete their education after a long absence from studies. Even in small towns, there are many fruitful avenues for earning money or engaging in a productive hobby.

A feeling of pride in accomplishment at a time when household chores and child-raising no longer require much daily attention is usually the best medicine for depressed spirits. Personally meaningful activities outside the home are also an excellent way to keep in touch with what's happening in the world. Nowadays there is no reason for a woman in her forties or fifties to feel restless, bored, or useless. The opportunities for self-expression and personal fulfillment are sufficiently varied to satisfy anyone's individual needs. All it takes is the genuine desire to find them.

More Than a Breadwinner: Vocation and Avocation

Everybody knows that it takes money to maintain a household and raise a family, and there is no doubt that during the middle years financial pressures reach their highest point, what with sending children through school, helping to support aging parents, and meeting increased medical and dental expenses. At this time, even those men who truly enjoy their work often feel they scarcely have the time or peace of mind to enjoy anything else.

Need for Other Outlets

Just as most women need personal outlets for their individuality away from home and family, so most men can achieve better emotional health if they find avenues of self-expression unrelated to their job or their role as husband and father. This does not mean becoming so passionately involved in playing golf or going fishing that the family

and gossip, who enjoy being a wife and mother and grandmother but also want an outlet that is their very own, disengaged from their role in the family. Such women might do some thinking about unfulfilled aspirations and the interests of their younger years, abandoned because of practical pressures.

Each one must find a way of spending leisure time in a way that is personally meaningful. Never mind that the children think it's funny for their mother to be going back to school for a college degree; or that the husband doesn't understand why his wife isn't taking it easy instead of taking a part-time job in a department store; or that the neighbors make remarks about the easel and paints that have suddenly appeared on the back porch.

Returning to Work or School

More middle-aged, middle-class women are taking jobs after years of housekeeping than ever before. Many companies are eager is constantly neglected. Nor does it mean spending excessive amounts of money on rare stamps at the expense of the family budget.

On the other hand, if a man chooses a hobby that doesn't include the family, such as singing in a choir or studying a foreign language, rather than choosing one that does—such as going on camping trips, or taking pictures—there is no reason for the rest of the household to be resentful. Togetherness is a good thing to strive for, but it isn't a hard and fast principle to be applied to all activities.

It's healthier for a man to take an occasional fishing trip with his cronies, enjoy every minute of it, and come home relaxed and refreshed, than to take along a wife who will be bored and children who will be restless. In such far-too-frequent cases, no one has a good time. Nor should a father insist on teaching his son how to play chess so that they can share a hobby when his son would rather spend his time otherwise.

Togetherness has its limitations; husbands and wives need personal outlets away from family.

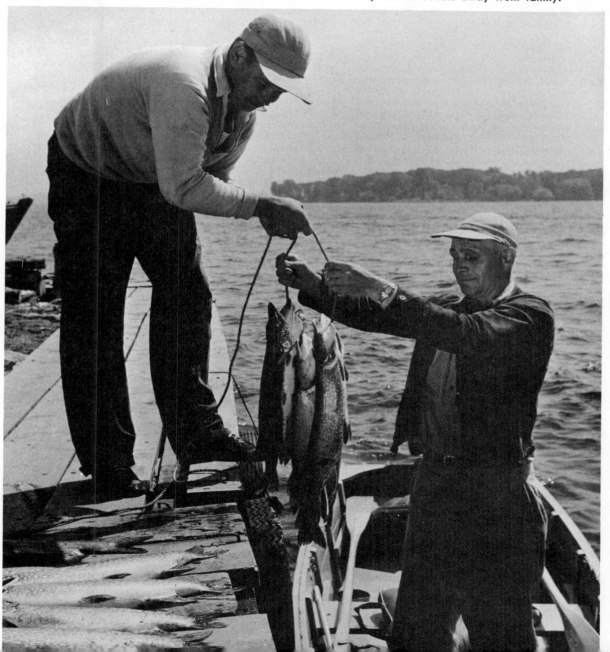

A Satisfying Hobby

The choice of a satisfying leisure-time activity is an entirely individual matter. Some men prefer a hobby that is sedentary, such as model-building. Others who have to sit in an office all day find the vigorous play of the handball court physically and emotionally exhilarating.

Some men, oppressed by constant association with other people, enjoy solitary hobbies such as long nature walks; others, whose jobs involve working alone, like to get together with a group for bowling or bridge playing. There are those who like competitive hobbies and those who want to escape the competitiveness of their work by puttering around in the basement or studying the fine points of the Civil War or experimenting in haute cuisine.

Many men as well as women find the idea of community service appealing as a productive way of using free time. The opportunities are endless: going into poorer neighborhoods and training athletic teams; starting a tutoring group as part of a church activity; getting involved in grass-roots politics and pressing for local reforms; organizing a block association for property maintenance and improvement.

Building a collection can be a gratifying hobby, and the collection need not involve much money. The pleasures usually come from finding a rare specimen—whether it's a matchbook cover or an old comic book—from satisfying a need to own something unique, and from learning in the process of looking for items of interest.

Flexing Mental Muscles

Healthy human beings, regardless of age, need a certain amount of intellectual stimulation to keep their spirits refreshed. The arteries of the body may harden slowly with age, but there are people whose minds remain young and limber in spite of their increasing years.

Housewives commonly complain that they do not get enough stimulation from their daily chores. Men talk about getting into a rut on their jobs—going stale. Yet stimulation for the mind is no farther away than the nearest library, if the mind is hungry for food for thought. There's plenty of mental exercise available for those in the middle years who are willing to review their old ideas and to examine some new ones.

Family discussions: Having relaxed discussions with teen-age children can be a fine source of intellectual refreshment if both generations can listen to each other with tolerance and mutual respect. Some parents get huffy and defensive if their views are challenged. This defensiveness—in some cases, downright hostility—results in closing the channels of communication.

This is not to suggest that every idea espoused by the young should be adopted by their elders. But opinions can be exchanged and challenges involving facts and figures can be met in the spirit of civilized discussion. There are areas in which parents can be educated by their children, and the areas can range all the way from trying out new recipes suggested by a venturesome daughter to getting a book on drugs from the library in order to answer a son who cheerfully calls his father a drug addict because he has to have three drinks when he comes home from work.

Community resources: Some families find they need go no farther than their own home for intellectual activity. For those who want broader opportunities to use their heads, there are community resources that can be explored. Church organizations, parent-teacher associations, or social clubs can be used as forums. These might include public discussions, film presentations, and meetings on problems of current interest, such as drug addiction and slum clearance.

For those looking for enlightenment of a specific kind, the facilities of schools in the area should be investigated. Many col-

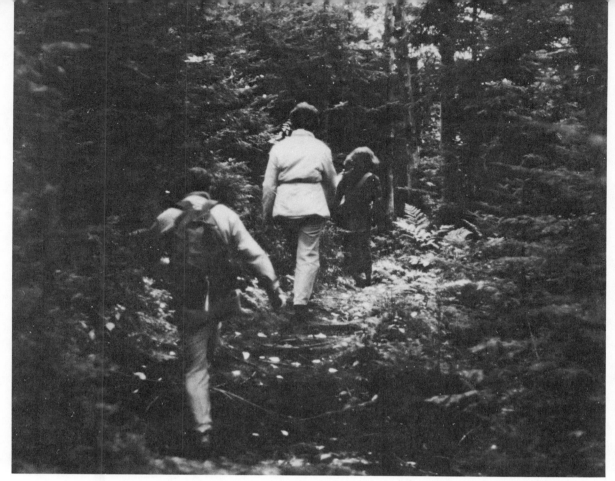

A hike in the woods on a weekend or during a family vacation gives parents and children a chance to spend some time together and to share their interest in nature.

leges and universities offer adult education programs that cover a wide range of subjects—from real estate evaluation to philosophy. It's also possible to set up a study group composed of friends and associates who want to find out more about American history or the history of art, to study anthropology or the behavior of social insects, and to hire a lecturer to meet with the group once or twice a week.

Travel

Travel is a wonderful way of broadening interests, even if the trip means going to a nearby city or dairy farm. When children are in their later teens and can safely be left on their own for a few days—with some neighborly supervision—a husband and wife can enjoy going places of special interest to them rather than having to take younger tastes into account.

The destination needn't be another continent to provide fascinating new sights and information. People who live in Chicago will find the small seacoast villages of New England a totally new world; Bostonians will find a way of life strange to them if they drive through the Smoky Mountains; people who live in a small town or a farm can get a big lift out of wandering about in a big city.

In traveling abroad, the more advance planning that is invested in the trip, the greater the rewards. Every effort should be made to learn at least a little of the language of the country to be visited, and instead of settling for a group tour in which each moment is planned, there's much pleasure to be gained from exploring a particular enthusiasm, whether it be food, architecture, history, or a return to the village of one's foreign-born ancestors.

Separation and Divorce

Marriage in this country is based on the highly personal concept of love rather than on such traditional foundations as a property merger between two families or an arrangement determined by the friendship of the young people's parents. It is often assumed, therefore, that if mutual love is the basis for embarking on a marriage, its absence is a valid reason for dissolving it, either by legal separation or divorce.

The idea of divorce is not particularly modern; in practically every time and place where a form of marriage has existed, so has some form of divorce, with reasons ranging from excessive wife-beating to failure to deliver a piece of land mentioned in the marriage contract.

The High Rate of Divorce

What is new is the high rate of divorce. Figures now indicate that in the United States as a whole, approximately one in every four marriages is terminated by legal arrangement. However, these figures by no means indicate that the family as an institution is on the way out, since a constantly increasing number of people who get divorced get married again.

There are many reasons for the growing rate of separation and divorce:

• Over the last 50 years, a continually increasing percentage of the population has been getting married.

• People marry at a much earlier age than in the past. (The number of divorces is highest among the poorly educated group who marry under the age of 21.)

• The legal requirements for separation and divorce are less rigid than formerly.

• With increasing independence and earning capacity, women are less frightened of the prospect of heading a family.

• The poorer groups in the population, in which desertion was a common practice, are more often obtaining divorces.

Contrary to popular belief, there are more divorces among the poor than among the rich, and more among the less well-educated than among the educated. Also, most divorces occur before the fifth year of marriage.

Telling the Truth to Children

Most people with children who are contemplating a breakup of their marriage generally make every effort to seek professional guidance that might help them iron out their differences. When these efforts fail and steps are taken to arrange for a separation or divorce, it is far healthier for parents to be honest with each other and with their children than to construct elaborate explanations based on lies.

A teen-ager who is given the real reason for a divorce is less likely to have something to brood about than one who is told lies that he can see through. If the real reason for a divorce is that the parents have tried their best to get along with each other but find it impossible, the child who is in his teens or older can certainly understand this. If the marriage is coming to an end because the husband or wife wants to marry someone else, the explanation to the child should avoid assigning blame. When the rejected parent tries to enlist the child's sympathy by blackening the character of the parent who is supposedly the cause of the divorce, results are almost always unpleasant. Under no circumstances and no matter what his age should a child be called on to take the side of either parent or to act as a judge.

Nor should children be told any more about the circumstances of the breakup of a marriage than they really want to know. Young people have a healthy way of protecting themselves from information they would find hurtful, and if they ask few questions, they need be told only the facts they are prepared to cope with. Of course, as they grow older and live through their

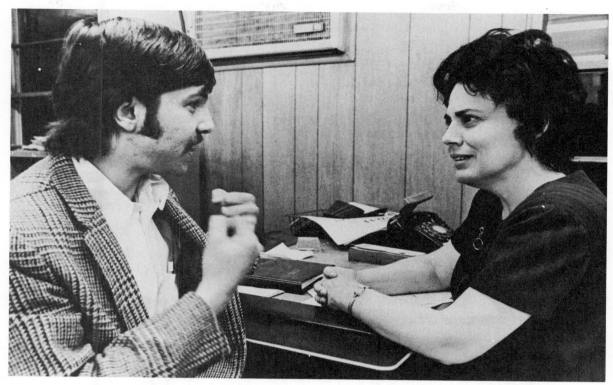

When a marriage is breaking up, any attempt on the part of one of the parents to gain the allegiance of the child by attacking the other parent is likely to backfire.

own problems, they will form their own view of what really happened between their parents.

After the Separation

In practically all separation and divorce proceedings, the children remain in the custody of the mother, with financial support arrangements and visiting rights spelled out for the father. This means that the mother must face the problems of single parenthood. (See below, p. 273.) Although teenage children may need some extra attention for a while, there is no need for a mother to make a martyr of herself, nor should she feel guilty when she begins to consider remarrying.

The father should be completely reliable in his visiting arrangements, and if he has remarried, should try to establish good relationships between the offspring of his former marriage and his new family.

Stepchildren

People who remarry during the middle years frequently find themselves in the role of stepparent. This is a role with many problems and many rewards; the chief requirements are patience and tact.

The stepchild has to deal with many complicated feelings: his sense of loss, either through death or divorce, of his own parent; his resentment against the parent who has remarried, and his hostility to the stranger who has become his new parent.

A stepparent should proceed affectionately but cautiously, and should not try to be accepted by the child as a replacement for the parent who has gone. If the child and stepparent have achieved a friendly rapport before the remarriage, they should build on the friendship rather than trying to transform it into a parent-child relationship immediately. When the child's trust

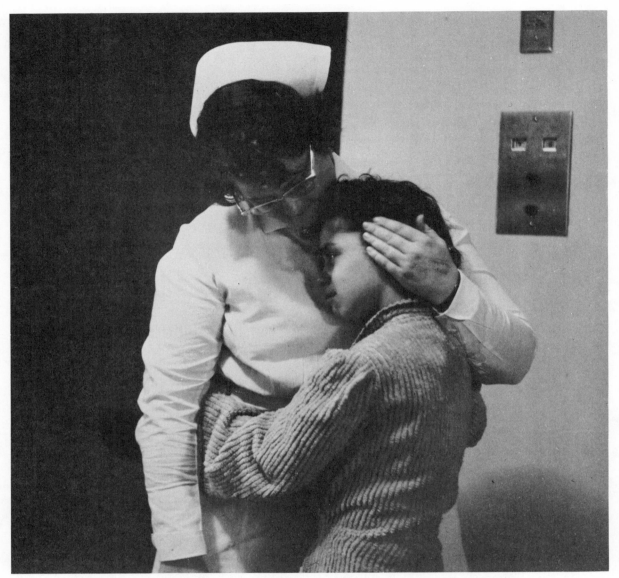

When a father or mother dies prematurely the child may go through a bewildering assortment of emotions, ranging from guilt toward the dead parent to resentment toward the remaining parent.

has been gained, the stepparent can gradually assume some of the authority of a true parent, always waiting for the child to indicate a desire and need for it first.

A Death in the Family

When a husband or wife dies during the middle years, there is a general feeling that the death is unnatural because it is in all ways premature: the normal life expectancy has been cut short, the one who remains is prematurely bereaved, and the children are deprived of a parent too soon.

There are a few consolations in the presence of death: some people are sustained by their religious beliefs, others by the rallying of relatives and friends, and still others by happy memories of the years spent together in a fulfilled relationship.

The bereft parent should share his grief with the children, but they should not be thought unfeeling if they seem to be going about their business almost in the usual way. They may be dealing with a tangle of feelings that will take some time to come to the surface—feelings of guilt about past thoughtlessness, of confusion about wishing that the parent who remains had died instead, and of fear connected with the thought of their own death.

When the time seems right, young people can be encouraged to talk about the parent who died. Remembering funny incidents and times of anger, reliving shared experiences—these can act as a restorative to the living and make family ties closer.

As for remarrying, although the children and the deceased's relatives may consider such a step a disloyalty to the memory of the dead, it is actually a tribute, since it implies that the state of marriage was a happy one.

The Single Parent

When the job of being a single parent has to be faced, either because of death or divorce, the problems may seem overwhelming. Although they differ considerably depending on whether the parent is the father or mother, they are nonetheless difficult to sort out, particularly at a time when morale may be at low ebb.

The Single Father

The single father with growing children usually feels helpless in dealing with household tasks and gains some insight into the number of tasks involved in keeping things running smoothly at home. If he has a teen-age daughter, he can depend on her to do part of the job, but young girls should not be burdened with all the responsibilities of housekeeping if some other arrangement can possibly be made. Perhaps a female relative can be called on to help out part-time, or a professional housekeeper can be engaged for a few hours a day. Outside help is particularly important if the care of younger children is involved.

A motherless girl in adolescence may seek out the companionship and occasional guidance of an older woman who was a friend of her mother's, or she may spend more and more time at the home of a friend whose mother she likes and respects. Such a transfer of affection should not be considered a disloyalty.

The Single Mother

The mother who is a single parent usually has to cope with problems of earning and managing money. Fortunately, the job opportunities for middle-aged women are varied, and if the family finances can be worked out on the basis of a part-time job, this is a good transitional solution for making the adjustment of handling a job and running the household. A widow should feel free to call on a male friend or relative to help her with such practical matters as income tax, mortgages, loans, or investments. If these matters can be handled by a family lawyer without the fees being prohibitive, so much the better.

A widow should avoid concentrating too much on her children, nor should she give a son in his teens the understanding that he is now the head of the family. He is and must remain her son and nothing more. If an authority figure is needed as partial replacement for the departed husband, he should be sought among neighbors or relatives for whom the children feel respect.

In many communities, single parents have formed groups for discussion and mutual help. Such groups can usually be located through local social work agencies. Parents Without Partners, Inc., 80 Fifth Avenue, New York, New York 10011, specializes in the problems of single parents and publishes literature of interest to them. For a discussion of physical problems that are associated with the middle years, see *Keeping Fit,* p. 165.   HMacL

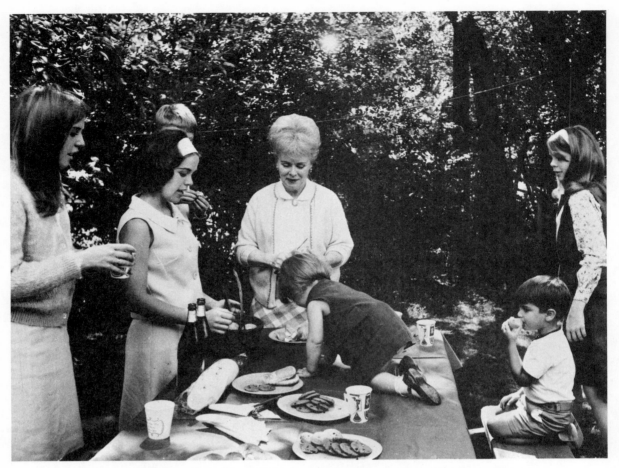

Picnicking and camping are popular recreation both before and after retirement because they are outdoor activities that permit families an inexpensive source of fun.

MEETING THE CHALLENGE OF LEISURE: THE LATER YEARS

Leisure Activities

In 10 years of retirement, you will have the leisure time equivalent of working 40 hours a week for 21 years. You cannot fish this time away and you cannot rest it away. Whatever you do for long must have meaning—must satisfy some basic need and want. Certain needs remain constant throughout life:

• Security—good health, income, and a recognized role in society

• Recognition—as an individual with your own abilities and personality

• Belonging—as a member of a family, social group, and community

• Self-expression—by developing abilities and talents in new areas and at new levels

• Adventure—new experiences, new sights, and new knowledge.

There are many activities that can satisfy these basic needs and wants and keep you mentally and physically in top shape.

Travel

Travel satisfies your need for adventure in many ways. If you travel off-season at bargain rates, you'll find that time truly is money. Most travel problems stem from rushing to meet a schedule. Making every minute count on a fast-paced European tour can be expensive and exhausting. For the same transatlantic fare, you can spend a full year in Europe at one-third the daily cost of a three-week vacation.

Wherever you travel, it isn't enough just to sight-see. Try to center your travel around an interest or a hobby. You can take art or music tours—tours that stress educa-

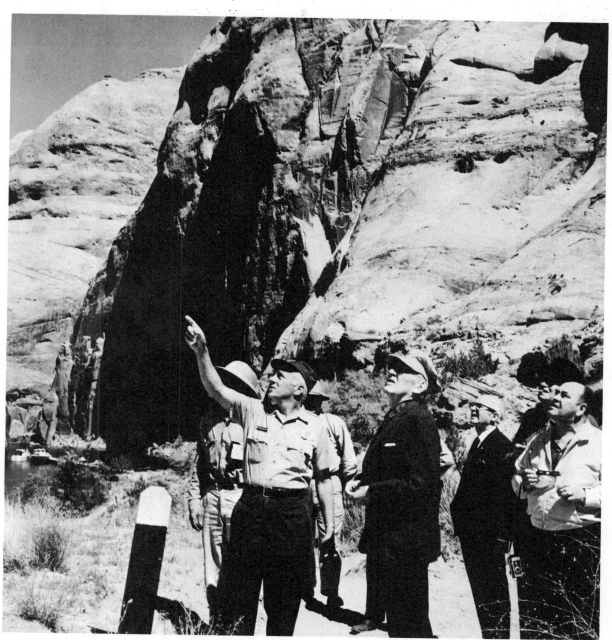

Today the retired can find adventure and stimulation for their interests by traveling, a pursuit that was previously available only to the wealthy, who could afford both the time and money.

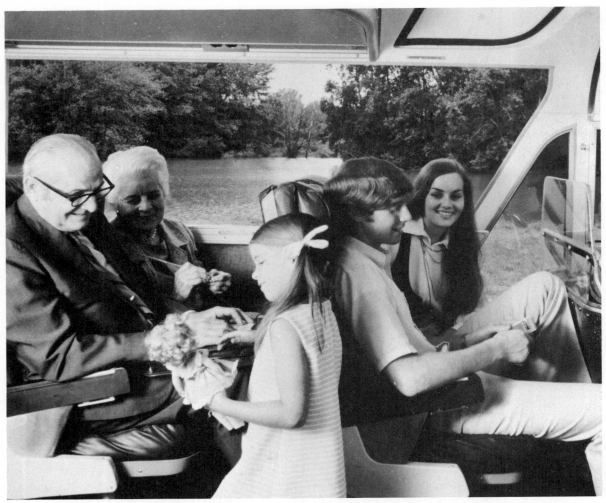

The traveler—whether alone or in groups—will get more out of his trips if he becomes an active participant in the tour rather than confining himself to the passive role of sightseer.

tion, night life, culture, or special interests. You can travel on your own or with a group. But whatever you do, participate; don't just observe.

Doing things instead of just observing adds new dimensions to the pleasure of going places. For people who participate, travel means the adventure of enjoying exciting new places, people, and experiences. To help plan your trip, write to the government tourist offices of foreign countries (ask your library for addresses); to the National Park Service, Washington, D.C.; to state or local chambers of commerce (no street addresses necessary); to major oil companies that supply free maps and routing services.

Gardening

Gardening satisfies one's need for self-expression in many ways. Being outside in the fresh air and planting living things can bring satisfaction and peace of mind.

Gardening is a many faceted hobby that offers many challenges. You can go into plant breeding, growing for resale, introducing new plants, collecting the rare and unusual, plant selecting, or simply cultivating what you find personally appealing and satisfying.

Your local library or bookstore has many books on the subject. There are local and national garden clubs that you can join to learn about your hobby and to meet other people who are interested in gardening. Write the Government Printing Office, Washington, D.C. 20420, for help and advice. In addition, state extension directors at state colleges and universities, county agricultural agents, and local plant nurseries can also give expert advice and information.

Reading

Reading offers excitement, adventure, pursuit of knowledge, and an introduction to new people and places. Your local library is the best place to launch a reading program—and you may be surprised to find that it offers more than books. Most libraries have art and music departments, audio-visual services (films and microfilm copies), foreign language departments, periodical rooms (newspapers and magazines), writ-

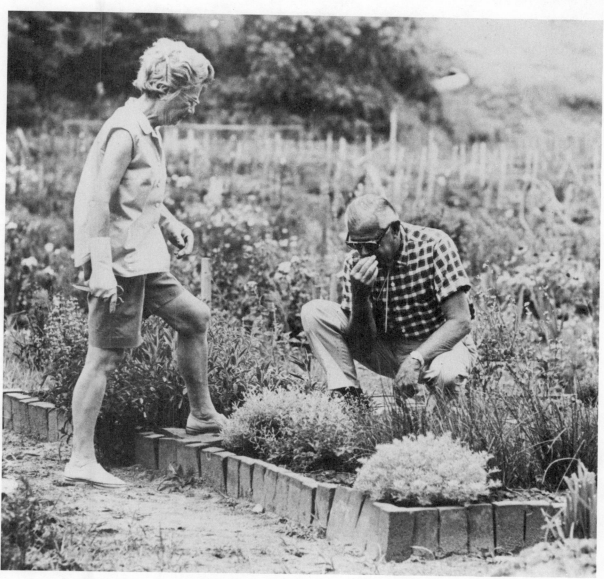

A healthful, relaxing recreation or an all-absorbing hobby, gardening knows no age limits.

ing classes, genealogy workshops, and special courses of general interest.

Hobbies

A hobby can be any physical or mental activity that gives you happiness, relaxation, and satisfaction. It should not be just a time killer—it should offer some tangible reward. Also, it should have continuity, not be too expensive, and not make undue demands on time and energy. Perhaps you would prefer a series of hobbies, some serious and some just for fun. They can be related to your work or completely unrelated. In any event, a hobby should be something you've always wanted to do.

Before selecting a hobby, consider these points:

• Do you like to do things alone? Consider arts, crafts, reading, sewing, fishing—activities that are not dependent on others, although you can enjoy them with others.

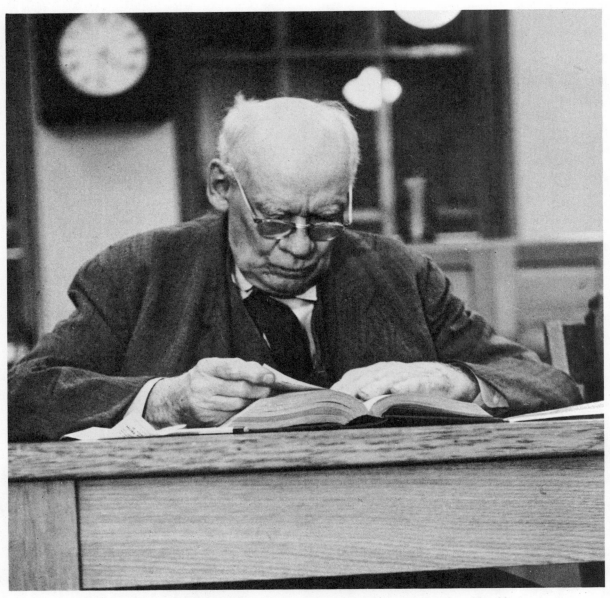

High adventure and knowledge at your fingertips, free: the local public library.

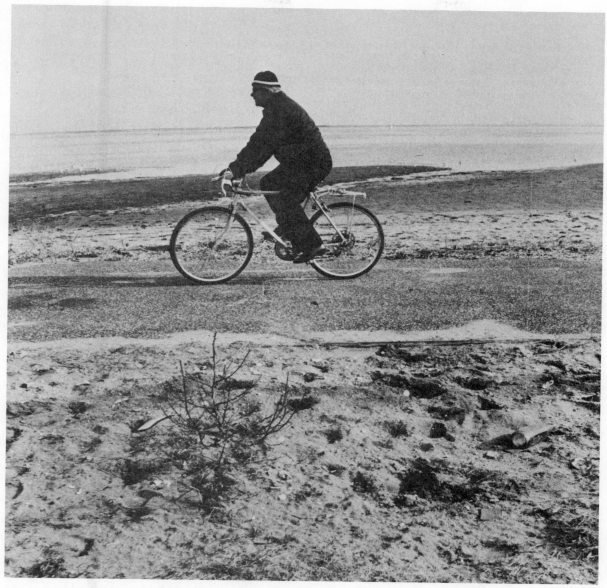

Cycling is a pleasant outdoor activity that older people can enjoy alone or with friends.

• Do you like groups? Seek hobbies that include other people—organizational, sport, game, or craft activities.

• Do you like to play to win? Try your luck in competitive or team games that stress winning.

• Do you have to be an expert? Too many of us are afraid to try new activities because we hate to fail or look clumsy. But be fair; judge your efforts in light of your past experience and present progress; do not compare yourself to someone who's been at it longer than you.

• Do you put a price tag on everything? Many people will not engage in an activity if it costs too much. Yet, many hobbies fail because they're tried on a shoestring without adequate equipment. Also, some people do not want to do anything unless it brings in money. If so, perhaps you should look for something that's an offshoot of the work or business you know best.

Creative Crafts

Creative crafts are difficult for most of us because we are conservative, afraid to make mistakes, sensitive because of buried and almost forgotten blunders. Yet creativity is essential to life. Without it we don't live fully; through creative skills we refurbish old interests and develop new ones.

Most of us are happiest with creative crafts that do not require intricate work or fine detail and that are not too demanding physically. Some crafts best suited to retirement years include weaving, rug making, sewing, ceramic work, knitting, plastic molding, woodwork, leathercraft, and lapidary.

You can learn these and other crafts and also market your products through senior centers, adult education classes, and senior craft centers.

Volunteer Work

Through community service and volunteer work, thousands are not only helping others but are serving themselves. Such activities keep time from hanging heavy, give purpose to retirement, and in some cases may lead to paying jobs and a second career.

Participating in community activities is not difficult. In some communities a call to the city clerk is enough to get started. In others, a letter to the mayor will bring

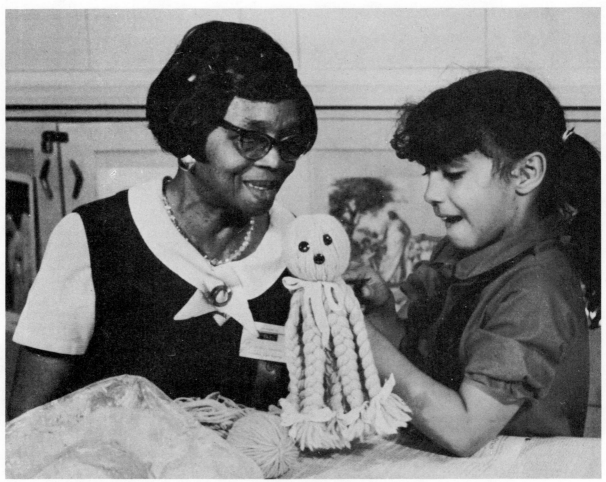

Volunteer work in community service activities can give a purpose to the retirement years.

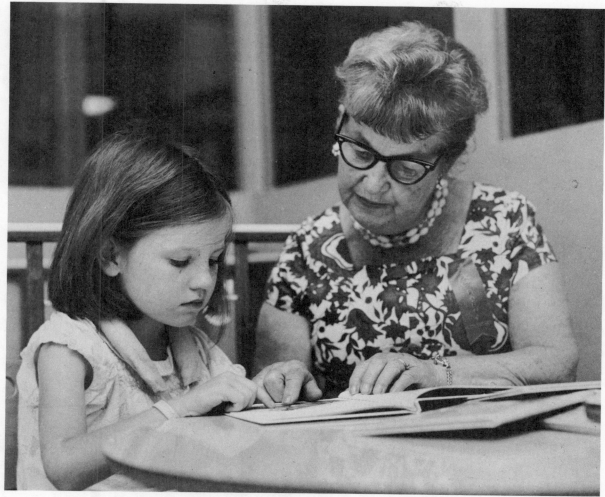

Volunteers In Service To America receive an allowance for working in poverty areas.

faster results. In larger cities, call the Volunteer Bureau in your area; this is a United Fund agency that acts as a clearing house for volunteer jobs.

If you wish to have the type of volunteer job that leads to a second career, you might consider doing work for one of the government programs utilizing the skills of older people. All of these programs have been recently assembled under the umbrella of one organization called ACTION. For additional information about any of the following programs, write to ACTION, Washington, D.C. 20525.

• The Foster Grandparent Program hires low income men and women over 60 to give love and attention to institutionalized and other needy children.

• The Peace Corps is seeking the skills of retirees. However, you must be skilled in some trade or profession, pass a tough physical examination, and complete a rigorous orientation and training program. For information, write to ACTION, Washington, D.C. 20525, and request a copy of *Older Volunteers in the Peace Corps*. It lists specific skills needed in the Peace Corps.

• Other programs within ACTION include the Retired Senior Volunteer Program, the Service Corps of Retired Executives, and the Active Corps of Executives,

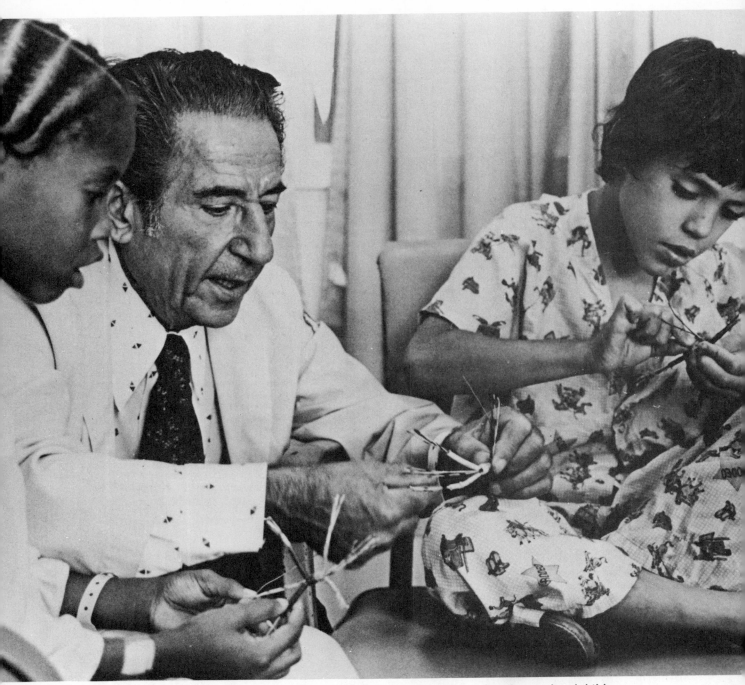

Many retired people enjoy volunteer work, such as teaching crafts to hospitalized children.

and VISTA (Volunteer in Service to America). Many of the workers in these programs are paid.

There are other volunteer jobs that may not pay a salary, but do fill a basic need by allowing you to pass along your skills and ideals to younger people. You can do this through the Boy Scouts, Girl Scouts, Boys Clubs of America, YMCA's and YWCA's, hospitals, schools for the handicapped and mentally retarded, and many other organizations.

Continuing Social and Intellectual Activities

The one organ we can depend upon in old age is the brain. At 80, a person can learn at approximately the same speed he could when he was 12 years old—and that's fast and keen. But like any organ, the brain must be kept active and alert by constant use.

One of the best ways to exercise the brain is through some process of continuing edu-cation. This does not have to mean going back to school or taking formal classes. Continuing education can take the form of participating in discussions in senior centers, "Y's", town meetings, or study courses. You can find out about educational opportunities and possibilities by contacting local, state, or national offices of education; state employment offices; the information service of your Community Council or Health and Welfare Federation; the Adult Education section of the U.S. Office of Education,

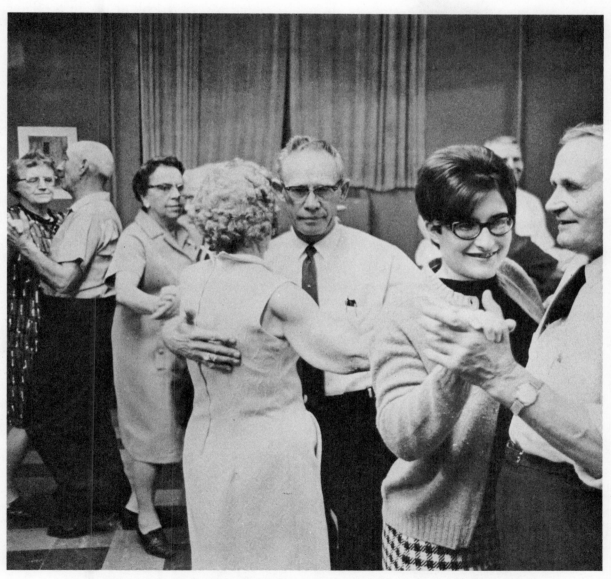

A continuing active social and intellectual program keeps body and mind healthy and alive.

Washington, D.C. 20202; the National Education Association, 1201 Sixteenth Street, N.W., Washington, D.C. 20036; the State Commission on Aging (write to your state capital).

Your local library may have some suggestions (and perhaps offers some classes), and your local "Y" is probably offering some programs.

Uncle Sam continues to be a prime source of educational literature. Each year the government prints about 50 million books, pamphlets, brochures, reports, and guidebooks on everything from astrology to zoology. For a free price list of specified subjects, write to the Superintendent of Documents, Government Printing Office, Washington, D.C. 20402.

Formal and informal learning situations can help you keep pace with change and the future. Continuing education prepares you to live contentedly with a free, independent spirit and mind—while providing you with the means for improved social integration, participation, and satisfaction.

Sexual Attitude and Activity in the Aged

We have come far since the Victorian era when talk about sex was taboo. Now science is taking a candid look at sex in the later years and is exploding old myths as well as exploring new truths. Such enlightenment can help reduce any remaining guilt in this area.

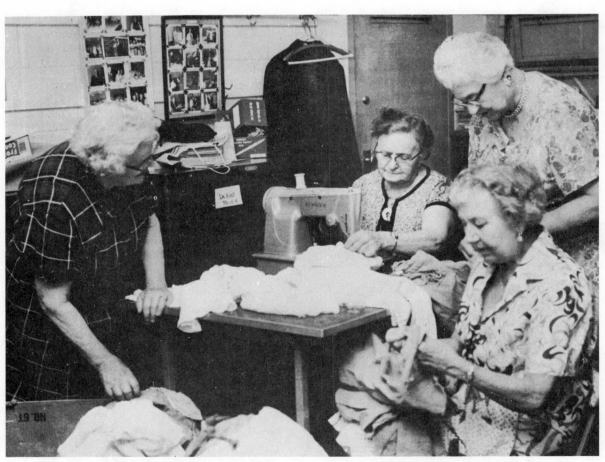

Making a contribution of time, skills, or talent to a worthwhile cause gives a sense of purpose to days that might otherwise be spent in empty loneliness.

After Age 60

In one study to determine the pattern of sexual behavior after 60, researchers at Duke University quizzed 250 people aged 60 to 93 about their sexual activities. Of the 149 who were married, 81 reported they were still sexually active; even in the single group, 7 of the 101 questioned reported "some sexual activity."

Dr. Gustave Newman, who conducted the study, reported 10 percent of the couples over 60 as having sexual relations more than once a week, though couples over 75 unanimously reported less activity.

"No age is an automatic cut-off point for sex," claims the late Dr. Isadore Rubin in his study, *Sexual Life After Sixty*. "But," he continues,

sexuality cannot flourish in a climate where rejection of aging as a worthwhile stage of life leads inevitably to self-rejection by many older persons . . . the men and women who 'act old' in their sexual activity before their bodies have really called a halt become sexually old long before their time.

Sexual Interest After Menopause

Actually, many women take a renewed interest in sex after menopause. Dr. William H. Masters and Mrs. Virginia E. Johnson in their study, *Human Sexual Response*, credit the tendency of many women to experience a second honeymoon in the early fifties to the fact that they no longer have to worry about pregnancy and usually have resolved most of the problems of raising a family.

On the other hand, they tell us:

Deprived of normal sexual outlets, women exhaust themselves physically in conscious or unconscious efforts to dissipate their accumulated and frequently unrecognized sexual tensions. Many demonstrate their basic insecurities by casting themselves unreservedly into their religion, the business world, volunteer social work, or overzealous mothering of their mature children or grandchildren.

Lessened Response of Men

While some women become more responsive as they grow older, Masters and Johnson point out, "There is no question that the human male's responsiveness wanes as he ages." They attribute this to attitudes arising from:

• Bordom—being taken for granted by his wife

• Economic pursuit—occupational competition becomes a demanding, all consuming activity

• Fatigue from unusual or excessive physical strain, such as that induced by sports; or mental fatigue induced by such factors as a "bad day at the office"

• Overindulgence in food and drink, usually alcohol

• Physical and mental infirmities

• Fear of failure.

Myths About Sex

One common reason for an older person's termination of sex life is the often mistaken idea that continued sexual activity in middle and old age may adversely affect health. Although the old myths that sex is weakening or speeds the aging process have been largely dismissed by doctors today, some people still cling to them; what sexual activity they do have is troubled by fear.

Heart patients: Today even cardiac patients are no longer admonished to lead sexless lives except in extreme cases. Even after a heart attack most are able to resume sexual activity within a few months, although patients with angina pectoris may be advised to proceed cautiously.

According to Dr. Philip Reichert, former executive secretary of the American College of Cardiology:

We must get rid of the notion that every heart patient lives under an overhanging sword and that he faces the constant threat of sudden death. The congenial married

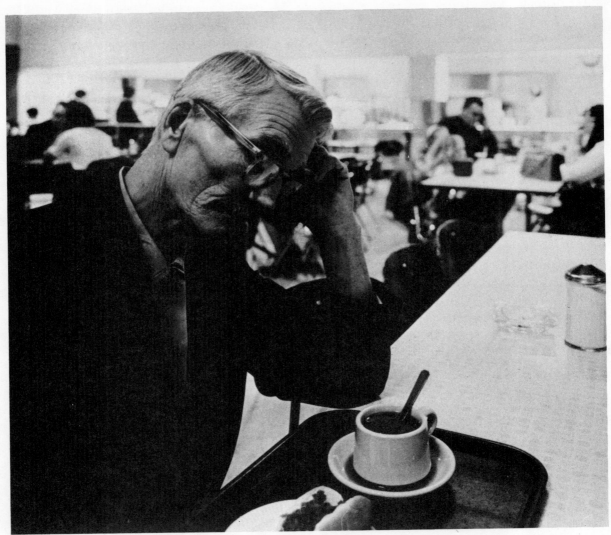

Loneliness can be a problem at any age, but is an especial source of apprehension among older people. By maintaining earlier interests and keeping up social activities, however, the retirement years can be as rich in satisfactions as any other period of life. For many it is the most rewarding time of all.

couple, accustomed to each other and whose technique is habituated through many years of companionship, can achieve sexual satisfaction without too great an expenditure of body energy or too severe a strain upon the heart. . . .

Today, even hypertension sufferers may sometimes indulge in a restricted form of sexual activity with medical supervision. And modern therapy and surgical methods can often prevent or delay impotence caused by prostate disease or diabetes.

Other health problems: But where any health problem is involved, it is best to analyze your sex needs and those of your partner; consult with your doctor and partner as to how you can both attain satisfaction without harm to your health; see your doctor regularly and report accurately distress symptoms and the conditions causing them.

Recent research has dispelled other long-held ideas about sex, too—among them the myth that masturbation is childish and harmful to health. Moreover, Rubin points out: "All studies of older persons have shown that autoerotic activity, while not as common as in the younger years, is far more prevalent in later years than most of us have imagined." He quotes a survey by *Sexology Magazine* which showed that of 279 married men studied, 1 out of every 4 masturbated after age 60.

Dr. Lester W. Dearborn, marriage consultant, in pointing out the role masturbation plays in the lives of the single or widowed, comments:

> It is to be hoped that those interested in the field of geriatrics will . . . encourage the aging to accept masturbation as a perfectly valid outlet when there is a need and other means of gratification are not available.

The "dirty old man" myth has run its course, too. Although society tends to picture both the child molester and the exhibitionist as older men, experts point out that both typically belong to much younger age groups. Donald Mulcock, child welfare specialist, in studying men who assaulted children sexually in England and Wales, found most offenses against boys were committed by men between the ages of 39 and 50, those against girls by men between 33 to 44. Only six percent of the men he studied were 63, and none was older.

Cellular Therapy and Hormone Treatment

To keep older people vigorous and active, some researchers have experimented with *cellular therapy* as a means of retarding aging. Dr. Paul Niehans, a Swiss physician, introduced the idea of cellular therapy in the 1930s with his theory that organs begin to deteriorate in old age when the body fails to replace the cells which compose it. He prescribed a treatment whereby a person is injected with cells from healthy embryonic animal organs. (He uses sheep, pigs, and calves.) He believed that the animal cells from a particular organ would migrate to the same organ in the aging body and re-

activate it. Thus, kidney troubles could be cured with cells from an embryonic animal kidney. Although such notables as Sir Winston Churchill, Pope Pius the XII, Somerset Maugham, and Dr. Konrad Adenauer submitted to it, cellular therapy is not widely accepted in the U.S. today as an effective agent against aging.

More to the point, most researchers feel, are the current experiments with hormones. Widely used today, hormones help women through the tensions of menopause and are used to treat impotence and loss of sexual desire, as well as to combat cancer and some types of heart problems. But because of side effects, hormones face many years of testing before they will be used extensively to retard aging.

Mental Outlook

Good health plus a romantic outlook promote sex appeal at any age. Being romantic and showing affection, whether sexually or not, keep you sparkling and lively no matter what your age.

A good wholesome attitude toward life, a hearty sense of humor, a sympathetic interest in other people—all help make up the indefinable something that makes us appealing to the opposite sex. Good grooming plays an important role, too. Cleanliness, neat suitable apparel, and good posture all add to the image we create of ourselves in other people's minds. So do the manners we reflect in the courtesies we show the people around us—the thoughtful little things we do for them, our reactions to the things they do for us.

If you're a woman over 65 who is looking for companionship, you'll probably find a good personality uplift will get you further than a face or bust lift. If you're a man who is hoping to find feminine companionship, you will probably find a good spiritual overhaul more image-enhancing than dyeing your hair. Also, a good night's sleep is the best aphrodisiac.

The Right Housing

Selecting retirement housing is like selecting a spouse: there are many possibilities, but few that are right.

Ideally, the right housing should take care of you rather than requiring you to take care of it. It should give you shelter, security, and privacy; allow you freedom; and keep you near friends, relatives, and a grocer who delivers.

To Move or Not To Move

What is the right housing for you—the one that you are in or some other place? The answer to this question depends upon

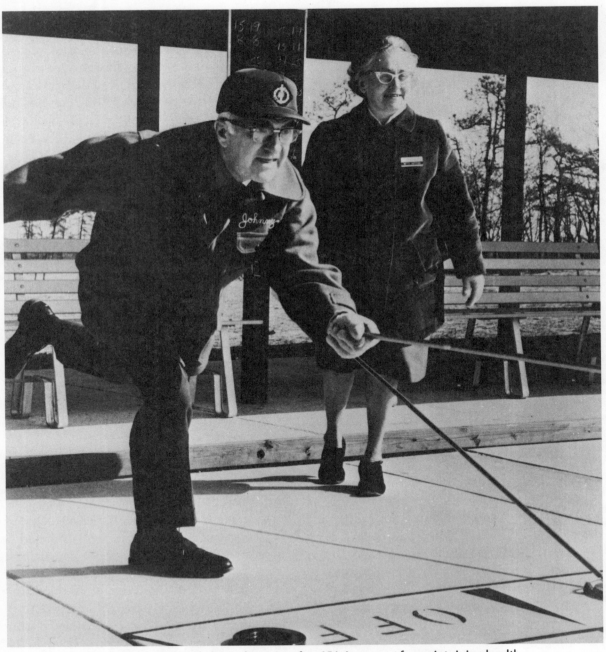

A regular program of physical activity after 65 is important for maintaining health.

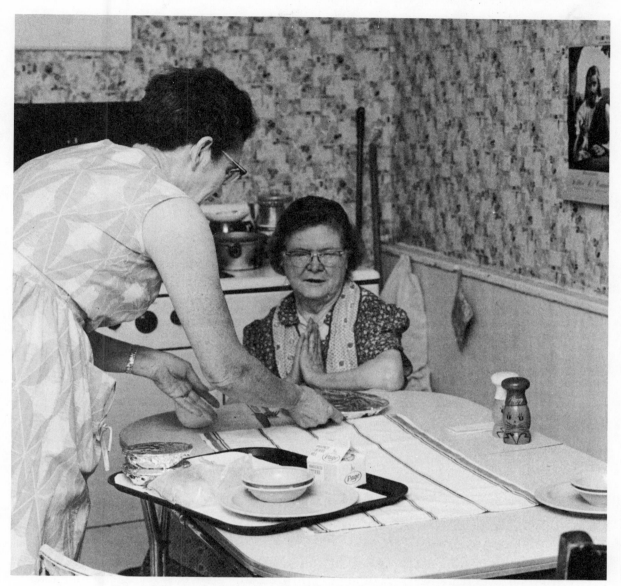

Home delivery of meals, both normal and therapeutic, is available in many areas for those who are unable to obtain or prepare their own food.

the state of your pocketbook and the state of your health.

Advantages of moving: Right now you might be in good health, but this could change. Would stairs become a problem? Could you keep up the house and garden? Would you want more adequate heat? Older people are more comfortable when the temperature is over 75° Fahrenheit. You might also need better lighting in the halls and bedroom.

If you are retired, you might find that you cannot keep up expenses on the old house. You might find that your larger, older house does not suit the reduced size of your family or your need for work or recreation. You could probably save money by living in a smaller place that requires less upkeep. You could also arrange to move nearer children and grandchildren, or into an area where you could find new opportunities for work and recreation.

Advantages of staying put: But by staying in your home you would remain in familiar surroundings and near old friends. You could maintain your comfortable routine and remain independent as long as possible. If you have unused space, you could move into the first floor and shut off the second floor to save on heat and maintenance. Or you could convert part of the house into apartments.

Requirements of Retirement Housing

Whatever you plan to do, your retirement housing should be located near or be easily accessible to shops and recreation centers by public transportation. To make living arrangements more pleasant, individual housing units should contain at least 400 square feet, and there should be two or more rooms.

The new dwelling unit should be equal to or better than the housing you have been used to in the past. It should be suitable for comfortable living in both health and sickness—easily adaptable to convalescent needs with either two bedrooms or a bedroom and sleeping alcove.

In addition, retirement housing should incorporate the following:

• All rooms on one floor, and that floor reached by few, if any, steps
• No thresholds or tripping hazards
• Nonslip surfaces in hallways, bedrooms, and kitchens
• Handrails by all steps and inclines
• Adequate illumination in halls, near steps, and in other potentially hazardous areas
• Fully automatic central heating
• Doors and halls wide enough to accommodate a wheelchair.

Public Housing

If you decide to move and to rent instead of buying, consider public housing projects. These projects are available to single men and women 62 or older, as well as to families whose head is 62 or older or has a spouse at least 62. Local housing authorities build, purchase, or lease the units and set entrance requirements and maximum income limits. Rents are low—averaging less than $40 per unit.

The Housing and Urban Development Agency also makes loans for nonprofit (and profit) sponsors that will build housing for senior citizens with moderate or higher incomes.

Retirement Hotels and Communities

You might also consider retirement hotels, which are especially numerous in Florida, California, and Texas. These hotels are usually refurbished former resorts that provide room and board at a fixed monthly rent—over $100 a month for one person and over $150 a month for a couple.

Retirement communities offer housing of various types, usually apartments, cooperatives, and individual units. It usually costs about $450 a month or more to cover mortgage payments, living, and maintenance expenses.

Would you like retirement community living? It's usually the life for people who like people and who enjoy being active. For those who don't, it can be a bit tiring. Some couples do not like the closeness and activity found in a retirement community and prefer living in a less social environment.

Lifetime Care Facilities

In contrast to the emphasis on independent living in retirement communities, many projects sponsored by church, union, and fraternal organizations stress lifetime care (room, board, and medical care for life), with fees based on actuarial tables of life expectancy at age of entry. Housing alone costs from $10,000 to $30,000, depending upon age and type of living accommodation, *plus* a monthly charge of around $250 per person to cover meals, medical care (exclusive of Medicare), maintenance, and

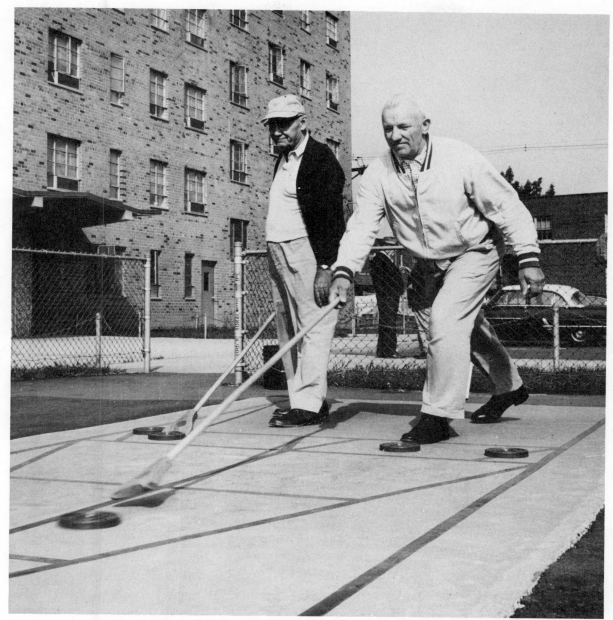

Public housing projects are an ideal solution for some senior citizens who prefer the excitement of living in a large community where friends and recreation are easily available.

other expenses. In many cases, lifetime care for a couple could cost around $90,000.

Cooperatives and Condominiums

In addition to lifetime care facilities, many church, fraternal, and union groups offer other types of housing. In the case of church-sponsored housing, residence usu- ally is not restricted to members of the sponsoring faith.

Some of these units are operated as *cooperatives;* others as *condominiums.* The major difference in the two is that condominium owners have titles to their units, while cooperative residents are stockholders in the cooperative association with occu-

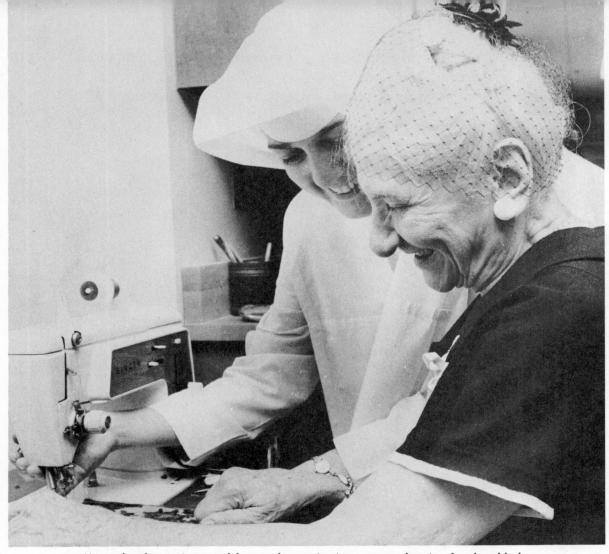

Many churches, unions, and fraternal organizations sponsor housing for the elderly.

pancy rights to specific units. Condominium owners pay their own taxes; cooperative residents pay taxes in their monthly charges.

Mobile Homes

You might also want to consider a mobile home. A suitable one, at least 10 feet wide and 50 feet long, would cost about $7,000.

What is it like to live in a mobile-home park? Certainly, there is a closeness in these parks that you would not have in a normal neighborhood. Typically, the mobile home is placed on a lot 25 to 30 feet wide and 75 feet deep. This means that you could have 12 families within a radius of 100 feet.

Residents visit back and forth and hold frequent picnics, barbecues, and other social activities. This would not be the way of life for someone who did not enjoy group activities.

Be Realistic

To find out what type of housing is best for you, look around the area to see where you want to live. Each community is different, shaped by the people who live there. Talk to the residents and do some serious thinking before you move, not forgetting to carefully consider your financial position in regard to the new locale. Try to be realistic; don't expect to find the perfect climate for health and happiness. The nearest thing to it would be a place that encourages outdoor life, is neither too hot nor too cold, has a relative humidity of around 55 percent, variety in the amount of cloudiness, and enough variety in weather, with frequent but moderate weather changes to be interesting and not too monotonous.

If you have any doubts about the location as far as health is concerned, check with your doctor.

When Faced With Ill Health

How can you help yourself or others when faced with a serious or terminal illness?

Alvin I. Goldfarb, M.D., former consultant on Services for the Aged, New York State Department of Mental Hygiene, notes the importance of self-esteem, self-confidence, sense of purpose, and well-being to a person who is seriously ill or dying. Supported by the idea, "I've led a good and full life," older people can face a serious or terminal illness with dignity. Sometimes this acceptance may be almost an unspoken and tacit understanding between the aging and society to help the separation process along.

When a person is terminally ill, the chances are that he is not in severe pain. With the increasing supply of pain-relieving drugs and the possibility of sedation, very few elderly patients suffer greatly with pain. While a fear of death probably exists in most people, when death is actually encountered the fear is seldom overwhelming, even though it may deeply affect others directly involved with the dying patient.

Most patients are at least aware of the possibility of dying soon; those with lingering conditions are particularly adept at self-diagnosis. But more often, they notice a change in social relationships with friends, family, and medical personnel.

Patient-doctor relationships can be vital in helping the seriously ill patient retain peace of mind. It is the doctor's responsibility to give compassion and recognize fear, even when it is hidden. Likewise, he should respond to a patient's hidden wish to discuss his illness. Of course, there is no set formula for communicating with seriously ill patients. Each individual needs a different approach, and most doctors are sensitive to this.

Many doctors report that death, except in unusual cases, is not accompanied by physical pain. Rather, there is often a sense of well-being and spiritual exaltation. Doctors think this feeling is caused by the anesthetic action of carbon dioxide on the central nervous system and by the effect of toxic substances. Ernest Hemingway wrote, "The pang of death, a famous doctor once told me, is often less than that of a toothache."

Stages of Death

According to doctors, man dies in stages —rapidly or slowly, depending on circumstances. First comes *clinical death,* when respiration and heartbeat cease. The brain dies as it is deprived of oxygen and circulating blood, and *biological death* occurs.

Life can be restored in the moments between clinical death and brain death if circulation and respiration are continued through the use of medical devices which stimulate the heart and lungs.

After the brain ceases to function, cellular death begins. Life is not considered to be completely lost until the brain stops functioning. It is possible for doctors to remove viable organs after biological death for transplant or other use.

Many clergymen and doctors insist that we need more honest communication about death, as such communication is probably the single most useful measure to avoid unnecessary suffering. Sound knowledge never made anyone afraid. And although death will probably always remain essentially a mystery to man, scientists will continue to search for a better understanding of its nature. By such means they may learn a great deal more about life.

For a discussion of physical problems associated with the later years, see *Aging and What To Do About It,* p. 188.   PAD

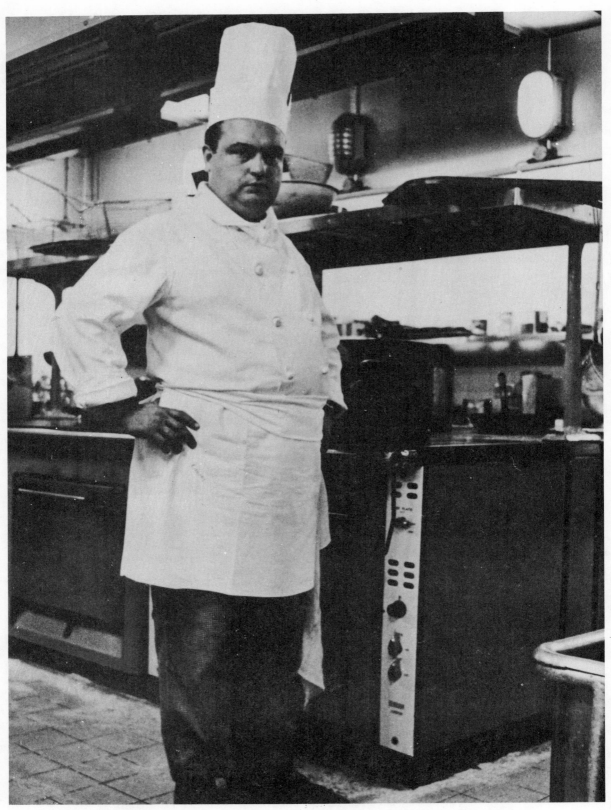

This chef stands in the grand tradition of fine food, one of civilization's oldest pleasures.

CHAPTER 4

Nutrition and Weight Control

Food and meals are man's best friends. His health and his social life are tied intimately and everlastingly to what he eats and how he eats it. Of all the physiological functions which maintain his life, eating and all that it entails is the one in which he most expresses his personal preferences and the cultural traditions of his ancestors.

Most people develop eating habits early in life that accord with family patterns and modify them only slightly over the years. Sometimes these habits conform to ideal food recommendations from the viewpoint of maintaining and fostering good health. More often, however, they do not.

Knowledge about food, eating, and their relationship to health is the best way to change inappropriate eating patterns of adults and to introduce youngsters to good eating habits that should last a lifetime.

Basic Nutritional Requirements

In a somewhat oversimplified way, a person can be compared with a working mechanism such as a car. The material of which each is made—tissue cells for the person, metal for the car—has to come from somewhere: the human's, from conception to birth comes from the food eaten by his mother; after birth, from what he himself eats.

During growth and thereafter, the person's cells must be repaired and replaced just as a car must have new tires, parts, and paint from time to time. And like the car, the human has an engine—his muscular activity—which requires fuel. This fuel is provided by food in the form of calories.

In humans, the process by which food is used by the body is called *metabolism*. It begins with chemical processes in the gastrointestinal tract which change plant and animal food into less complex components so that they can be absorbed to fulfill their various functions in the body.

Protein

Of the several essential components of food, *protein* is in many ways the most important. This is so because much of the body's structure is made up of proteins.

295

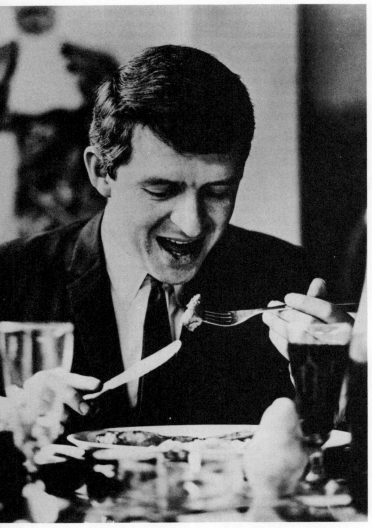

Food is the raw material that is chemically altered by digestion to supply the body with the nutrients needed to replace cells and to fuel the muscles with enough energy to carry out their activities.

For example, the typical 160-pound man is composed of about 100 pounds of water, 29 pounds of protein, 25 pounds of fat, 5 pounds of minerals, 1 pound of carbohydrate, and less than an ounce of vitamins. Since the muscles, heart, brain, lungs, and gastrointestinal organs are made up largely of protein, and since the protein in these organs is in constant need of replacement, its importance is obvious.

Chemically, proteins are mixtures of amino acids which contain various elements, including nitrogen. There are 20 different amino acids that are essential for the body's protein needs. Eight of these must be provided in the diet; the rest can be synthesized by the body itself.

Meat, fish, eggs, and milk or milk products are the primary protein foods and contain all of the necessary amino acids. Grains and vegetables are partly made up of protein, but more often than not, they do not provide the whole range of amino acids required for proper nourishment.

Carbohydrates

Carbohydrates are another essential food component. They are also called *starches* or *sugars* and are present in large quantities in grains, fruits, and vegetables. They serve as the primary source of calories for muscle contraction and must be available in the body constantly for this purpose.

It takes one pound of carbohydrates to provide a 160-pound man with fuel for about half a day. Therefore, if he isn't getting new carbohydrate supplies during the day from his food, he will begin to convert his body fat or protein into sugar. This isn't desirable unless he has an excess of body fat, and in any event, could not go on indefinitely.

Fats

Fats are a chemically complex food component composed of *glycerol* (a sweet, oily alcohol) and fatty acids. Fats exist in several forms and come from a variety of sources. One way to think of them is to group them as visible fats, such as butter, salad oil, or the fat seen in meat, and as invisible fats, which are mingled, blended, or absorbed into food, either naturally, as in nuts, meat, or fish, or during cooking. Another way is to think of them as solid at room temperature (fats), or as liquid at room temperature (oils).

Saturated and unsaturated: Fats are also classified as *saturated* or *unsaturated.* This is a chemical distinction based on the differences in molecular structure of different kinds of fat. If the carbon atoms in a fat molecule are surrounded or boxed in by hydrogen atoms, they are said to be saturated. This type of fat seems to increase the cholesterol content of the blood. *Polyunsaturated* fats, such as those found in fish and vegetable oils, contain the least number of hydrogen atoms and do not add to the blood cholesterol content. In general, fats in foods of plant origin are more unsaturated than in those of animal origin.

Fats play several essential roles in the metabolic process. First of all, they provide more than twice the number of calories on a comparative weight basis than do proteins and carbohydrates. They also can be stored in the body in large quantities and used as a later energy source. They serve as carriers of the fat-soluble vitamins A, D, E, and K, and—of no little importance—they add to the tastiness of food.

Vitamins

Vitamins, which are present in minute quantities in foods in their natural state, are essential for normal metabolism and for the development and maintenance of tissue structure and function. In addition to the fat-soluble vitamins noted above, there are a number of B vitamins, as well as vitamin C, also called ascorbic acid. If any particular vitamin is missing from the diet over a sufficiently long time, a specific disease will result.

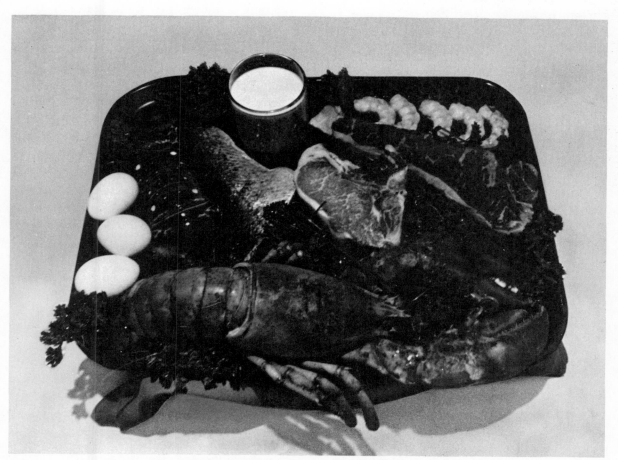

Meat, fish, eggs, and milk are examples of foods that are rich sources of protein, which is perhaps the most important of all the body's nutritional requirements.

The understanding of the subtle and complicated role of vitamins in maintaining life and health has come about during this century with the development of highly refined research methods. It is likely that continuing research will shed more light on their importance.

Minerals

Minerals are another component of basic nutritional needs. All living things extract them from the soil, which is their ultimate source. Like vitamins, they are needed for normal metabolism and must be present in the diet in sufficient amounts for the maintenance of good health. The essential minerals are copper, iodine, iron, manganese, zinc, molybdenum, fluorine, and cobalt.

When the normal diet is deficient in certain minerals, these minerals need to be specially added to the diet: iodine for thyroid function, and fluorine for protection against dental cavities. Additional iron for hemoglobin formation may be indicated when the diet is deficient in it, or when there has been an excessive loss of red blood cells, as some women experience with their menstrual periods.

Water

Water is not really a food in the fuel or calorie-producing sense, but it is in many ways a crucial component of nutrition. It makes up from 55 to 65 percent of the body's weight, and is constantly being eliminated in the form of urine, perspiration, and expired breath. It must therefore be replaced regularly, for while a person can live for weeks without food, he can live for only a few days without water.

NUTRIENTS IN COMMON FOODS

	Food energy	Protein	Fat	Carbohydrate
	Calories	Grams	Grams	Grams
Milk and Milk Products				
Milk; 1 cup:				
Fluid, whole	165	9	10	12
Fluid, nonfat (skim)	90	9	Trace	13
Buttermilk, cultured (from skim milk)	90	9	Trace	13
Evaporated (undiluted)	345	18	20	24
Dry, nonfat	290	29	1	42
Yoghurt (from partially skimmed milk); 1 cup	120	8	4	13
Cheese; 1 ounce:				
Cheddar, or American	115	7	9	1
Cottage:				
From skim milk	25	5	Trace	1
Creamed	30	4	1	1
Cream cheese	105	2	11	1
Swiss	105	7	8	1
Desserts (largely milk):				
Custard, baked; 1 cup, 8 fluid ounces	285	13	14	28
Ice cream, plain, factory packed:				
1 slice or individual brick, ⅐ quart	165	3	10	17
1 container, 8 fluid ounces	295	6	18	29
Ice milk; 1 cup, 8 fluid ounces	285	9	10	42

Adapted from *Food: The Yearbook of Agriculture 1959*, U.S. Department of Agriculture, pp. 243–265. The cup measure used in the following table refers to the standard 8-ounce measuring cup of 8 fluid ounces or one-half liquid pint. When a measure is indicated by ounce, it is understood to be by weight—1/16 of a pound avoirdupois—unless a fluid ounce is indicated.

NUTRITION AND WEIGHT CONTROL

Normally, the best guide to how much water a person needs is his sense of thirst. The regulating mechanism of excretion sees to it that an excessive intake of water will be eliminated as urine. The usual water requirement is on the order of two quarts a day in addition to whatever amount is contained in the solids which make up the daily diet. Information on the protein, fat, and carbohydrate content in specific foods, as well as the number of calories, may be obtained by consulting the table *Nutrients in Common Foods,* pp. 298–319.

Basic Daily Diets

Everyone should have at least the minimal amount of basic nutrients for resting or basal metabolism. The specific needs of each individual are determined by whether

he is still growing, and by how much energy is required for his normal activities. All those who are still growing—and growth continues up to about 20 years of age—have relatively high food needs.

For Infants

That food needs of an infant are especially acute should surprise no one. The newborn baby normally triples his birth weight during his first year and is very active in terms of calorie expenditure.

For his first six months, breast milk or formula, or a combination of both, fills his nutritional needs. The amount of milk he should get each day is about two and a half ounces per pound of his body weight. This provides 50 calories per pound, and in the early months is usually given in six feedings a day at four-hour intervals.

NUTRIENTS IN COMMON FOODS

	Food energy	Protein	Fat	Carbohydrate
	Calories	Grams	Grams	Grams
Eggs				
Egg, raw, large:				
1 whole	80	6	6	Trace
1 white	15	4	Trace	Trace
1 yolk	60	3	5	Trace
Egg, cooked; 1 large:				
Boiled	80	6	6	Trace
Scrambled (with milk and fat)	110	7	8	1
Meat, Poultry, Fish, Shellfish				
Bacon, broiled or fried, medium done; 2 slices	95	4	9	Trace
Beef, cooked without bone:				
Braised, simmered, or pot-roasted; 3-ounce portion:				
Entire portion, lean and fat	340	20	28	0
Lean only, approx. 2 ounces	115	18	4	0
Hamburger patties, made with				
Regular ground beef; 3-ounce patty	245	21	17	0
Lean ground round; 3-ounce patty	185	23	10	0
Roast; 3-ounce slice from cut having relatively small amount of fat:				
Entire portion, lean and fat	255	22	18	0
Lean only, approx. 2.3 ounces	115	19	4	0

BEEF CHART

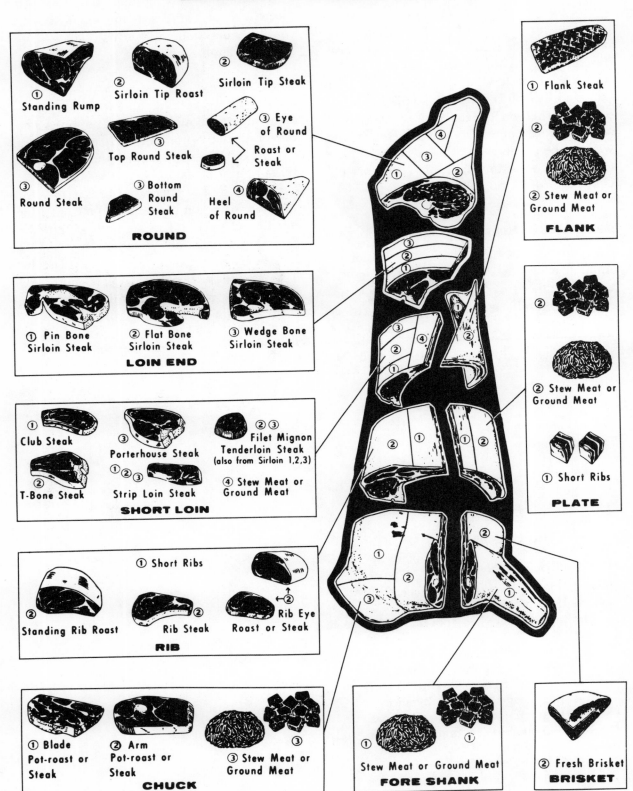

ROUND
① Standing Rump
② Sirloin Tip Roast
② Sirloin Tip Steak
③ Eye of Round
Roast or Steak
③ Round Steak
③ Top Round Steak
③ Bottom Round Steak
④ Heel of Round

LOIN END
① Pin Bone Sirloin Steak
② Flat Bone Sirloin Steak
③ Wedge Bone Sirloin Steak

SHORT LOIN
① Club Steak
③ Porterhouse Steak
②③ Filet Mignon Tenderloin Steak (also from Sirloin 1,2,3)
② T-Bone Steak
①②③ Strip Loin Steak
④ Stew Meat or Ground Meat

RIB
① Short Ribs
② Standing Rib Roast
② Rib Steak
② Rib Eye Roast or Steak

CHUCK
① Blade Pot-roast or Steak
② Arm Pot-roast or Steak
③ Stew Meat or Ground Meat

FLANK
① Flank Steak
② Stew Meat or Ground Meat

PLATE
② Stew Meat or Ground Meat
① Short Ribs

FORE SHANK
Stew Meat or Ground Meat

BRISKET
② Fresh Brisket

If his weight gain is adequate and he appears healthy, and if his stomach is not distended by swallowed air, his appetite is normally a satisfactory guide to how much he needs. The formula-fed baby should get a supplement of 35 milligrams of ascorbic acid each day and 400 international units of vitamin D if the latter has not been added to the milk during its processing.

Solid foods: Between two and six months of age, the baby should begin to eat solid foods such as cooked cereals, strained fruits and vegetables, egg yolk, and homogenized meat. With the introduction of these foods, it is not really necessary to calculate the baby's caloric intake. Satisfaction of appetite, proper weight gain, and a healthy appearance serve as the guides to a proper diet.

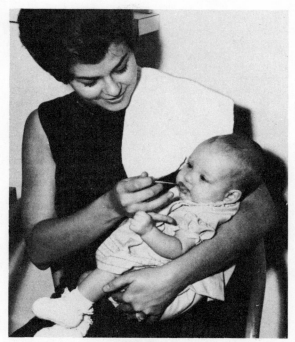

Babies begin eating solid foods between 2–6 months.

NUTRIENTS IN COMMON FOODS

	Food energy Calories	Protein Grams	Fat Grams	Carbohydrate Grams
Steak, broiled; 3-ounce portion:				
Entire portion, lean and fat	375	19	32	0
Lean only, approx. 1.8 ounces . . .	105	17	4	0
Beef, canned: corned beef hash: 3 ounces . . .	120	12	5	6
Beef and vegetable stew: 1 cup	250	13	19	17
Chicken, without bone: broiled; 3 ounces . . .	115	20	3	0
Lamb, cooked:				
Chops; 1 thick chop, without bone, 4.8 ounces:				
Lean and fat, approx. 3.6 ounces . . .	450	24	39	0
Lean only, 2.4 ounces	130	19	5	0
Roast, without bone:				
Leg; 3-ounce slice:				
Entire slice, lean and fat	265	20	20	0
Lean only, approx. 2.3 ounces . . .	120	19	5	0
Shoulder; 3-ounce portion, without bone:				
Entire portion, lean and fat . . .	300	18	25	0
Lean only, approx. 2.2 ounces . . .	125	16	6	0
Liver, beef, fried; 2 ounces	120	13	4	6
Pork, cured, cooked:				
Ham, smoked; 3-ounce portion, without bone .	340	20	28	Trace
Luncheon meat:				
Boiled ham; 2 ounces	170	13	13	0
Canned, spiced; 2 ounces	165	8	14	1

LAMB CHART

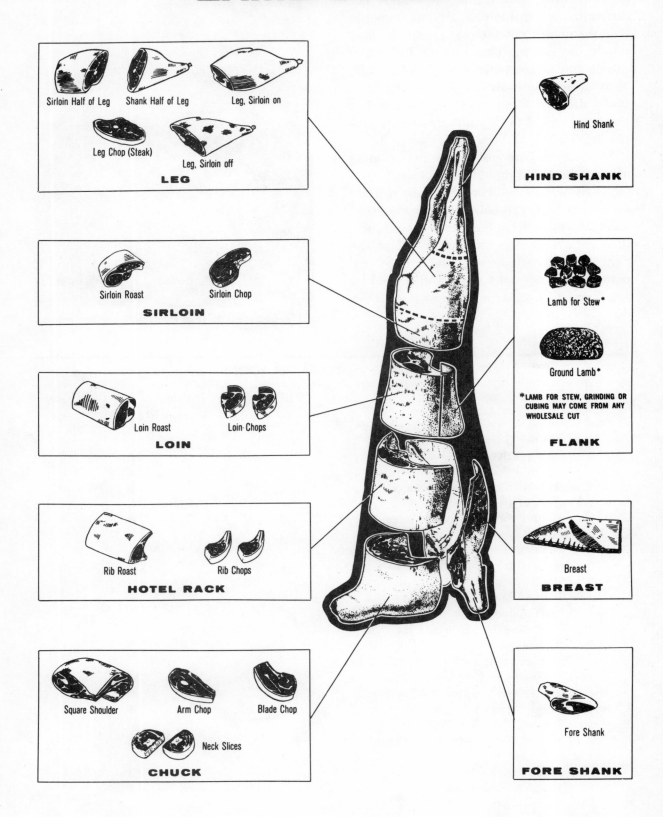

LEG
Sirloin Half of Leg   Shank Half of Leg   Leg, Sirloin on
Leg Chop (Steak)
Leg, Sirloin off

SIRLOIN
Sirloin Roast   Sirloin Chop

LOIN
Loin Roast   Loin Chops

HOTEL RACK
Rib Roast   Rib Chops

CHUCK
Square Shoulder   Arm Chop   Blade Chop
Neck Slices

HIND SHANK
Hind Shank

FLANK
Lamb for Stew*
Ground Lamb*

*LAMB FOR STEW, GRINDING OR CUBING MAY COME FROM ANY WHOLESALE CUT

BREAST
Breast

FORE SHANK
Fore Shank

By one year of age, a baby should be getting three regular meals a day, and as his teeth appear, his food no longer needs to be strained. By 18 to 24 months, he should no longer need baby foods. For further information on the care and feeding of infants, see under *Birth, Infancy, and Maturation*, p. 99.

Basic Food Groups

The recommended daily amounts of food for people over the age of two have been established with reasonable accuracy. They are called minimal daily amounts, but they always contain a fairly generous safety factor.

The four group division: In general, foods are divided into four major groups:

• Meat, fish, eggs
• Dairy products
• Fruits and vegetables
• Breads and cereals.

The seven group division: For purposes of planning daily requirements, a more detailed way of considering food groupings is the following:

• Leafy green and yellow vegetables
• Citrus fruits, tomatoes, and raw cabbage
• Potatoes and other vegetables and fruits
• Milk, cheese, and ice cream
• Meat, poultry, fish, eggs, dried peas, and beans
• Bread, flour, and cereals
• Butter and fortified margarine.

The *Daily Food Guide* (see p. 305) is a general guide to planning nutritionally balanced meals for pre-teens, teens, and adults of any age.

NUTRIENTS IN COMMON FOODS

	Food energy	Protein	Fat	Carbohydrate
	Calories	Grams	Grams	Grams
Pork, fresh, cooked:				
Chops; 1 chop, with bone, 3.5 ounces:				
Lean and fat, approx. 2.4 ounces	295	15	25	0
Lean only, approx. 1.6 ounces	120	14	7	0
Roast; 3-ounce slice, without bone:				
Entire slice, lean and fat	340	19	29	0
Lean only, approx. 2.2 ounces	160	19	9	0
Sausage:				
Bologna; 8 slices (4.1 by 0.1 inches each), 8 ounces	690	27	62	2
Frankfurter; 1 cooked, 1.8 ounces	155	6	14	1
Tongue, beef, boiled or simmered; 3 ounces	205	18	14	Trace
Veal, cutlet, broiled; 3-ounce portion, without bone	185	23	9	0
Fish and shellfish:				
Bluefish, baked or broiled; 3 ounces	135	22	4	0
Clams: raw, meat only; 3 ounces	70	11	1	3
Crabmeat, canned or cooked; 3 ounces	90	14	2	1
Fishsticks, breaded, cooked, frozen; 10 sticks (3.8 by 1.0 by 0.5 inches each), 8 ounces	400	38	20	15
Haddock, fried; 3 ounces	135	16	5	6
Mackerel: broiled; 3 ounces	200	19	13	0
Oysters, raw, meat only; 1 cup (13–19 medium-size oysters, selects)	160	20	4	8

PORK CHART

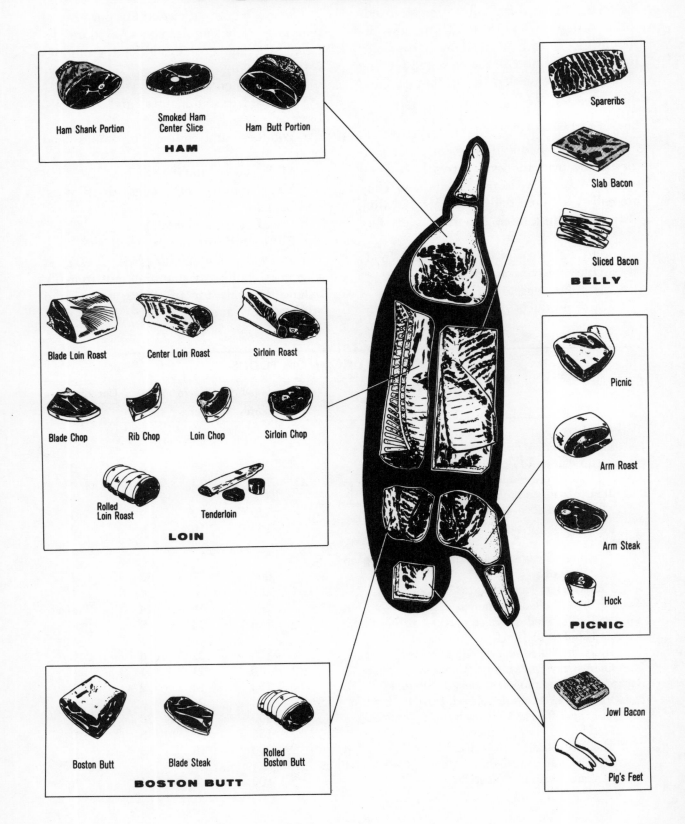

HAM
- Ham Shank Portion
- Smoked Ham Center Slice
- Ham Butt Portion

LOIN
- Blade Loin Roast
- Center Loin Roast
- Sirloin Roast
- Blade Chop
- Rib Chop
- Loin Chop
- Sirloin Chop
- Rolled Loin Roast
- Tenderloin

BOSTON BUTT
- Boston Butt
- Blade Steak
- Rolled Boston Butt

BELLY
- Spareribs
- Slab Bacon
- Sliced Bacon

PICNIC
- Picnic
- Arm Roast
- Arm Steak
- Hock

- Jowl Bacon
- Pig's Feet

DAILY FOOD GUIDE

	Child	Pre-teen and Teen	Adult	Aging Adult
Milk or milk products (*cups*)	2–3	3–4 or more	2 or more	2 or more
Meat, fish, poultry, and eggs (*servings*)	1–2	3 or more	2 or more	2 or more
Green and yellow vegetables (*servings*)	1–2	2	2	at least 1
Citrus fruits and tomatoes (*servings*)	1	1–2	1	1–2
Potatoes, other fruits, and vegetables (*servings*)	1	1	1	0–1
Bread, flour, and cereal (*servings*)	3–4	4 or more	3–4	2–3
Butter or margarine (*tablespoons*)	2	2–4	2–3	1–2

1. The need for the nutrients in 1 or 2 cups of milk daily can be satisfied by cheeses or ice cream. (1 cup of milk is approximately equivalent to 1½ cups of cottage cheese or 2–3 large scoops of ice cream.)

2. It is important to drink enough fluid. The equivalent of 3–5 cups daily is recommended.

3. The recommended daily serving of meat, fish, and poultry (3 oz.) may be alternated with eggs or cheese, dried peas, beans, or lentils.

4. Iron-rich foods should be selected as frequently as possible by teen-age and adult females to help meet their high requirement for this mineral (liver, heart, lean meats, shellfish, egg yolks, legumes, green leafy vegetables, and whole grain and enriched cereal products).

From *Your Age and Your Diet* (1971), reprinted with permission from the American Medical Association

NUTRIENTS IN COMMON FOODS

	Food energy	Protein	Fat	Carbohydrate
	Calories	Grams	Grams	Grams
Oyster stew: 1 cup (6–8 oysters)	200	11	12	11
Salmon, canned (pink); 3 ounces	120	17	5	0
Sardines, canned in oil, drained solids; 3 ounces	180	22	9	1
Shrimp, canned, meat only; 3 ounces . . .	110	23	1	—
Tuna, canned in oil, drained solids; 3 ounces . .	170	25	7	0

Mature Beans and Peas, Nuts

Beans, dry seed:

Common varieties, as Great Northern, navy, and others, canned; 1 cup:

	Food energy	Protein	Fat	Carbohydrate
Red	230	15	1	42
White, with tomato or molasses:				
With pork	330	16	7	54
Without pork	315	16	1	60
Lima, cooked; 1 cup	260	16	1	48
Cowpeas or black-eyed peas, dry, cooked; 1 cup . .	190	13	1	34
Peanuts, roasted, shelled; 1 cup	840	39	71	28
Peanut butter; 1 tablespoon	90	4	8	3
Peas, split, dry, cooked; 1 cup	290	20	1	52

Vegetables

Asparagus:

	Food energy	Protein	Fat	Carbohydrate
Cooked; 1 cup	35	4	Trace	6

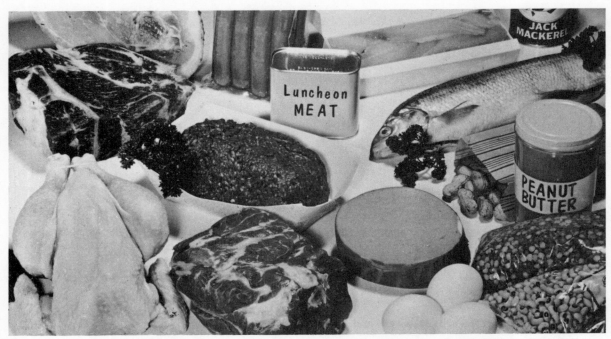

One of the four basic food groups: meat, fish, eggs, nuts, and dried peas.

NUTRIENTS IN COMMON FOODS

	Food energy	Protein	Fat	Carbohydrate
	Calories	Grams	Grams	Grams
Asparagus:				
Canned; 6 medium-size spears:	20	2	Trace	3
Beans:				
Lima, immature, cooked; 1 cup	150	8	1	29
Snap, green:				
Cooked; 1 cup	25	2	Trace	6
Canned: solids and liquid; 1 cup . . .	45	2	Trace	10
Beets, cooked, diced; 1 cup	70	2	Trace	16
Broccoli, cooked, flower stalks; 1 cup	45	5	Trace	8
Brussels sprouts, cooked; 1 cup	60	6	1	12
Cabbage; 1 cup:				
Raw, coleslaw	100	2	7	9
Cooked	40	2	Trace	9
Carrots:				
Raw: 1 carrot (5½ by 1 inch) or 25 thin strips .	20	1	Trace	5
Cooked, diced; 1 cup	45	1	1	9
Canned, strained or chopped; 1 ounce . . .	5	Trace	0	2
Cauliflower, cooked, flower buds; 1 cup	30	3	Trace	6
Celery, raw: large stalk, 8 inches long	5	1	Trace	1
Collards, cooked; 1 cup	75	7	1	14
Corn, sweet:				
Cooked; 1 ear 5 inches long	65	2	1	16
Canned, solids and liquid; 1 cup	170	5	1	41

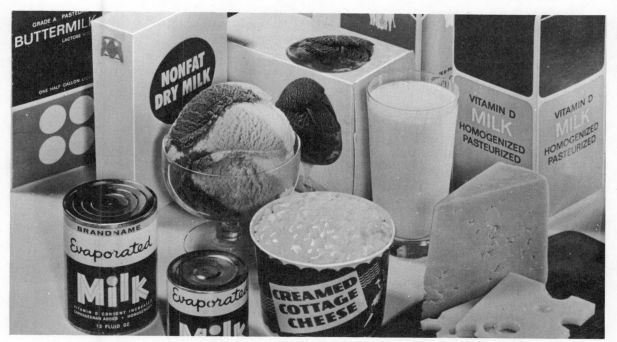

One of the four basic food groups: milk, cheese, ice cream, and other dairy products.

NUTRIENTS IN COMMON FOODS

	Food energy	Protein	Fat	Carbohydrate
	Calories	Grams	Grams	Grams
Cucumbers, raw, pared; 6 slices (⅛-inch thick, center section)	5	Trace	Trace	1
Lettuce, head, raw:				
2 large or 4 small leaves	5	1	Trace	1
1 compact head (4¾-inch diameter)	70	5	1	13
Mushrooms, canned, solids and liquid; 1 cup	30	3	Trace	9
Okra, cooked; 8 pods (3 inches long, ⅝-inch diameter)	30	2	Trace	6
Onions: mature raw; 1 onion (2½-inch diameter)	50	2	Trace	11
Peas, green; 1 cup:				
Cooked	110	8	1	19
Canned, solids and liquid	170	8	1	32
Peppers, sweet:				
Green, raw; 1 medium	15	1	Trace	3
Red, raw; 1 medium	20	1	Trace	4
Potatoes:				
Baked or boiled; 1 medium, 2½-inch diameter (weight raw, about 5 ounces):				
Baked in jacket	90	3	Trace	21
Boiled; peeled before boiling	90	3	Trace	21
Chips; 10 medium (2-inch diameter)	110	1	7	10
French fried:				
Frozen, ready to be heated for serving; 10 pieces (2 by ½ by ½ inch)	95	2	4	15

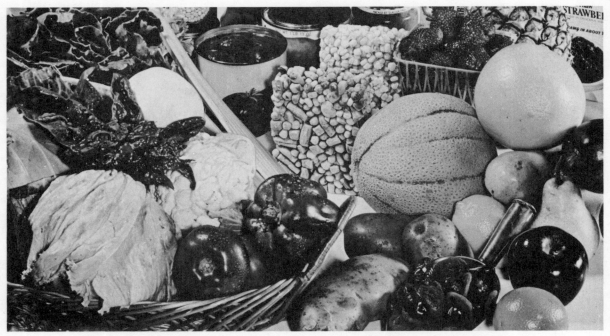

One of the four basic food groups: fruits and vegetables, including potatoes.

NUTRIENTS IN COMMON FOODS

	Food energy	Protein	Fat	Carbohydrate
	Calories	Grams	Grams	Grams
Potatoes:				
French fried:				
Ready-to-eat, deep fat for entire process; 10 pieces (2 by ½ by ½ inch) . . .	155	2	7	20
Mashed; 1 cup:				
Milk added	145	4	1	30
Milk and butter added	230	4	12	28
Radishes, raw; 4 small	10	Trace	Trace	2
Spinach:				
Cooked; 1 cup	45	6	1	6
Canned, creamed, strained; 1 ounce	10	1	Trace	2
Squash:				
Cooked, 1 cup:				
Summer, diced	35	1	Trace	8
Winter, baked, mashed	95	4	1	23
Canned, strained or chopped; 1 ounce . . .	10	Trace	Trace	2
Sweet potatoes:				
Baked or boiled; 1 medium, 5 by 2 inches (weight raw, about 6 ounces):				
Baked in jacket	155	2	1	36
Boiled in jacket	170	2	1	39
Candied; 1 small, 3½ by 2 inches	295	2	6	60
Canned, vacuum or solid pack; 1 cup . . .	235	4	Trace	54

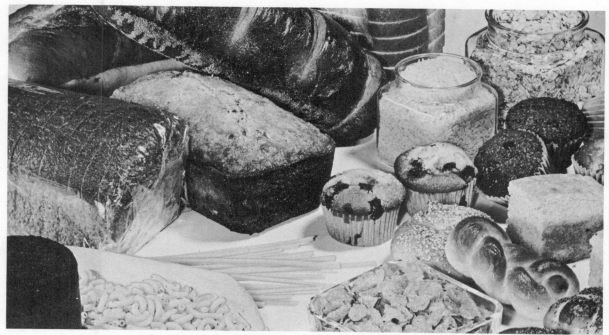

One of the four basic food groups: breads and cereals, including rice and pasta.

NUTRIENTS IN COMMON FOODS

	Food energy	Protein	Fat	Carbohydrate
	Calories	Grams	Grams	Grams
Tomatoes:				
Raw; 1 medium (2 by 2½ inches), about ⅓ pound	30	2	Trace	6
Canned or cooked; 1 cup	45	2	Trace	9
Tomato juice, canned; 1 cup	50	2	Trace	10
Tomato catsup; 1 tablespoon	15	Trace	Trace	4
Turnips, cooked, diced; 1 cup	40	1	Trace	9
Turnip greens, cooked; 1 cup	45	4	1	8
Fruits				
Apples, raw; 1 medium (2½ inch diameter), about ⅓ pound	70	Trace	Trace	18
Apple juice, fresh or canned; 1 cup	125	Trace	0	34
Apple sauce, canned:				
Sweetened; 1 cup	185	Trace	Trace	50
Unsweetened; 1 cup	100	Trace	Trace	26
Apricots, raw; 3 apricots (about ¼ pound)	55	1	Trace	14
Apricots, canned in heavy sirup; 1 cup	200	1	Trace	54
Apricots, dried: uncooked; 1 cup (40 halves, small)	390	8	1	100
Avocados, raw, California varieties: ½ of a 10-ounce avocado (3½ by 3¼ inches)	185	2	18	6
Avocados, raw, Florida varieties: ½ of a 13-ounce avocado (4 by 3 inches)	160	2	14	11

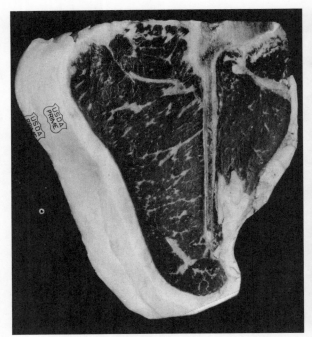 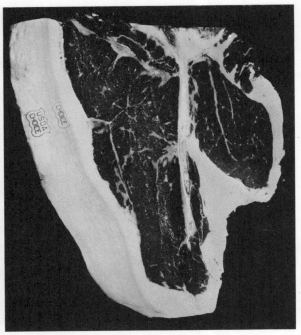

Prime and choice grades of beef are the best in tenderness, juiciness, and flavor.

NUTRIENTS IN COMMON FOODS

	Food energy	Protein	Fat	Carbohydrate
	Calories	Grams	Grams	Grams
Bananas, raw; 1 medium (6 by 1½ inches), about ⅓ pound	85	1	Trace	23
Blueberries, raw; 1 cup	85	1	1	21
Cantaloupes, raw, ½ melon (5-inch diameter) . .	40	1	Trace	9
Cherries, sour, sweet, and hybrid, raw; 1 cup . . .	65	1	1	15
Cranberry sauce, sweetened; 1 cup	550	Trace	1	142
Dates, "fresh" and dried, pitted and cut; 1 cup . .	505	4	1	134
Figs:				
Raw; 3 small (1½-inch diameter), about ¼ pound	90	2	Trace	22
Dried; 1 large (2 by 1 inch)	60	1	Trace	15
Fruit cocktail, canned in heavy sirup, solids and liquid; 1 cup	175	1	Trace	47
Grapefruit:				
Raw; ½ medium (4¼-inch diameter, No. 64's) .	50	1	Trace	14
Canned in sirup; 1 cup	165	1	Trace	44
Grapefruit juice:				
Raw; 1 cup	85	1	Trace	23
Canned:				
Unsweetened; 1 cup	95	1	Trace	24
Sweetened; 1 cup	120	1	Trace	32
Frozen concentrate, unsweetened:				
Undiluted; 1 can (6 fluid ounces) . . .	280	4	1	72

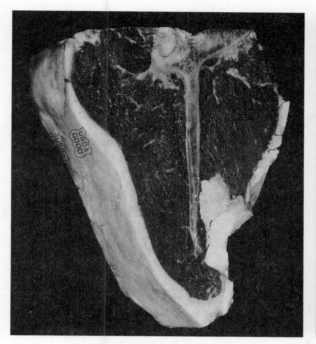 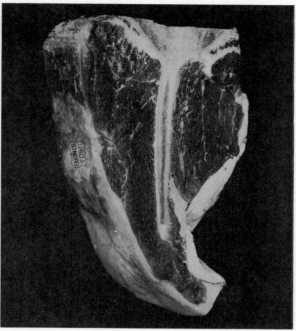

Good and Standard grades of beef are leaner, with less marbling, than the top grades.

NUTRIENTS IN COMMON FOODS

	Food energy	Protein	Fat	Carbohydrate
	Calories	Grams	Grams	Grams
Grapefruit juice:				
Frozen concentrate, unsweetened:				
Diluted, ready-to-serve; 1 cup	95	1	Trace	24
Frozen concentrate, sweetened:				
Undiluted; 1 can (6 fluid ounces) . . .	320	3	1	85
Diluted, ready-to-serve; 1 cup	105	1	Trace	28
Grapes, raw; 1 cup:				
American type (slip skin)	70	1	1	16
European type (adherent skin)	100	1	Trace	26
Grape juice, bottled; 1 cup	165	1	1	42
Lemonade concentrate, frozen, sweetened:				
Undiluted; 1 can (6 fluid ounces) . . .	305	1	Trace	113
Diluted, ready-to-serve; 1 cup	75	Trace	Trace	28
Oranges, raw; 1 large orange (3-inch diameter) . .	70	1	Trace	18
Orange juice:				
Raw; 1 cup:				
California (Valencias)	105	2	Trace	26
Florida varieties:				
Early and midseason	90	1	Trace	23
Late season (Valencias)	105	1	Trace	26
Canned, unsweetened; 1 cup	110	2	Trace	28
Frozen concentrate:				
Undiluted; 1 can (6 fl. ounces) . . .	305	5	Trace	80

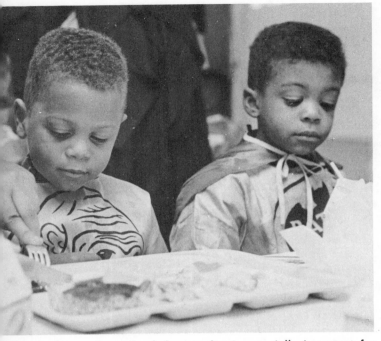

A good, wholesome diet is especially important for young children during the years of rapid growth.

The Years of Growth

Even though a child will never again triple his weight in a single year as he did during his first, a proper diet is crucial during the years from 2 to 18, since this is a period of tremendous growth.

Other food goals that should be realized during the childhood and adolescent years are an awareness of what a balanced diet is, a reasonable tolerance for a variety of foods, decent manners at the table, and a sense of timing about when to eat and when not to eat.

These are also the years that a young person should begin to learn something about how to buy and prepare food, how to serve it attractively, and how to clean up after a meal.

Creating a pleasant atmosphere at mealtime: Although a child's behavior about

NUTRIENTS IN COMMON FOODS

	Food energy	Protein	Fat	Carbohydrate
	Calories	Grams	Grams	Grams
Orange juice:				
Frozen concentrate:				
Diluted, ready-to-serve; 1 cup	105	2	Trace	27
Peaches:				
Raw:				
1 medium (2½ by 2-inch diameter), about ¼ pound	35	1	Trace	10
1 cup, sliced	65	1	Trace	16
Canned (yellow-fleshed) in heavy sirup; 1 cup .	185	1	Trace	49
Dried: uncooked; 1 cup	420	5	1	109
Pears:				
Raw; 1 pear (3- by 2½-inch diameter) . . .	100	1	1	25
Canned in heavy sirup; 1 cup	175	1	Trace	47
Plums:				
Raw; 1 plum (2-inch diameter), about 2 ounces .	30	Trace	Trace	7
Canned (Italian prunes), in sirup; 1 cup . .	185	1	Trace	50
Prunes, dried:				
Uncooked; 4 medium prunes	70	1	Trace	19
Cooked, unsweetened; 1 cup (17–18 prunes and ⅓ cup liquid)	295	3	1	78
Prune juice, canned; 1 cup	170	1	Trace	45
Raisins, dried; 1 cup	460	4	Trace	124

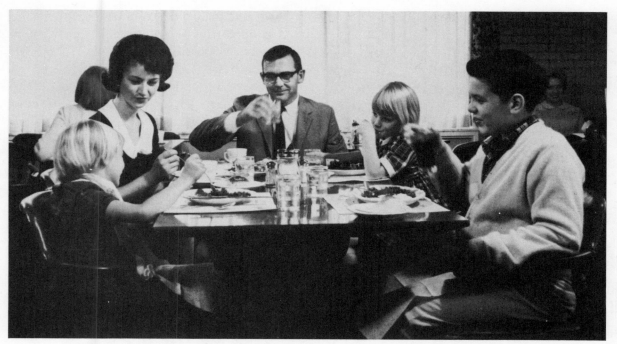

Eating should be a pleasant family experience, not an ordeal to be gotten over with as soon as possible. Food should never be used as a punishment or reward.

NUTRIENTS IN COMMON FOODS

	Food energy	Protein	Fat	Carbohydrate
	Calories	Grams	Grams	Grams
Raspberries, red:				
Raw; 1 cup	70	1	Trace	17
Frozen; 10-ounce carton	280	2	1	70
Strawberries:				
Raw; 1 cup	55	1	1	12
Frozen; 10-ounce carton	300	2	1	75
Tangerines; 1 medium (2½-inch diameter), about ¼ pound	40	1	Trace	10
Watermelon: 1 wedge (4 by 8 inches), about 2 pounds (weighed with rind)	120	2	1	29
Grain Products				
Biscuits, baking powder, enriched flour; 1 biscuit (2½-inch diameter)	130	3	4	20
Bran flakes (40 percent bran) with added thiamine; 1 ounce	85	3	1	22
Breads:				
Cracked wheat:				
1 pound (20 slices)	1,190	39	10	236
1 slice (½ inch thick)	60	2	1	12
Italian; 1 pound	1,250	41	4	256

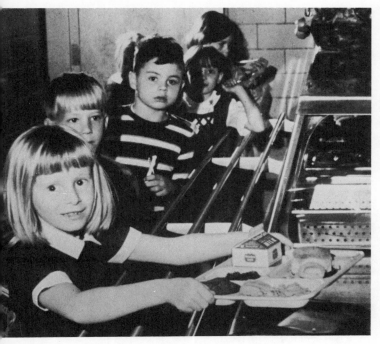

Because many a child's diet at home is deficient, wholesome school lunches are especially important.

food and eating can often be exasperating, it is up to the parent to make mealtime as pleasant as possible, and above all, to avoid any battles of will.

If a young child is too tired, too excited, or too hungry to cope with a meal without ending up in tears or a tantrum, he should not be forced to eat. There are several ways to help children develop a wholesome attitude towards food and eating; here are a few suggestions:

• Children should never be bribed with candy, money, or the promise of special surprises as a way of getting them to eat properly.

• They should not be given the idea that dessert is a reward for finishing the earlier part of the meal.

• Relatively small portions should be served and completely finished before anything else is offered.

NUTRIENTS IN COMMON FOODS

	Food energy	Protein	Fat	Carbohydrate
	Calories	Grams	Grams	Grams
Breads:				
Rye:				
American (light):				
1 pound (20 slices)	1,100	41	5	236
1 slice (½ inch thick)	55	2	Trace	12
Pumpernickel; 1 pound	1,115	41	5	241
White:				
1–2 percent nonfat dry milk:				
1 pound (20 slices)	1,225	39	15	229
1 slice (½ inch thick)	60	2	1	12
3–4 percent nonfat dry milk:				
1 pound (20 slices)	1,225	39	15	229
1 slice (½ inch thick)	60	2	1	12
5–6 percent nonfat dry milk:				
1 pound (20 slices)	1,245	41	17	228
1 slice (½ inch thick)	65	2	1	12
Whole wheat, graham, or entire wheat:				
1 pound (20 slices)	1,105	48	14	216
1 slice (½ inch thick)	55	2	1	11
Cakes:				
Angelfood: 2-inch sector (¹⁄₁₂ of cake, 8-inch diameter)	110	3	Trace	23

• Between-meal snacks should be discouraged if they cut down on the appetite at mealtime.

• From time to time, the child should be allowed to choose the foods that he will eat at a meal.

Parents should keep in mind that the atmosphere in which a child eats and the attitudes instilled in him toward food can be altogether as basic as the nourishment for his body.

Teen-age diet: From the start of a child's growth spurt, which begins at age 10 or 11 for girls and between 13 and 15 for boys, and for several years thereafter, adolescent appetites are likely to be unbelievably large and somewhat outlandish. Parents should try to exercise some control over the youngster who is putting on too much weight as well as over the one who is attracted by a bizarre starvation diet.

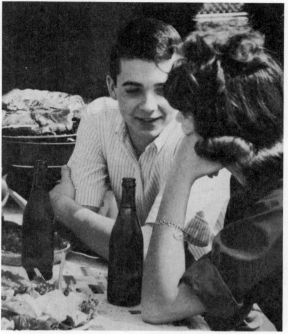

Since the teen-ager's appetite is likely to be very large, care should be taken to avoid overweight.

NUTRIENTS IN COMMON FOODS

	Food energy	Protein	Fat	Carbohydrate
	Calories	Grams	Grams	Grams
Cakes:				
Butter cakes:				
Plain cake and cupcakes without icing:				
1 square (3 by 2 by 1½ inches) . .	180	4	5	31
1 cupcake (2¾-inch diameter) . .	130	3	3	23
Plain cake with icing:				
2-inch sector of iced layer cake (1/16 of cake, 10-inch diameter) . . .	320	5	6	62
Rich cake:				
2-inch sector of layer cake, iced (1/16 of cake, 10-inch diameter) . . .	490	6	19	76
Fruit cake, dark; 1 piece (2 by 2 by ½ inches) .	105	2	4	17
Sponge; 2-inch sector (1/12 of cake, 8-inch diameter)	115	3	2	22
Cookies, plain and assorted; 1 cookie (3-inch diameter)	110	2	3	19
Cornbread or muffins made with enriched, degermed cornmeal; 1 muffin (2¾-inch diameter) . . .	105	3	2	18
Cornflakes: 1 ounce	110	2	Trace	24
Corn grits, degermed, cooked: 1 cup	120	3	Trace	27
Crackers:				
Graham; 4 small or 2 medium	55	1	1	10
Saltines; 2 crackers (2-inch square)	35	1	1	6

Adult Nutrition

Adult nutrition is concerned with more than 50 years of an individual's life span. In typical cases, there is a slow but inevitable weight gain, and for some, there is an obesity problem that begins at about age 40.

Since it is never easy to lose weight, it is especially important for adults to eat sensibly and avoid excess calories. See under *Weight,* p. 320, for a discussion of weight control and obesity.

For older people: People over 60 tend to have changes in their digestive system that are related to less efficient and slower absorption. Incomplete chewing of food because of carelessness or impaired teeth can intensify this problem. Avoiding haste at mealtimes ought to be the rule.

In cases where a dental disorder makes proper chewing impossible, food should be chopped or pureed. Older people occasionally have difficulty swallowing and may choke on a large piece of unchewed meat.

Food for older people should be cooked simply, preferably baked, boiled, or broiled rather than fried, and menus excessively rich in fats should be avoided. A daily multivitamin capsule is strongly recommended for those over 60. A poor appetite can be stimulated by an ounce or two of sherry before a meal unless there are medical reasons for avoiding alcoholic beverages of any kind. See under *Aging and What to Do About It,* p. 188, for a discussion of diet and eating habits in the later years.

During pregnancy: A pregnant woman needs special foods to maintain her own health as well as to safeguard the health of

NUTRIENTS IN COMMON FOODS

	Food energy	Protein	Fat	Carbohydrate
	Calories	Grams	Grams	Grams
Crackers:				
Soda, plain: 2 crackers (2½-inch square) . .	45	1	1	8
Doughnuts, cake type; 1 doughnut	135	2	7	17
Farina, cooked; 1 cup	105	3	Trace	22
Macaroni, cooked; 1 cup:				
Cooked 8–10 minutes (undergoes additional cooking as ingredient of a food mixture) . .	190	6	1	39
Cooked until tender	155	5	1	32
Noodles (egg noodles), cooked: 1 cup	200	7	2	37
Oat cereal (mixture, mainly oat flour), ready-to-eat; 1 ounce	115	4	2	21
Oatmeal or rolled oats, regular or quick cooking, cooked; 1 cup	150	5	3	26
Pancakes, baked; 1 cake (4-inch diameter):				
Wheat (home recipe)	60	2	2	7
Buckwheat (with buckwheat pancake mix) . .	45	2	2	6
Pies; 4-inch sector (⅐ of 9-inch diameter pie):				
Apple	330	3	13	53
Cherry	340	3	13	55
Custard	265	7	11	34
Lemon meringue	300	4	12	45
Mince	340	3	9	62
Pumpkin	265	5	12	34

her baby. She should have additional vitamin D and iron, usually recommended as dietary supplements. More important for most women is the provision of adequate protein in the diet to prevent toxemia of pregnancy or underweight babies. Between 70 and 85 grams of protein a day should be eaten during pregnancy, even if this results in a weight gain of as much as 25 pounds. Adequate nutrition is more important than restricting weight gain to 20 pounds or less.

Nursing mothers: A nursing mother has special dietary needs in addition to those satisfied by the normal adult diet. She should drink an extra quart of milk and eat two more servings of citrus fruit or tomatoes, one more serving of lean meat, fish, poultry, eggs, beans, or cheese, and one more serving of leafy green or yellow vegetables.

Malnutrition

The classic diseases of nutritional deficiency, or malnutrition, such as scurvy and pellagra, are now rare, at least in the United States. The chief reason for their disappearance is the application of scientific knowledge gained in this century of the importance of vitamins and minerals in the diet. Thus most bread is fortified with vitamins and minerals, and in addition, commercial food processing has made it possible for balanced diets of an appealing variety to be eaten all year round.

Many people do not get an adequate diet, either through ignorance or because they simply cannot afford it. A number of food programs have been created to assist them, but unfortunately, the programs don't reach everyone who needs help.

NUTRIENTS IN COMMON FOODS

	Food energy	Protein	Fat	Carbohydrate
	Calories	Grams	Grams	Grams
Pretzels; 5 small sticks	20	Trace	Trace	4
Rice, cooked; 1 cup:				
Converted	205	4	Trace	45
White	200	4	Trace	44
Rice, puffed or flakes; 1 ounce	110	2	Trace	25
Rolls:				
Plain, pan (16 ounces per dozen); 1 roll	115	3	2	20
Hard, round (22 ounces per dozen); 1 roll	160	5	2	31
Sweet, pan (18 ounces per dozen); 1 roll	135	4	4	21
Spaghetti, cooked until tender; 1 cup	155	5	1	32
Waffles, baked, with enriched flour: 1 waffle (4½ by 5½ by ½ inches)	215	7	8	28
Wheat, puffed: 1 ounce	100	4	Trace	22
Wheat, rolled, cooked; 1 cup	175	5	1	40
Wheat flakes; 1 ounce	100	3	Trace	23
Wheat flours:				
Whole wheat; 1 cup, sifted	400	16	2	85
All purpose or family flour: 1 cup, sifted	400	12	1	84
Wheat germ; 1 cup, stirred	245	17	7	34

Fats, Oils, Related Products

Butter; 1 tablespoon	100	Trace	11	Trace

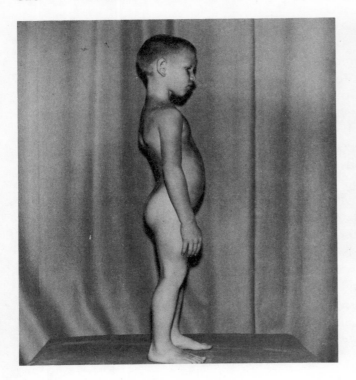

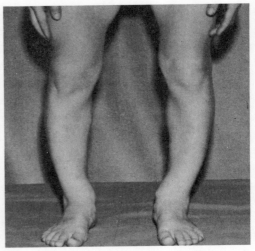

A badly curved spine (*left*) and bowed legs (*above*) are characteristics of rickets, a childhood nutritional disease. A deficiency of vitamin D prevents the bones from hardening (ossifying) properly. Fortunately, now that milk and other foods are commonly fortified with vitamin D, the disorder is relatively rare.

NUTRIENTS IN COMMON FOODS

	Food energy	Protein	Fat	Carbohydrate
	Calories	Grams	Grams	Grams
Fats, cooking:				
Vegetable fats:				
1 cup	1,770	0	200	0
1 tablespoon	110	0	12	0
Lard:				
1 cup	1,985	0	220	0
1 tablespoon	125	0	14	0
Margarine; 1 tablespoon	100	Trace	11	Trace
Oils, salad or cooking; 1 tablespoon	125	0	14	0
Salad dressings; 1 tablespoon:				
Blue cheese	90	1	10	1
Commercial, plain (mayonnaise type)	60	Trace	6	2
French	60	Trace	6	2
Mayonnaise	110	Trace	12	Trace
Thousand Island	75	Trace	8	1
Sugars, Sweets				
Candy; 1 ounce:				
Caramels	120	1	3	22
Chocolate, sweetened, milk	145	2	9	16
Fudge, plain	115	Trace	3	23
Hard	110	0	0	28
Marshmallow	90	1	0	23

Causes of Malnutrition

Some people, either because of ignorance or food fadism, do not eat a balanced diet even though they can afford to. There are also large numbers of people who have nutritional deficiency diseases who can be described as abnormal, at least in regard to eating. Some are alcoholics; others live alone and are so depressed that they lack sufficient drive to feed themselves properly. Combinations of any of these factors can exist with health-damaging consequences.

Disease: People can also develop nutritional deficiencies because they have some disease that interferes with food absorption, storage, and utilization, or that causes an increased excretion, usually in the urine, of substances needed for nutrition. These are generally chronic diseases of the gastro-intestinal tract including the liver, or of the kidneys or the endocrine glands.

Medications: Nutritional deficiencies can also result from loss of appetite caused by medications, especially when a number of different medications are taken simultaneously. This adverse affect on the appetite is a strong reason for not taking medicines unless told to do so by a doctor for a specific purpose.

Most people are not aware of inadequacies in their diet until there are some dramatic consequences. Nor is it easy to recognize the presence of a disorder that might be causing malnutrition. A doctor should be consulted promptly when there is a persistent weight loss, especially when the diet is normal. He should also be informed of any changes in the skin, mucous membranes of the mouth or tongue, or ner-

NUTRIENTS IN COMMON FOODS

	Food energy	Protein	Fat	Carbohydrate
	Calories	Grams	Grams	Grams
Jams, marmalades, preserves; 1 tablespoon . . .	55	Trace	Trace	14
Jellies; 1 tablespoon	50	0	0	13
Sugar; 1 tablespoon	50	0	0	12
Syrup, table blends; 1 tablespoon	55	0	0	15
Miscellaneous				
Beverages, carbonated, kola type; 1 cup . . .	105	—	—	28
Bouillon cubes; 1 cube	2	Trace	Trace	0
Chocolate, unsweetened; 1 ounce	145	2	15	8
Gelatin dessert, plain, ready-to-serve; 1 cup . . .	155	4	0	36
Sherbet, factory packed; 1 cup (8-fluid-ounce container)	235	3	Trace	58
Soups, ready-to-serve; 1 cup:				
Bean	190	8	5	30
Beef	100	6	4	11
Bouillon, broth, and consomme	10	2	—	0
Chicken	75	4	2	10
Clam chowder	85	5	2	12
Cream soup (asparagus, celery, or mushroom) .	200	7	12	18
Noodle, rice, or barley	115	6	4	13
Tomato	90	2	2	18
Vegetable	80	4	2	14
Vinegar; 1 tablespoon	2	0	—	1

TABLE 1

Desirable Weights for Men and Women Aged 25 and Over[1]							
(in pounds by height and frame, in indoor clothing)							
MEN (in shoes, 1-inch heels)				WOMEN (in shoes, 2-inch heels)			
Height	Small Frame	Medium Frame	Large Frame	Height	Small Frame	Medium Frame	Large Frame
5 ft. 2 in.	112–120	118–129	126–141	4 ft. 10 in.	92– 98	96–107	104–119
5 ft. 3 in.	115–123	121–133	129–144	4 ft. 11 in.	94–101	98–110	106–122
5 ft. 4 in.	118–126	124–136	132–148	5 ft. 0 in.	96–104	101–113	109–125
5 ft. 5 in.	121–129	127–139	135–152	5 ft. 1 in.	99–107	104–116	112–128
5 ft. 6 in.	124–133	130–143	138–156	5 ft. 2 in.	102–110	107–119	115–131
5 ft. 7 in.	128–137	134–147	142–161	5 ft. 3 in	105–113	110–122	118–134
5 ft. 8 in.	132–141	138–152	147–166	5 ft. 4 in.	108–116	113–126	121–138
5 ft. 9 in.	136–145	142–156	151–170	5 ft. 5 in.	111–119	116–130	125–142
5 ft. 10 in.	140–150	146–160	155–174	5 ft. 6 in.	114–123	120–135	129–146
5 ft. 11 in.	144–154	150–165	159–179	5 ft. 7 in.	118–127	124–139	133–150
6 ft. 0 in.	148–158	154–170	164–184	5 ft. 8 in.	122–131	128–143	137–154
6 ft. 1 in.	152–162	158–175	168–189	5 ft. 9 in.	126–135	132–147	141–158
6 ft. 2 in.	156–167	162–180	173–194	5 ft. 10 in.	130–140	136–151	145–163
6 ft. 3 in.	160–171	167–185	178–199	5 ft. 11 in.	134–144	140–155	149–168
6 ft. 4 in.	164–175	172–190	182–204	6 ft. 0 in.	138–148	144–159	153–173

[1]Adapted from Metropolitan Life Insurance Co., New York. New weight standards for men and women. *Statistical Bulletin* 40:3, Nov.-Dec., 1959

vous system function, since such symptoms can be a warning of dietary deficiency.

The family or friends of a person with a nutritional deficiency can often detect his condition because they become aware of changes in his eating patterns. They can also note early signs of a deficiency of some of the B vitamins, such as cracks in the mucous membranes at the corners of the mouth, or some slowing of intellectual function.

Correction of Nutritional Deficiencies

Nutritional deficiencies are among the most easily preventable causes of disease. It is important to realize that even mild deficiencies can cause irreparable damage, particularly protein deprivation in young children, which can result in some degree of mental retardation. Periodic medical checkups for everyone in the family are the best way to make sure that such deficiencies are corrected before they snowball into a

chronic disease. In most cases, all that is required is a change in eating habits.

Weight

Probably the most important dietary problem in the United States today is obesity. It is certainly the problem most talked about and written about, not only in terms of good looks, but more important, in terms of good health.

All studies indicate that people who are obese have a higher rate of disease and a shorter life expectancy than those of average weight. From a medical point of view, people who are too fat may actually suffer from a form of malnutrition, even though they look overnourished.

Being too fat and being overweight are not necessarily the same. Heavy bones and muscles can make a person overweight in terms of the charts, but only an excess amount of fat tissue can make someone

TABLE 2

Average Weights for Men and Women[1]

(in pounds by age and height, in paper gown and slippers)

MEN

Height	18–24 years	25–34 years	35–44 years	45–54 years	55–64 years	65–74 years	75–79 years
5 ft. 2 in.	137	141	149	148	148	144	133
5 ft. 3 in.	140	145	152	152	151	148	138
5 ft. 4 in.	144	150	156	156	155	151	143
5 ft. 5 in.	147	154	160	160	158	154	148
5 ft. 6 in.	151	159	164	164	162	158	154
5 ft. 7 in.	154	163	168	168	166	161	159
5 ft. 8 in.	158	168	171	173	169	165	164
5 ft. 9 in.	161	172	175	177	173	168	169
5 ft. 10 in.	165	177	179	181	176	171	174
5 ft. 11 in.	168	181	182	185	180	175	179
6 ft. 0 in.	172	186	186	189	184	178	184
6 ft. 1 in.	175	190	190	193	187	182	189
6 ft. 2 in.	179	194	194	197	191	185	194

WOMEN

Height	18–24 years	25–34 years	35–44 years	45–54 years	55–64 years	65–74 years	75–79 years
4 ft. 9 in.	116	112	131	129	138	132	125
4 ft. 10 in.	118	116	134	132	141	135	129
4 ft. 11 in.	120	120	136	136	144	138	132
5 ft. 0 in.	122	124	138	140	149	142	136
5 ft. 1 in.	125	128	140	143	150	145	139
5 ft. 2 in.	127	132	143	147	152	149	143
5 ft. 3 in.	129	136	145	150	155	152	146
5 ft. 4 in.	131	140	147	154	158	156	150
5 ft. 5 in.	134	144	149	158	161	159	153
5 ft. 6 in.	136	148	152	161	164	163	157
5 ft. 7 in.	138	152	154	165	167	166	160
5 ft. 8 in.	140	156	156	168	170	170	164

[1] Adapted from National Center for Health Statistics: Weight by Height and Age of Adults, United States, 1960–1962. *Vital Health Statistics.* PHS Publication No. 1000—Series 11, No. 14., May 1966, pp. 16–17

obese. However, height and weight tables are generally used to determine obesity.

Table 1 lists standard desirable weights for people of various heights, calculated with indoor clothing and shoes on. Frame sizes are estimated in a general way. This table applies to anyone over the age of 25, indicating that weight gain for the rest of the life span is unnecessary for biological normalcy.

Table 2 gives average weights of American men and women, according to height and age. These measurements are made without clothing or shoes. Note that the weights are considerably higher than the corresponding ones of Table 1. There is a modest weight gain until the middle years and then a gradual loss.

To determine whether a person is obese according to the tables, the percent that he is overweight has to be calculated. An individual is usually considered obese in the clinical sense if he weighs 20 percent more than the standard tables indicate for his size and age.

The pinch test: Another method of determining obesity is to use the "pinch" test. In most adults under 50 years of age, about they have the time for nibbling at all hours, especially when sitting in front of the television screen.

These patterns usually begin in childhood. Youngsters rarely walk to school any more; they get there by bus or car. They often have extra money for snacks and soft drinks, and frequently parents encourage them to overeat without realizing that such habits do them more harm than good.

Most overweight children remain overweight as adults. They also have greater difficulty losing fat, and if they do lose it, tend to regain it more easily than overweight adults who were thin as children. Many adults become overweight between the ages of 20 and 30. Thus, by age 30, about 12 percent of American men and women are 20 percent or more overweight, and by age 60, about 30 percent of the male population and 50 percent of the female are at least 20 percent overweight. As indicated above, the phenomenon of weight

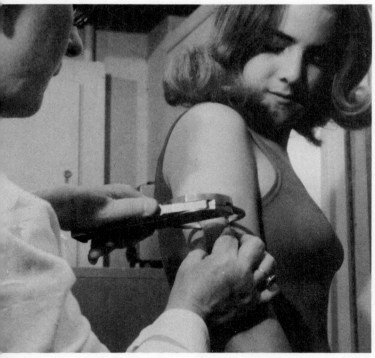

The pinch test for obesity: a fold of skin and fat of the upper arm should be no thicker than one inch.

half of the body fat is located directly under the skin. There are various parts of the body, such as the side of the lower torso, the back of the upper arm, or directly under the shoulder blade, where the thumb and forefinger can pinch a fold of skin and fat away from the underlying bone structure.

If the fold between the fingers—which is, of course, double thickness when it is pinched—is thicker than one inch in any of these areas, the likelihood is that the person is obese.

The Problem of Overweight

The percentage of overweight people in this country has been increasing steadily, chiefly because people eat more and use less physical energy than they used to. Americans do very little walking because of the availability of cars; they do very little manual labor because of the increasing use of machines. They may eat good wholesome meals, but

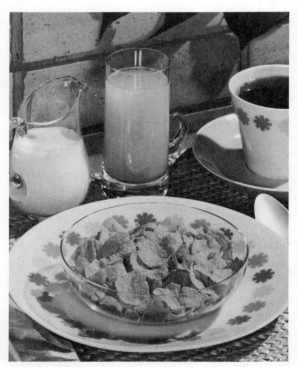

Weight reduction depends upon the simple arithmetic of food intake vs. caloric expenditure. In other words, if you take in more calories (continued next page)

gain while aging does not represent biological normalcy.

Why People Put On Weight

Why does weight gain happen? Excess weight is the result of the imbalance between caloric intake as food and caloric expenditure as energy, either in maintaining the basic metabolic processes necessary to sustain life or in performing physical activity. Calories not spent in either of these ways become converted to fat and accumulate in the body as fat, or *adipose* tissue.

A *calorie* is the unit of measurement that describes the amount of energy potentially available in a given food. It is also used to describe the amount of energy the body must use up to perform a given function.

An ounce of protein contains 130 calories, as does an ounce of carbohydrate. An ounce of fat, by contrast, contains 270 calories. This biochemical information isn't too helpful in calculating the calories in a particular piece of meat, slice of bread, or pat of butter. For such practical figures, there are useful pocket guides, such as *Calories and Weight*, a U.S. Government publication that can be obtained by sending $1.00 to the Superintendent of Documents, U.S. Government Printing Office, Washington, D.C. 20401, and asking for the Agriculture Information Bulletin No. 364.

Counting Calories

If an adult gets the average 3,000 calories a day in his food from the age of 20 to 70, he will have consumed about 55 million calories. About 60 percent of these calories will have been used for his basic metabolic processes. The rest—22 million calories—might have resulted in a gain of about 6,000 pounds of fat, since each group of 3,500 extra calories could have produced one pound of fat.

In some ways, it's a miracle that people don't become more obese than they do. The

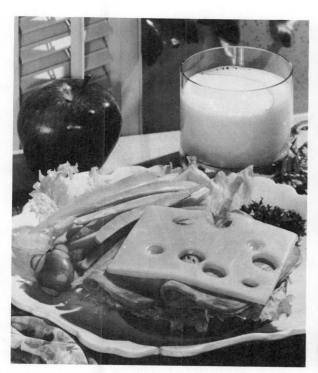 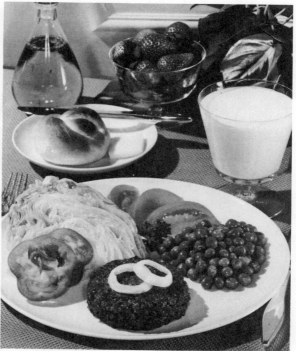

in food than your body can use up (e.g., in respiration, digestion, muscular exertion), you gain weight. Pictured here are three meals that are part of a low-calorie (1400-calorie) weight-reducing diet. See also page 331 for three sample low-calorie menus.

		Calories
	Sedentary	2,500
	Moderately active	3,000
	Active	3,500
	Very active	4,250
	Sedentary	2,100
	Moderately active	2,500
	Active	3,000
	Very active	3,750

Some rough guidelines of daily average consumption of calories by men and women. With the increasing reliance on the automobile and other labor-saving devices, most people in the U.S. today would fall into the sedentary category in caloric expenditure.

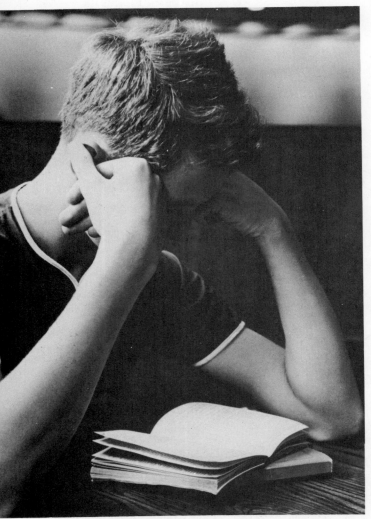

A sedentary activity such as reading, watching TV, or driving a car consumes 30–100 calories per hour.

reason of course is that most or all of these extra calories are normally used to provide energy for physical activity. Here are some examples of calorie expenditure during various activities:

TYPE OF ACTIVITY	CALORIES PER HOUR
Sedentary: reading, sewing, typing, etc.	30–100
Light: cooking, slow walking, getting dressed, etc.	100–170
Moderate: sweeping, light gardening, making beds, etc.	170–250
Vigorous: fast walking, hanging out clothes, golfing, etc.	250–350
Strenuous: swimming, bicycling, dancing, etc.	350 and more

A reasonably good way for an adult to figure his daily caloric needs for moderate activities is to multiply his desirable weight (as noted in Table 1) by 18 for men and by 16 for women. If the typical day includes vigorous or strenuous activities, extra calories will, of course, be required.

Parental Influences and Hereditary Factors

Although there are exceptions, almost all obese people consume more calories than they expend. The reasons for this imbalance are complex. One has to do with parental weight. If the weight of both parents is normal, there is only a 10 percent likelihood that the children will be obese. If one parent is obese, there is a 50 percent probability that the children will be too, and if both are, the probability of obese offspring is 80 percent.

No one knows for certain why this is so. It is probably a combination of diet habits acquired in youth, conditioning during early years to react to emotional stress by eating, the absence of appropriate exercise patterns, and genetic inheritance.

Some obese people seem to have an impairment in the regulatory mechanism of the area of the central nervous system that governs food intake. Simply put, they do not know when to stop eating. Others, particularly girls, may eat less than their nonobese counterparts, but they are considerably less active. Some researchers think that obese people have an inherent muscle rhythm deficiency. A few people appear to have an abnormality in the metabolic process which results in the accumulation of fat even when the calorie balance is negative and should lead to weight loss.

Obesity and Health

There are many reasons why obesity is a health hazard. The annual death rate for obese people between the ages of 20 and 64 is half again as high as that for people whose weight is close to normal. This statistical difference is due primarily to the increased likelihood that the obese person will suffer from diabetes mellitus and from diseases of the digestive and circulatory systems, especially of the heart.

One possible reason for the increased possibility of heart disease is that there are about two-thirds of a mile of blood vessels in each pound of adipose tissue. Thus 20

A moderate activity such as taking care of a youngster in a playground requires in the neighborhood of 170–250 calories per hour.

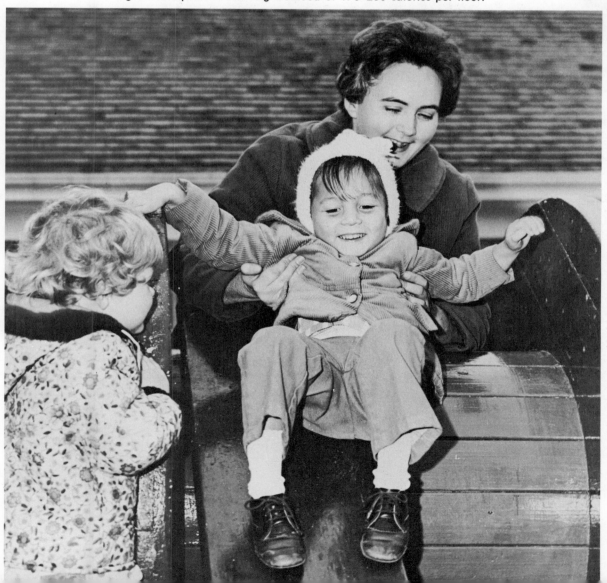

or more pounds of excess weight are likely to impose a great additional work load on the heart.

Obese people are also poorer surgical risks than the nonobese, and it is often more difficult to diagnose and therefore to treat their illnesses correctly.

Permanent loss of excess weight makes the formerly obese person come closer to matching the life expectancy of the nonobese. However, losing and regaining weight as a repeated pattern is even more hazardous in terms of health than consistent obesity.

Psychological Consequences of Obesity

In ways that are both obvious and subtle, obesity often has damaging psychological consequences. This is particularly true for obese children, who tend to feel isolated and rejected by their peers. They may consider themselves victims of prejudice and blame their obesity for everything that goes wrong in their lives. In many cases, the destructive relationship between obesity and self-pity keeps perpetuating itself.

Obese adults are likely to experience the same feelings, but to a somewhat lesser

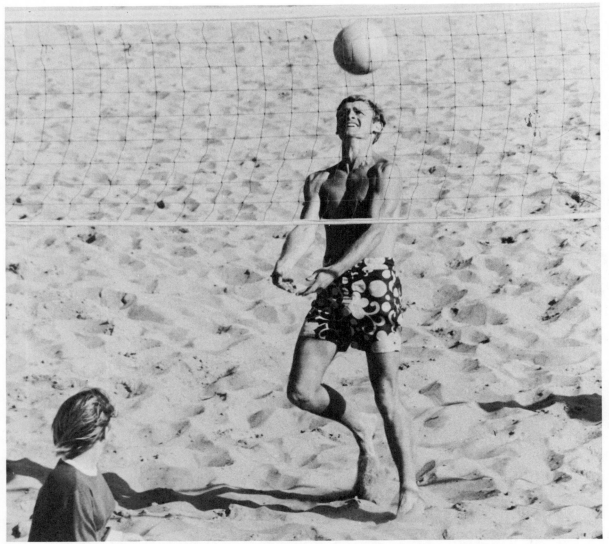

The strenuous activity of a sport involving running can consume more than 350 calories per hour.

degree. For some, obesity is an escape which consciously or unconsciously helps them to avoid situations in which they feel uncomfortable—those that involve active competition or relationships with the opposite sex.

Avoiding Excess Weight

Clearly, obesity is a condition that most people would like to avoid. Not putting on extra pounds does seem to be easier, in theory at least, than taking them off. One possible explanation for this is that additional adipose tissue consists of a proliferation of fat cells. Shrinking these cells is one thing, eliminating them is another. Our present lack of fundamental knowledge about the regulatory and metabolic mechanisms relating to obesity limits the technique of preventing overweight to recommending a balance between caloric intake and expenditure.

The real responsibility for preventing the onset of obesity in childhood rests with parents. All of the fundamentals of good nutrition and healthy eating habits are of the utmost importance in this connection. Caloric expenditure in the form of regular exercise is equally important.

Exercising by habit: This does not necessarily mean that exercise should be encouraged for its own sake. What it does mean is making a habit of choosing an active way of approaching a situation rather than a lazy way: walking upstairs rather than taking the elevator; walking to school rather than riding; walking while playing golf rather than riding in a cart; running to get the ball that has rolled away rather than ambling toward it. These choices should be made consistently and not just occasionally if obesity is to be avoided. Those people who naturally enjoy the more active way of doing things are lucky. Those who don't should make an effort to develop new patterns, especially if obesity is a family problem.

Anyone with the type of physical handicap that makes a normal amount of exercise impossible should be especially careful about caloric intake.

Weight Reduction

The treatment of obesity is a complicated problem. In the first place, there is the question of who wants or needs to be treated and how much weight should be lost. Except in unusual situations, anyone who wants to lose weight should be encouraged to do so. Possible exceptions are teen-agers who are not overweight but who want to be as thin as they can possibly be—the boy who is involved in an athletic event such as wrestling, or the girl who has decided she wants to look like a fashion model.

Crash dieting is usually unwise if the goal is to lose too much weight too rapidly and should be undertaken only after consulting a doctor about its advisability. As for adolescents who have become slightly overweight during puberty, they may be ill-advised to try to take off the extra pounds that probably relate to a temporary growth pattern.

Losing Weight Must Be Self-Motivated

Unless there are compelling medical reasons for not doing so, anyone weighing 20 percent or more over the normal limit for his age and body build should be helped to slim down. It is extremely important, however, for the motivation to come from the person himself rather than from outside pressure.

Unless an overweight person really wants to reduce, he will not succeed in doing so, certainly not permanently, even though he appears to be trying. He must have convinced himself—intellectually and emotionally—that the goal of weight loss is truly worth the effort.

It is very difficult not only for his friends and family but for the person himself to

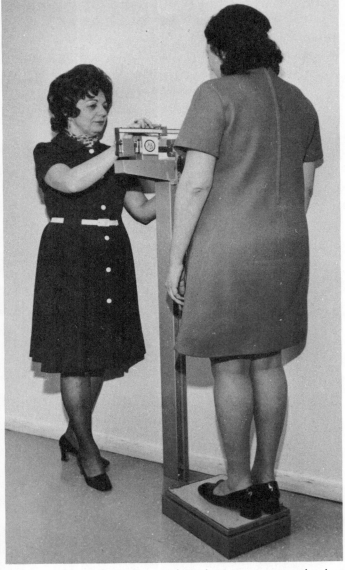

No program for weight reduction can succeed unless the overweight person is self-motivated. The psychological effort to reduce demands determination.

the emotional desire is absent, or that there are emotional conflicts that stand in the way.

It is very possible that such a person could be harmed psychologically by losing weight, since he might need to be overweight for some deep-seated reason. This can be true for both children and adults. Occasionally it is possible for a psychiatrist or psychologist to help the patient remove a psychological block, and then weight reduction can occur if the caloric balance is straightened out.

Effective Planning for Weight Loss

The ultimate key to successful weight reduction is proper eating combined with proper physical activity. This balance is extremely difficult for many people to achieve because it involves a marked change in attitudes and behavior patterns that are generally solidly established and of long duration. Furthermore, once the changes are made, they will have to endure for a lifetime if the weight that has been lost is not to be regained.

It is therefore important that the reducing diet should be somewhat similar to the person's usual eating pattern in terms of style and quality. Ideally, only the caloric content should be changed, and probably the word "dieting" should not be used to describe the process, since most people don't find the idea of permanent dieting congenial.

Similarly, the increased physical activity that must accompany the new eating style should be of a type that the person enjoys. It is virtually impossible for an overweight person to reduce merely by restricting his caloric intake, or merely by increasing his caloric expenditure. The two must go together.

Cutting Down Step By Step

The first thing to determine when planning to lose weight is the number of pounds

be absolutely sure about the depth of his motivation. A doctor treating an overweight patient has to assume that the desire to reduce is genuine and will try to reinforce it whenever he can. However, if a patient has made a number of attempts to lose weight over a period of years and has either been unable to reduce to any significant degree, or has become overweight again after reducing, it is probably safe to assume that

that have to go. A realistic goal to set is the loss of about one pound a week. This may seem too slow, but remember that at this rate, fifty pounds can be lost in a year.

Getting started: Start by weighing yourself on arising, and then for two weeks try to eat in your customary manner, but keep a careful record of everything that you eat, the time it is eaten, and the number of calories it contains. During this period, continue to do your usual amount of physical activity.

When the two weeks are over, weigh yourself again at the same time of day as before. If you haven't gained any weight, you are in a basal caloric state. Then check over your food list to see what might be eliminated each day without causing discomfort.

Try to think in terms of eliminating fats and carbohydrates first, because it is essential that you continue to get sufficient vitamins and minerals which are largely found in proteins. The foods described in the chart on page 305 should all continue to be included in your daily food consumption. If you are in the habit of having an occasional drink, remember that there are calories in alcohol but no nutrients, and that most alcoholic beverages stimulate the appetite. See *Low Calorie Diet* sample menus on page 331, and *Nutrients in Common Foods*, pp. 298–319, for estimating calories in particular foods.

Planning meals: When you replan your meals, keep in mind that the items you cut down on must add up to between 300 and 400 calories a day if you are going to lose one pound a week.

Your total daily food intake should be divided among at least three meals a day, more if you wish. If you need to eat more food or to eat more often, try snacking on low calorie foods such as cabbage, carrots, celery, cucumber, and cauliflower. All of these can be eaten raw between meals.

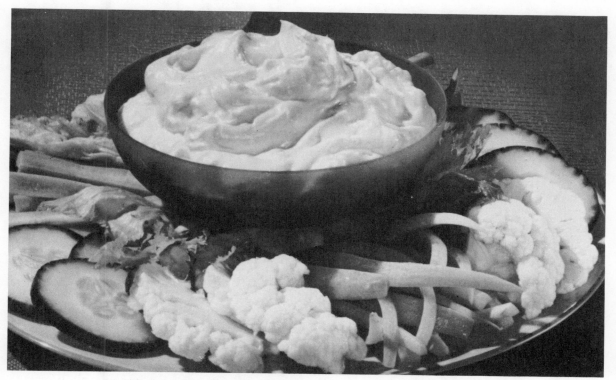

If dieters must snack, raw cauliflower, carrots, and cucumbers are relatively harmless, but they should avoid the sour cream dip at all costs.

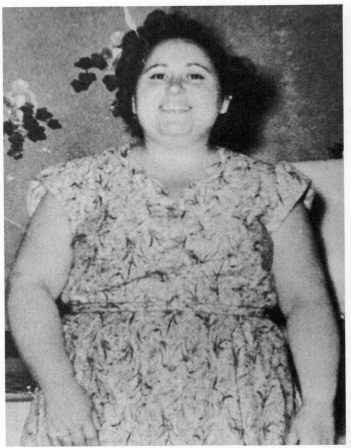
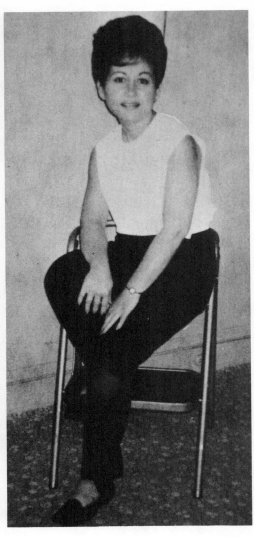

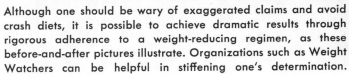

Although one should be wary of exaggerated claims and avoid crash diets, it is possible to achieve dramatic results through rigorous adherence to a weight-reducing regimen, as these before-and-after pictures illustrate. Organizations such as Weight Watchers can be helpful in stiffening one's determination.

There is definitely something to be said in favor of having breakfast every morning, or at least most mornings. This may be psychologically difficult, but try to do it, because it will be easier to control your urge to eat too much later in the day.

Increasing exercise: At the same time that you begin to cut down on your food intake, start to increase your daily exercise in whatever way you find congenial so that the number of calories expended in increased exercise plus the number of calories eliminated from your diet comes to 500 or more. This is your daily caloric loss compared with your so-called basal caloric state.

Achieving your goal: You may wish to double your daily caloric loss so that you lose two pounds a week. Do not try to lose any more than that unless you are under close medical supervision. Also, do not reduce your daily caloric intake below 1500 if you are a man, or below 1000 if you are a woman.

If you gained weight during your two-week experimental period, you will have to increase your daily caloric loss by 500 for every pound gained per week. Thus, if you gained one pound during the two weeks, you will have to step up your daily caloric loss to 750 to lose a pound a week.

LOW CALORIE DIET

Sample Menus

	800 calories		1,200 calories		1,600 calories	
	Weight grams	Household measure	Weight grams	Household measure	Weight grams	Household measure
Breakfast						
Orange, sliced	125	1 medium	125	1 medium	125	1 medium
Soft cooked egg	50	One	50	One	50	One
Toast	25	1 slice	25	1 slice	25	1 slice
Butter	5	1 teaspoon	5	1 teaspoon	5	1 teaspoon
Coffee or tea	—	As desired	—	As desired	—	As desired
Milk	240	1 cup skimmed	240	1 cup skimmed	240	1 cup whole
Luncheon						
Clear broth	—	As desired	—	As desired	—	As desired
Salad (cottage cheese, tomato, plain lettuce leaf)	90	½ cup	90	½ cup	90	½ cup
Egg			50	One	50	One
Green peas					100	½ cup
Baked apple, unsweetened	80	1 small	80	1 small	80	1 small
Bread			25	1 slice	25	1 slice
Butter			5	1 teaspoon	5	1 teaspoon
Milk	240	1 cup skimmed	240	1 cup skimmed	240	1 cup whole
Coffee or tea	—	As desired	—	As desired	—	As desired
Dinner						
Roast beef, lean	60	2 ounces	90	3 ounces	120	4 ounces
Carrots, plain	100	½ cup	100	½ cup	100	½ cup
Tossed vegetable salad with vinegar	50	¾ cup	50	¾ cup	50	¾ cup
Pineapple, unsweetened	80	½ cup	80	½ cup	80	½ cup
Bread			25	1 slice	25	1 slice
Butter			5	1 teaspoon	10	2 teaspoons
Coffee or tea	—	As desired	—	As desired	—	As desired
Nourishment						
Peach					100	1 medium

These diets contain approximately 800, 1,200, and 1,600 calories. The 800 calorie diet, even with variations in selections of food, will not meet the recommended daily allowances in iron and thiamine. The approximate composition is as follows:

	800 calories	1,200 calories	1,600 calories
Protein	60 gm.	75 gm.	85 gm.
Fat	30 gm.	50 gm.	80 gm.
Carbohydrate	75 gm.	110 gm.	130 gm.

From the *Clinical Center Diet Manual*, revised edition, prepared by the Nutrition Department, The Clinical Center, National Institutes of Health, Public Health Service, U.S. Department of Health, Education, and Welfare (Public Health Service Publication No. 989), pp. 67–68.

You'll have to keep slugging away to achieve your goal. It will be trying and difficult in many ways. You may get moody and discouraged and be tempted to quit. Don't. You'll probably go on periodic food binges. All this is natural and understandable, so try not to brood about it. Just do the best you can each day. Don't worry about yesterday, and let tomorrow take care of itself.

In many ways it can help, and in some cases it's essential, to have the support and encouragement of family and friends, particularly of those with whom you share meals. You may find it helpful to join a group that has been formed to help its members lose weight and maintain their weight loss. This is good psychological support.

Maintaining your weight loss: Once you have achieved your desired weight, you can test yourself to see what happens if you increase your caloric intake. Clearly, anyone who can lose weight in the manner described can't stay in a state of negative caloric imbalance indefinitely. But you will have to be careful, or you'll become overweight again. It's a challenge, but people who stick to a disciplined program can be rewarded by success.

Special Problems

If you do not succeed in losing weight in spite of carrying out the program described above, you may need professional help because of some special problem. A qualified physician may try some special diets, or he may even suggest putting you into a hospital so that he can see to it that you have no caloric food at all for as long as three weeks.

Perhaps the situation is complicated by a metabolic abnormality that can be corrected or helped by medication. Although such conditions are rare, they are not unheard of.

Obesity is almost never caused by a "glandular" problem—which usually means an underactive thyroid. Do not take thyroid pills to reduce unless your thyroid has been found to be underactive on the basis of a specific laboratory test.

The indiscriminate use of pills to reduce, even when prescribed, is never helpful in the long run, although it may appear to be at first. The unsupervised use of amphetamines, for example, can be extremely dangerous. See *Stimulant Drugs,* p. 652, for further information about the dangers of amphetamine abuse.

Because so many people are eager to reduce, and because losing weight isn't easy, there are many unethical professionals who specialize in the problem. Avoid them. All they are likely to do for you is take your money and make your situation worse than it was to begin with.

Underweight

Weighing too little is a problem which is considerably less common than weighing too much. In fact, in many cases, it isn't accurate to call it a problem at all, at least not a medical one.

There are some circumstances, however, when underweight may indicate the presence of a disease, especially when a person rather suddenly begins and continues to lose weight, even though there has been no change in his eating habits. This is a situation that calls for prompt medical evaluation. Such a person may already be under a doctor's care at the time the weight loss is first noticed.

More often, however, underweight is a chronic condition that is of concern to the person who feels his looks would improve if he could only add some extra pounds. This is especially true in the case of adolescent girls and young women.

What To Do About Weighing Too Little

Chronic underweight is rarely a reflection of underlying disease. It is rather an expression of individual heredity or eating patterns, or a combination of both. Treatment for the condition is the opposite of the treatment for overweight. The achievement of a positive caloric balance comes first; more calories have to be consumed each day than are expended. An underweight person should record his food history over a two-week period in the manner described for an overweight one. Once this has been done, various adjustments can be made.

First of all, he should see that he eats at least three meals a day and that they are eaten in a leisurely way and in a relaxed frame of mind. All of the basic foods should be represented in the daily food intake, with special emphasis on protein. The daily caloric intake should then be gradually increased at each meal and snacks added, so long as the snacks don't reduce the appetite at mealtimes.

Carbohydrate foods are the best ones to emphasize in adding calories. Since the extra food intake may cause a certain amount of discomfort, encouragement and support from family and friends can be extremely helpful. Just as there may be psychological blocks against losing weight, there may be a complicated underlying resistance to adding it.

Anyone trying to gain weight should remain or become reasonably active physically. Adding a pound or two a month for an adult—and a little more than that for a growing youngster—is an achievable goal until the desired weight is reached. When this happens, there will probably have to be some adjustments in eating and exercise patterns so that a state of caloric balance is achieved.

How Food Relates To Disease

Just as proper food is essential in the prevention of some diseases, it is helpful in the treatment of others. It also plays an impor-

tant role in protecting and fortifying the general health of a patient while a specific illness is being treated.

The components of therapeutic diets are usually prescribed by the physician in charge, but some general principles will be presented here. Remember that diets designed to treat a given disease must also supply the patient's basic nutritional requirements.

Ulcers

Special diet is a major treatment consideration in the case of peptic ulcer, whether located in the stomach (gastric) or in the small intestine (duodenal). A major aim of such a diet is the neutralizing of the acidity of gastric juices by the frequent intake of high protein foods such as milk and eggs. Foods which irritate an ulcer chemically, such as excessive sweets, spices, or salt, or mechanically, such as foods with sharp seeds or tough skins, and foods that are too hot or too cold, should be avoided. It is also advisable to eliminate gravies, coffee, strong tea, carbonated beverages, and alcohol, since all of these stimulate gastric secretion. Such a diet is called a *bland* diet. See *Soft and Bland Soft Diets*, pp. 334–337. A soft diet is recommended for some forms of gastrointestinal distress and for those people who have difficulty chewing. It is often combined with the bland diet recommended for peptic ulcer patients to reduce the likelihood of irritation. See under *Diseases of the Digestive System*, p. 522, for further information about ulcers.

Diabetes

As the section on diabetes mellitus indicates (see *Diabetes Mellitus*, p. 573), the major objectives of the special diet are weight control, control of the abnormal carbohydrate metabolism, and as far as possible, psychological adjustment by the patient to his individual circumstances. To some extent, he must calculate his diet

SOFT AND BLAND SOFT DIETS

Type of food	Foods included	Foods excluded	Modifications required to convert soft to bland soft diet
Beverages	Coffee, decaffeinated coffee, tea, carbonated beverages, cereal beverages, cocoa, milk.	None	Omit coffee, tea and cola drinks.
Breads	White; whole wheat, finely ground; rye (without seeds), finely ground; white or whole wheat rolls or muffins, finely ground; plain crackers.	Coarse whole wheat breads; breads, rolls, and muffins with seeds, nuts, raisins, etc.	Omit all whole grain breads, rolls, muffins.
Cereals	Cooked or prepared cereals, such as corn flakes, strained oatmeal, cream of rice or wheat, farina, hominy grits, cornmeal, puffed rice, other rice cereals.	Cooked or prepared coarse cereals, such as bran, shredded wheat.	Omit all whole grain cereals.
Desserts	Plain cake and cookies, sponge cake; custards, plain puddings, rennet desserts; gelatin desserts with allowed fruits; plain ice cream, sherbets (except pineapple), fruit ices.	Pies; pastries; desserts made with coconut, nuts, pineapple, raisins, etc.	None.
Fats	Butter, cream, fortified fats, plain gravies, mayonnaise, cream sauces.	Fried foods; rich highly seasoned sauces and gravies with mushrooms, pimento, etc.	Omit all gravies and salad dressings.
Fruits	Raw ripe bananas; canned or cooked fruits without skins or small seeds, such as applesauce, baked apple without skin, apricots, sweet cherries, peaches, pears; fruit juices as desired.	Raw fruits except bananas; canned or cooked fruits with skins, coarse fibers, or seeds, such as figs, raisins, berries, pineapple, etc.	None.
Meat, poultry, fish	Bacon, beef, ham, lamb, pork, veal, poultry, and fish that has been baked, boiled, braised, broiled, or roasted.	Fried meat, poultry, or fish; highly seasoned meats; stews containing celery, onions, etc.; cold cuts, sausages.	Omit meat extractives and pork.

From the *Clinical Center Diet Manual*, revised edition, prepared by the Nutrition Department, The Clinical Center, National Institutes of Health, Public Health Service, U.S. Department of Health, Education, and Welfare (Public Health Service Publication No. 989), pp. 45–52.

SOFT AND BLAND SOFT DIETS (continued)

Type of food	Foods included	Foods excluded	Modifications required to convert soft to bland soft diet
Cheese	All except strongly flavored cheeses.	Cheeses with pimento, caraway seeds, etc.; strongly flavored cheeses.	None.
Eggs	Any raw, soft cooked, hard cooked, soft scrambled, poached; omelets made with allowed foods.	Fried eggs, omelets containing mushrooms, etc.	None.
Potato or substitute	Hominy, macaroni, noodles, rice, spaghetti; white or sweet potatoes without skins.	Fried potatoes; potato chips; highly seasoned sauces for spaghetti, macaroni, etc.	None.
Soups	Broth, strained soups; cream soups made with allowed vegetables.	All others	Omit broth and soups made with meat base. Use only strained cream soups.
Sweets	Hard candies, simple chocolate candies without nuts or fruit; strained honey, jelly, sugar, syrup.	Candies with whole fruit, coconut, or nuts; jam, marmalade.	None. Limit quantities of jelly, sugar, and hard candies.
Vegetables	Cooked or canned asparagus tips, string beans, wax beans, beets, carrots, chopped spinach, winter squash; tomato puree, tomato juice; raw lettuce leaf as garnish.	Cooked broccoli, brussels sprouts, cabbage, cauliflower, celery, corn, mustard greens, turnip greens, mushrooms, onions, fresh and dried peas, summer squash, whole tomatoes; dried beans, lima beans, lentils. All raw vegetables except lettuce as a garnish.	Omit lettuce.
Miscellaneous	Salt; small amounts of white or black pepper used in cooking; creamy peanut butter.	Hot seasonings, such as chili sauce, red pepper, etc.; coconut, nuts, olives, pickles; spiced fruit.	Omit all seasonings and spices except salt.

Soft diet. Foods allowed on this diet are left whole. The fiber content is modified by using only cooked or canned fruits and vegetables (with skins and seeds removed); refined or finely ground cereals and breads are included. Some restrictions have been placed on highly seasoned and rich foods because of the specific needs for which the soft diet is usually ordered.

Bland soft diet. If further restrictions on seasonings and food items are necessary, a bland soft diet may be ordered. This diet follows the same pattern as the soft diet outlined above but is further modified to eliminate all stimulants, such as meat extractives, spices, condiments (except salt), strongly flavored foods, and beverages that contain caffeine. Extremely hot or cold foods are avoided. The foods allowed may be divided into five or six small meals with each feeding containing a good source of protein.

SOFT DIET

Sample Menu

Breakfast
    Orange juice . . . ½ cup
    Corn flakes . . . . ½ cup
    Poached egg . . . . One
    Whole wheat toast . . 1 slice
    Butter or fortified fat . . 1 teaspoon
    Milk, whole . . . . 1 cup
    Coffee or tea . . . . As desired
    Cream . . . . . As desired
    Sugar . . . . . As desired

Luncheon
    Creamed chicken on toast ½ to ¾ cup
    Mashed potato . . . ½ cup
    Buttered carrots . . . ½ cup
    Bread, enriched . . . 1 slice
    Butter or fortified fat . . 1 teaspoon
    Canned pear halves . . 2 halves
    Milk, whole . . . . 1 cup
    Coffee or tea . . . . As desired
    Cream . . . . . As desired
    Sugar . . . . . As desired

Dinner
    Roast beef, gravy . . 2 to 3 ounces
    Baked potato . . . 1 medium
    Buttered asparagus spears 1 serving
    Bread, enriched . . . 1 slice
    Butter or fortified fat . . 1 teaspoon
    Vanilla ice cream . . ½ cup
    Coffee or tea . . . . As desired
    Cream . . . . . As desired
    Sugar . . . . . As desired

mathematically. First, his daily caloric needs have to be determined in terms of his activities:

TYPE OF ACTIVITY	CALORIES PER POUND OF BODY WEIGHT
Sedentary	13.5
Moderate	16
Marked	18

If he is overweight or underweight, the total calories per pound of body weight will have to be adjusted downward or upward by about five calories per pound.

After his total daily caloric needs have been figured out, he can calculate the number of grams of carbohydrate he should have each day by dividing his total calories by 10. The number of grams of protein per day as well as the number of grams of fat should be half the number of grams of carbohydrate.

This will mean that 40 percent of his daily calories will come from carbohydrate,

BLAND SOFT DIET

Sample Menu
(six small meals)

Breakfast
Egg, poached   .   .   .   One
White toast, enriched.   .   1 slice
Butter or fortified fat .   .   1 teaspoon
Hot cocoa   .   .   .   1 cup

10:00 a.m.
Orange juice.   .   .   ½ cup
Corn flakes   .   .   .   ½ cup
Cream   .   .   .   .   ¼ cup
Sugar   .   .   .   .   2 teaspoons

Luncheon
Creamed chicken on toast   ½ cup
Mashed potato   .   .   .   ½ cup
Buttered carrots .   .   .   ½ cup
Milk   .   .   .   .   1 cup
Canned pears   .   .   .   1 half

2:30 p.m.
Milkshake   .   .   .   1 cup
Soda crackers   .   .   .   Three

Dinner
Roast beef   .   .   .   .   2 ounces
Baked potato   .   .   .   1 medium
Buttered asparagus   .   .   1 serving
Butter or fortified fat .   .   1 teaspoon
Milk   .   .   .   .   1 cup
Vanilla ice cream   .   .   ½ cup

8:30 p.m.
Baked custard   .   .   .   ½ cup
Vanilla wafers   .   .   .   Two

40 percent from fat, and 20 percent from protein. One-fifth of the total should be obtained at breakfast and the rest split between lunch and dinner. Snacks that are taken during the day should be subtracted equally from lunch and dinner.

It is important that meals and planned snacks be eaten regularly and that no food servings be added or omitted. Growing children from 1 to 20 years of age who have diabetes will require considerably more daily calories. A rough estimation is 1,000 calories for a one-year-old child and 100 additional calories for each year of age.

Salt-Free Diets

There are a number of chronic diseases which are treated in part by restricting the amount of sodium in the diet. These are diseases which are associated with fluid retention in the body. They include congestive heart failure, certain types of kidney and liver diseases, and hypertension or high blood pressure.

SODIUM RESTRICTED DIETS

DIETS MODERATELY RESTRICTED IN SODIUM

If only a moderate sodium restriction is necessary, a normal diet *without added salt* may be ordered. Such an order is interpreted to mean that the patient will be offered the regular salted food on the general selective menu with the following exceptions:

1. No salt will be served on the tray.
2. Soups that are salted will be omitted.
3. Cured meats (ham, bacon, sausage, corned beef) and all salted cheeses will be omitted.
4. Catsup, chili sauce, mustard, and other salted sauces will be omitted.
5. Salt-free gravies, sauces, and salad dressings will be substituted for the regular salted items.
6. Salted crackers, potato chips, nuts, pickles, olives, popcorn, and pretzels will be omitted.

This diet contains approximately 3 grams of sodium or 7.5 grams of sodium chloride, depending on the type and quantity of the food chosen.

LOW SODIUM DIETS[1]
(1,000 mg. Sodium and 800 mg. Sodium Diets)

Type of food	Foods included	Foods excluded
Beverages	Coffee, tea, carbonated beverages, cereal beverages; milk, cream, or cocoa within stated milk limitations.	All others.
Breads	Any unsalted yeast bread or rolls; quick breads made with "sodium-free" baking powder; unsalted matzoth.	All bread and rolls containing salt, baking powder or baking soda; salted or soda crackers; pretzels.
Cereals	Any cereal that is cooked without salt; puffed rice, puffed wheat; shredded wheat; specially prepared "sodium-free" corn flakes and rice flakes; unsalted popcorn.	All prepared cereals containing salt; hominy grits.
Desserts	Any unsalted dessert; custards and puddings made with allowed milk; puddings made without milk; unflavored gelatin	Desserts made with salt, baking powder, or baking soda; flavored gelatin desserts.

[1] Approximate composition is indicated in the following table. 1,000 milligrams (abbreviated *mg.*) equals 1 gram. The 500, 800, and 1,000 milligram sodium diets meet the recommended nutrient levels of the normal diet.

Nutrient	Unit	500 mg. sodium	800 mg. sodium	1,000 mg. sodium
Sodium	Milligrams	485	775	970
Protein	Grams	70	95	95
Fat	Grams	90	90	90
Carbohydrate	Grams	185	250	250
Calories*		1,830	2,190	2,190

*Calories can be augmented by using additional salt-free fats and oils, white sugar, and pure jellies.

From the *Clinical Center Diet Manual*, revised edition, prepared by the Nutrition Department, The Clinical Center, National Institutes of Health, Public Health Service, U.S. Department of Health, Education, and Welfare (Public Health Service Publication No. 989), pp. 77–86.

LOW SODIUM DIETS (continued)

Type of food	Foods included	Foods excluded
Desserts (continued)	desserts; fruit ices; unsalted fruit pie and fruit whips.	
Fats	Any unsalted fat or oil, vegetable or animal; unsalted salad dressings.	Salted butter, salted margarine; commercial salad dressings; bacon drippings.
Fruits	Any fresh, canned, or frozen fruit or juice.	Dried fruits prepared with sodium preservatives.
Meat, poultry, fish.	Prepared without salt: beef, lamb, fresh pork, veal; poultry; fresh-water fish;[2] liver (limit to one serving per week).	Salted meats; bacon; smoked or canned meats or fish; shellfish; all glandular meats except liver as allowed.
Cheese	Unsalted cottage cheese; specially prepared "sodium-free" yellow cheese.	All other.
Eggs	Limit to one daily, prepared without salt.	Any prepared with salt.
Potato or substitute.	Dried beans (navy, pea), macaroni, noodles, potato, rice, spaghetti, sweet potato, all prepared without salt.	Salted potato chips, hominy.
Soups	Unsalted meat broth; cream soups prepared with allowed milk and allowed vegetables.	Bouillon; all soups prepared with salt.
Sweets	Hard candies, honey, jam, jelly, white sugar, syrup.	Commercial candy prepared with sodium salts; brown sugar.
Vegetables, cooked and raw.	Two servings (½ cup) of vegetables listed below, fresh, frozen, or canned without salt: asparagus, lima beans,[3] navy beans, snap beans (green or yellow wax), broccoli, brussels sprouts, cabbage, carrots, cauliflower, corn, cucumbers, eggplant, dried lentils, lettuce, mushrooms, okra, onions, parsley, parsnips, black-eyed peas, green peas,[3] green peppers, radishes, rutabaga, squash, tomatoes, turnips, turnip greens.	Beets, beet greens, celery, dandelion greens, kale, frozen lima beans, mustard greens, frozen peas, sauerkraut, spinach, frozen succotash, swiss chard.
Miscellaneous	Herbs and spices, except salt. Unsalted peanut butter.	Salt, celery salt, garlic salt; celery seed, parsley flakes; sauces containing salt, such as catsup, chili sauce, mustard, steak sauces; salted nuts and popcorn; olives, pickles; monosodium glutamate.

[2] Unsalted salt-water fish is usually avoided because of the difficulty of obtaining a consistently unsalted supply.

[3] Use only fresh or canned without salt.

LOW SODIUM DIETS (continued)

Sample Menus

	500 mg. Sodium		800 mg. Sodium	
	Weight —Gms.	Household measure	Weight —Gms.	Household measure
Breakfast				
Orange, sliced	125	1 medium	125	1 medium
Soft cooked egg	50	One	50	One
Unsalted oatmeal	100	½ cup	100	½ cup
Unsalted toast	25	1 slice	25	1 slice
Unsalted butter	10	2 teaspoons	10	2 teaspoons
Jelly	As desired		As desired	
Milk, low sodium	None		None	
Milk (or cream)	240	1 cup	240	1 cup
Coffee or tea	As desired		As desired	
Sugar	As desired		As desired	
Luncheon				
Unsalted beef patty	60	2 ounces	60	2 ounces
Unsalted fried potatoes	100	½ cup	100	½ cup
Unsalted asparagus	100	½ cup	100	½ cup
Lettuce and tomato salad	100	1 small	100	1 small
Unsalted French dressing	15	1 tablespoon	15	1 tablespoon
Unsalted chocolate cookies	None			1 serving
Canned peaches	100	1 serving	As desired	
Unsalted bread	25	1 slice	25	1 slice
Unsalted butter	10	2 teaspoons	10	2 teaspoons
Jelly	As desired		As desired	
Milk, low sodium	None		None	
Milk	240	1 cup	240	1 cup
Coffee or tea	As desired		As desired	
Sugar	As desired		As desired	
Dinner				
Unsalted roast chicken	60	2 ounces	90	3 ounces
Unsalted gravy	30	2 tablespoons	30	2 tablespoons
Unsalted mashed potatoes	100	½ cup	100	½ cup
Unsalted green beans	100	½ cup	100	½ cup
Banana salad	100	One	100	One
Unsalted mayonnaise	15	1 tablespoon	15	1 tablespoon
Fresh fruit cup	100	½ cup	100	½ cup
Unsalted bread	25	1 slice	25	1 slice
Unsalted butter	10	2 teaspoons	10	2 teaspoons
Jelly	As desired		As desired	
Milk, low sodium	As desired		None	
Milk	None		240	1 cup
Coffee or tea	As desired		As desired	
Sugar	As desired		As desired	
Nourishment				
Orange juice	240	1 cup	As desired	
Milk	None		240	1 cup

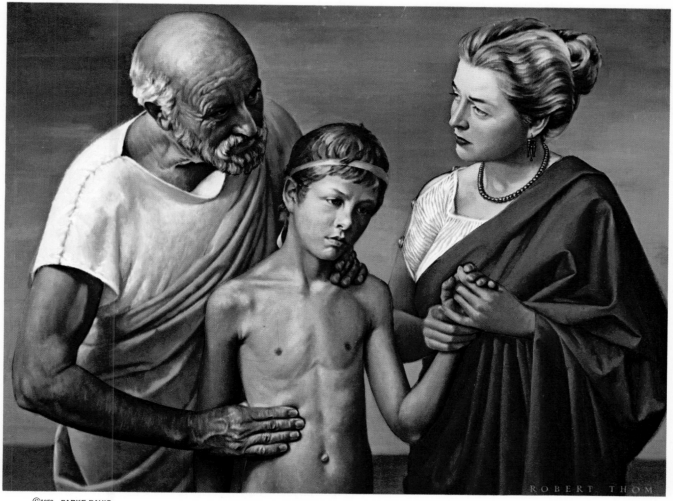

HIPPOCRATES: MEDICINE BECOMES A SCIENCE

The art of medicine in the ancient world developed to its highest point in Greece, during the millennium between 500 B.C. and 500 A.D. This creative period is symbolized by Hippocrates, the "Father of Medicine," whose name has come to represent the beauty, value, and dignity of medicine for all times. Hippocrates' kindliness and concern are embodied in his aphorism, "Where there is love for mankind, there is love for the art of healing." These qualities are reflected in the face of this great practitioner, scientist, and teacher, as he palpates a young patient and attempts to soothe a worried mother sometime late in the fifth century B.C. His name is still revered in medical circles.

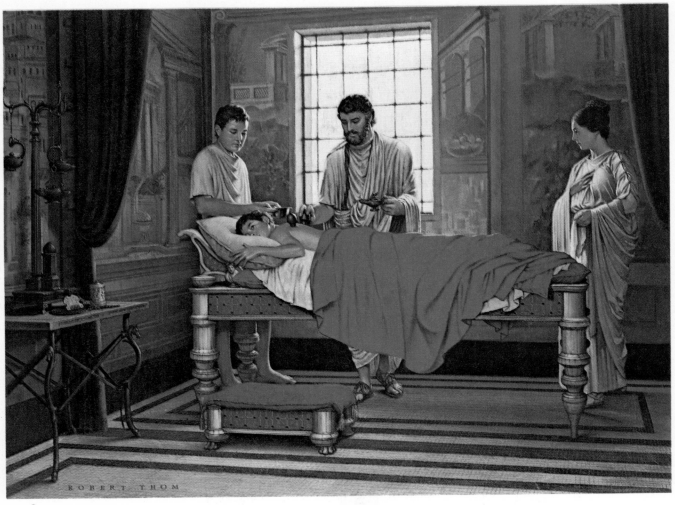

ROBERT THOM

GALEN, INFLUENCE FOR FORTY-FIVE GENERATIONS

Galen was a pillar of medicine; the last important pillar in the millennium of Greek domination of the medical world. Physician to emperors as well as commoners in the Roman Empire, Galen (130-200 A.D.) traveled extensively, lectured widely, wrote prolifically. The great Greek was a shrewd observer who gained much experience through experimentation. Cupping was among the forms of treatment which he advocated. Pharmacy as well as medicine benefited from his formulas, called "galenicals;" he was a leader in the health sciences of his day. Galen's teachings were accepted as dogma by both teachers and practitioners of medicine for fifteen hundred years.

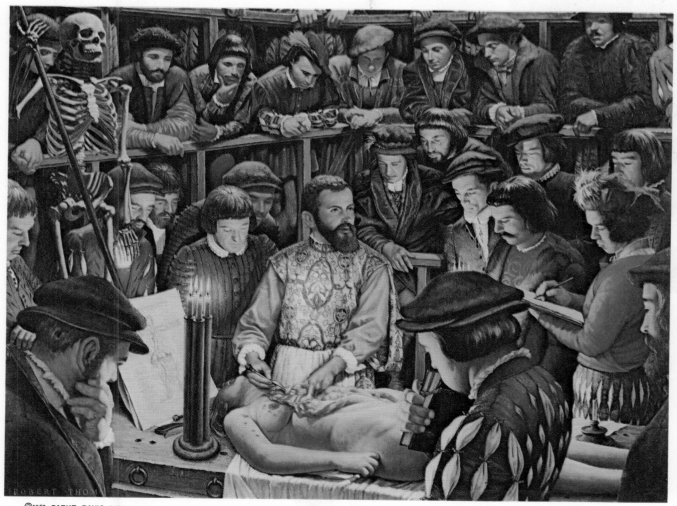

VESALIUS—AND THE ANATOMY OF MAN

Andreas Vesalius of Brussels, first great teacher of anatomy from natural observations, conducted many anatomical demonstrations on human bodies while Professor of Surgery and of Anatomy at the University of Padua, 1537-1543. Highly successful, these were attended by medical students, physicians, interested civic officials, sculptors, and artists. First to break with Galen's 1400-year-old anatomical texts, Vesalius published Tabulae Anatomicae Sex *in 1538, and the monumental* De Humani Corporis Fabrica *in 1543. Though reviled and ridiculed by Galenists, the validity of Vesalius' works soon overcame detractors and they became classic in medical literature.*

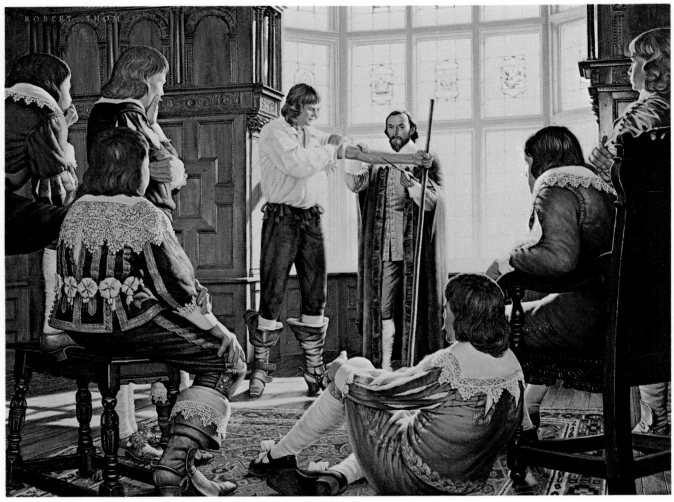

HARVEY AND THE CIRCULATION OF THE BLOOD

William Harvey, slight, energetic, scientific English physician of the seventeenth century, with his famed pointer in hand, used demonstrations to prove his revolutionary theory of the circulation of blood, during his anatomical lectures before the College of Physicians of London. His book De Motu Cordis, *published in 1628, upset traditional followers of Galen, brought entirely new concepts of circulation and of anatomy to medicine. Harvey, a graduate in medicine from Padua and Cambridge, physician to Kings James I and Charles I, was unperturbed by criticism, dedicated to research and to hard work. He died in 1657, after having seen his theory generally accepted by physicians.*

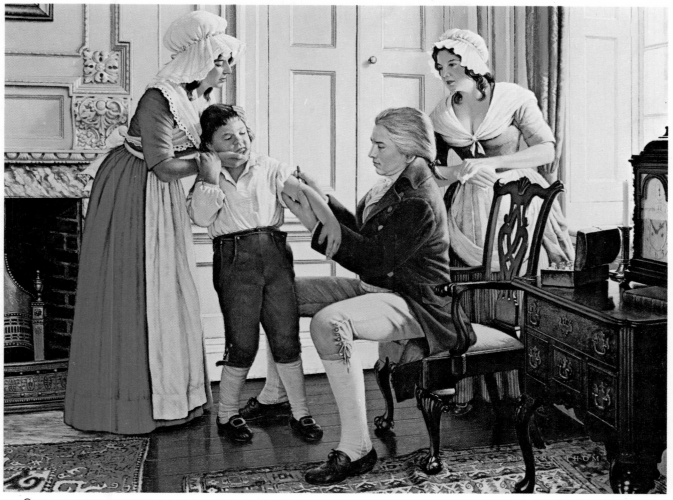

JENNER: SMALLPOX IS STEMMED

The first vaccination against smallpox was performed by Edward Jenner, English rural physician, in his apartment in the Chantry House, Berkeley, Gloucestershire. Exudate from a cowpox pustule on the hand of dairymaid, Sarah Nelmes, was inserted in scratches on the arm of eight-year-old James Phipps, May 14, 1796. The vaccination was effective, for two later attempts to induce infection with smallpox pus were unsuccessful. After proving his discovery, Jenner published his vaccination findings in 1798. Despite opposition, vaccination became accepted practice during Jenner's lifetime.

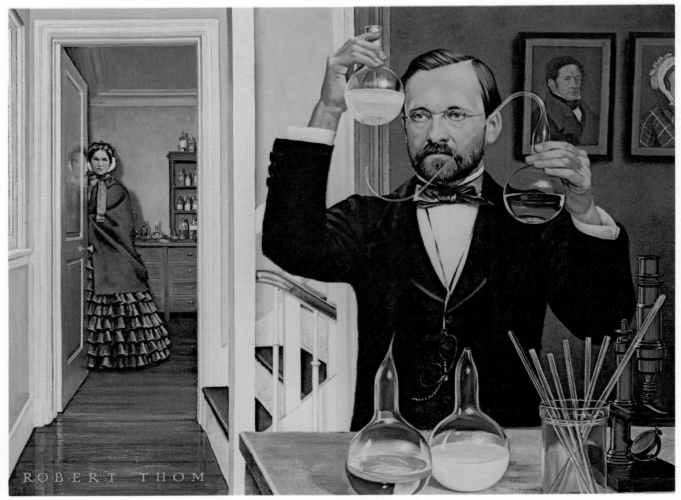

ROBERT THOM

PASTEUR: THE CHEMIST WHO TRANSFORMED MEDICINE

Proof that microbes are reproduced from parent organisms, and do not result from spontaneous generation, came from careful experiments in makeshift laboratories of France's famed chemist and biologist, Louis Pasteur (1822-1895), at the Ecole Normale, Paris. Behind him are portraits of his father and mother, which he painted during his youth. Mme. Pasteur waits patiently for him to complete an observation. From basic work in these laboratories came proof of the germ theory of disease, which transformed medical practice; vaccines for virulent diseases, including anthrax and rabies; solution of many industrial biochemical problems; and founding of the Pasteur Institute.

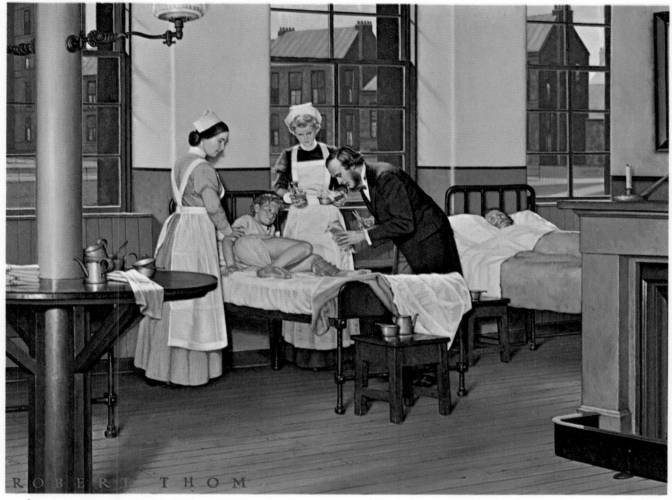

LISTER INTRODUCES ANTISEPSIS

When Surgeon Joseph Lister (1827-1912) of Glasgow Royal Infirmary removed dressings from James Greenlees' compound fracture, the wound had healed without infection—something unheard of before. For six weeks, beginning August 12, 1865, Lister had treated the boy's wound with carbolic acid. Now, Lister had proof of success of his principle of antisepsis—which was to revolutionize methods of treatment and to open new vistas in practice of surgery, of medicine, and of environmental sanitation. Hospitals were turned from "houses of torture and death" to "houses of healing and cure." In 1897, Lister became the first British surgeon to be elevated to peerage.

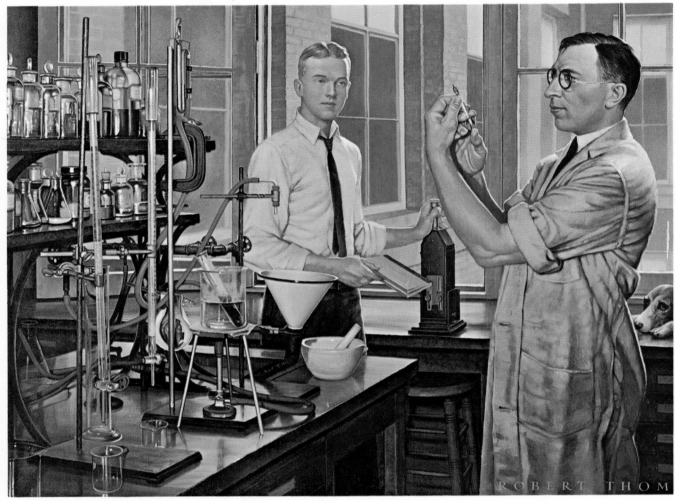

BANTING, BEST, AND DIABETES

During the summer of 1921, Charles H. Best, youthful biologist, and Dr. Frederick G. Banting experimented in laboratories loaned by Professor J. J. R. Macleod of the Physiology Department, University of Toronto. The inexperienced Canadian investigators found what trained research men before them had missed—an extract of the pancreas that controlled the high blood sugar of diabetes mellitus. Proved and reproved on laboratory animals, their extract was tried on a human diabetic in February, 1922. Best developed mass production methods while studying for a medical degree. Banting and Best's discovery of insulin gave hope of life to millions of diabetics who otherwise would have been doomed.

The restriction of sodium intake helps to reduce or avoid the problem of fluid retention. The normal daily diet contains about seven or more grams of sodium, most of it in the form of sodium chloride or table salt. This amount is either inherent in the food or added during processing, cooking, or at mealtime. Half the weight of salt is sodium.

For people whose physical condition requires only a small restriction of the normal sodium intake, simply not salting food at the table is a sufficient reduction. They may decide to use a salt substitute, but before doing so should discuss the question with their physician.

A greater sodium restriction, for example, to no more than 5 grams a day, requires the avoidance of such high salt content foods as ham, bacon, crackers, catsup, and potato chips, as well as almost entirely eliminating salt in the preparation and serving of meals. Severe restriction—1 gram or less a day—involves special food selection and cooking procedures, as well as the use of distilled water if the local water has more than 20 milligrams of sodium per quart. In restricting sodium to this extent, it is important to make sure that protein and vitamins are not reduced below the minimum daily requirements. See *Sodium Restricted Diets*, pp. 338–340.

Other Diseases Requiring Special Diets

There are several other disorders in which diet is an important consideration: all chronic gastrointestinal disorders, such as ulcerative colitis, enteritis, gall bladder stones, and diverticulitis; a variety of hereditary disorders such as phenylketonuria, and galactosemia; atherosclerosis, especially when it is associated with elevated blood levels of cholesterol or triglycerides or both; liver disease such as cirrhosis; many of the endocrine diseases; kidney stones; and sometimes certain neurological diseases such as epilepsy. Diet also plays a special role in convalescence from most illnesses and in post-surgical care. The *Modified Fat Diet* (pp. 342–344) and *Low Fat Diet* (pp. 348–349) are recommended for some diseases of the liver and gall bladder. The *Minimal Residue Diet* (pp. 350–351) is recommended for some digestive troubles and before and after gastrointestinal surgery.

Diet and Individual Differences

Most discussions about food and eating tend to suggest that all normal people have identical gastrointestinal and metabolic systems. This is simply not true. There are many individual differences that explain why one man's meat is another man's poison. A person's intolerance for a given food may be caused by a disorder, such as an allergy or an ulcer, and it is possible that many of these intolerances will ultimately be related to enzyme deficiencies or some other biochemical factor.

More subtle are the negative physical reactions to particular foods as a result of psychological conditioning. In most such cases, the choice is between avoiding the food that causes the discomfort or eating it and suffering the consequences. Of course, compulsive overeating can also cause or contribute to discomfort. Practically no one can eat unlimited quantities of anything without having gastrointestinal discomfort or *dyspepsia*.

The establishment of so-called daily minimum food requirements suggests that every day's intake should be carefully balanced. Although this is beneficial, it is by no means necessary. Freedom from such regimentation can certainly be enjoyed during a holiday, or a trip to another country, or on a prolonged visit to relatives with casual food habits.

Sometimes a change in diet is dictated by a cold or an upset stomach or diarrhea. Liquids containing carbohydrates, such as tea with sugar and light soups, should be emphasized in treating a cold, while at the

MODIFIED FAT DIET

Type of food	Foods included	Foods excluded
Beverages	Coffee, tea, carbonated beverages, cereal beverages; skimmed milk, nonfat dried milk and buttermilk (made from skimmed milk).	Cream, evaporated milk, whole milk, whole milk beverages.
Breads	Whole wheat, rye, or enriched white bread; plain yeast rolls.	All others, including biscuits, cornbread, French toast, muffins, sweet rolls.
Cereals	Any; whole grain or enriched preferred.	None.
Desserts	Angel food cake; plain puddings made with skimmed milk; gelatin desserts; fruit ices, sherbets; fruit whips; meringues.	Cakes except angel food; cookies; ice cream; pastries; rich desserts.
Fats	Oils: corn, cottonseed, olive, peanut, safflower, soy bean. (If calories permit, 1½ to 3 ounces will be included daily.) Specially prepared margarines.	Bacon drippings, butter, coconut oil, regular fortified fats, salt pork, vegetable shortenings, commercial salad dressings.
Fruits	Any fresh (except avocado), canned, frozen, or dried fruit or juice (one citrus fruit to be included daily).	Avocado.
Meat, poultry, fish, cheese	Limit to 4 ounces daily from Group I or the equivalent from Groups II or III (below). Lean meat trimmed of all visible fat.	Fried meats; fat meats, such as bacon, cold cuts, duck, goose, pork, sausage; fish canned in oil; all other fish except those allowed. All cheese except dry cottage cheese.
Eggs	Egg whites as desired; whole eggs (a maximum of one per day or about 3 per week) poached, soft or hard cooked, fried in allowed oil.	Eggs or egg whites cooked with fat, except those fats allowed.
Potato or substitute	Hominy, macaroni, noodles, popcorn (prepared with allowed oil), potato, rice, spaghetti.	Potato chips; any of these items fried or creamed unless prepared with allowed fats.
Group I	7 gms. fat per 30 gms. (1 ounce).	Lean beef, ham, lamb, and pork; tongue; veal; trout.
Group II	3 gms. fat per 30 gms. (1 ounce).	Beef liver, heart, kidney, dried or chipped beef; chicken, turkey; lean fish, such as codfish, haddock, halibut, mackerel, shad, salmon, tuna, whitefish.
Group III	Less than 1 gm. fat per 90 gms. (3 ounces).	Crab, clams, flounder, lobster, oysters, perch, scallops, shrimp.

From the *Clinical Center Diet Manual*, revised edition, prepared by the Nutrition Department, The Clinical Center, National Institutes of Health, Public Health Service, U.S. Department of Health, Education, and Welfare (Public Health Service Publication No. 989), pp. 69–72.

	MODIFIED FAT DIET *(continued)*	
Type of food	Foods included	Foods excluded
Soups	Bouillon, clear broth, vegetable soup; cream soups made with skimmed milk.	All others.
Sweets	Hard candies, jam, jelly, sugar, syrup; chocolate syrup made only with cocoa, sugar, and water.	All other candies; chocolate.
Vegetables	Any fresh, frozen, or cooked without added fat (one green or yellow vegetable should be included daily).	Buttered, creamed, or fried vegetables unless prepared with allowed fats.
Miscellaneous	Condiments, pickles, salt, spices, vinegar.	Gravies, nuts, olives, peanut butter.

This diet is planned to reduce the intake of fats containing a high degree of either saturated or short-chain fatty acids and to avoid the excessive carbohydrate intake associated with a very low fat diet. This is done through replacement of saturated fat sources with those containing higher quantities of poly-unsaturated fatty acids. The fats ordinarily used are corn oil, cottonseed oil, safflower oil, olive oil, peanut oil, and soybean oil. Fats containing large amounts of saturated fatty acids are restricted to approximately 30 grams daily. Carbohydrate and protein are planned to conform to normal levels, with approximately 300–350 grams carbohydrate and approximately 70–80 grams protein. The modified fat diet is planned to meet normal dietary allowances. Calories can be adjusted to fit the needs of the individual. If normal or higher than normal calories are required, fats containing a high percentage of unsaturated fatty acids, such as corn oil, cottonseed oil, etc., may be added.

same time solid food intake should be somewhat reduced. In the case of an upset stomach or diarrhea, the discomfort may be eased by not eating or drinking anything at all for a whole day. This form of treatment may be helpful for an adult, but since children with diarrhea can become dehydrated in a day or so, professional advice is indicated when cutting down liquid intake.

Diet and Disease Prevention

Whether or not diet can be helpful in preventing various diseases other than those caused by nutritional deficiency is an unsettled question. Some specialists think that a diet low in cholesterol and saturated fats can help prevent cardiovascular disease caused by atherosclerosis, but the evidence for this point of view is not yet definitive.

It has been said for years that vitamin C is helpful in preventing the common cold, and this point of view has recently received a great deal of publicity, but the evidence is not conclusive.

Food-borne diseases: There are several ways in which food can be the *cause* of disease, most commonly when it becomes contaminated with a sufficient amount of harmful bacteria, bacterial toxin, viruses, or other poisonous substances. The gastrointestinal diseases typically accompanied by nausea, vomiting, diarrhea, or stomach cramps that are produced in this way are not, strictly speaking, caused by the foods themselves, and are therefore called food-borne diseases.

Most food-borne illnesses are caused by a toxin in food contaminated by staphylococcal or salmonella bacteria. In general,

MODIFIED FAT DIET (continued)

Sample Menu

Household measure[1]

Breakfast

Orange juice	½ cup
Oatmeal	½ cup
Nonfat milk[2]	1 cup
Sugar	2 teaspoons
Poached egg	One
Toast, enriched or whole grain	2 slices
Jelly	1 tablespoon
Coffee or tea	As desired

Luncheon

Clear broth, fat free	As desired
Lean roast beef	2 ounces
Baked potato	1 medium
Green beans	½ cup
Lettuce and tomato salad, oil dressing	1 serving
Bread, enriched or whole grain	1 slice
Jelly	1 tablespoon
Canned peach halves	2 halves
Nonfat milk[2]	1 cup
Coffee or tea	As desired
Sugar	1 teaspoon

Dinner

Roast chicken (no skin)	4 ounces
Diced potato	½ cup
Green peas	½ cup
Head lettuce salad, oil dressing	1 serving
Bread, enriched or whole grain	1 slice
Jelly	1 tablespoon
Nonfat milk[2]	1 cup
Fruited gelatin	½ cup
Coffee or tea	As desired
Sugar	1 teaspoon

[1] Household measure is given to indicate the quantity of food necessary to supply 2,200 calories.
[2] As an example of the manner in which oil can be incorporated into the modified fat diet, a recipe for nonfat milk with oil follows:

For one quart of nonfat milk including one and one-half ounces of oil:

Dried powdered skim milk*	3¼ ounces (1⅓ cup)
Corn oil	1½ ounces
Water	to make 1 quart

Blend water with powdered skimmed milk in food blender until thoroughly mixed. Add corn oil and blend at a high speed until fully blended. Fresh skimmed milk may be substituted in the recipe for the powdered skimmed milk and water. The skimmed milk should be served cold, and the addition of flavoring is not recommended.

*Dried skimmed milk powders vary in weight. They may be reliquefied according to the directions on each package.

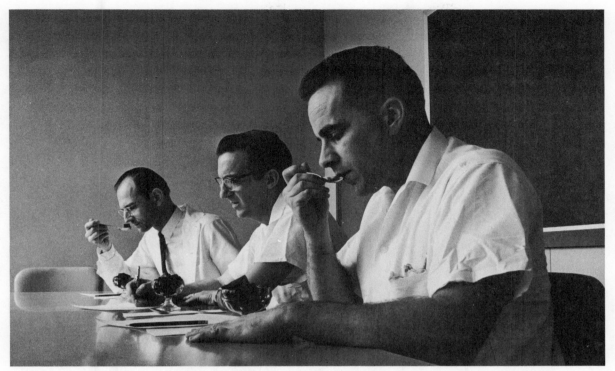

A team of tasters from private industry evaluates an additive's effect on the flavor of a gelatin dessert. Additives are used to enhance the appearance, taste, or nutritive value of food.

milk, milk products, raw shellfish, and meats are the foods most apt to be contaminated. This is most likely to happen when such foods are left standing at room temperature for too long between the time they are prepared and the time they are eaten. However, food can also become contaminated at many different points in time and at various stages of processing. Various standards enforced by federal and local government agencies provide good protection for the consumer both for the foods bought for preparation at home as well as for those served in restaurants.

Food Storage

Food is best protected from contamination when it is stored below 40 degrees Fahrenheit or heated to 145 degrees or more. Cold slows bacterial growth; cooking kills it. Bacteria present in food can double in number every 15 minutes at room temperature.

All food stored in the refrigerator should be covered except ripe fruits and vegetables. Leftover foods cannot be kept indefinitely, nor can frozen foods be stored beyond a certain length of time. Specific information about these time periods for individual items is available from the Agricultural Extension Service in each state.

Commercially processed foods sold in the United States are under government control and generally are safe. However, any food can spoil or become contaminated at any point in time, and the consumer should not buy or serve food whose container (package or can) has been broken, cracked, or appears unusual.

Food Additives

From time to time, concern is expressed about one or another food additive as a hazard to health. Most of these additives are put into foods during processing in order to increase their nutritional value, or to

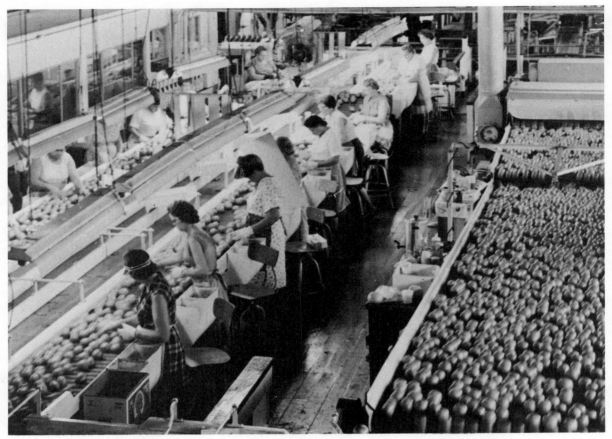

Oranges move from the conveyor at right onto the two conveyors at left, where defective fruit are withdrawn. Inspectors periodically test samples for pesticide residue.

improve their chemical or physical characteristics, such as taste and color.

Perhaps as many as 2,000 different substances are used in this way in the United States. Some are natural products such as vanilla, others are chemicals derived from other foods, and a few, like saccharin, are synthetic.

Other additives are referred to as indirect, since they are residues in the food from some stage of growing, processing, or packaging. Since food additives, which are generally used in tiny amounts, are controlled and approved by agencies such as the federal Food and Drug Administration, there is little or no need to be concerned about them as health hazards. The risks of an inadequate diet should really take top priority as a health consideration.

Organic Foods

Some people feel that industrial methods of food farming and processing introduced during the past century, and more particularly in the last four or five decades, have resulted in foods that are deficient in nutritional value. They have recommended a return to the techniques of food production of an earlier era, in which only organic fertilizers were used. Foods so produced are called *organic foods*. Standard, commercially prepared foods, they feel, lack the health benefits and better tastes of organic foods and may even be damaging to health.

The damage, they believe, is caused because chemical fertilizers, pesticides, and food additives make foods toxic in some way or other. These toxins include female hormones, antibiotics, and an inordinate number of organic and inorganic chemicals. They are thought to cause or contribute to the development of some cancers, arteriosclerosis, and other degenerative diseases, the causes of which really are unknown.

Organic foods are also said to make people less susceptible to viral infections such as common colds, and to tooth decay. All of these claimed health benefits could also be the result of having preserved in organically prepared foods various substances that are eliminated in normal commercial processing.

The organic food philosophy calls for growing your own foods, using only organic fertilizers such as compost or animal (not human) manure, and without using pesticides or herbicides. For those unable to grow their own foods, commercial sources of organic foods are becoming more and more readily available.

Typical Organic Foods

Whole grain cereals such as brown rice, and wheat, beans, vegetables, and fruits are the major sources of organic foods. Unsulfured molasses and natural honey are the primary sweeteners. Sea salt and herbs are used for flavoring. Organic meat is available, but many organic food people are vegetarians. Fertile eggs, cheeses, especially those from raw goat or cow milk, and yogurt also are basic parts of an organic diet. Cold pressed vegetable oils, filtered in a special way, and made from sesame, corn germ, or soy are used regularly; they are not only unsaturated fats and therefore have low cholesterol contents but also contain many natural vitamins. Herb teas, fruit juices, and raw milk are among the preferred liquids. Ideally, all organic foods should be eaten when fresh or in season, since canning or freezing requires the addition of chemicals.

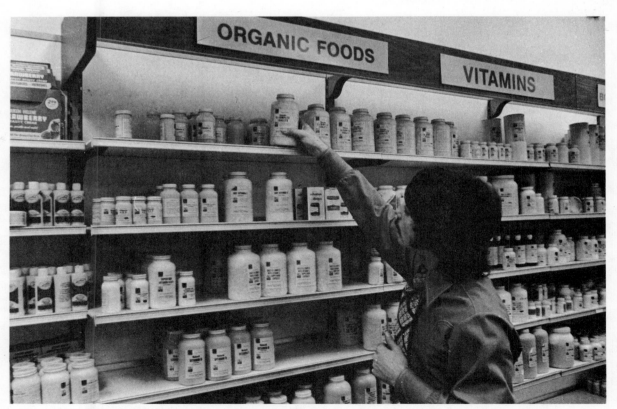

Organic food stores, often featuring vitamins as well as foods, are on the increase.

LOW FAT DIET		
Type of food	Foods included	Foods excluded
Beverages	Coffee, tea, carbonated beverages, cereal beverages, skimmed milk or nonfat buttermilk.	Cream, whole milk, whole milk beverages.
Breads	Whole wheat, rye, or enriched white bread; plain yeast rolls.	Muffins, biscuits, sweet rolls, cornbread, pancakes, waffles, french toast.
Cereals	Any: whole grain or enriched preferred.	None.
Desserts	Plain angel food cake; custards and puddings made with skimmed milk and egg allowances; fruit puddings; gelatin desserts; ices; fruit whips made with egg white.	Rich desserts, pastries; sherbets, ice cream; cakes, except angel food.
Fats	None	All fats and oils; salad dressings.
Fruits	Any fresh (except avocado), canned, frozen, or dried fruit or juice (one citrus fruit to be included daily).	Avocado.
Meat, poultry, fish, cheese.	Limit to 5 ounces daily: lean meat, such as lean beef, lamb, liver, veal; chicken, turkey; canned salmon or tuna (canned without oil); shellfish, lean whitefish; dry cottage cheese.	Fried meats; fat meats, such as bacon, cold cuts, duck, goose, pork, sausage; fish canned in oil. All cheese except dry cottage cheese.
Eggs	Any poached, soft or hard cooked; limit to one egg daily.	Fried eggs; eggs scrambled with fat.
Potato or substitute.	Hominy, macaroni, noodles, potatoes, rice, spaghetti.	Any of these items fried or creamed; potato chips.
Soups	Bouillon, clear broth, vegetable soup; cream soups made with skimmed milk.	All others.
Sweets	Hard candies, jam, jelly, sugar, syrup; chocolate syrup made only with cocoa, sugar, and water.	All other candies or chocolate.
Vegetables	Any fresh, frozen or cooked without added fat (one green or yellow vegetable should be included daily).	Buttered, creamed or fried vegetables.
Miscellaneous	Condiments, pickles, salt, spices, vinegar.	Gravies, nuts, olives, peanut butter.

This diet contains approximately 40 grams of fat. To maintain normal calorie intake with fat restricted, it has a high carbohydrate content. The low fat diet is adequate in all nutrients. Calories can be adjusted to fit the needs of the individual patient. Approximate composition is as follows:

Protein	85 gm.
Fat	40 gm.
Carbohydrate	325 gm.
Calories	2,000

From the *Clinical Center Diet Manual*, revised edition, prepared by the Nutrition Department, The Clinical Center, National Institutes of Health, Public Health Service, U.S. Department of Health, Education, and Welfare (Public Health Service Publication No. 989), pp. 73–75.

LOW FAT DIET (continued)	
Sample Menu	

	Household measure[1]
Breakfast	
Orange juice	½ cup
Oatmeal	½ cup
Skimmed milk	1 cup
Sugar	1 tablespoon
Poached egg	One (limit to one daily)
Toast, enriched or whole grain	2 slices
Jelly	1 tablespoon
Coffee or tea	As desired
Luncheon	
Beef broth, fat free . . .	As desired
Sliced chicken	2 ounces
Baked potato	1 small
Peas	½ cup
Lettuce and tomato salad . .	1 serving
Lemon ice	½ cup
Bread, enriched or whole grain	1 slice
Jelly	1 tablespoon
Skimmed milk	1 cup
Coffee or tea	As desired
Sugar	1 tablespoon
Nourishment	
Pineapple juice	1 cup
Dinner	
Lean roast beef	3 ounces
Steamed potato	1 small
Carrots	½ cup
Mixed fruit salad	1 serving
Angel food cake	1 serving
Bread, enriched or whole grain	1 slice
Jelly	1 tablespoon
Coffee or tea	As desired
Sugar	1 tablespoon
Nourishment	
Tomato juice	1 cup
Crackers	Five

[1] Household measures are given to indicate the quantity of food necessary to supply 2,000 calories.

Natural Foods

Several other food styles are associated with organic foods. *Natural foods* are not necessarily grown organically, but are not processed very much. *Macrobiotics* is a special natural food concept, oriental in origin, and based upon the idea of maintaining an equilibrium between foods that make one active (*Yang*) and foods that make one relax (*Yin*). A proper mixture of grain and vegetables contains an excellent balance of Yin and Yang. Yoga diets center around such natural foods as fruits and nuts.

	MINIMAL RESIDUE DIET	
Type of Food	Foods included	Foods excluded
Beverages	Black coffee, tea, carbonated beverages, cereal beverages.	Milk, milk drinks.
Breads	Salted and soda crackers.	All breads.
Cereals	Cooked rice cereals or refined wheat cereals, made with water.	Whole grain cereals.
Desserts	White angel food cake, arrowroot cookies; ices; clear gelatin dessert.	Custards, puddings; desserts made with milk; ice cream.
Fats	Bacon, butter, fortified fats.	Cream.
Fruits	Strained fruit juices only.	All fruits.
Meat, fish, poultry, eggs, cheese	Beef, lamb, veal; chicken, turkey; whitefish; eggs.	Fried meats, poultry, or fish; all cheese.
Potato or substitute	Macaroni, noodles, rice, spaghetti.	Potatoes, hominy.
Soups	Bouillon, broth.	Cream soups.
Sweets	Hard candies without nuts or fruit; honey, jelly, sugar, syrup.	Candies with fruit or nuts; jam, marmalade.
Vegetables	Tomato juice only.	All other vegetables.
Miscellaneous	Salt, small amounts of pepper used in cooking.	All other spices; condiments; nuts, olives, pickles, etc.

Minimal residue diet. The foods included on the minimal residue diet are selected on the basis of the small amount of residue left in the intestines after digestion. Since milk, milk products, fruits, and vegetables are thought to leave a large residue, these foods (except fruit and vegetable juices) have been omitted from the diet. The minimal residue diet is adequate in protein and calories. All other nutrients are below the recommended allowances.

From the *Clinical Center Diet Manual*, revised edition, prepared by the Nutrition Department, The Clinical Center, National Institutes of Health, Public Health Service, U.S. Department of Health, Education, and Welfare (Public Health Service Publication No. 989), pp. 45, 56–57.

Psychological Aspects of Food and Meals

Food and meals play an important role in emotional well-being and interpersonal relationships as well as in physical health and appearance.

During Infancy

The infant whose needs are attended to by a loving family develops a general sense of trust and security. The major contribution to his emotional contentment is probably made at mealtimes, and perhaps in a special way if he is breast-fed.

For most infants, food comes to be identified with love, pleasure, protection, and the satisfaction of basic needs. If there is an atmosphere of tension accompanying his feeding times, his digestion can be impaired in such a way as to cause vomiting, fretting, or signs of colic. If the tension and

MINIMAL RESIDUE DIET (continued)

Sample Menu

Breakfast
Orange juice	½ cup
Cream of wheat (cooked in water with butter)	½ cup; 1 teaspoon butter
Poached egg	One
Salted crackers	4 to 5
Butter	2 teaspoons
Jelly	1 tablespoon
Coffee or tea	As desired
Sugar	As desired

Luncheon
Roast beef	3 ounces
Buttered noodles	½ cup
Tomato juice	½ cup
Salted crackers	4 to 5
Butter	2 teaspoons
Jelly	1 tablespoon
Plain gelatin dessert	½ cup
Coffee or tea	As desired
Sugar	As desired

Dinner
Grapefruit juice	½ cup
Clear broth	As desired
Baked chicken	4 ounces
Buttered rice	½ cup
Salted crackers	4 to 5
Butter	2 teaspoons
Fruit ice	½ cup
Coffee or tea	As desired
Sugar	As desired

Nourishment
Strained fruit juices	As desired
Plain gelatin desserts	As desired
Fruit ices	As desired

the baby's reaction to it—and inevitably the mother's increasing tension as a consequence—become a chronic condition, the result may be a failure to gain weight normally, and in extreme cases, some degree of mental retardation. Throughout life, good nutrition depends not only on eating properly balanced meals that satisfy the body's physiological requirements, but also on a reasonable degree of contentment and relaxation while eating.

Everybody develops individual emotional reactions and attitudes about food and its role as a result of conditioning during the years of infancy and childhood. These attitudes relate not only to food itself and to mealtimes in general, but also to other aspects of eating, including the muscle activities of sucking, chewing, and swallowing.

If food symbolized contentment during the early years, it probably will have the same role later on. If it was associated with conflict, then it may be associated throughout life with strife and neurotic eating patterns.

During Childhood

For the preschool child, mealtimes should provide the occasion for the development of interpersonal relationships, since they are a daily opportunity for both verbal and nonverbal self-expression. The child who eats with enthusiasm and obvious enjoyment is conveying one message; the one who dawdles, picks at food, and challenges his mother with every mouthful is conveying quite a different one.

Meals can become either positive or negative experiences depending in large part on how the adults in the family set the stage. Communication can be encouraged by re-

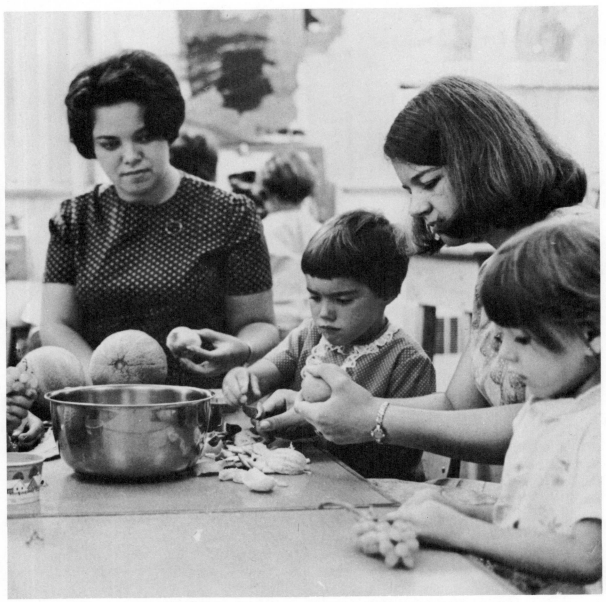

Many nursery schools use food as the subject of a learning experience. Meals are made more meaningful if the preparation as well as the eating of food is shared.

laxed conversation and a reasonably leisurely schedule. It can be discouraged by watching television or reading while eating, by not eating together, or by eating and running.

Reasonably firm attitudes about eating a variety of foods in proper quantities at proper times and avoiding excessive catering to individual whims can also help in the development of wholesome eating patterns.

The person who selects and prepares the food can transmit special messages of love and affection by serving favorite dishes, by setting the table attractively, and by creating an atmosphere of grace and good humor. Or she can show displeasure and generate hostility by complaining about all the work involved in feeding everyone, or by constant criticism of table manners, or by bringing up touchy subjects likely to cause arguments at the table.

How Food Can Relieve Tension

Food can be instrumental in relieving individual tension as well as in smoothing over minor family conflicts. Most people are familiar with the type of individual who is grumpy before a meal and who visibly brightens when he begins to eat. Sometimes this is due to the condition of *hypoglycemia* in which the blood sugar is too low for comfort. More often, the good spirits come from the psychological uplift brought about by the comradeship of eating.

People often turn to food as a way of relieving tension, thus reverting to a pattern established in childhood. Milk, for example, is often sought in times of stress. The relationship between food and anxiety is a complex one, and if it becomes so distorted that neurosis results, the physical consequences can be extremely unpleasant. Gastrointestinal disorders such as ulcers, bloating, belching, passing gas, diarrhea, and constipation are more often than not emotional rather than purely physical in origin.

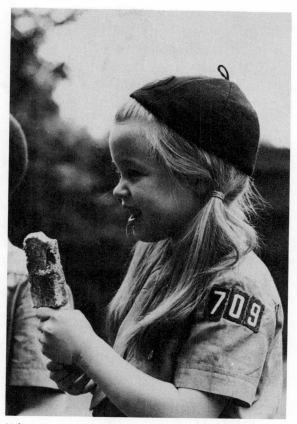

When you've had to wait impatiently while the ice cream pops were being handed out, the joy of taking that first bite is really something to remember.

The Symbol of Food

Food has many symbolic aspects: it can transmit and reinforce ethnic traditions either regularly or on special holidays. It can be used at lavish dinner parties as an expression of economic success; it can denote worldliness and sophistication in the form of complicated gourmet dishes of obscure origin.

A great deal can be learned about a person by knowing something about his attitudes toward food—not only what, how, when, and where he eats, but also how the groceries are bought, how the refrigerator and pantry shelves are stocked, how the cooking is organized, and how the dishes are cleaned up. In many significant ways, all of us are not only *what* we eat; we truly express who we are by *how* we eat.   DST

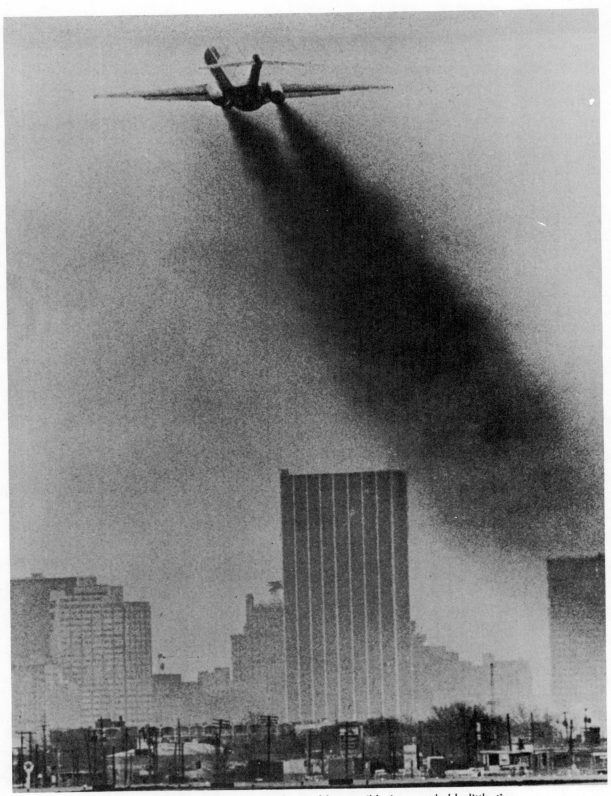

Jet travel has made any place in the world accessible in remarkably little time, but it has also contributed to the problems of air pollution and noise pollution.

CHAPTER 5

The Environment
and Health

"Ecology . . . pollution . . . deterioration of the environment . . . the quality of life. . . ."

These words are with us constantly, in the news, political speeches, informed conversation. Heated controversy flairs over just how contaminated the globe is, the extent of the danger, the cost of cleaning up the mess, and whether any solution is realistically possible.

One thing is clear and incontestable: the quality of the environment is crucial to health, perhaps more important than any individual personal health measures you can employ. According to the federal Task Force on Research Planning in Environmental Health Science: ". . . the environment plays a predominant role in man's health; . . . rapid technologic change, increased population, and greater concentration of people into urban centers are compounding the problems of maintaining the environment at a healthful level."

Kinds of Pollution

Harmful ingredients in the environment are often the result of pollution; however, nat-

ural components—ultraviolet radiation in sunlight, for example—can also be contributing factors. These pollutants and the occasional natural counterparts can damage health in a variety of ways; even though there is as yet no scientific proof linking some of these pollutants with a specific malady, the statistical, or circumstantial evidence is impressive. Most health experts believe, for example, that there is a direct connection between air pollution and various forms of respiratory illness.

Excessive noise, sometimes referred to as the "third pollution," after air and water pollution, is known to cause temporary and permanent hearing loss, anxiety, tension, and insomnia; it is strongly suspected of contributing to cardiovascular disease.

Many of the products of the technological age are toxic. Quantities of them find their way into the air, water, and food. Apart from outright poisoning, some of these contaminants are implicated in the development of cancer. Others are thought to cause mutations in the consumer, resulting in abnormal and sometimes nonviable offspring.

Occupational disease: Because of our jobs, some of us are vastly more exposed to

355

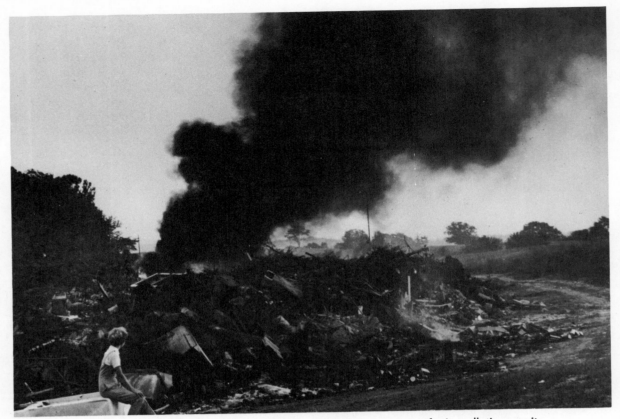

The improper burning of garbage, one of the major causes of air pollution, emits poisonous ash and chemicals. Many experts link air pollution with respiratory diseases.

these dangerous contaminants than others. Occupational disease linked to specific pollutants has a long and unpleasant history. Chimney sweeps in 18th-century London developed cancer of the scrotum from long exposure to coal soot, which contained potent cancer-producing agents (*carcinogens*). The malady was called "soot-wart." The Mad Hatter in Lewis Carroll's *Alice in Wonderland* represents a well-known type, a victim of "hatter's disease"—chronic mercury poisoning. (Mercury was used in the preparation of felt for hats.) During the latter part of the 19th century, skin cancer was a frequent hazard of work in the coal tar, paraffin, oil, and lignite tar industries. Bladder cancer began to appear among workers in the new aniline dye industry; it wasn't until 1938 that the carcinogen responsible was identified.

Today, miners contract *black lung disease* and *silicosis* from inhaling coal and other dusts. Cotton workers suffer chest-tightening *byssinosis* ("white lung disease") from inhaling cotton dust. Asbestos workers have seven times more lung cancer than the general population, and risk several other lung diseases, among them silicosis. Recently, some clothing workers were exposed to similar risks when they unknowingly manufactured 100,000 women's coats from a cloth containing eight percent asbestos fiber. One authority advised any woman in possession of such a coat to "bury it." Merely rubbing or brushing the coat would produce asbestos levels in the air 10,000 times higher than normal. See also *Lung Disease*, p. 555.

Added to all these and other traditional occupational hazards are those from a bewildering new profusion of synthetic chemicals whose dangerous properties may become known only long after they are in production.

Radiation: Finally, there is a category of contaminants about which so little is known that they are provoking raging debate: ionizing radiation (such as that from nuclear reactors and other radioactive sources), microwave radiation (such as that from microwave ovens), and laser radiation. The Task Force quoted earlier points out with some asperity that the United States allows a level of microwave radiation for occupational exposure that is 1,000 times higher than the maximum set by Soviet Russia and other Eastern European countries. Microwaves, similar to radio waves and used in communications as well as ovens, are measurable in the environment of one-half the U.S. population.

Air Pollution

Most air pollution results from the incomplete burning of fuels and other materials, such as garbage. There are hundreds of different pollutants; some are visible as the yellowish brown haze that hangs over most large cities, but most are invisible. There is some debate over the precise relation between these various contaminants and the level of respiratory disease among the general population, although many experts think that the evidence now linking them with asthma, emphysema, and bronchitis is very strong.

Inversions

No one can doubt that high concentrations of air pollution are deadly. Modern history has seen some appalling examples. They usually occur in a region that is subject to a freak weather condition called an *inversion,* during which a mass of warm air sits like a lid on top of cool air, trapping it and preventing the pollutants that are produced daily from being ventilated. The

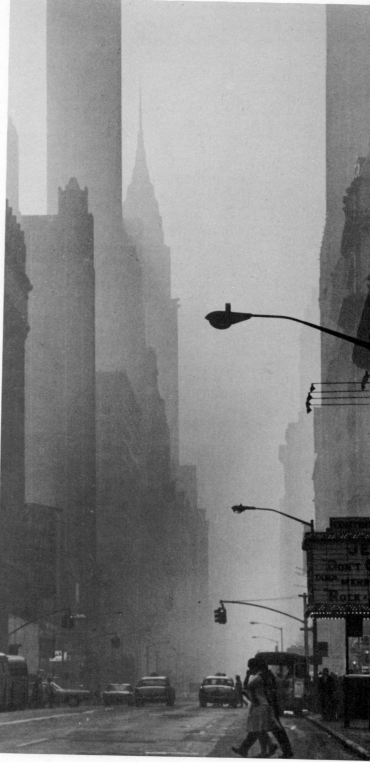

A temperature inversion occurs when a layer of warm air traps a mass of cool air beneath it, thus preventing the pollutants from being dispersed as usual.

pollutants accumulate in this stagnant air until they sometimes reach high concentrations, with lethal results.

The Meuse valley in Belgium, a center of heavy industry with many coal-burning factories, experienced an inversion in 1930 that trapped the smoke for five days. Some 60 people died as a result and 6,000 were sickened.

A killer smog brought a new menace to London's notorious pea-soupers in December, 1952. For five days an impenetrable, smoky fog paralyzed the city. Hospitals were jammed with people gasping for breath. When the smog finally lifted, medical statisticians calculated that 4,000 deaths during and immediately after the siege could be attributed to the smog.

The United States has known its share of such tragedies. Perhaps the worst and most famous was the inversion that hit Donora,

Pennsylvania, in October, 1948, in a valley similar in topography and in pollution-creating industry to the Meuse. The inversion lasted six days—six days of even more unhealthy air. At its peak, more than half of the valley's 14,000 persons had been stricken; at least 20 deaths were blamed on the pollution. Many more persons suffered irreversible damage to their health, according to a U.S. Public Health Service study.

Sulfur Dioxide

Today, increasing numbers of cities report unsatisfactory or unhealthy air conditions with growing frequency. New York City's Environmental Protection Administration has stated that between 1,000 and 2,000 deaths a year there probably result from sulfur dioxide—the main toxic component of killer smogs—and other particles suspended in the air. Sulfur dioxide is spewed into the air—more than 23 million tons in the country, and 380,000 tons in New York City alone—when heavy fuel oil and coal are burned to provide heat, generate electricity, and provide industrial power. These fuels are generally rich in sulfur. Recently, some localities have passed legislation requiring the use of low-sulfur coal and oil for certain uses.

No one knows exactly how sulfur dioxide affects the respiratory tract. The likelihood is that it irritates the lungs and contributes to a reduction of the lungs' oxygen-handling capacity. Persons especially vulnerable to smogs are those suffering from bronchial asthma, chronic bronchitis (some studies show 13 percent of U.S. men have the disease) and emphysema, because their respiratory capacity is already defective. In emphysema, for example, the elasticity of the air sacs in the lungs has progressively broken down, usually after prolonged infection or repeated bronchial irritation (such as is produced by cigarette smoking). Deaths from emphysema are twice as high in cities as in rural areas.

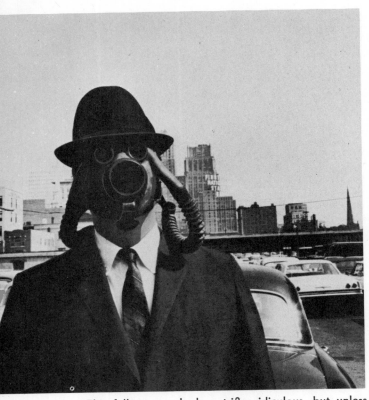

This fellow may look a trifle ridiculous, but unless effective measures are taken soon to reduce air pollution, we may all wish we had gas masks, too.

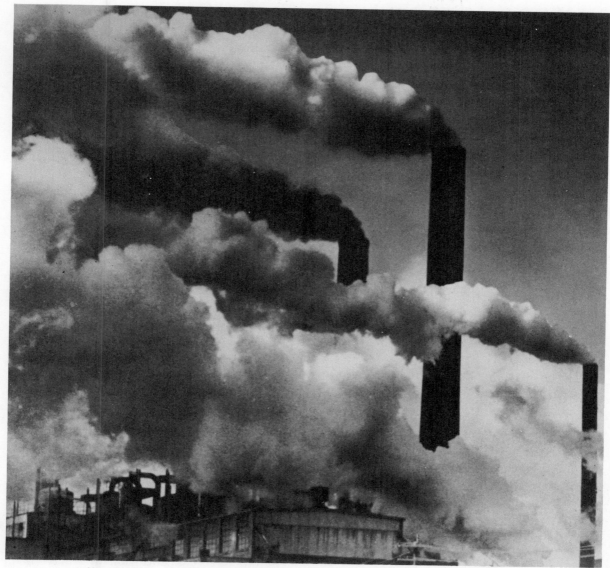

Sulfur dioxide, a by-product of the burning of heavy fuel oil or coal, can be lethal. Emissions of power plants and industrial smokestacks contribute to this health hazard.

Other Contaminants

Other major contaminants that have been identified as dangerous are nitrogen oxides, lead, carbon monoxide, hydrocarbons, and soot—the visible particles of carbon suspended in the air.

Dust may be harmful by transporting corrosive chemicals or other irritants to the lungs. Ordinarily, particles in the air are trapped in the nasal passages, but very small ones can slip past into the lungs. These tiny motes are called submicron particles—less than one twenty-five-thousandth of an inch in size.

Auto Exhausts

The major contributor of these harmful agents is the automobile. Auto exhausts contribute more than one-half the total of all atmospheric contaminants; in large cities, the figure is much higher. For example, in

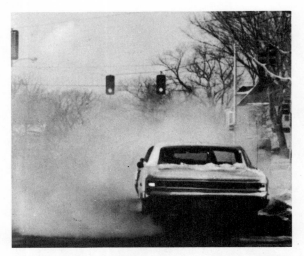

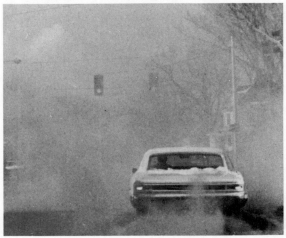

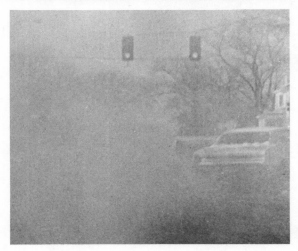

This remarkable sequence of photographs graphically demonstrates the buildup of auto exhaust pollution from a single car. Add to this the other 90,000,000 motor vehicles operating in the U.S., and you will begin to understand the seriousness of the problem.

New York City in 1970, cars, buses, and trucks contributed 77% by weight of all air pollution.

How can these substances affect your health? Nitrogen oxides irritate the eyes and the respiratory tract. Moreover, when nitrogen oxide and hydrocarbons mix in the presence of sunlight, they form other noxious substances in what is called a photochemical smog that has a typical yellowish cast. The new ingredients produced include ozone—a poisonous form of oxygen—and peroxyacl nitrate (PAN), which is intensely irritating to the eyes. Los Angeles was the first city to experience these smogs; they have lately spread elsewhere.

Auto exhaust hydrocarbons include varieties that are suspected of being carcinogens, that is, of contributing to the development of cancer in susceptible individuals. This link so far has been proven only in animals. Dr. Ernest Wynder of the Sloan-Kettering Institute for Cancer Research, however, got some provocative results by painting the skin of laboratory mice with the residues collected from filters exposed to New York air. The mice developed cancer.

Carbon monoxide is an odorless, colorless gas that is lethal even in very small concentrations because it combines with hemoglobin readily and thus replaces oxygen in the blood. In concentrations that have been measured in heavy city traffic, it can make you tired, headachy, drowsy, and careless.

Lead poisoning: Lead is an extremely poisonous substance. Acute cases of lead poisoning suffer headache, nausea, cramps, anemia, numbness, loss of control of wrist and ankle, and finally, coma and death. The symptoms of chronic lead poisoning are much more subtle and harder to pinpoint. Test animals that have consumed lead in amounts comparable to those ingested by men over long periods have suffered life spans reduced by 20 percent, increased infant mortality rates, sterility, and birth

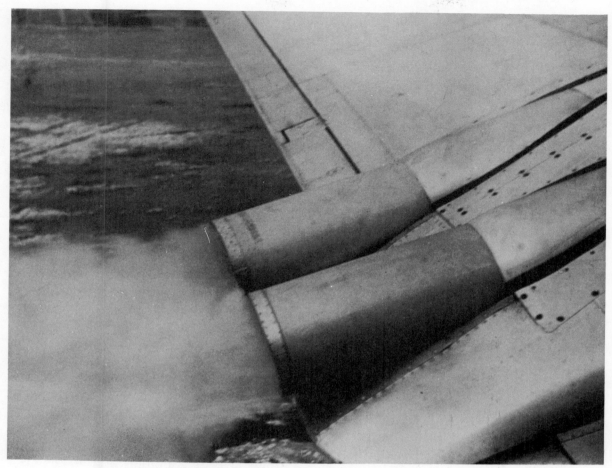

Although motor vehicles contribute far more to the national air pollution problem than jet planes, jet exhaust is a major pollution factor in communities near airports.

defects. In 1971, testifying before the Senate Subcommittee on Energy, Natural Resources and the Environment, Carl L. Klein, an assistant Secretary of the Interior, said that "there can be little doubt that exposure of mothers to lead has a damaging effect upon fertility, the course of pregnancy, and the development of the fetus."

One expert estimated that auto exhausts were releasing 300,000 tons of lead annually into the air, some of which winds up in the water supply. Industrial users also vent large quantities of lead into lakes and rivers.

Experts are now debating exactly how much airborne lead can be tolerated. But a strange phenomenon is occurring in big cities such as New York. The tragedy of

slum children developing lead poisoning has been explained readily because it is known that they nibble lead-bearing paint peeling from their walls. Yet a number of instances of high lead levels in the blood of middle-class children have been discovered. These children live in dwellings painted with modern house paints containing no lead. Some doctors have concluded that the children have been poisoned by auto exhausts. Lead levels in high traffic areas of New York are sometimes 25 times higher than the legal limit in California.

The outlook for any drastic improvements in the air pollution scene is not good. The federal government has given auto manufacturers until 1975 or 1976 to reduce

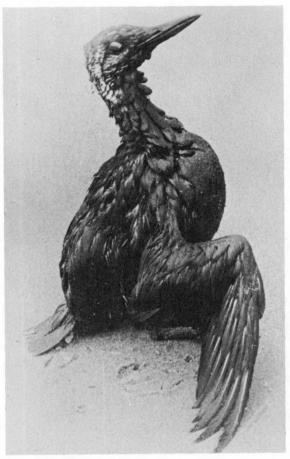

This bird was one of the thousands of victims of a ruptured oil well off the California coast in 1969.

exhaust emissions by 90%, but the manufacturers express doubt that this goal is reachable. In any event, the pollution contribution of older cars will continue into the '80s.

Energy production, the other major air polluter, also offers little hope for immediate improvement, because it will be many years before we can rely heavily on other than fossil fuels such as coal and oil. Supplies of nonpolluting natural gas are in too short supply to do us much good, and it will be at least a decade before nuclear plants make a dent in the energy crisis. See under *Lung Disease,* p. 555, for additional information about the effects of air pollution on health.

Water Pollution

The quality of water is intimately tied to our physical well-being, and we have, therefore, come to expect high standards of cleanliness and purity in the water we drink and bathe in. Public health authorities are increasingly concerned, however, at the progressive deterioration of this country's water supply. This deterioration results

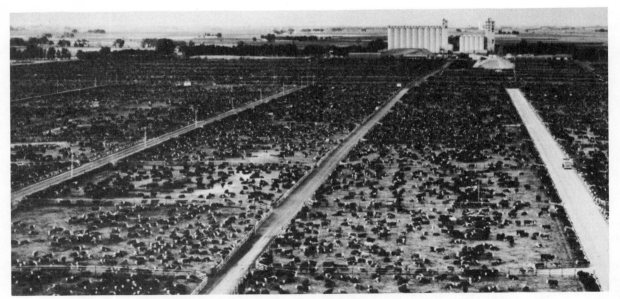

Wastes of these beef cattle will be washed by rain into nearby streams, thus polluting them.

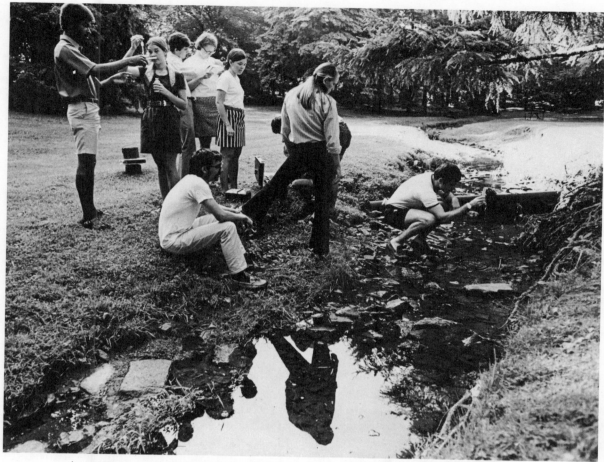

An environmental biology class checks a river for its nitrate and phosphate content.

from years of abuse in which natural water-ways were inundated with quantities of raw sewage, waste products of industrial and chemical plants and slaughterhouses, petroleum residues, poisonous herbicides and insecticides—the list is almost endless, but our water supply is not. In 1970, the Division of Water Hygiene, part of the federal Environmental Protection Agency, concluded that some 969 of the nation's individual water supplies were substandard.

Many householders do not need to be told that their water is less than sparkling and delicious. Bad tastes and odors, off colors and cloudiness plague many regions and make water drinking distasteful, even if it is not yet dangerous. In Suffolk County on New York's Long Island, for example,

water in the region's wells has become so infiltrated with detergents that a glass of water was likely to have a head of detergent foam. After much controversy, the County banned the sale of all laundry products containing detergents.

The problem is that some synthetic detergents are not *biodegradable*—they are not broken down by microorganisms in the soil and water, and thus become water pollutants. Even biodegradable synthetic detergents may add another pollutant—phosphates—to water. Phosphates overstimulate the growth of the primitive water plants called algae, which overrun lakes and streams, consume vast quantities of oxygen, and choke out other life, such as game and food fish.

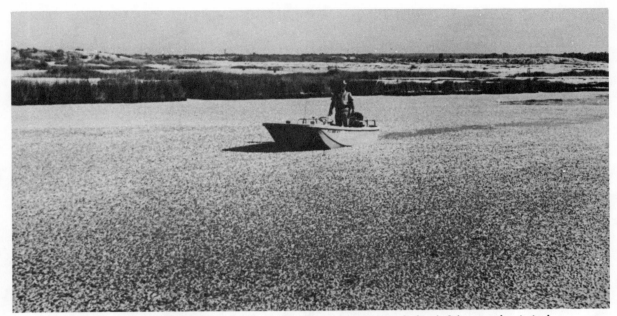

This Florida Marine Patrol boat is cruising through millions of dead fish—mostly six-inch menhaden—killed by deoxygenation of the water, a process stimulated by phosphates.

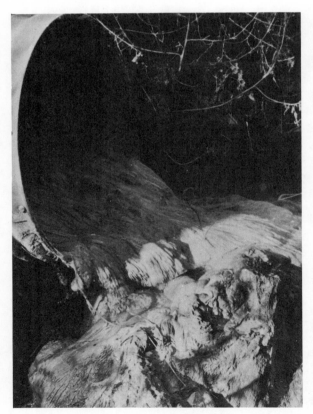

The dumping of raw sewage or of sludge, as seen here, creates "dead seas" where no aquatic life can exist. It may also make nearby beaches unsafe for swimming.

Microbes in Sewage

The risk to health from drinking contaminated water depends on the contaminant. It is fairly rare in this country for cases of typhoid, for example, caused by a pathogenic bacillus, to be contracted through an impure water supply. But you may risk gastrointestinal upsets caused by other organisms if you swim at a beach that is posted "Polluted Waters," as so many beaches now are. The cause is generally the dumping of raw sewage nearby, or of sludge, the solid mass that is left after some kinds of sewage treatment. In New York Harbor there is a dead sea 21 miles square where nothing can live.

Chemical Contamination

In addition to the danger of infection from viral and microbial agents in polluted water, there is mounting danger from chemical contamination. Literally hundreds of chemical compounds find their way into the water supply, some of them in potentially dangerous quantities. Attention has

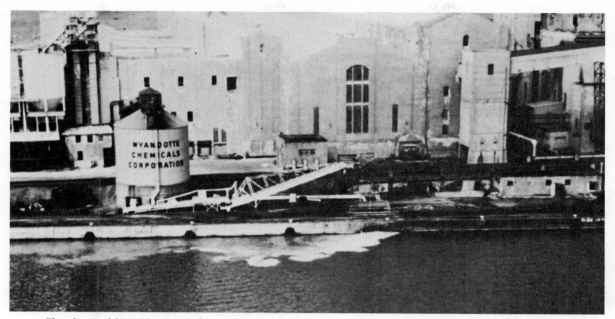

The disposal by industry of chemical wastes by dumping them in a convenient body of water may be dangerous, since communities depend upon these rivers and lakes for their water supply.

focused most recently on the heavy metals and especially mercury. In March, 1971, the U.S. Geological Survey reported that small amounts of seven toxic metals were present in many of the country's lakes and streams, with dangerous concentrations seemingly rare. The metals are mercury, arsenic, cadmium, chromium, cobalt, lead, and zinc. Aside from being generally poisonous, some of these metals are implicated in specific health problems. Cadmium, for example, has been linked to hypertension due to kidney malfunction. In Taiwan, skin cancer has been proved to rise with the quantity of arsenic in well water.

The Dangers of Mercury

Mercury represents a special case. For years, experts thought that since mercury was heavier than water and couldn't dissolve in it, it was therefore safe to dump large quantities of the metal into the waterways on the assumption that it would simply lie quiescent on the bottom. They were, however, wrong. Bacteria can convert some of the metallic form of the element into a water-soluble form, which enters the food chain and eventually winds up, concentrated, in fish. When dangerous levels of this form of mercury were found in some waters and in food fish, the boom was lowered. There was a scare over canned tuna (the government later said that 97 percent of the canned tuna on the market was safe to eat) and swordfish. Lakes and rivers across the country were closed to commercial and sport fishing, and some remain closed.

The reason is not hard to understand. Mercury is an exceedingly toxic substance. The U.S. Food and Drug Administration has established the safe limit of mercury in food at half a part per million, comparable to a thimbleful in an Olympic-sized swimming pool. Even infinitesimal amounts absorbed by the body over a period of time can produce blindness, paralysis, and brain damage.

Swordfish: In an extremely unusual action, the Food and Drug Administration in 1971 advised the public to stop eating swordfish. The FDA had no power to ban

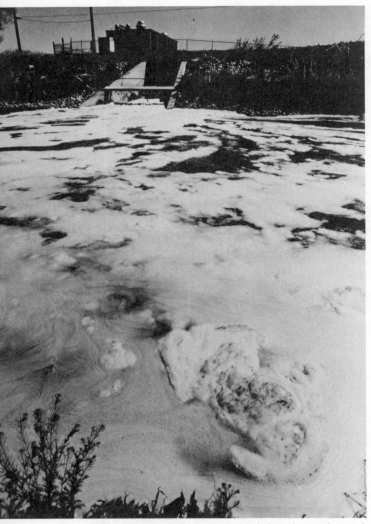

Contamination of rivers and lakes by industrial wastes has become a serious problem in recent years. Fish from polluted waters are often unfit to eat.

The population of Minimata, a Japanese coastal town, was afflicted in 1953 by a strange malady that killed 40, crippled 70. The Minimatans had eaten the local fish and shellfish, which had absorbed mercury discharged into the water in a water soluble form by a nearby plastics factory. Similar cases of mass mercury poisoning have occurred in Italy, Guatemala, and Pakistan.

Pollution experts are particularly worried about mercury because even if we stopped producing mercury compounds and discharging mercury wastes into the country's waters today, the problem would continue to worsen. The enormous store of metallic mercury already discharged and sitting on river and lake bottoms continues to be converted slowly into soluble forms. One chemist has estimated that in the St. Clair River system alone (between Detroit and southwestern Ontario), about 200,000 pounds of metallic mercury have been discharged in the last 20 years.

Recently, high amounts of selenium, an element considered more toxic than mercury, have been found in microscopic animal life in Lake Michigan downwind from Chicago and Milwaukee.

Food Hazards

Contaminants found in water often make their way into food products in the cooking and packaging processes, so that many of the comments on water apply here. Some dilute water pollutants become highly concentrated as they pass up the food chain and end in fish or other foods for man. Mercury was cited earlier as one example. Contamination of food with harmful microorganisms is an everpresent concern wherever standards of cleanliness and sanitation are low.

Additives

Food entails a whole new set of problems because of the thousands of new ingredients

the fish legally, but the move probably meant the end of swordfish as a food in this country. FDA investigators had discovered that only 42 of 853 samples of the fish contained acceptable levels of mercury. The average level of the remaining samples was twice the permissible amount. Soon after the announcement, doctors disclosed the first death in this country attributable to eating mercury-contaminated swordfish— that of a woman who had been eating large quantities of the fish on a weight-reducing diet.

that have been added to it, directly and indirectly, in recent years. These substances include many that have been deemed necessary because of the revolution in food technology—the rise of packaged convenience foods of all kinds. Labels on today's convenience foods list preservatives, thickeners, mold inhibitors, fillers, emulsifiers, and artificial colors and flavors. The trouble with food additives is that we have had little time to learn about their properties in the body, especially over a long period of time. The Food and Drug Administration does set standards in this area; but in the opinion of many experts, these safeguards are inadequate. According to Bess Myerson, Commissioner of New York City's Department of Consumer Affairs, "The food that we eat is becoming as polluted as the air we breathe. Inadequate federal regulations allow manufacturers of prepared foods to ignore potential health hazards. No reasonable person would knowingly drink a glass full of the chemicals he unwittingly consumes in his daily diet."

What are some of these chemicals, and how could they be dangerous? One that was imbibed freely by large numbers of Americans and in great quantities was sodium cyclamate, the artificial sweetener used in diet drinks and foods. It was eventually withdrawn after it was linked to cancer and chromosome damage in experimental animals. The controversy continues, however, and some accused the government of acting precipitately in this case. Cyclamates are still recommended for diabetics and dieters.

Nitrates and nitrites are used in enormous quantities as preservatives in food. Recently, Food and Drug Administration chemists found that these chemicals had apparently given rise to substances called nitrosamines in samples of fish. Nitrosamines are powerful carcinogenic agents,

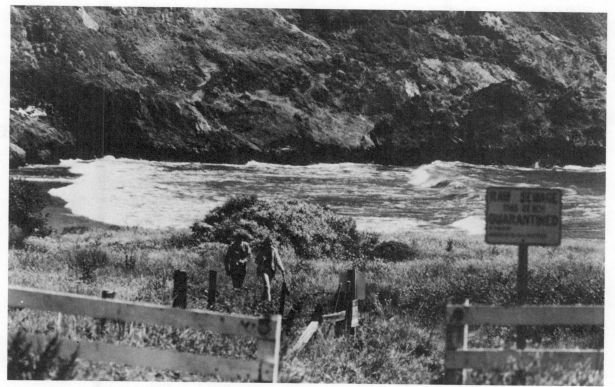

This California beach has been closed to swimmers because of raw sewage in the water. People who ignore quarantine signs at polluted beaches risk contracting serious diseases.

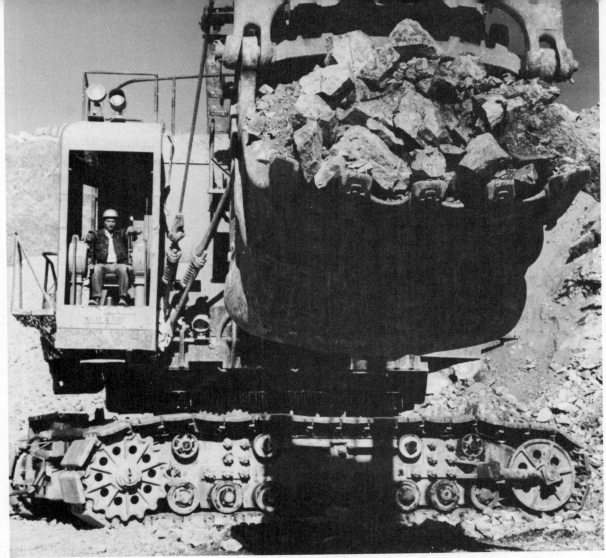

Constant noise from heavy machinery such as power shovels may be harmful to health.

even in small amounts. The amounts found in the fish were minuscule, up to 26 parts per billion. These chemicals are also thought to be capable of producing genetic and birth defects.

In Sweden, a geneticist and microbiologist named Dr. Bjorn Gillsberg has warned that unless we start to screen potentially mutagenic (causing changes in the genes) substances from our food we face an epidemic of birth defects, loss of fertility, and other genetic damage. He cited sodium bisulphate, a chemical used to prevent peeled potatoes from darkening, as a potentially dangerous additive.

The federal Task Force on Research Planning in Environmental Health Science estimates there are some 10,000 of these chemicals—additives and residues—to be found in our foods, and it holds that "only a portion . . . have been studied thoroughly enough to meet exacting, present-day standards."

Pesticide Residues

Every year until recently, synthetic organic pesticides have drenched the territory of the United States in an amount equivalent to 220 pounds for every square mile. American mother's milk now contains four times the level of DDT that is permitted in cow's milk. We know that DDT and similar compounds have had devastating effects on many forms of wildlife, especially fish and birds. Some scientists fear the genetic and other effects of these compounds on human beings. As the result of widespread clamor, the use of DDT and related pesticides is on the wane in many parts of the world.

Noise Pollution

Most people are aware that their health may be threatened by the contamination of the air they breathe or the water they drink or swim in. Some know that dangerous substances may pollute the food they eat. But few realize that we are all adversely affected by a pollutant so common it tends to be overlooked—noise.

Noise is generally defined as any unwanted sound. It is the most widespread form of pollution in the United States. Who has not been driven to distraction by the wail of sirens, the din of construction noise, cars, trucks, and buses? The old joke about city-dwellers being so used to noise that they were kept awake by the silence of a vacation retreat in the country is an expression of just how much noise most of us have accepted as inevitable.

The joke has a new twist now, because rural and suburban areas are plagued by their own varieties of noise. Farms have become increasingly more mechanized, and agricultural machinery contributes its ear-splitting toll. The once-inviolate stillness of snow-blanketed wilderness is now ruptured by the buzz of snowmobiles. Suburban homes are filled with the newest gadgets, such as power lawn mowers, garbage disposals, electric tools—all potent noise makers.

Worst of all is the situation of some workers, who, in addition to all this domestic noise, must suffer high noise levels on the job. Boilermakers and jackhammer operators are obvious examples, but cab drivers, bookkeeping machine operators, and mothers of young children are all subject to special, if less conspicuous, hazards.

For noise is not just annoying, it is potentially dangerous, both physically and mentally. Dr. Vern Knudsen, a specialist in sound and chancellor emeritus at UCLA, has said, "Noise, like smog, is a slow agent of death. If it continues to increase for the next 30 years as it has for the last 30, it could become lethal."

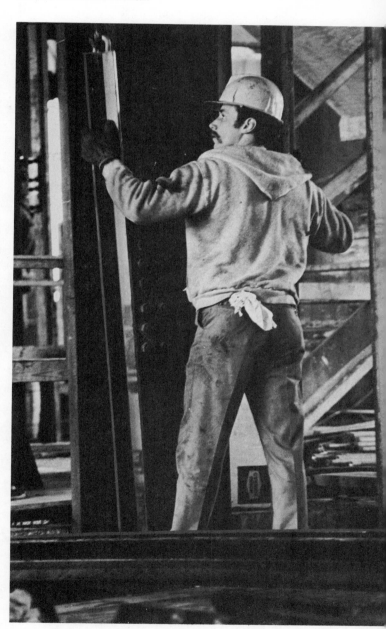

Construction noise is often at a very high level of intensity. Both workers and pedestrians suffer, and street noises such as auto horns only add to the din.

Effect of Sound on the Eardrum

How can mere sound have such dire effects? Sound is a form of energy, and energy can be destructive as well as constructive. Sound is caused by anything that moves back and forth—vibrates. For us to hear sound over a distance, the energy of this vibrating motion must be transmitted to our ears over a distance, via sound waves. A sound wave in air is a succession of regions of compressed air and partial vacuums, or areas of high and low air pressure. (Sound waves can also travel through liquids and solids.) We hear sound because our eardrums are moved back and forth by these changes in air pressure. The eardrum, or *tympanic membrane,* can be incredibly delicate, perceiving a sound that moves it only one billionth of a centimeter—the threshold of hearing—equivalent, perhaps,

to the rustle of one blade of grass against another. If the intensity of sound pressure becomes too great, at something like a billion billion times the energy at the threshold of hearing, we experience pain, and the eardrum or the delicate structures inside the ear may be damaged.

The intensity of sounds is often measured in units called *decibels,* or *db.* These units are logarithmic—that is, 10 db is ten times as powerful as 1 db, 20 db is 100 times as powerful, 30 db is 1,000 times as powerful, and so on. On this scale, 0 db is at the threshold of hearing; rustling leaves, 20 db; a quiet office, about 50 db; conversation, 60 db; heavy traffic, 90 db; a pneumatic jackhammer six feet away, 100 db; a jet aircraft 500 feet overhead, 115 db; a Saturn rocket's takeoff, 180 db.

For most people, the pain threshold is about 120 db; deafening ear damage will

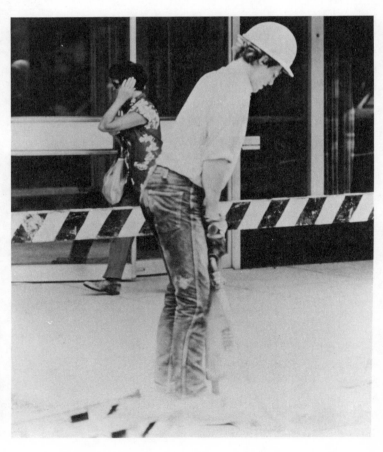

A pneumatic jackhammer produces 100 decibels of sound, enough to cause acute discomfort and even temporary hearing impairment to anyone within six feet of it.

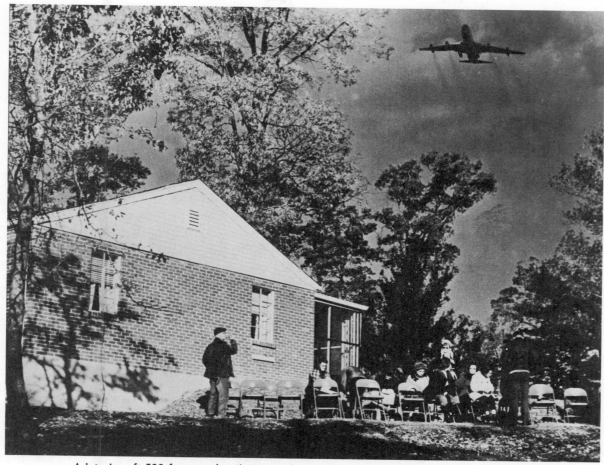

A jet aircraft 500 feet overhead can produce 115 decibels of noise to someone on the ground. Sound intensities of 85–95 decibels and over are regarded as dangerous.

result at 150 db. But damage of various kinds can come from much lower exposures. Temporary hearing impairment can result from sounds over 85 db now found in modern kitchens with all appliances going. If the ears don't get a chance to recover, the impairment will become permanent.

Damage to the Inner Ear

Although very loud noise can damage the eardrum, most physiological damage from noise occurs in the snail-shaped, liquid-filled cochlea, or inner ear. Sound transmitted to the cochlea produces waves in the liquid, which in turn move delicate and minute structures called hair cells or *cilia* in that part of the cochlea known as the organ of Corti. The motion of the cilia is transformed into electrical impulses that conduct the sensation of sound to the brain.

The cilia can easily be fatigued by noise, causing a temporary loss of hearing, or a shift in the threshold of hearing. If they are not given a chance to recuperate, they will be permanently damaged, and irreversible hearing loss will result. There are some 23,000 cilia in the average cochlea; different sets of cilia respond to different frequency bands. The cilia responding to sound frequencies of 4,000 to 6,000 cps (cycles per second) are especially vulnerable to damage. The region of 85–95 db is generally regarded as the beginning of dangerous sound intensities. In general, the louder the noise, the longer it lasts, the higher it is, and the purer in frequency, the more dangerous it is. Thus jet engines and powerful sirens are particularly hazardous.

Noise and Mental Illness

Moreover, noise has a definite effect on mental well-being. No one knows exactly how, but noise can produce irritability, tension, and nervous strain. Extreme noise conditions can cause, or at least contribute to, mental illness. British medical authorities have reported a significantly higher incidence of mental illness among people exposed to aircraft noise.

Dr. Jack C. Westman, Director of the Child Psychiatry Division of the University of Wisconsin Medical School, thinks that unwanted noise in the home is contributing to divorce and the generation gap:

We scapegoat, take out our tensions in other ways. Mothers yell at the youngsters, and parents bicker and fight between themselves. The average kitchen is like a boiler room, and what we thought was our friendly dishwasher is adding to the unhealthy surroundings by contributing to the noise.

Dr. Westman said that one of the prime causes of the "tired mother syndrome," being seen by more and more physicians, is constant exposure to noise. He compares this syndrome to combat fatigue (an analogy many mothers will heartily endorse): "The mother is worn out, irritable, depressed, tense, and experiences headaches and upset stomachs."

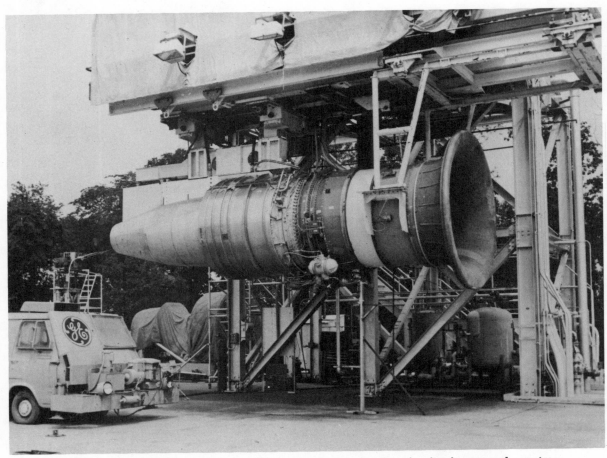

The National Aeronautics and Space Administration is sponsoring the development of a quieter jet engine. Here a prototype of a quieter engine is tested to measure the smoke it produces.

A Growing Problem

Unfortunately, the noise problem seems to be getting worse. The U.S. Surgeon General states that as many as 16 million citizens are now losing their hearing from on-job noise. In March, 1971, the U.S. Department of Commerce's Panel on Noise Abatement observed that noise pollution in the United States is reaching a serious level—a conclusion that most authorities had reached some time ago. Noise experts generally agree that the over-all sound level in this country is rising at the rate of 1 db per year—or doubling every decade. There is every reason to believe that the rate of increase will rise in the coming years. Some scientists predict that even at the current rate, everyone in America will be deaf by the year 2,000. Measurements conducted in average American towns show that noise levels have boomed four times higher than 1956 values and 32 times those in 1938. A New York City task force on noise control found that noise had reached a level "intense, continuous and persistent enough to threaten basic community life." The Federal Council for Science and Technology reckons that this major health hazard costs the nation $4 billion a year in decreased efficiency and lost compensation.

Some experts have linked the rise in diseases of the cardiovascular system to this steady increase in noise pollution. Noise elevates blood pressure and raises the amount of cholesterol in the blood. A group of Africans living in the hushed environment of the Southeast Sudan retain acute hearing and youthful arteries into advanced old age. But when they move to their noisy capital, their hearing deteriorates, and their rate of heart disease goes up.

Protection Against Noise

What can you do to protect yourself and your family from the effects of noise pollution? You can't do much to control some

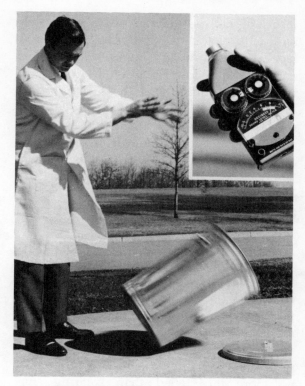

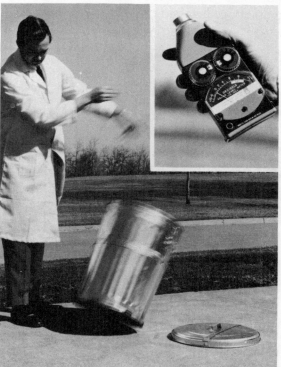

Relative noise levels of the conventional galvanized steel garbage can (*top*) and its sound-deadened counterpart (*above*) are reflected in the sound-meter readings. Noise of the treated can is greatly reduced.

forms of noise—such as traffic noise—directly. But you can support local, state, and federal legislation that seeks to control or eliminate some forms of noise. For example, many communities have laws that forbid blowing car horns except in emergencies; regrettably, such laws are poorly enforced, and the noise contribution from impatient drivers in our metropolitan areas is staggering. Yet, European cities have shown that such anti-honking ordinances can be effective if an aroused citizenry demands strict enforcement.

You have at your constant command two effective noise-control instruments—your hands. Cupping your ears with them during noise of extraordinary pitch and intensity may help preserve your hearing. If you regularly encounter loud or irritating noise on your job or travels, buy a pair of ear protectors and wear them. This solution is no more far-fetched than wearing sunglasses on dazzling days at the beach.

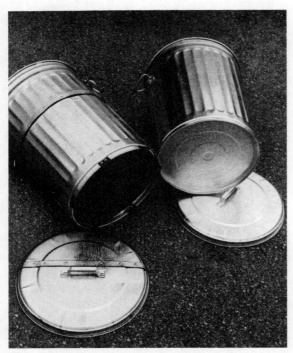

Sound-deadening materials of the garbage can at left include six rubber feet at base and a belt of galvanized steel with a felt lining around the barrel wall.

If you're responsible for the running of an office or plant, seek professional sound engineers' advice to make sure that you've taken advantage of the latest techniques and materials to cut noise to a minimum.

One of the most important things you can do is to stay clear of avoidable dangerous noise. A prevalent source of this kind of sound is rock music played or reproduced at damaging levels. If you or your children pooh-pooh this threat, here are the facts: listening to the new music at levels typical of those now current may blow not only your mind, but your hearing, too.

Dr. Ralph R. Rupp, head of the audiology division of the speech clinic of the University of Michigan, together with his assistant, Larry J. Koch, measured sound levels produced by a rock combo. In the rehearsal room, these averaged 120–130 db during loud passages. All members of the combo reported ringing in their ears or other uncomfortable symptoms for from eight hours to several days after their get-togethers—signs of temporary or permanent hearing damage. Dr. Rupp says that people who either play or listen to music at such high levels may pay an enormous price in terms of eventual hearing loss. He suggests that rock musicians wear ear protectors that could reduce the sound levels at the ear by 20 or 30 db. He also proposes that local governments set safe maximum allowable noise limits for electronic amplification in clubs and discothèques.

In another test, Dr. Kenneth Pollock of the University of Florida found that the sound levels at a swinging teen club dropped to a safe 90 db only when he moved his equipment 40 feet outside the club. Ten teen-agers suffered hearing losses after dancing for three hours near the bandstand, where the din averaged 120 db. Listening to music via earphones offers a particularly effective means of going deaf—all it takes is a twist of the dial and you are

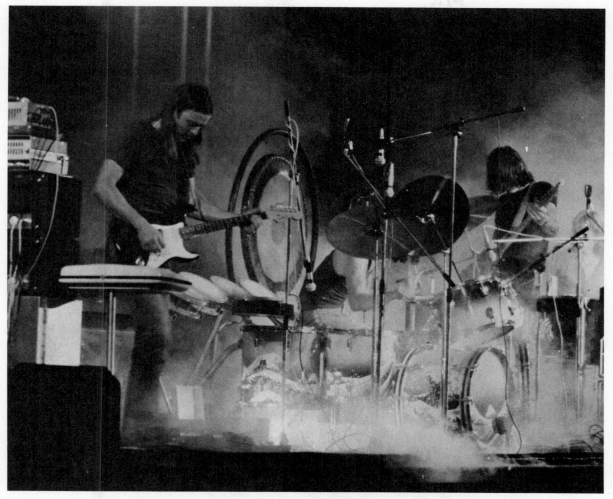

Amplified rock music sometimes reaches 120–130 decibels, a level of sound intensity that can eventually cause permanent hearing loss, say some investigators.

instantly assaulted with sound levels that are practically unbearable. Dr. David M. Lipscomb of the University of Tennessee says, "We are apparently reaching the point where young people are losing sufficient hearing to jeopardize their occupational potential."

Yet another form of noise introduced to our novelty-hungry society is that from snowmobiles—those off-road vehicles that have enjoyed an amazing boom in recent years. Some ranch hands, foresters, and Arctic Indians and Eskimos have found the snowmobile literally a lifesaver in their harsh, snowbound winters, but most snow-mobiles are used for recreational purposes. If you ride a snowmobile for any reason, you should know that its snarl is a definite hazard to your hearing, and wear special ear protectors. John G. Bollinger, a professor of mechanical engineering at the University of Wisconsin, measured snowmobile noise in a project to determine how they might be quietened. He recorded levels of about 110 db at a point six inches in front of the driver's head. Noise of this intensity can cause temporary hearing loss for an occasional rider, and permanent hearing loss for someone who spends several hours a day on the snowmobile during a winter. AF

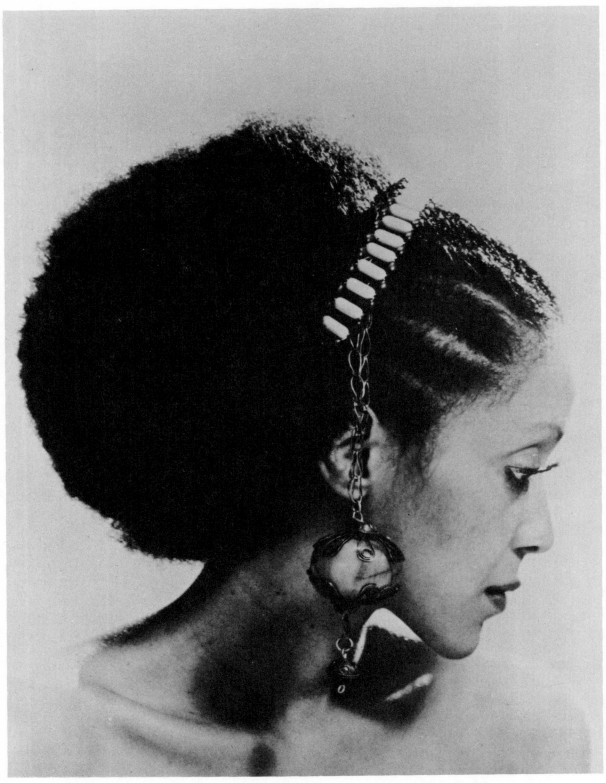

Not everyone can have the elegant beauty of this professional model, but anyone can maintain attractive skin and hair by developing habits of cleanliness and good grooming.

CHAPTER 6

Skin and Hair

Not many people have perfectly proportioned faces and bodies, but practically anyone, at any age, can present an attractive appearance if skin is healthy-looking and glowing and hair is clean and shining. Healthy skin and hair can be achieved through good health habits, cleanliness, and personal grooming. Expensive skin-and-hair products may boost self-confidence, but they are a poor substitute for proper diet, exercise, enough sleep, and soap and water or cleansing creams.

The condition of skin and hair reflects a person's physical and emotional health. Of course, general appearance is determined not only by what is going on inside the body, but by outward circumstances, such as extremes of temperature or the use of harsh soaps. Appearance can also be altered temporarily by cosmetics and permanently by surgery.

The Skin

The skin is one of the most important organs of the body. It serves as protection against infection by germs and shields delicate underlying tissue against injury. Approximately one-third of the bloodstream flows through the skin, and as the blood vessels contract or relax in response to heat and cold, the skin acts as a thermostat that helps control body temperature. The two million sweat glands in the skin also regulate body temperature through the evaporation of perspiration. The many delicate nerve endings in the skin make it a sense organ responsive not only to heat and cold, but to pleasure, pain, and pressure.

Certain cells in the skin produce a protective pigmentation that determines its color and guards against overexposure to the ultraviolet rays of the sun. By absorption and elimination, the skin helps regulate the body's chemical and fluid balance. One of the miracles of the skin is that it constantly renews itself.

Structure of the Skin

The skin is made up of two layers. The outer layer or *epidermis* has a surface of horny, nonliving cells that form the body's protective envelope. These cells are constantly being shed and replaced by new ones which are made in the lower or inner layer of the epidermis.

ANATOMY OF THE SKIN

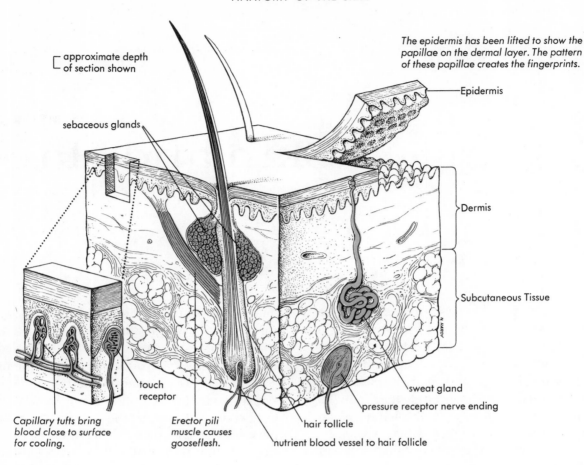

approximate depth
of section shown

The epidermis has been lifted to show the
papillae on the dermal layer. The pattern
of these papillae creates the fingerprints.

Epidermis

sebaceous glands

Dermis

Subcutaneous Tissue

N. HARDY

touch
receptor

sweat gland

pressure receptor nerve ending

Capillary tufts bring
blood close to surface
for cooling.

Erector pili
muscle causes
gooseflesh.

hair follicle

nutrient blood vessel to hair follicle

Underneath the epidermis is the *dermis,* the thicker part of the skin. It contains blood vessels, nerves, and connective tissue. The sweat glands are located in the dermis, and they collect fluid containing water, salt, and waste products from the blood. This fluid is sent through tiny canals that end in pores on the skin's surface.

The oil or *sebaceous* glands that secrete the oil which lubricates the surface of the skin and hair are also located in the dermis. They are most often associated with hair *follicles.* Hair follicles and oil glands are found over most of the body, with the exception of the palms of the hands and the soles of the feet.

The layer of fatty tissue below the dermis, called *subcutaneous* tissue, acts as an insulator against heat and cold and as a shock absorber against injury.

Skin Color

The basic skin color of each person is determined at birth, and is a part of his heritage that cannot be changed.

Melanin: There are four pigments in the normal skin that affect its color: melanin, oxygenated hemoglobin, reduced hemoglobin, and various carotenes. Of these, *melanin* is the most powerful. The cells that produce it are the same in all races, but there is wide variation in the amount produced, and wide variation in its color, which ranges from black to light tan. Every adult has about 60,000 melanin-producing cells in each square inch of skin.

Melanin cells also affect eye color. When the cells are deep in the eye, the color produced is blue or green. When they are close to the surface, the eye is brown. An *albino*, a person with no melanin, has eyes that appear pink because the stronger pigment that ordinarily masks the blood vessels is lacking.

Hemoglobin: The pigment that gives blood its color, called hemoglobin, has the next greatest effect on skin color. When it is combined with oxygen, a bright red is the result, and this in turn produces the rosy complexion associated with good health in light-skinned people. When such people suffer from reduced hemoglobin due to anemia, they appear to be excessively pale. A concentration of reduced hemoglobin gives the skin a bluish appearance. Since hemoglobin has a weaker coloring effect than the melanin that determines basic skin color, these variations are more visible in lighter-skinned individuals.

Carotenes: The weakest pigments in the skin are the *carotenes*. These produce a yellowish tone that is increased by eating excessive amounts of carrots and oranges. In people with black or brown skin, excess carotene is usually masked by the melanin pigment.

Aging Skin

Skin appearance is affected by both internal and external factors. The silken quality of a baby's skin is due mainly to the fact that it has not yet begun to show the effects of continued exposure to sun and wind. The skin problems associated with adolescence reflect the many glandular changes that occur during the transition to adulthood. As the years pass, the skin becomes the most obvious indicator of aging.

Heredity, general health, and exposure to the elements are some of the factors that contribute to aging skin. Because people with darker skin have built-in protection against the ravages of the sun, their skin usually has a younger appearance than that of lighter-skinned people of comparable age.

In general, the skin of an older person is characterized by wrinkles and shininess. It feels thinner when pinched because it has lost its elasticity and part of the underlying fat that gives firmness to a younger skin.

Constant exposure to sunlight is now thought to play a more important role in the visible aging of skin than the aging process itself. Such exposure also appears to be directly related to the greater frequency of skin cancer among farmers, sailors, and others who spend most of their working hours out-of-doors.

Care of the Skin

Healthy, normal skin should be washed regularly with mild soap and warm water to remove grease, perspiration, and accumulated dirt. For those with a limited water supply or inadequate bath and shower facilities, sponge baths are a good substitute if the sponge or washcloth is thoroughly rinsed as various parts of the body are washed. Many people feel that a shower is a much more efficient way of getting clean than a bath, since the bath water becomes the receptacle for the dirt washed from the body, instead of its being rinsed away.

No matter what method is used, all soap should be thoroughly rinsed off the skin after washing. Unless specifically prescribed by a doctor, medicated or germicidal soaps should not be used, since they may be an irritant. Skin should be dried with a fluffy towel, and bath towels should never be shared. Hands should be washed several times a day, and fingernails kept clean.

Facial skin requires special care because of its constant exposure. The face should be cleaned in the morning and before bedtime. Some women may prefer to use a cleansing cream rather than soap and water. Everyone should avoid massaging soap into the skin, since this may cause drying.

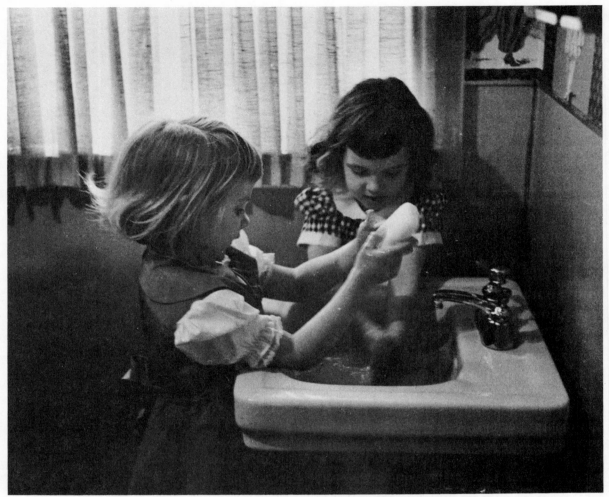

Washing the hands several times a day to rid them of accumulated dirt and grease, particularly before meals, is an important health habit that should be established in the early years.

Dry and Oily Skin

Both heredity and environment account for the wide variation in the amount of oil and perspiration secreted by the glands of different people. Also, the same person's skin may be oily in one part of the body and dry in another.

Dry skin: This condition is the result of loss of water from the outer surface of the epidermis and its insufficient replacement from the tissues below. Some causes of the moisture loss are too frequent use of soap and detergents, and constant exposure to dry air. Anyone spending a great deal of time in air-conditioned surroundings in which the humidity has been greatly lowered is likely to suffer from dry skin.

To correct the condition, the use of soap and water should be kept to a minimum for those parts of the body where the skin is dry. Cleansing creams or lotions containing lanolin should be used on the face, hands, elbows, and wherever else necessary. If tub baths are taken, a bath oil can be used in the water or applied to the skin after drying. Baby oil is just as effective and much cheaper than glamorously packaged and overadvertised products. Baby oil or a protective lotion should also be used on any parts of the body exposed to direct sunlight for any extended length of time. Applying oil to the skin will not, however, prevent wrinkles.

Oily skin: The amount of oil that comes to the surface of the skin through the sebaceous glands is the result not only of heredity, but also of temperature and emotional state. In warm weather, when the skin perspires more freely, the oil spreads like a film on the surface moisture. Non-oily foundation lotions can be helpful in keeping the oil spread to a minimum, and so can frequent washing with soap and water. When washing is inconvenient during the day, cleansing pads packaged to fit in pocket or purse are a quick and efficient solution for both men and women.

Too much friction from complexion brushes, rough washcloths, or harsh soaps may irritate rather than improve an oily skin condition.

Deodorants and Antiperspirants

Sweat glands are present almost everywhere in the skin, except for the lips and a few other areas. Most of them give off the extremely dilute salt water known as sweat, or perspiration. Their purpose is to cool the body by evaporation of water. Body odors are not produced by perspiration itself, but by the bacterial activity that takes place in the perspiration. The activity is most intense in warm, moist parts of the body from which perspiration cannot evaporate quickly, such as the underarm area.

Deodorants: The basic means of keeping this type of bacterial growth under control is through personal cleanliness of both skin and clothing. Deodorant soaps containing antiseptic chemicals are now available. Though they do not kill bacteria, they do reduce the speed with which they multiply.

Underarm deodorants also help to eliminate the odor. They are not meant to stop the flow of perspiration, but rather to slow down bacterial growth and mask body odors with their own scent. Such deodorants should be applied immediately after bathing. They are usually more effective if the underarm area is shaved, since the hair in this unexposed area collects perspiration and encourages bacterial growth.

Antiperspirants: Antiperspirants differ from deodorants in that they not only affect the rate of bacterial growth, but also reduce the amount of perspiration that reaches the skin surface. Since the action of the chemical salts they contain is cumulative, they seem to be more effective with repeated use. Antiperspirants come under the category of drugs, and their contents must be printed on the container. Deodorants are considered cosmetics, and may or may not name their contents on the package.

No matter what the nature of the advertising claim, neither type of product completely stops the flow of perspiration, nor would it be desirable to do so. Effectiveness of the various brands differs from one person to another. Some may produce a mild allergic reaction; others might be too weak to do a good job. It is practical to experiment with a few different brands, using them under similar conditions, to find the type that works best for you.

Creams and Cosmetics

The bewildering number of creams and cosmetics on the market and the exaggerated claims of some of their advertising can be reduced to a few simple facts. In most cases, the higher price of such products is an indication of the amount of money spent on advertising and packaging rather than on the ingredients themselves. Beauty preparations should be judged by the user on their merits rather than on their claims.

Cold creams and cleansing creams: These two products are essentially the same. They are designed to remove accumulated skin secretions, dirt, and grime, and should be promptly removed from the skin with a soft towel or tissue.

Lubricating creams and lotions: Also called night creams, moisturizing creams, and conditioning creams, these products are supposed to prevent the loss of moisture from the skin and promote its smoothness. They are usually left on overnight or for an extended length of time. Anyone with dry skin will find it helpful to apply a moisturizer under foundation cream. This will help keep the skin from drying out even further, and protect it against the effects of air conditioners.

Vanishing creams and foundation creams: These products also serve the purpose of providing the skin with moisture, but are meant to be applied immediately before putting on makeup.

Rejuvenating creams: There is no scientific proof that any of the "royal jelly," "secret formula," or "hormone" creams produce a marked improvement on aging skin. They cannot eliminate wrinkles, nor can they regenerate skin tissue.

Medicated creams and lotions: These products should not be used except on the advice of a doctor, since they may cause or aggravate skin disorders of various kinds.

Lipsticks: Lipsticks contain lanolin, a mixture of oil and wax, a coloring dye, and pigment, as well as perfume. Any of these substances can cause an allergic reaction in individual cases, but such reactions are uncommon. Sometimes the reaction is caused by the staining dye, in which case a "nonpermanent" lipstick should be used.

Cosmetics and the sensitive skin: Anyone with a cosmetic problem due to sensitive skin should consult a *dermatologist,* a physician specializing in the skin and its diseases. Cosmetic companies will inform a physician of the ingredients in their products, and he can then recommend a brand that will agree with the patient's specific skin problems. He may also recommend a special nonallergenic preparation.

Eye makeup: Eye-liner and mascara brushes and pencils—and lipsticks for that matter—can carry infection and should never be borrowed or lent. *Hypoallergenic* makeup, which is specially made for those who get allergic reactions to regular eye makeup, is available and should be used by anyone so affected.

Suntanning lotions: See under *Aches, Pains, Nuisances, Worries,* p. 417, for a discussion of sunburn.

Hair

Hair originates in tiny sacs or follicles deep in the dermis layer of skin tissue. The part of the hair below the skin surface is the root; the part above is the shaft. Hair follicles are closely connected to the sebaceous glands which secrete oil to the scalp and give hair its natural sheen.

Hair grows from the root outward, pushing the shaft farther from the scalp. Depending on its color, there may be as many as 125,000 hairs on an adult's head. The adult male may have as many as 300 hairs on each square inch of chin. The palms of the hands, the soles of the feet, and the lips are the only completely hairless parts of the surface of the body.

Texture

Each individual hair is made up of nonliving cells that contain a tough protein called *keratin.* Hair texture differs from one part of the body to another. In some areas, it may be soft and downy; in others, tough and bristly. Hair texture also differs between the sexes, among individuals, and among the different races.

If an individual hair is oval in cross-section, it is curly along its length. If the cross-section is round, the hair is straight. Thick, wiry hair is usually triangular or kidney-shaped. The fineness or coarseness of hair texture is related to its natural color.

Curling: Anyone using a home preparation should read and follow instructions with great care. If a new brand is tried, the

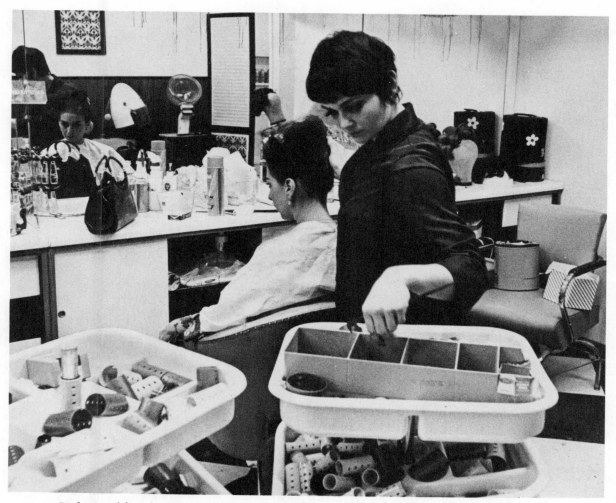

Professional hairdressers are better equipped than amateurs to give permanent waves or to straighten or color the hair, but any hair can be damaged by too vigorous treatment.

instructions should be read all over again, since they may be quite different from the accustomed ones.

Electric curling irons are not safe because they may cause pinpoint burns in the scalp which are hardly noticeable at the time but may lead to permanent small areas of baldness. The danger can be minimized, however, if instructions for use are followed exactly and the recommended moisturizing lotions are used. It is especially important that the iron not be hot enough to singe the hair. The results, even if there is no damage, are not long lasting and are adversely affected by dampness. Setting lotions used

with rollers or clips have a tendency to dull the hair unless they are completely brushed out.

Straightening: The least harmful as well as the least effective way of straightening the hair temporarily is the use of pomades. They are usually considered unsatisfactory by women because they are too greasy, but are often used by men with short unruly hair. Heat-pressing the hair with a metal comb is longer-lasting but can cause substantial damage by burning the scalp. When this method is used, humidity or scalp perspiration will cause the hair to revert to its natural curl. The practice of ironing the

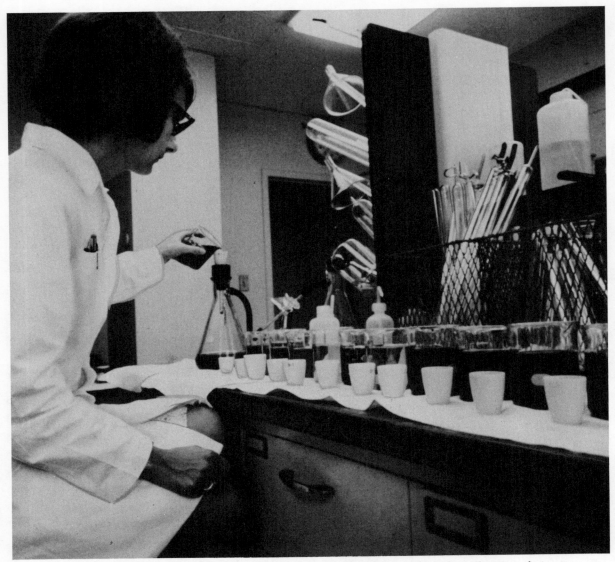

This chemist is using a method called chromatography for separating the colors in a hair tint preparation in order to determine the number and identity of the basic colors.

hair should be discouraged since it causes dryness and brittleness, with resultant breakage. Chemical straighteners should be used with great care since they may cause serious burns. Special efforts must be made to protect the eyes from any contact with these products.

Hair Color

In the same way that melanin colors the skin, it also determines hair color. The less melanin, the lighter the hair. As each hair loses its melanin pigment, it gradually turns gray, then white. It is assumed that the age at which hair begins to gray is an inherited characteristic and therefore can't be postponed or prevented by eating special foods, by taking vitamins, or by the external application of creams. The only way to recolor gray hair is by the use of a chemical dye.

Dyes and tints: Anyone wishing to make a radical change in hair color should consult a trained and reliable hairdresser. Trying to turn black hair bright red or dark red hair to blonde with a home preparation can sometimes end up with unwanted purplish or greenish results. When tints or dyes are used at home to lighten or darken the hair color by one or two shades, instructions accompanying the product must be followed carefully. Anyone with a tendency to contract contact dermatitis (see page 391) should make a patch test on the skin to check on possible allergic reactions. Hair should be tinted or dyed no more often than once a month.

Dye stripping: The only safe way to get rid of an unwanted dye color that has been used on the hair is to let it grow out. The technique known as stripping takes all color from the hair and reduces it to a dangerously weak mass. It is then redyed its natural color. Such a procedure should never be undertaken by anyone except a trained beautician, if at all.

Bleaching: Hydrogen peroxide is mixed with a hair-lightener to prebleach hair before applying blond tints. Bleaching with peroxide alone can cause more damage to the hair than dyeing or tinting it with a reliable commercial preparation, because it causes dryness, brittleness, and breakage.

General Hair Care

Properly cared for hair usually looks clean, shiny, and alive. Unfortunately, too many people mask the natural good looks of their hair with unnecessary sprays and "beauty" preparations.

Washing the hair: Hair should be washed about once a week—more often if it tends to be oily. The claims made by shampoo manufacturers need not always be taken too seriously, since most shampoos contain nothing more than soap or detergent and a perfuming agent. No shampoo can restore the natural oils to the hair at the same time that it washes it. A castile shampoo is good for dry hair, and one containing tincture of green soap is good for oily hair.

Thorough rinsing is essential to eliminate any soap deposit. If the local water is hard, a detergent shampoo can be rinsed off more easily than one containing soap.

Drying the hair: Drying the hair in sunlight or under a heat-controlled dryer is more satisfactory than trying to rub it dry with a towel. Gentle brushing during drying reactivates the natural oils that give hair its shine. Brushing in general is excellent for the appearance of the hair. Be sure to wash both brush and comb as often as the hair is washed.

Hair pomades should be avoided or used sparingly, since they are sometimes so heavy that they clog the pores of the scalp. A little bit of olive oil or baby oil can be rubbed into dry hair after shampooing. This is also good for babies' hair.

There is no scientific evidence that creme rinses, protein rinses, or beer rinses accomplish anything for the hair other than making it somewhat more manageable if it is naturally fine and flyaway.

Dandruff

Simple dandruff is a condition in which the scalp begins to itch and flake a few days after the hair has been washed. There is no evidence that the problem is related to germ infection.

Oiliness and persistent dandruff may appear not only on the scalp, but also on the sides of the nose or the chest. In such cases, a dermatologist should be consulted. Both light and serious cases often respond well to prescription medicines containing tars. These preparations control the dandruff, but there is no known cure for it.

Nits

Head lice sometimes infect adults as well as children. These tiny parasites usually live on the part of the scalp near the nape of the neck, and when they bite, they cause itching. They attach their eggs, which are called *nits,* to the shaft of the hair, and

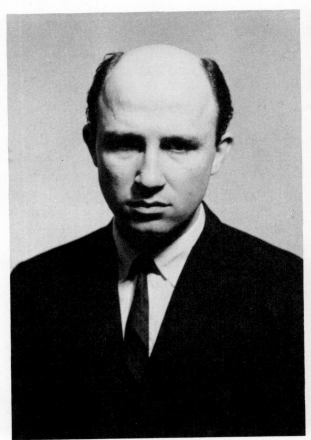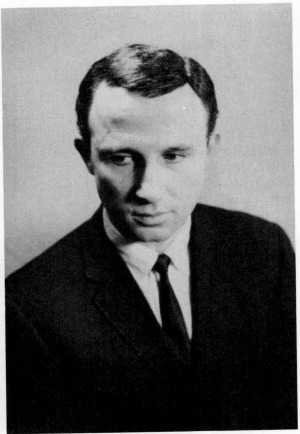

For those men concerned about their baldness, a wig can be a relatively inexpensive and effective means of achieving a more youthful appearance, as these before-and-after pictures demonstrate.

when they are plentiful, they can be seen by a trained eye as tiny, silvery-white ovals. This condition is highly contagious and can be passed from one head to another by way of combs, brushes, hats, head scarfs, and towels. A doctor can be consulted for information on effective ways of eliminating nits—usually by the application of chemicals and the use of a fine-toothed comb.

Baldness

Under the normal circumstances of combing, brushing, and shampooing, a person loses anywhere from 25 to 100 hairs a day. Because new hairs start growing each day, the loss and replacement usually balance each other. When the loss rate is greater than the replacement rate, thinning and baldness are the result.

Alopecia: The medical name for baldness is *alopecia,* the most common form of which is *male pattern baldness.* Dr. Eugene Van Scott, Professor of Dermatology of Temple University's Health Sciences Center, sums up the opinion of medical authorities on the three factors responsible for this type of baldness: sex, age, and heredity. Unfortunately, these are three factors over which medical science has no control.

Other causes of baldness: Other forms of baldness may be the result of bacterial or fungus infections, allergic reactions to particular medicines, radiation, or continual friction. It has also been suggested that constant stress from hair curlers or tightly pulled ponytails can cause loss of hair. These forms of baldness usually disappear when the cause is eliminated.

Although diet has very little to do with baldness, poor nutrition can result in hair that is dry, dull, and brittle enough to break easily. Any serious illness can lead to hair loss as well. It is thought that vitamin A taken in grossly excessive amounts can contribute to hair loss.

Women ordinarily lose some of their hair at the end of pregnancy, after delivery, and during the menopause, but regrowth can be expected in a few months.

It is now possible for anyone suffering from temporary baldness or from male pattern baldness to choose from a wide variety of inexpensive, attractively styled wigs and hairpieces.

A surgical procedure for treating male pattern baldness called *hair transplantation* is discussed under *Plastic and Cosmetic Surgery*, p. 402.

Hair Removal

Over the centuries and around the world, fashions in whiskers and beards come and go, but the average American male still subjects at least part of his face to daily shaving. Although feminine shaving practices are a more recent phenomenon, most American women now consider it part of good grooming to remove underarm and leg hair with a razor as often as twice a week. Shaving removes not only the dead skin cells that make up the protective layer of the body's surface, but also some of the living skin underneath. Instead of being harmful, this appears to stimulate rather than damage new skin growth.

Male Shaving

The average beard grows about two-tenths of an inch a day. However, the density of male face hair varies a great deal depending on skin and hair color. In all races, the concentration is usually greatest on the chin and in the area between the nose and upper lip.

There is no proof that an electric razor is safer or better for all types of skin than a safety razor. Both types result in nicks and cuts of the living skin tissue, depending on the closeness of the shave.

Twice as many men prefer wet shaving to dry because the use of soap and hot water softens the hair stubble and makes it easier to remove. Shaving authorities point out that thorough soaking is one of the essentials of easy and safe shaving. Leaving the shaving lather on the face for at least two minutes will also soften whiskers a good deal.

The razor should be moistened with hot water throughout the process, and the chin and upper lip left for last so that the heavier hair concentration in these areas has the longest contact with moisture and lather.

Oily skin: Men with oily skin should use an aerosol shaving preparation or a lather type applied with a brush. These are really soaps, and are therefore more effective in eliminating the oils that coat the face hair, thus making it easier to shave.

Dry skin: A brushless cream is more advisable since it lubricates the skin rather than further depriving it of oil.

Ingrown hairs: One of the chief problems connected with shaving is that it often causes ingrown hairs, which can lead to pore-clogging and infection. Hair is more likely to turn back into the skin if it is shaved against the grain, or if the cutting edge of the blade is dull and rough rather than smooth. Men with coarse, wiry, curly hair may find that whisker ends are more likely to become ingrown than men with fine hair. The problem is best handled by shaving with the grain, using a sharp blade, and avoiding too close a shave, particularly in the area around the neck.

Shaving and skin problems: For men with acne or a tendency to skin problems, the following advice is offered by Dr. Howard T. Behrman, Director of Dermatological Research, New York Medical College:

• Shave as seldom as possible, perhaps only once or twice a week, and always with the grain.

• If wet shaving is preferred, use a new blade each time, and shave as lightly as possible to avoid nicking pimples.

• Wash face carefully with plenty of soap and hot water to make the beard easy to manage, and after shaving, rinse with hot water followed by cold.

• Use an antiseptic astringent face lotion.

• Instead of plucking out ingrown hairs, loosen them gently so that the ends do not grow back into the skin.

• Although some people with skin problems find an electric shaver less irritating, in most cases, a wet shave seems best.

Female Shaving

About 60 million American women regularly shave underarm and leg hair, and most of them do so with a blade razor. In recent years, various types of shavers have been designed with blade exposure more suited to women's needs than the standard type used by men. To make shaving easier and safer, the following procedures are recommended:

• Since wet hair is much easier to cut, the most effective time to shave is during or immediately following a bath or shower.

• Shaving cream or soap lather keeps the water from evaporating, and is preferred to dry shaving.

• Underarm shaving is easier with a contoured razor designed for this purpose. If a deodorant or antiperspirant causes stinging or irritation after shaving, allow a short time to elapse before applying it.

• Light bleeding from nicks or scrapes can be stopped by applying pressure to a sterile pad placed on the injured area.

Unwanted Hair

The technical word for excess or unwanted hair on the face, chest, arms, and legs is *hirsutism.* This condition varies greatly among different ethnic strains, and so does the attitude toward it. Women of southern European ancestry are generally hairier than those with Nordic or Anglo-Saxon ancestors. Caucasoid peoples are hairier than Negroid peoples. The sparsest amount of body hair is found among the Mongolian races and American Indians.

Although heredity is the chief factor in hirsutism, hormones also influence hair growth. If there is a sudden appearance of coarse hair on the body of a young boy or girl or a woman with no such former tendency, a glandular disturbance should be suspected and investigated by a doctor.

A normal amount of unwanted hair on the legs and under the arms is usually removed by shaving. When the problem involves the arms, face, chest, and abdomen, other methods of removal are available.

Temporary Methods of Hair Removal

Bleaching: Unwanted dark fuzz on the upper lip and arms can be lightened almost to invisibility with a commercially prepared bleach or with a homemade paste consisting of baking soda, hydrogen peroxide (bleaching strength), and a few drops of ammonia. Soap chips can be used instead of baking soda. The paste should be left on the skin for a few minutes and then washed off. It is harmless to the skin, and if applied repeatedly, the hair will tend to break off as a result of constant bleaching.

Chemical depilatories: These products contain alkaline agents that cause hair to detach easily at the skin surface. They can be used on and under the arms, and on the legs and chest. However, they should not be used on the face unless the label says it is safe to do so. Timing instructions should be followed carefully. If skin irritation results, this type of depilatory should be discontinued in favor of some other method.

Abrasives: Devices which remove hair from the skin surface by rubbing are cheap but time-consuming. However, if an abrasive such as pumice is used regularly, the offending hairs will be shorter with each application. A cream or lotion should be applied to the skin after using an abrasive.

Waxing: The technique of applying melted wax to the skin for removal of excess facial hair is best handled by an experienced cosmetician. The process involves pouring hot wax onto the skin and allowing it to cool. The hairs become embedded in the wax, and are plucked out from below the skin surface when the wax is stripped off. Since this method is painful and often causes irritation, it is not very popular, although the results are comparatively long-lasting.

Plucking: The use of tweezers for removing scattered hairs from the eyebrows, face, and chest is slightly painful but otherwise harmless. It is not a practical method for getting rid of dense hair growth, however, since it takes too much time.

Permanent Hair Removal by Electrolysis

The only permanent and safe method of removing unwanted hair is by *electrolysis.* This technique destroys each individual hair root by transmitting electric current through fine wire needles into the opening of the hair follicle. The hair thus loosened is then plucked out with a tweezer. The older type of electrolysis machine uses galvanic current. The newer type, sometimes called an electrocoagulation machine, uses modified high frequency current. In either case, the efficiency and safety of the technique depends less on the machine than on the care and skill of the operator.

Since the process of treating each hair root is expensive, time-consuming, and uncomfortable, it is not recommended for areas of dense hair growth such as the arms or legs. Before undertaking electrolysis either at a beauty salon or at a home, it would be wise to consult a dermatologist about individual skin reaction.

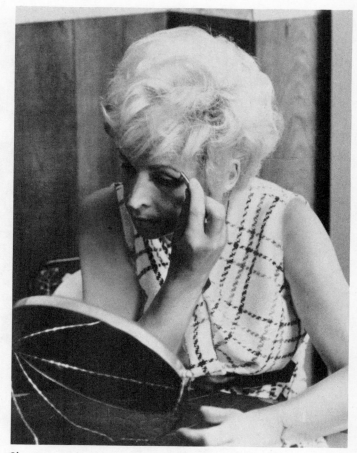

Shaping eyebrows by plucking hairs with tweezers is harmless, but it is impractical for more dense hair growth. Bleaching unwanted hair is another method.

Nails

Fingernails and toenails are an extension of the epidermis or outer layer of the skin. They are made of elastic tissue formed from keratin, the substance that gives hair its strength and flexibility.

Some of the problems associated with fingernails are the result of too much manicuring. White spots, for example, are often caused by too much pressure at the base of the nail when trying to expose the "moon"— the white portion which contains tissue not yet as tough as the rest of the nail.

Splitting: Infection or injury of the tissue at the base of the nail may cause its surface to be rigid or split. Inflammation of the finger joints connected with arthritis will

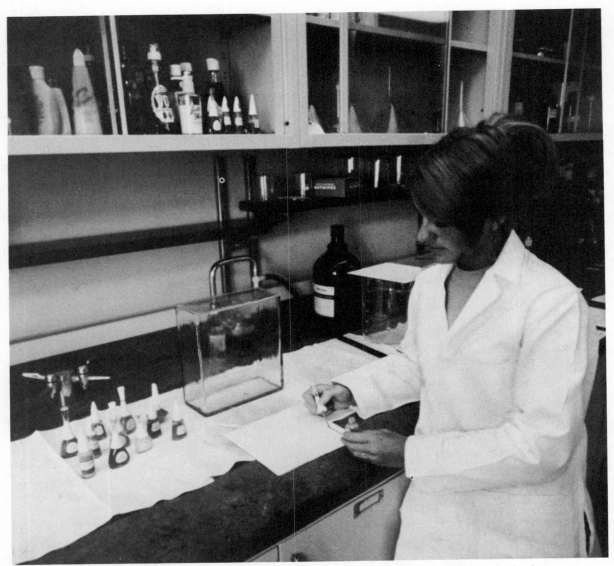

Nail polish should not be worn constantly, nor should it be applied right down to the base of the nail. Here a chemist is separating the several colors in a nail polish for identification.

also cause nail deformity. For ordinary problems of splitting and peeling, the nails should be kept short enough so that they don't catch and tear during daily activities. For practical purposes, the top of the nail should not be visible when the palm is held about six inches from the eye. As the nails grow stronger, they can be grown longer without splitting.

Brittleness: This condition seems to be caused by external factors such as the chemicals in polish removers, soaps, and deter-gents. It is also a natural consequence of aging. Commercial nail-hardening prepara-tions that contain formaldehyde are not recommended, since they are known to cause discoloration, loosening, or even loss of nails in some cases.

Nail damage can be reduced by wearing rubber gloves while doing household chores. Hand cream massaged into the skin around the nails will counteract dryness and lessen the possibility of hangnails. Although nail polish provides a shield against damage, it should not be worn all the time, particularly if the nail is polished right down to the base, since this prevents live tissue from "breathing."

Toenails

To ensure the health of toenails, feet should be bathed once a day and the nails cleaned with a brush dipped in soapy water. Shoes should fit properly so that the toenails are not subjected to pressure and distortion. In order to avoid ingrown toenails, trimming should be done straight across rather than by rounding or tapering the corners.

Disorders of the Skin

The skin is subject to a large number of disorders, most of which are not serious even though they may be temporarily uncomfortable. A disorder may be caused by one or another type of allergy; by excessive heat or cold; or by infection from fungi, bacteria, viruses, or parasites. There are also many skin ailments that are the result of emotional disturbances.

The symptoms and treatment of the more common disorders are discussed in the following pages. Any persistent change in skin condition should be brought to the attention of a doctor.

Allergies and Itching

Dermatitis: Dermatitis is the term used for an inflammation of the skin. The term for allergic reactions of the skin resulting from surface contact with outside agents is *contact dermatitis*. This condition is characterized by a rash and may be brought on by sensitivity to cosmetics, plants, cleaning materials, metal, wool, and so on. Other forms of dermatitis can be caused by excesses of heat or cold, by friction, or by sensitivity to various medicines. Dermatitis is usually accompanied by itching at the site of the rash.

Poison ivy: This common plant, unknown in Europe, but widespread everywhere in the United States except in California and Nevada, produces an allergic reaction on the skin accompanied by a painful rash and blisters. Some people are so sensitive to it that they are affected not only by contact with the plant itself, but with animal fur or clothing that might have picked up the sap weeks before.

A mild attack of poison ivy produces a rash and small watery blisters that get progressively larger. The affected area of the skin becomes crusty and dry, and after a few weeks, all symptoms vanish. If the exposed area is thoroughly washed with laundry soap immediately after contact, the poison may not penetrate the skin.

If the symptoms do develop, they can be relieved with Burow's solution—one part

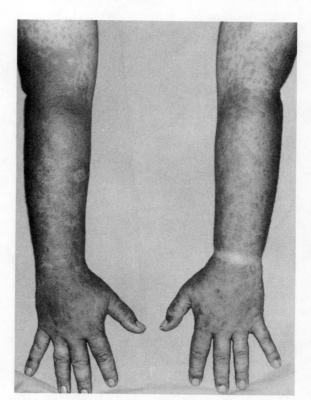

Dermatitis can be caused by sensitivity to medicines, as illustrated by this patient's reaction to the smallpox vaccine. The vaccine induced a hypersensitivity to sunlight, which led to the inflammation.

solution to fifteen parts of cool water—or with the application of calomine lotion. If the symptoms are severe, and especially if the area around the eyes is involved, a doctor should be consulted. He may prescribe an application or an injection of cortisone.

The best way to avoid the unpleasantness of a poison ivy attack is to learn to recog-

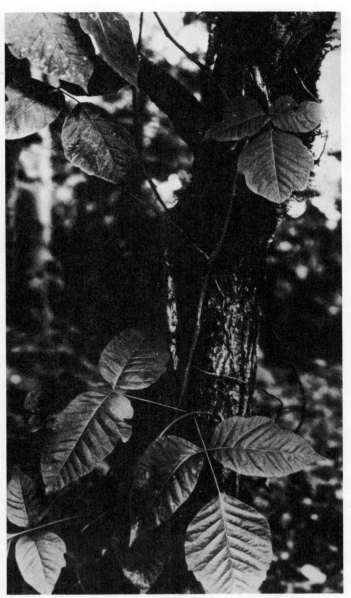

The characteristic three-leaf clusters of the poison ivy plant are easy to recognize. The leaves are glossy and often have irregularly-shaped notches.

nize the plant and stay away from it. Children especially should be warned against putting the leaves and berries in their mouths.

Poison oak and poison sumac produce somewhat the same symptoms and should also be avoided.

Under no circumstances should these plants be burned in order to eliminate them, since the inhaling of the contaminated smoke even from a distance can cause a serious case of poisoning. The application of special sprays, if the instructions are followed carefully, will get rid of the plants without affecting people or the neighborhood greenery.

Hives: These are large, irregularly shaped swellings on the skin that burn and itch. The cause is unknown, but allergic reactions to certain foods and medicine or to insect bites have been suggested as possible causes. The swellings of hives usually disappear within a day or so, but they can be very uncomfortable while they last. The itching and burning can often be relieved by applying cold water and a calomine solution. Commercial preparations containing surface anesthetics are seldom effective and may cause allergic reactions.

If the outbreak of hives can be traced to a specific food such as shellfish or strawberries, the food should be eliminated from the diet. If a medicine such as penicillin or a sulfa drug is the cause, the doctor should be told about the reaction.

Eczema: This condition is an allergic reaction that produces itching, swelling, blistering, oozing, and scaling of the skin. It is more common among children than among adults and may sometimes cover the entire body, although the rash is usually limited to the face, neck, and the folds of the knees and elbows. Unlike contact dermatitis, it is likely to be caused by an allergy to a food or a pollen or dust. Advertised cures for eczema cannot control the cause and sometimes make the condition worse. A doctor should be consulted if the symptoms are severe, particularly if the patient is an infant or very young child.

Itching: The technical name for the localized or general sensation on the skin which can be relieved by scratching is *pruritus*. Itching may be caused by many skin disorders, by infections, by serious diseases such as nephritis or leukemia, by medicines, or by psychological factors such as tension. A doctor should always be consulted to find the cause of persistent itching, since it may be the symptom of a basic disorder. Repeated scratching may provide some relief, but it can also lead to infection.

Anal pruritus: If itching in the anal area is so severe that only painful scratching will relieve it, the condition is probably *anal pruritus*. It is often accompanied by excessive rectal mucus that keeps the skin irritated and moist. This disorder is most commonly associated with hemorrhoids, but many other conditions, such as reactions to drugs, can cause it. Anxiety or tension can also contribute to it. Sitz baths with warm water are usually recommended. Every effort should be made to reduce scratching and to keep the anal skin clean and dry. Cortisone cream may be prescribed in persistent cases.

Other Skin Irritations

Chapping: In cold weather, the sebaceous glands slow down the secretions that lubricate the skin, causing it to become dry. When dry skin is exposed to wintry weather, it becomes irritated and is likely to crack, particularly around the lips. Chapped skin is especially sensitive to harsh soaps. During such periods of exposure, the skin can be protected with a mild cream or lotion. A lubricating ointment should be used on the lips to prevent them from cracking. Children who lick their lips constantly no matter what the weather can benefit from this extra protection. Chapped hands caused by daily use of strong soaps and detergents can

be helped by the use of a lubricating cream and rubber gloves during housework.

Frostbite: Exposure to extreme cold for a prolonged period may cause freezing of the nose, fingers, toes, or ears, thus cutting off the circulation to the affected areas. Frostbitten areas look white or grayish-yellow, and are numb. They should not be rubbed with snow or exposed to intense heat. Areas should be thawed gradually, and a doctor should be consulted for aftercare in extreme cases.

Chilblains: A localized inflammation of the skin, called *chilblains,* is common among people who are particularly sensitive to cold because of poor circulation. Chilblains may occur in the ears, hands, feet, and face, causing itching, swelling, and discoloration of the skin. Anyone prone to chilblains should dress protectively during the cold weather and use an electric pad or blanket at night. Affected parts should not be rubbed or massaged, nor should ice or extreme heat be applied directly, since these measures may cause additional damage. Persistent or extreme attacks of chilblains should be discussed with a doctor.

Chafing: This condition is an inflammation of two opposing skin surfaces caused by the warmth, moisture, and friction of their rubbing together. Diabetics, overweight people, and those who perspire heavily are particularly prone to chafing. Chafing is accompanied by itching and burning, and sometimes infection can set in if the superficial skin is broken. Parts of the body subject to chafing are the inner surfaces of the thighs, the anal region, the area under the breasts, and the inner surfaces between fingers and toes.

To reduce the possibility of chafing, cool clothing should be worn and strenuous exercise avoided during hot weather. Vaseline or a Vitamin A and D ointment may be applied to reduce friction. In general, the treatment is the same as that for diaper rash in infants. If the condition becomes acute,

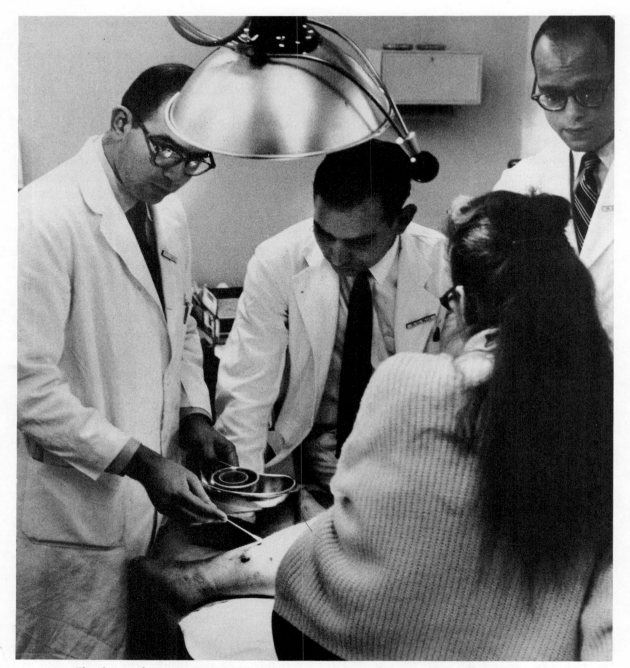

The dermatologist is treating a disorder marked by pustules—pus-filled, inflamed pimples.

a doctor can prescribe more effective remedies.

Prickly heat: This skin rash is usually accompanied by itching and burning. It is caused by an obstruction of the sweat ducts so that perspiration does not reach the surface of the skin, but backs up and causes pimples the size of a pinhead. If the obstruction is superficial, the pimples are white; if it is deeper, they are red. The condition can be brought on by other minor skin irritations, by continued exposure to moist heat such as a compress, or by exercise in humid weather. Infants and people who are overweight are especially prone to prickly heat.

The discomfort can be eased by wearing lightweight, loose-fitting clothing, especially at night, and keeping room temperature low. Alcoholic beverages, which tend to dehydrate the body, should be avoided. Tepid baths and the application of cornstarch to the affected skin areas will usually relieve itching. If the rash remains for several days, a doctor should be consulted to make sure it does not arise from some other cause.

Calluses and corns: As a result of continued friction or pressure in a particular area, the skin forms a tough, hard, self-protecting layer known as a *callus.* Calluses are common on the soles of the feet, the palms of the hands, and, among guitarists and string players, on the tips of the fingers. A heavy callus which presses against a bone in the foot because of poorly fitted shoes can be very painful. The hard surface can be reduced somewhat by the use of pumice, or by gently paring it with a razor blade that has been washed in alcohol.

Corns are a form of callus that appear on or between the toes. They usually have a hard inner core that causes pain when pressed against underlying tissue by badly fitted shoes. A hard corn that appears on the surface of the little toe can be removed by soaking for about ten minutes and applying a few drops of ten percent salicylic acid in collodion. The surface should be covered with a corn pad to reduce pressure, and the corn lifted off when it is loose enough to be released from the skin. Anyone suffering from a circulatory disease and particularly from diabetes should avoid home treatment of foot disturbances. Those with a tendency to callus and corn formations should be especially careful about the proper fit of shoes and hose. A *chiropodist* or *podiatrist* is a trained specialist in foot care who can be visited on a regular basis to provide greater foot comfort.

Fungus Infections

Fungi are plantlike parasitic growths found in the air, in water, and in the soil. They comprise a large family that includes mushrooms, and are responsible for mildew and mold. Only a small number cause disease.

Ringworm: This condition is not caused by a worm, but by a group of funguses that live on the body's dead skin cells in those areas that are warm and damp because of accumulated perspiration. One form of ringworm attacks the scalp, arms, and legs, especially of children, and is often spread by similarly affected pets. It appears as reddish patches that scale and blister and frequently feel sore and itchy. Ringworm is highly contagious and can be passed from person to person by contaminated objects such as combs and towels. It should therefore be treated promptly by a doctor. Ringworm can best be prevented by strict attention to personal cleanliness.

Athlete's foot: Another form of ringworm, *athlete's foot,* usually attacks the skin between the toes and under the toenails. If not treated promptly, it can cause an itching rash on other parts of the body. Athlete's

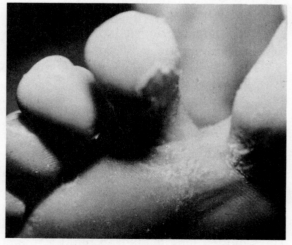

Athlete's foot, a form of ringworm, is marked by a cracking of the skin between the toes or under the toenails. Itching and soreness are usual symptoms.

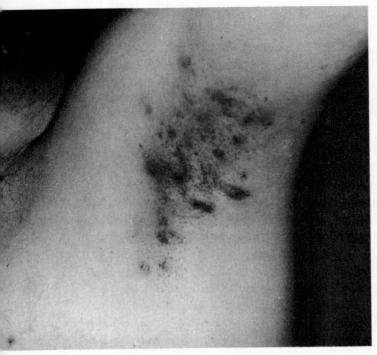

Skin is susceptible to many kinds of bacterial infection. Shown is hydradenitis suppurativa, a disease of the sweat glands affecting the underarm area.

foot causes the skin to itch, blister, and crack, and as a result, leaves it vulnerable to more serious infection from other organisms. The disorder can be treated at home by gently removing the damaged skin, and, after soaking the feet, thoroughly drying and dusting between the toes with a medicated foot powder. Some of the powder should be sprinkled into shoes. If the condition continues, a fungicidal ointment can be applied in the morning and at night. Persistent cases require the attention of a doctor.

Scabies

An insectlike parasite causes the skin irritation called *scabies,* otherwise known as "the itch." The female itch mite burrows a hole in the skin, usually in the groin or between the fingers or toes, and stays hidden long enough to build a tunnel in which to deposit her eggs. The newly hatched mites then work their way to the skin surface and begin the cycle all over again. There is little discomfort in the early period of infestation, but in about a week, a rash appears accompanied by extreme itching, which is usually most severe at night. Constant scratching during sleep can lead to skin lesions that invite bacterial infection.

Scabies is very contagious and can spread rapidly through a family or through a community, such as a summer camp or army barracks. It can also be communicated by venereal contact.

Treatment by a doctor involves the identification of the characteristic tunnels from which sample mites can be removed for examination. Hot baths and thorough scrubbing will expose the burrows, and medical applications as directed by the doctor usually clear up the condition in about a week.

Bacterial Infections

Boils: These abscesses of the skin are caused by bacterial infection of a hair follicle or a sebaceous gland. The pus that accumulates in a boil is the result of the encounter between the bacteria and the white blood cells that fight them. Sometimes a boil subsides by itself and disappears; sometimes the pressure of pus against the skin surface may bring the boil to a head. It will then break, drain, and heal if washed with an antiseptic and covered with a sterile pad. Warm water compresses can be applied for ten minutes every hour to relieve the pain and to encourage the boil to break and drain. A fresh dry pad should be applied after each period of soaking.

Anyone with a serious or chronic illness who develops a boil should consult a doctor. Since the bacteria can enter the bloodstream and cause a general infection with fever, a doctor should also be consulted for a boil on the nose, scalp, upper lip, or in the ear, groin, or armpit.

Carbuncles: This infection is a group of connected boils and is likely to be more painful and less responsive to home treatment. Carbuncles may occur as the result of poor skin care. They tend to occur in the back of the neck where the skin is thick, and the abscess tends to burrow into deeper tissues. A doctor usually lances and drains a deep-seated carbuncle, or he may prescribe an antibiotic remedy.

Impetigo: This skin infection is caused by staphylococcal or streptococcal bacteria, and is characterized by blisters that break and form yellow crusted areas. It is spread from one person to another and from one part of the body to another by the discharge from the sores. Impetigo occurs most frequently on the scalp, face, and arms and legs. The infection often is picked up in barber shops, swimming pools, or from body contact with other infected people or household pets.

Special care must be taken, especially with children, to control the spread of the infection by keeping the fingers away from infected parts. Bed linens should be changed daily, and disposable paper towels as well as paper plates and cups should be used during treatment. A doctor should be consulted for proper medication and procedures to deal with the infection.

Barber's itch: Sycosis, commonly called *barber's itch,* is a bacterial infection of the hair follicles accompanied by inflammation, itching, and the formation of pus-filled pimples. People with stiff, curly hair are prone to this type of chronic infection, since their hair is more likely to curve back and reenter the skin. The infection should be treated promptly to prevent scarring and the destruction of the hair root. In some cases, doctors recommend antibiotics. If these are not effective, it may be necessary to drain the abscesses and remove the hairs from the inflamed follicles. During treatment, it is best to avoid shaving, if possible. If one must shave, the sterilization of all shaving equipment and the use of a brushless shaving cream are recommended.

Erysipelas: An acute streptococcal infection of the skin, *erysipelas* can be fatal, particularly to the very young or very old, if not treated promptly. One of its symptoms is the bright redness of the affected areas of the skin. These red patches enlarge and spread, making the skin tender and painful. Blisters may appear nearby. The patient usually has a headache, fever, chills, and nausea. Erysipelas responds well to promptly administered antibiotics, particularly penicillin. The patient is usually advised to drink large amounts of fluid and to eat a nourishing, easily digested diet.

Virus Infections

Cold sores: Also called fever blisters, *cold sores* are technically known as *herpes simplex.* They are small blisters that appear most frequently in the corners of the mouth, and sometimes around the eyes and on the genitals. The presumed cause is a virus that lies dormant in the skin until it is activated by infection or by excessive exposure to sun or wind. There is no specific cure for cold sores, but the irritation can be eased by applying drying or cooling agents such as camphor ice or cold water compresses. Recurrent cold sores, especially in infants, should be called to a doctor's attention.

Shingles: The virus infection of a sensory nerve, accompanied by small, painful blisters that appear on the skin along the path of the nerve—usually on one side of the chest or abdomen—is called *shingles.* The medical name for the disorder, which is caused by the chicken pox virus, is *herpes zoster,* Latin for "girdle of blisters." When a cranial nerve is involved, the blisters appear on the face near the eye. The preliminary symptom is neuritis with severe pain and, sometimes, fever. The blisters may take from two to four weeks to dry up and disappear. Although there is no specific cure, the pain can be alleviated by aspirin. In severe cases, or if the area near the eye is involved, a doctor should be seen.

Warts: These growths are caused by a virus infection of the epidermis. They never become cancerous, but can be painful when found on the soles of the feet. In this location, they are known as *plantar warts,* and they cause discomfort because constant pressure makes them grow inward. Plantar warts are most likely to be picked up by children because they are barefooted so much of the time, and by adults when their feet are moist and they are walking around in showers, near swimming pools, and in locker rooms. Warts can be spread by scratching, by shaving, and by brushing the hair. They are often transmitted from one member of the family to another. Since warts can spread to painful areas, such as the area around or under the fingernails, and since they may become disfiguring, it is best to consult a doctor whenever they appear.

In many ways, warts behave rather mysteriously. About half of them go away without any treatment at all. Sometimes, when warts on one part of the body are being treated, those in another area will disappear. The folklore about "witching" and "charming" warts away has its foundation in fact, since apparently, having faith in the cure, no matter how ridiculous it sounds, sometimes brings success. This form of suggestion therapy is especially successful with children.

There are several more conventional ways of treating warts. Depending on their size and the area involved, electric current, dry ice, or various chemicals may be employed. A doctor should be consulted promptly when warts develop in the area of the beard or on the scalp, since they spread quickly in these parts of the body and thus become more difficult to eliminate.

Sebaceous Cysts

When a sebaceous gland duct is blocked, the oil which the gland secretes cannot get to the surface of the skin. Instead, it accumulates into a hard, round, movable mass contained in a sac. This mass is known as a *sebaceous cyst.* Such cysts may appear on the face, back, ears, or in the genital area. A sebaceous cyst that forms on the scalp is called a *wen,* and may become as large as a billiard ball. The skin in this area will become bald, because the cyst interferes with the blood supply to the hair roots.

Some sebaceous cysts just disappear without treatment. However, those that do not are a likely focus for secondary infection by bacteria, and they may become abscessed and inflamed. It is therefore advisable to have cysts examined by a doctor for possible removal. If such a cyst is superficial, it can be punctured and drained. One that is deeper is usually removed by simple surgical procedure in the doctor's office.

Acne

About 80 percent of all teen-agers suffer from the skin disturbance called *acne.* It is also fairly common among women in their twenties. Acne is a condition in which the skin of the face, and often of the neck, shoulders, chest, and back, is covered to a greater or lesser extent with pimples, blackheads, whiteheads, and boils.

The typical onset of acne in adolescence is related to the increased activity of the glands, including the sebaceous glands. Most of the oil that they secrete gets to the surface of the skin through ducts that lead into the pores. When the surface pores are clogged with sebaceous gland secretions and keratin, or when so much extra oil is being secreted that it backs up into the ducts, the result is the formation of the skin blemishes characteristic of acne. Dirt or make-up does not cause acne.

The blackheads are dark not because they are dirty, but because the fatty material in the clogged pore is oxidized and discolored by the air that reaches it. When this substance is infected by bacteria, it turns into a pimple. Under no circumstances should

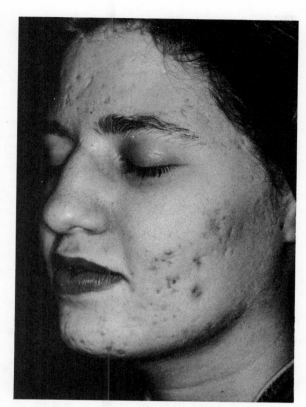

A typical case of common acne, a condition marked by pimples, blackheads, whiteheads, and boils. Acne is not caused by dirt or make-up. Skin pores are either plugged by keratin and sebaceous gland secretions, or excess secretions back up into the ducts.

Creams and cosmetics: Nonprescription medicated creams and lotions may be effective in reducing some blemishes, but if used too often, they make the skin dry. They should be applied according to the manufacturer's instructions and should be discontinued if they cause additional irritation. If makeup is used, it should have a non-oily base and be completely removed at night.

Forbidden foods: Although acne is not caused by any particular food, it can be made worse by a diet overloaded with candy, rich pastries, and fats. Chocolate and cola drinks must be eliminated entirely in some cases.

Professional treatment: A serious case of acne, or even a mild one that is causing serious emotional problems, should receive the attention of a doctor. He may prescribe antibiotics, usually considered the most effective treatment, or recommend sunlamp treatments. He can also be helpful in dealing with the psychological aspects of acne that are so disturbing to teen-agers.

Psoriasis

Psoriasis is a noncontagious chronic condition in which the skin on various parts of the body is marked by bright red patches covered with silvery scales. The areas most often affected are the knees, elbows, scalp, and trunk, and less frequently, the areas under the arms and around the genitals.

The specific cause of psoriasis has not yet been discovered, but it is thought to be an inherited abnormality in which the formation of new skin cells is too rapid and disorderly. In its mild form, psoriasis responds well to a variety of long-term treatments. When it is acute, the entire skin surface may be painfully red, and large sections of it may scale off. In such cases, prompt hospitalization and intensive care are recommended.

Conditions that can bring on an outbreak: It has been observed that the onset or ag-

such pimples be picked at or squeezed, since the pressure can rupture the surrounding membrane and spread the infection further.

Although a mild case of acne usually clears up by itself when the glands calm down, it is often helpful to get the advice of a doctor so that it does not get any worse.

Cleanliness: Although surface dirt does not cause acne, it can contribute to its spread. Therefore, the affected areas should be cleansed with a medicated soap and hot water twice a day. Hair should be shampooed frequently and brushed away from the face. Boys who are shaving should soften the beard with soap and hot water. The blade should be sharp and should skim the skin as lightly as possible to avoid nicking pimples.

gravation of psoriasis can be triggered by some of the following factors:

• Bruises, burns, scratches, and overexposure to the sun

• Sudden drops in temperature—a mild, stable climate is most beneficial

• Sudden illness from another source, or unusual physical or emotional stress

• Infections of the upper respiratory tract, especially bacterial throat infections and the medicines used to cure them.

Treatment: Although there is no specific cure for psoriasis, these are some of the recommended treatments:

• Controlled exposure to sunlight or an ultraviolet lamp

• The application of creams or lotions based on tar derivatives or those containing cortisone

• The direct injection of medicines containing cortisone and steroids

• In extremely severe cases, taking *antimetabolites,* chemicals that interfere with cell metabolism, by pill or injection.

Pigment Disorders

The mechanism which controls skin coloration is described above under *Skin Color.* Abnormalities in the creation and distribution of melanin result in the following disorders, some of which are negligible.

Freckles: These are small spots of brown pigment which frequently occur when fairskinned people are exposed to the sun or to ultraviolet light. For those whose skin gets red rather than tan during such exposure, freckles are a protective device. In most cases, they recede in cold weather. A heavy freckle formation that is permanent can be covered somewhat by cosmetic preparations. No attempt should be made to remove freckles with commercial creams or solutions unless supervised by a doctor.

Liver spots: Flat, smooth, irregularly placed markings on the skin, called *liver spots,* often appear among older people, and result from an increase in pigmentation.

They have nothing to do with the liver and are completely harmless. Brownish markings of similar appearance sometimes show up during pregnancy or as a result of irritation or infection. They usually disappear when the underlying cause is eliminated. Liver spots are permanent, and the principal cause is not aging, but the accumulated years of exposure to sun and wind. They can be disguised and treated in the same way as freckles. A liver spot that becomes hard and thick should be called to the doctor's attention.

Moles: Clusters of melanin cells, called *moles,* may appear singly or in groups at any place on the body. They range in color from light tan to dark brown; they may be raised and hairy or flat and smooth. Many moles are present at birth, and most make their appearance before the age of twenty. They rarely turn into malignancies, and require medical attention only if they become painful, if they itch, or if they suddenly change in size, shape, or color.

There are several ways of removing moles if they are annoying or particularly unattractive. They can be destroyed by the application of an electric needle, by cauterizing, and by surgery. A mole that has been removed is not likely to reappear. The hairs sometimes found in moles can be clipped close to the surface of the skin, or they can be permanently removed. Hair removal often causes the mole to get smaller.

Vitiligo: The condition called *vitiligo* stems from a loss of pigment in sharply defined areas of the skin. There is no known cause for this abnormality of melanin distribution. It may affect any part of the body and may appear any time up to middle age. It is particularly conspicuous when it occurs among blacks, or when a lighter skinned person becomes tanned except around the paler patches. There is no cure for vitiligo, but cosmetic treatment with pastes and lotions can diminish the contrast between affected areas and the rest of the skin.

Birthmarks

About one-third of all infants are born with the type of birthmark called a *hemangioma,* also known as a vascular birthmark. These are caused by a clustering of small blood vessels near the surface of the skin. The mark, which is flat, irregularly shaped, and either pink, red, or purplish, is usually referred to as "port wine stain." There is no known way to remove it, but with cosmetic covering creams, it can usually be successfully masked.

The type of hemangioma which is raised and bright red—called a strawberry mark —spontaneously disappears with no treatment in most cases during early childhood. If a strawberry mark begins to grow rather than fade, or if it begins to ulcerate, a physician should be promptly consulted.

See under *Cancer,* p. 609, for a discussion of skin cancer; see under *Puberty and Growth,* p. 122, for a discussion of adolescent skin problems; see under *Aches, Pains, Nuisances, Worries,* p. 409, for further discussion of minor skin problems.   HMacL

CHAPTER 7

Plastic and Cosmetic Surgery

The use of surgical techniques for the correction of physical deformities is by no means a modern development. The practice goes back to ancient India, where as early as the sixth century B.C. Hindu specialists were reconstructing noses, reshaping ears, and grafting skin for reducing scar tissue.

Through the centuries, improvements in procedure and new types of operations became part of the common fund of information. During World War I, great technical advances were made when the Medical Corps of the United States Army created a special division of *plastic surgery* to treat the deformities caused by battle injuries. Today's plastic surgery is based on many of the procedures perfected then and during World War II.

In recent years, attention has been focused not only on birth and injury deformities, but on lesser irregularities as well. Surgeons in the field of *cosmetic surgery* perform such procedures as nose reconstruction, face lifting, reshaping of breasts, removal of fatty tissue from upper arms and

legs, and the transplanting of hair to correct baldness.

There is no longer any reason for someone to suffer from the emotional and professional problems caused by abnormalities in appearance. No child should be expected to live with the disability of a cleft lip or crossed eyes. A young woman tormented by what she considers to be a grotesque nose can have it recontoured to her liking. An older woman who finds wrinkles a social liability can have them removed. Anyone interested in undergoing *any* form of cosmetic surgery should stay away from so-called "beauty experts," and deal only with a reputable surgeon or physician.

Some surgical specialists, called *plastic surgeons,* perform cosmetic or plastic surgery exclusively. Other surgeons and physicians, including general surgeons, dermatologists, ophthalmologists, and others are qualified to do some kinds of plastic surgery, usually the techniques related to their particular specialties. The kind of surgery desired should first be discussed with the family doctor, who can then evaluate the problem and recommend a qualified surgeon to deal with it.

Before undergoing any kind of plastic surgery, the prospective patient should realize that it is neither inexpensive nor totally painless. Most cosmetic surgery is performed in hospitals, which means that in addition to the surgeon's fees there can be a bill for the anesthetist, use of the operating and recovery rooms, and for the hospital stay itself. Also, because cosmetic surgery is often *elective surgery,* surgery not needed to ensure the patient's physical health, it may not be covered by a health-insurance policy. Getting one's nose fixed, for example, may cost between $500 and $1,500.

Crossed Eyes

The condition technically known as *strabismus,* in which one eye drifts so that its position is not parallel with the other, is caused by a congenitally weak muscle. Infants often appear to have crossed eyes, but in most cases the drifting corrects itself by the time the baby is six months old. If the condition persists beyond that time, a doctor should be consulted. He may recommend the use of an eye patch over the stronger eye so that the weaker one will be exercised. If this does not achieve the desired result, he may prescribe special glasses and eye exercises as the child gets older so that there is no impairment of vision.

If corrective surgery proves necessary after these measures, it is usually done before the child enters school. The operation is a simple one involving the muscle and not the inside of the eye itself. Crossed eyes should receive professional attention early enough to prevent a permanent visual handicap.

Cleft Palate and Cleft Lip

A *cleft palate* is a split in the roof of the mouth sometimes extending to the lip and into the nose. The split is caused by the failure of the two sides of the face to unite properly during prenatal development. The

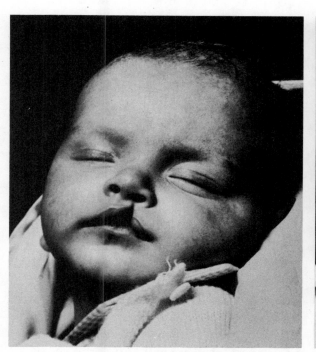 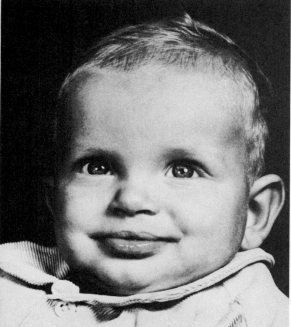

Cleft palate and cleft lip interfere with the infant's ability to suck and, if uncorrected, would later cause speech impairment. These pictures show how surgery can correct the disfigurement.

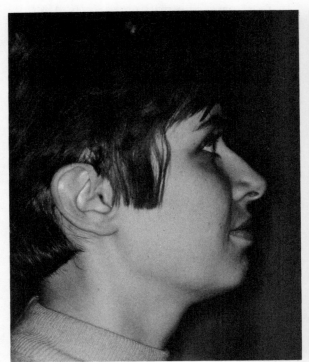 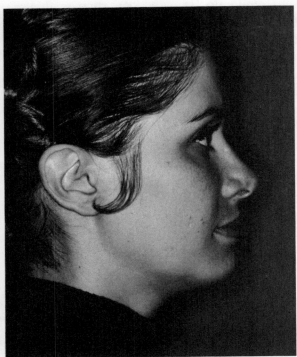

A rhinoplasty, or surgical reconstruction of the nose, is done by way of the nostrils to avoid facial scarring. The skin is loosened from the underlying bone and cartilage and reshaped.

condition occurs in about 1 out of 1,000 births and is sometimes associated with a foot or spine deformity. It is in no way related to mental retardation.

An infant born with a cleft palate cannot suck properly unless a special device, called an *obturator,* is inserted into the split to close it against the flow of air. Where this is undesirable, feeding may be done with a spoon or a dropper.

Since the condition eventually causes speech distortion, it should be corrected at about 18 months of age, before the child begins to talk. The surgery consists of reconstructing the tissue. Sometimes even at this early age, the child may need some corrective speech therapy following the operation.

If the split occurs only in the lip, commonly called a *harelip,* surgery may be recommended when the infant weighs about 15 pounds, usually at the age of 12 to 15 months. When the operation is performed

this early, there is no danger of speech impairment, and the result is only a thin scar.

Reshaping the Nose

Known technically as a *rhinoplasty,* the operation for the reconstruction of the nose is not only one of the oldest, but also one of the most common forms of cosmetic surgery. Depending on the demands of facial symmetry and individual taste, the nose can be shortened, straightened, narrowed, or even lengthened. If a nose deformity has caused breathing problems, the surgeon will take the correction of this situation into account in planning the reconstruction.

Barring accidents, most children's noses are perfectly adequate until they enter their teens, when the facial bones begin to take on the contours determined by inheritance. Teen-agers are especially sensitive about their looks. If nose surgery seems advisable, therefore, it is usually undertaken when the child is between 14 and 16 years of age, though the operation is also performed on adults.

In many cases, parents agree with the youngster about the need for surgery. In some families, however, the parent who has lived with a nose very similar to the one which the child finds so objectionable, may take a negative view of the need for correction. If a serious disagreement results, it may be necessary to seek family counseling from a professional source to resolve it.

Surgical procedures: When a nose reconstruction is being planned, the surgeon requires photographs of both the left and right profiles as well as front and under views of the nose. Transparent paper is placed on top of the photos, and the recommended changes are drawn over the original nose structure. The patient's preferences are always taken into account, but the surgeon has the final say in determining the suitability of the new shape in terms of appearance and function. In some cases, facial surgery to build up an underdeveloped chin, called a *mentoplasty,* is recommended so that better balance of the features is achieved.

The surgery itself is performed under local anesthesia in a hospital. It is done through the nostrils so that there is no scarring of facial tissue. The skin is loosened from the bone and cartilage, and these are reshaped to the desired specifications. The skin then resettles on its new frame, and the new shape is retained by packing the nostrils and splinting the nose.

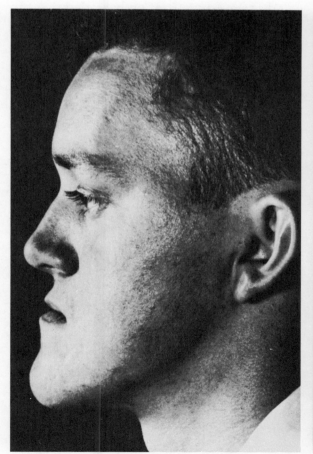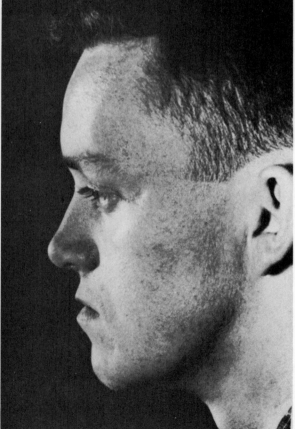

Prognathism, the condition of having a protruding jaw, can be corrected by removing part of the bone or grinding it down. Orthodontic treatment is often required to align the jaws properly.

The healing process: The packing is left in place for about three to five days or until it can be removed without sticking. The total dressing stays on for about a week. During the healing period, the nose is cleaned with cotton swabs. All swelling in the area vanishes in about a month, and within a year the reconstructed nose is as strong if not stronger than its original counterpart.

Cosmetic Breast Surgery

Inverted nipples: The condition in which the nipples are turned back into the breasts rather than projecting from them can be corrected by a simple operation. The breast tissue is cut to release the nipple so that it can be pulled outward to the normal position. This surgical procedure is sometimes recommended to facilitate the nursing of a newborn baby.

Breast lifting: Breasts that sag even though they are not too large can be lifted to a more attractive contour by an operation that consolidates the tissue. The surgical procedure consists of removing strips of skin from the base of the breasts and bringing the rest of the skin together under tension so that it is tight enough to support the tissue in an upward position.

Breast reduction: In spite of all the publicity given to breast augmentation, most cosmetic surgery involving the breasts is concerned with reducing rather than enlarging them. Breast reduction is frequently undertaken not only to improve appearance, but also for purposes of health and comfort.

The operation, called a *mastoplasty,* is performed under general anesthesia and consists in cutting out fatty tissue and skin. Although the incision may be large, the resulting scars are no thicker than a hairline and are hidden in the fold below the breasts.

The most remarkable thing about this type of surgery—and the reason for its being considerably more complicated than breast enlargement—is the repositioning of the nipples so that they are properly placed relative to the newly proportioned breast contours.

Breast enlargement: The techniques used in this operation, called a *mammoplasty,* have changed over the years. Early operations to augment the size of the breasts involved the injection of paraffin, but this was soon abandoned as unsatisfactory. Considerable experimentation with the use of various synthetics as well as with the use of fatty tissue taken from the buttocks didn't provide good results either.

Silicone—a form of man-made plastic material of great versatility—was first used in this connection in the form of sponges, and later was injected in liquid form directly into the tissue. However, the federal Food and Drug Administration has ruled that the use of liquid silicone is unsafe and illegal, since its presence would mask signs of malignancy. Another problem with liquid silicone is that it has a tendency to drift to other parts of the body.

In the latest techniques of breast augmentation, a silicone gel or saline solution is placed in a flexible silicone bag shaped to resemble the breast. The bags are inserted through incisions under the breast tissue, and to date appear to be the safest and most satisfactory solution to the problem of breast enlargement.

Face Lift

Face lifting, or *rhytidoplasty,* is a form of cosmetic surgery designed to eliminate as far as possible signs of aging such as wrinkles, pouches under the chin and eyes, and sagging tissue generally. About 7,000 such operations are performed each year with satisfactory results.

In deciding on the advisability of a face lift, a reputable surgeon will take into account the person's age, emotional stability, and physical condition. The main procedure involves tightening the skin after the

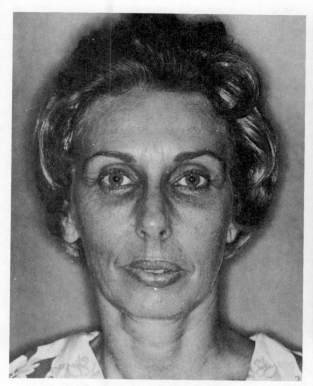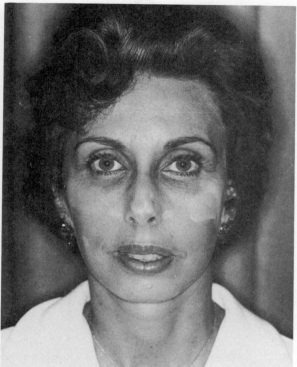

Face lift, or rhytidoplasty, removes wrinkles by tightening facial skin and removing the excess. Scars are hidden under hair and behind the ears. Wrinkles will, however, reappear in time.

surplus has been removed. The resulting scars are usually hidden in the hair and behind the ears. Those directly in front of the ears are visible only under very close scrutiny. Even after a face lift, however, the same wrinkles will eventually reappear because of the characteristic use of the individual's facial muscles.

Body Lift

Recently there has been considerable interest in the application of cosmetic surgery to the problem of removing surplus fat from various parts of the body. This operation is still considered controversial, however, and most doctors prefer to recommend controlled diet and suitable exercise as the best way to deal with excess weight. It is usually done in the United States only when the person who desires to have the operation is rendered grotesque by a huge amount of fat.

To reduce the size of the upper arms or legs, the abdomen, or the buttocks, an incision is made in a natural fold of the body area in question. The surrounding skin is loosened, the surplus fatty tissue and the excess skin are removed, and the remaining skin is then stretched tight and sutured. Because such a large area is covered, the procedure usually leaves a long scar.

Eyelids

The shape and size of the eyelids can be changed by an operation called a *blepharoplasty*. In this procedure, an incision is made in the fold of the upper eyelid, and excess skin and fat are removed. The technique can be used to correct congenital deformities such as hanging upper eyelids that do not fully open. When a comparable incision is made below the lash line on the lower lid, the surgeon can remove the fat which causes bags under the eyes.

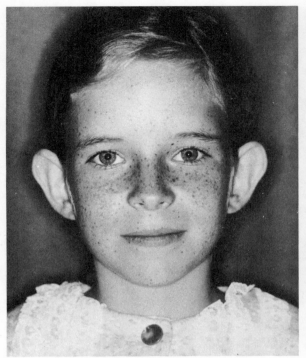 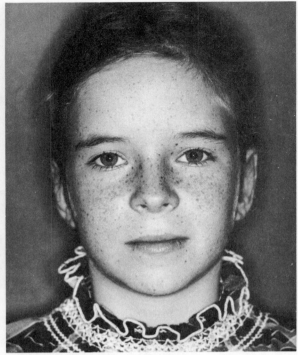

In an otoplasty, an operation to correct protruding ears, cartilage behind each ear is cut and the ears are repositioned closer to the skull, as this pair of photographs illustrates.

Ears

Surgery to correct protruding or over-large ears is called *otoplasty*. Though it can be performed on adults, it is usually performed on children before they enter school to prevent the psychological problems that often result from teasing. In the procedure, an incision is made behind the ear, cartilage is cut, and the ear is repositioned closer to the skull. Otoplasty can also build up or replace an ear missing because of a birth defect or accident.

Scar Reduction

Unsightly scars that are the result of a birth defect or an injury can usually be reduced by plastic surgery to thin hairlines. The procedure is effective only if there has been no extensive damage to surrounding areas of underlying tissue, as sometimes occurs in severe burns. The operation involves the removal of the old scar tissue, under-mining the surrounding skin, and pulling it together with very fine stitches.

Hair Transplant

A comparatively new solution to the problem of baldness is the technique called hair transplantation. This involves the surgical grafting of hair-bearing skin taken from the back part and sides of the scalp onto the bald areas of the head. The transplanting is usually done in the surgeon's office. The patient usually receives between 10 and 30 transplants per session.

Within about a month, the hairs in the grafted skin fall out, but the roots remain, and most of these eventually produce new hair. The areas from which the grafts are taken remain hairless, but since each transplant is very small, about 150 to 200 graftings can be done without creating any conspicuous bald spots. Transplanted hair has the same thickness and appearance that it had in its former location.   HMacL

CHAPTER 8

Aches, Pains, Nuisances, Worries

And Other Things You Can Live With But Could Get Along Very Well Without

None of the variety of discomforts discussed in this chapter is a laughing matter. The best thing about most of them is that they will pass, given your common-sense attention, or will disappear if you follow your doctor's advice. This includes taking the medications prescribed by your doctor exactly as directed. In a few cases, such as allergies or gout, long-term drug therapy may be necessary on a self-supervised basis, once treatment has been established by a doctor. Of course, when symptoms of any kind persist or get worse, you should waste no time in seeking a professional diagnosis.

There may be somebody, somewhere, who has never felt rotten a day in his life. But most of us are not so fortunate. Among the most common nuisance ailments are:

- Upper respiratory infections
- Allergies
- Occasional headaches
- Backaches
- Weight problems
- Weather discomforts
- Disturbances of normal sleep patterns
- Aching feet
- Indigestion.

The unpleasant feeling associated with any of these common disorders can almost always be banished with a modicum of care and thought. For example, allergic reactions to particular foods can be avoided by identifying the offending food and avoiding it. Self-diagnosis and self-discipline can often cope with weight problems. A backache may be cured by attention to posture, or adjusting your office chair. A sensible approach to clothing and exposure can often do away with weather discomforts.

But when symptoms do not respond to self-help—as when sporadic difficulty in sleeping burgeons into a string of near-sleepless nights, or when abdominal pain you interpret as indigestion is intense or frequent in spite of avoiding rich or heavy foods, it's time to see a doctor.

409

The Common Cold and Upper Respiratory Infections

"Common cold" is the label attached to a group of symptoms that can be caused by one or more of some 20 different viruses. Colds are considered highly contagious, but some doctors think that people don't entirely catch others' colds—in a sense they catch their own. While the viruses that carry the infection are airborne and practically omnipresent, somebody in good health is usually less susceptible to a cold than someone who is run down. Both environmental factors (such as air pollution) and emotional ones (such as anxiety or depression) seem to increase susceptibility.

Symptoms: Symptoms differ from person to person and from cold to cold with the same person. Generally, a cold starts with sneezes, a running nose, teary eyes, and a stuffed head. Sometimes the nasal membranes become so swollen that a person can only breathe through the mouth; sometimes the senses of smell and taste simply disappear. The throat may be sore; a postnasal drip may cause a constant cough when lying down at night.

When these symptoms are acute and are accompanied by fever and aching joints, the illness is usually referred to as influenza or "the flu." There are many different viruses that cause influenza, and new ones are always turning up, most recently the one

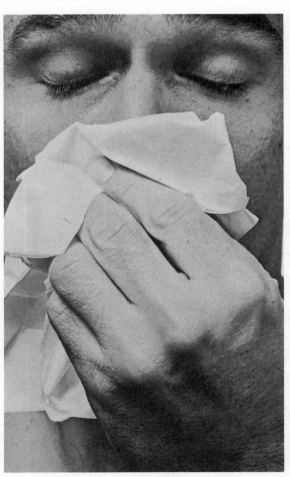

The common cold, with its familiar symptoms of sneezing and a runny nose, can be caused by many viruses.

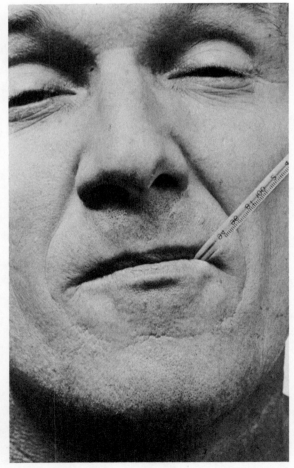

Severe cold symptoms and fever accompany influenza. Persistent symptoms require a doctor's attention.

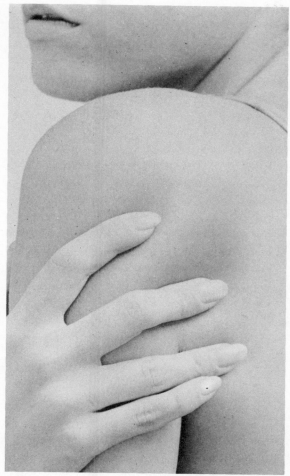

Aching joints are another common influenza symptom. Since influenza is viral, antibiotics will not help.

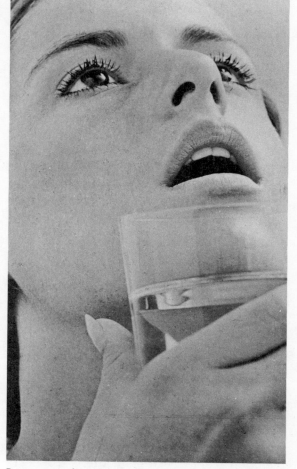

Rest, extra liquids, and aspirin to relieve discomfort are recommended for treating the common cold.

causing Asian flu. Unfortunately, there is as yet no medicine that can cure either a cold or a flu attack, although many people do get relief from symptoms by taking various cold remedies. Antibiotics are sometimes prescribed by doctors to prevent more serious bacterial diseases, such as pneumonia, from developing, but antibiotics are not effective against the cold viruses.

Treatment: Some people can get away with treating a cold with contempt and an occasional aspirin, and go about their business. Others are laid low for a few days. If you are the type who is really hit hard by a cold, it isn't coddling yourself to stay home for a couple of days. In any event, a

simple cold usually runs its course, lasting anywhere from a few days to two weeks.

Discomfort can be minimized and recovery speeded by a few simple steps: extra rest and sleep, drinking more liquids than usual, and taking one or two aspirin tablets every four hours. Antihistamine preparations or nose drops should be avoided unless specifically prescribed by a physician.

A painful sore throat accompanied by fever, a persistent earache, a dry hacking cough, or pains in the chest are symptoms that should be brought to the attention of a physician.

Prevention: Although taking massive doses of vitamin C at the first sign of a cold

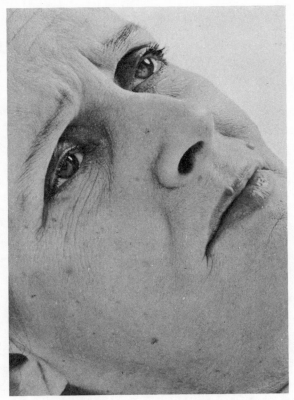

Itching and tearing eyes are a common symptom of allergy caused by airborne substances such as pollen.

is said by some authorities to prevent the infection from developing, there is not yet general agreement on the effectiveness of this treatment.

Actually, there are several common-sense ways of reducing the risk of infection, particularly for those people who are especially susceptible to catching a cold. For most people, getting a proper amount of sleep, eating sensibly, avoiding exposure to sudden chill, trying to stay out of crowds, and trying to keep emotional tensions under control can increase resistance to colds and other minor respiratory infections.

Inoculation against particular types of viruses is recommended by many physicians in special cases: for pregnant women, for the elderly, and for those people who have certain chronic heart and lung diseases. Flu shots are effective against a particular virus or viruses for a limited period.

Allergies

Discomforts of various kinds are considered allergies when they are brought on by substances or conditions that ordinarily are harmless. Not too long ago, perturbed allergy sufferers would say things like:

"I can't use that soap because it gives me hives."

"Smelling roses makes me sneeze."

"Eating almonds gives me diarrhea."

Nowadays, such complaints are commonly recognized as allergies.

Symptoms: Allergic symptoms can range from itching eyes, running nose, coughing, difficulty in breathing, welts on the skin, nausea, cramps, and even going into a state of shock, depending upon the severity of the allergic individual's response. Almost any part or system of the body may be affected, and almost anything can pose an allergic threat to somebody.

Allergens: Substances that trigger an allergic reaction are called *allergens.* The system of an allergic individual reacts to such substances as if they were germs, producing *antibodies* whose job it is to neutralize the allergens. But the body's defense mechanism overreacts: in the process of fighting off the effects of the allergens, various chemicals, particularly *histamines,* are dumped indiscriminately into the bloodstream. It is the overabundance of these "good" chemicals that causes the discomforts associated with allergies.

Allergens are usually placed in the following categories:

• Those that affect the respiratory tract, or *inhalants,* such as pollens, dust, smoke, perfumes, and various airborne, malodorous chemicals. These bring on sneezing, coughing, and breathing impairment.

• Food substances that affect the digestive system, typically eggs, seafood, nuts, berries, chocolate, and pork. These may not only cause nausea and diarrhea, but hives and skin rashes.

• Medicines and drugs, such as penicillin, or a particular serum used in inoculations.

• Agents that act on the skin and mucous membranes, such as insecticides, poison oak, and poison ivy, particular chemical dyes, cosmetics, soaps, metals, leathers, and furs.

• Environmental agents such as sunlight, excessive cold, light, and pressure.

• Microbes, such as particular bacteria, viruses, and parasites.

Treatment: Some allergic reactions are outgrown; some don't develop until adulthood. In many cases, the irritating substance is easy to identify and then avoid; in others, it may take a long series of tests before the allergen is finally tracked down.

As soon as the source of the allergen is identified, the best thing for the allergic person to do is avoid it—if possible. But a person may find it more convenient to be relieved of the allergy by desensitization treatments administered by a doctor. Some-

times allergies that resist these treatments are kept under control by medicines such as adrenaline, ephedrine, cortisone, or the antihistamines.

Any person subject to severe, disabling allergy attacks by a known allergen should carry a card describing both the allergic reactions and the allergen. Detailed information on the latest developments in the treatment of allergies is available from the Allergy Foundation of America, 801 Second Avenue, New York, New York 10017.

Headaches

The common headache is probably as ancient as primitive man. The headache, a pain or ache across the forehead or within the head, may be severe or mild in character, and can last anywhere from under half an hour to three or four days. It may be accompanied by dizziness, nausea, nasal

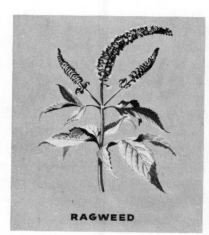
RAGWEED

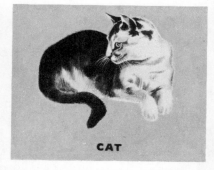
CAT

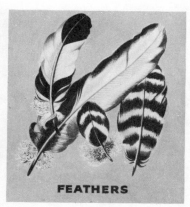
FEATHERS

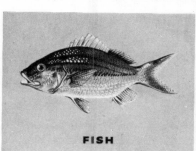
FISH

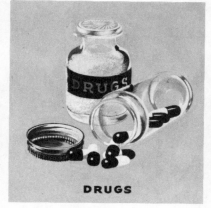
DRUGS

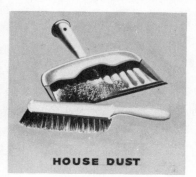
HOUSE DUST

All of the creatures and substances illustrated here can cause allergic reactions in susceptible individuals. Once the cause is known, the best advice is to avoid it as much as possible.

stuffiness, or difficulty in seeing or hearing. It is not a disease or illness, but a symptom.

Causes: Headaches in today's modern world can arise from any of a number of underlying causes. These include excessive drinking or smoking, lack of sleep, hunger, drug abuse, and eye strain. Eye strain commonly results from overuse of the eyes, particularly under glaring light, or from failure to correct defective vision.

Headaches can also be caused by exposure to toxic gases such as carbon monoxide and sulfur dioxide, which are common components in polluted air. Some headaches are symptoms of illness or disease, including pneumonia, constipation, allergy, high blood pressure, and brain tumor. Finally, emotional strain or tension can cause headache by unconsciously constricting the head and neck muscles. Many of these causes give rise to the common physiological cause of headache—dilation of the blood vessels in the head.

Migraine: Headaches may be suffered on an occasional basis, or they may be chronic. Chronic headaches are usually *tension headaches* or *migraine.* Migraine, also called *sick headache,* is a particularly severe, intense kind of headache. An attack may last several days and necessitate bed rest. Dizziness, sensitivity to light, and chills may accompany migraine.

The exact cause of migraine is unknown, but researchers suspect a hereditary link, since the majority of migraine patients have one or more close relatives with migraine. Migraine headaches can be precipitated by changes in body hormone balance, sudden changes in temperature, shifts in barometric pressure, or by the intake of alcoholic beverages or the abuse of drugs. Anyone suffering from very severe or chronic headaches should see a doctor and get a complete physical checkup.

Tension headaches: Tension headaches can be avoided by getting adequate amounts of sleep and exercise and by learning to cope with frustrations and anxieties. Find time to relax each day, and resist the temptation to be a perfectionist or overachiever in all things. Tension headaches can be helped by neck massage, use of a heating pad, or a long, hot bath.

Headache relief: Aspirin is often effective against headaches, but should be taken according to directions. A double dose is dangerous, and is not doubly effective. A cup of coffee or other caffeine beverage may prove helpful, since caffeine helps con-

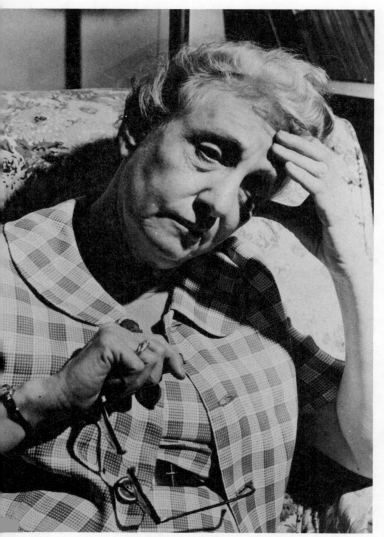

Headaches are usually brought on by the dilation of blood vessels in the head. Typical causes of this condition are tension, eye strain, and lack of sleep.

strict blood vessels. In some cases headaches can be helped by nothing more than a few deep breaths of fresh air. Excess use of alcohol and tobacco should be avoided. If you must skip a meal, have a candy bar, piece of fruit, or some soup to prevent or relieve a hunger headache.

Take care of your eyes. Do not read in dim or glaring light. Have your eyes checked regularly, and if you have glasses, wear them when you need them.

Backaches

"Oh, my aching back" is probably the most common complaint among people past the age of 40. Most of the time, the discomfort—wherever it occurs, up or down the backbone—can be traced to some simple cause. However, there are continuous backaches which have their origin in some internal disorder that needs the attention of a physician. Among the more serious causes are kidney or pancreas disease, spinal arthritis, and peptic ulcer.

Some common causes: Generally a backache is the result of strain on the muscles, nerves, or ligaments of the spine. It can occur because of poor posture, carelessness in lifting or carrying heavy packages, sitting in one position for a long time in the wrong kind of chair, or sleeping on a mattress that is too soft. Backache often accompanies menstruation, and is common in the later stages of pregnancy. Emotional tension can also bring on back pain.

Prevention: In general, maintaining good posture during the waking hours and sleeping on a hard mattress at night—if necessary, inserting a bedboard between the mattress and bedsprings—are the first line of defense against backaches. Anyone habitually carrying heavy loads of books or groceries, or even an overloaded attaché case, should make a habit of shifting the weight from arm to arm so that the spine doesn't always get pulled in one direction.

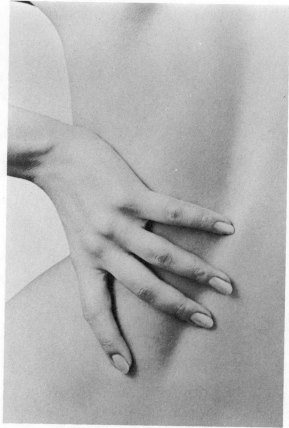

Backaches are often caused by weak muscles that are subjected to unusual strain. A supervised program of exercises can help strengthen the back muscles.

Workers who are sedentary for most of the day at a desk or factory table should be sure that the chair they sit in provides firm support for back muscles and is the right height for the working surface.

Treatment: Most cases of simple backache respond to rest, aspirin, and the application of heat, applied by a hot water bottle or heating pad. In cases where the pain persists or becomes more acute, a doctor should be consulted. He may find that the trouble is caused by the malfunctioning of an internal organ, or by pressure on the sciatic nerve (*sciatica*). With X rays he may also locate a slipped disk or other abnormality in the alignment of the vertebrae of the spine. See *Back Pain and Its Causes*, p. 459.

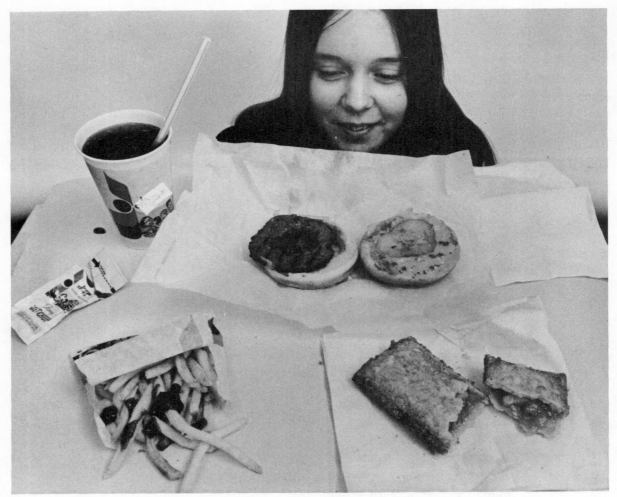

This young office worker may well wonder why she's putting on weight if this is her usual lunch—rich in fried, fatty foods and carbohydrates and poor in other nutrients.

Weight Problems

A few people can maintain the weight that is right for their body build without ever having to think about it. However, most experts believe that just about half the people in the United States may be risking shorter lives because they are too heavy. By one estimate, approximately one out of five American men and one out of four American women are ten percent or more overweight, a group that may be called the borderline obese.

There is no longer any reasonable doubt that, if you are overweight, you have statis-tically a greater chance of high blood pressure, diabetes, and *atherosclerosis*, (lumpy deposits in the arteries). And since athero-sclerotic heart disease alone accounts for 20 percent of deaths among adults in the United States, it is understandable why doctors consider weight truly a national problem.

Causes: In practically all cases, weighing too much is the result of eating too much and exercising too little. In many cases, the food eaten is of the wrong kind and leisure time is used for riding around in a car rather than walking, or for watching television rather than playing tennis.

Many people like to think that they weigh too much only because they happen to like good food; but the real explanations may be considerably more complicated. In some cases, overeating has been found to have emotional sources: feelings of inadequacy; the need to compensate for a lack of affection or approval, or an unconscious desire to ward off the attention of the opposite sex. Psychological weight problems of this kind can be helped by consulting a psychiatrist or psychologist.

Treatment: There are many overweight people who merely need the support and encouragement that comes from participating in a group effort, and for them, joining one of the various weight-control organizations can be extremely beneficial in taking off extra pounds and keeping them off.

Permanent results are rarely achieved by crash diets, faddish food combinations, or reducing pills. Not only are such solutions usually temporary, they may actually be harmful. See *Weight,* p. 320, for further information about weight problems.

Weather Discomforts

Using good sense about clothing, exercise, and proper diet is probably our best protection against the discomforts caused by extremes of temperature. Sometimes circumstances make this exercise of good sense impossible, with unpleasant but rarely serious results, if treatment is promptly administered. Following are some of the more common disorders resulting from prolonged exposure to excessive heat or cold, and what you can do to alleviate them.

Heat Cramps

In a very hot environment, a person may drink great quantities of water while "sweating buckets" of salty perspiration. Thus, the body's water is replaced, but its salt is not. This salt-water imbalance results in a feeling of faintness and dizziness accompanied by acute stomach cramps and muscle pains in the legs. When the symptoms are comparatively mild, they can be relieved by taking coated salt tablets in five to ten grain doses with a full glass of tepid or cool—not iced—water. Salt tablets should be taken regularly as a preventive measure by people who sweat a great deal during hot weather.

Sunburn

If you have not yet been exposed to much sun, as at the beginning of summer, limit your exposure at first to a period of 15 or 20 minutes, and avoid the sun at the hours around mid-day even if the sky is overcast. Remember, too, that the reflection of the sun's rays from water and beach sand intensifies their effect. Some suntan lotions give effective protection against burning, and some creams even prevent tanning; but remember to cover all areas of exposed skin and to reapply the lotion when it's been washed away after a swim.

Treatment: A sunburn is treated like any other burn, depending upon its severity. See *Burns,* p. 677. If there is blistering, take care to avoid infection. Extensive blistering requires a physician's attention.

Heat Exhaustion

This condition is different from heatstroke or sunstroke, discussed below. Heat exhaustion sets in when large quantities of blood accumulate in the skin as the body's way of increasing its cooling mechanism during exposure to high temperatures. This in turn lowers the amount of blood circulating through the heart and decreases the blood supply to the brain. If severe enough, fainting may result. Other symptoms of heat exhaustion include unusual pallor and profuse cold perspiration. The pulse may be weak and breathing shallow.

Treatment: A person suspected of having heat exhaustion should be placed in a reclining position, his clothing loosened or

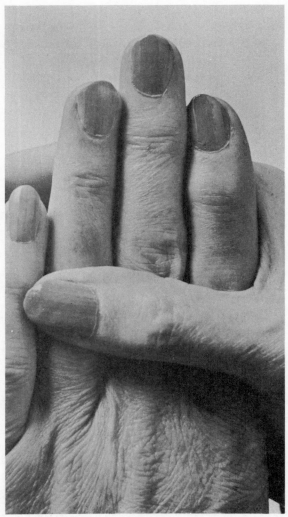

Chapped skin is caused by dryness resulting from the effect of cold weather on the sebaceous glands. The glands' secretions are reduced at low temperatures.

removed, and his body cooled with moist cloths applied to his forehead and wrists. If he doesn't recover promptly from a fainting spell, smelling salts can be held under his nose to revive him. As soon as he is conscious, he can be given salt tablets and a cool sugary drink—either tea or coffee—to act as a stimulant. Don't give the patient any alcoholic beverages.

Sunstroke or Heatstroke

Sunstroke is much more of an emergency than heat exhaustion and requires immediate attention. The characteristic symptom is extremely high body temperature brought on by cessation of perspiration. If hot, dry, flushed skin turns ashen gray, a doctor must be called immediately. Too much physical activity during periods of high temperature and high humidity is a direct contributing cause.

Treatment: See *Sunstroke*, p. 680, for a description of the emergency treatment recommended for this condition.

Chapped Skin

One of the most widespread discomforts of cold weather is chapped skin. In low temperatures, the skin's sebaceous glands produce less of the oils that lubricate and protect the skin, causing it to become dry. Continued exposure results in reddening and cracking. In this condition, the skin is especially sensitive to strong soaps.

Treatment: During cold, dry weather, less soap should be used when washing, a bath oil should be used when bathing, and a mild lotion or cream should be applied to protect the skin from the damaging effects of wind and cold. A night cream or lotion containing lanolin is also helpful, and the use of cleansing cream or oil instead of soap can reduce additional discomfort when cleansing chapped areas. The use of a colorless lip pomade is especially recommended for children when they play out of doors in cold dry weather for any length of time.

Chilblain

A *chilblain* is a local inflammation of the skin brought on by exposure to cold. The condition commonly affects people overly sensitive to cold because of poor circulation. When the hands, feet, face, and ears are affected, the skin in these areas itches and burns, and may swell and turn reddish blue.

Treatment: The best way to avoid chilblains is to wear appropriate clothing during cold weather, especially warm socks, gloves, and ear coverings. The use of bed socks and a heating pad at night is also advisable. Cold wet feet should be dried promptly, gently, and thoroughly, once indoors. Rubbing or massaging should be avoided, since these can cause further irritation. People who suffer from repeated attacks of chilblains should consult a doctor for diagnosis of circulatory problems.

Frostbite

Frostbite is a considerably more serious condition than chilblains, since it means that a part or parts of the body have actually been frozen. The fingers or toes, the nose, and the ears are most vulnerable. If frostbitten, these areas turn numb and pale, and feel cold when touched. The dangerous thing about frostbite is that pain may not be a warning. If the condition is not treated promptly, the temperature inside the tissues keeps going down and eventually cuts off blood circulation to the overexposed parts of the body. In such extreme cases, there is a possible danger of gangrene.

Treatment: In mild cases, prompt treatment can slowly restore blood circulation.

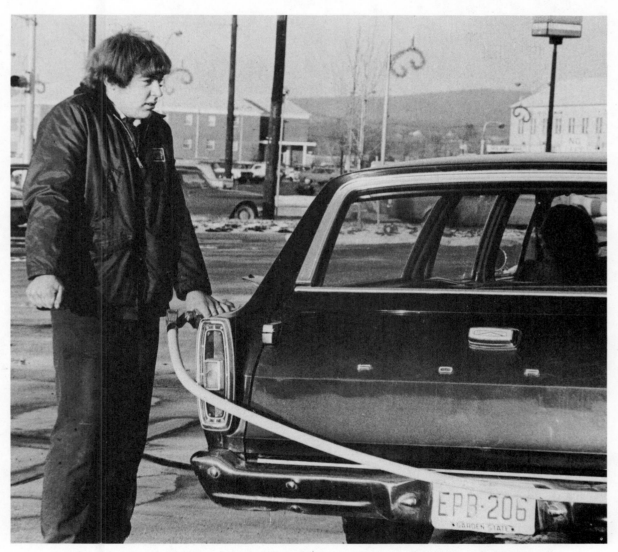

People with poor circulation are especially subject to chilblain, a local skin inflammation. Anyone who must work outdoors in cold weather is well advised to wear gloves and ear coverings.

The frozen parts should be rewarmed *slowly* by covering them with warm clothing or by soaking them in lukewarm water. Nothing hot should be applied—neither hot water nor a heating pad. Nor should the patient be placed too close to a fireplace or radiator. Since the affected tissues can be easily bruised, they should not be massaged or rubbed. If you are in doubt about restoring circulation, a doctor should be called promptly or the patient taken to a hospital for emergency treatment.

Sleep and The Lack of It

Until rather recently, it was assumed that sleep was the time when the body rested and recovered from the activities of wakefulness. Although there is still a great deal to learn about why we sleep and what happens when we are sleeping, medical researchers have now identified several different phases of sleep, all of them necessary over the long run, but some more crucial than others.

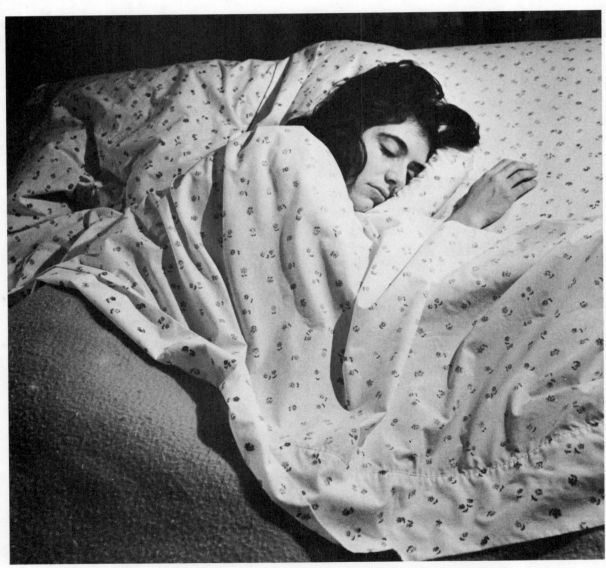

Recent studies have demonstrated the importance of different phases of sleep, but little is known about how sleep reinvigorates the body or why some people need more sleep than others.

How much sleep a person needs varies a great deal from individual to individual; and the same individual may need more or less at different times. Children need long periods of unbroken sleep; the elderly seem to get along on very little. No matter what a person's age, too little sleep over too long a time leads to irritability, exhaustion, and giddiness.

Insomnia

Almost everybody has gone through periods when it is difficult or impossible to fall asleep. Excitement before bedtime, temporary worries about a pressing problem, spending a night in an unfamiliar place, changing to a different bed, illness, physical discomfort because of extremes of temperature—any of these circumstances can interfere with normal sleep patterns.

But this is quite different from *chronic insomnia,* when a person consistently has trouble falling asleep for no apparent reason. If despite all your common-sense approaches insomnia persists, a doctor should be consulted about the advisability of taking a tranquilizer or a sleeping pill. Barbiturates should not be taken unless prescribed by a physician.

The Vulnerable Extremities

Aches and pains in the legs and feet occur for a wide variety of reasons, some trivial and easily corrected, others serious enough to require medical attention. Those that originate in such conditions as arthritis and rheumatism can often be alleviated by aspirin or some of the newer prescription medications.

Gout

Gout, which is actually a metabolic disorder, is a condition that especially affects the joint of the big toe, and sometimes the ankle joint, causing the area to become swollen, hot, and acutely painful. Although

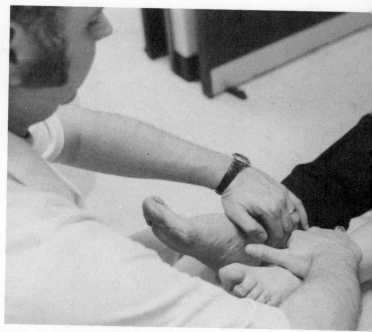

Occasional aches of the feet are almost universal, but persistent pain can indicate a serious condition and should be brought to the attention of a physician.

the specific cause of gout is not yet clearly understood, the symptoms can be alleviated by special medication prescribed by a physician. An attack of gout can be triggered by a wide variety of causes: wearing the wrong shoes, eating a diet too rich in fats, getting a bad chill, surgery in some other part of the body, or chronic emotional anxiety, as well as the use of certain medicines such as diuretics ("water-pills").

Fallen Arches

Fallen arches can cause considerable discomfort because the body's weight is carried on the ligaments of the inside of the foot rather than on the sole. When the abnormality is corrected by orthopedic shoes with built-in arches for proper support, the pressure of the ligaments is relieved. A doctor rather than a shoe salesman should be consulted for a reliable diagnosis. In some cases, the doctor may also recommend special exercises to strengthen the arch.

Flat Feet

Flat feet can usually be revealed by a simple test—making a footprint on level earth or hard-packed sand. If the print is solid rather than indented by a curve along the big-toe side of the foot, the foot is flat. Aching ligaments in the area of the instep are often a result, but can be relieved by proper arch supports inside the shoes. Corrective arch supports are particularly important for young children, for anyone who is overweight, and for anyone who has to stand a great deal of the time.

Blisters

Although blisters are sometimes a sign of allergy, fungus infection, or sunburn, they most commonly appear on the feet because of the friction of a shoe or of hosiery

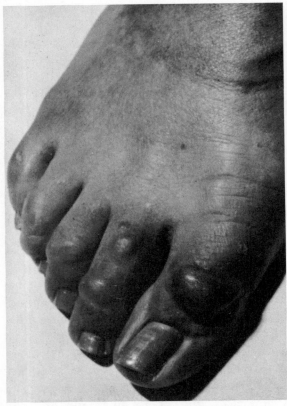

Blisters are often the result of ill-fitting shoes or hosiery. "Water" blisters actually contain lymph. Blood blisters collect blood from broken capillaries.

that does not fit properly. A *water blister* is a collection of lymph that forms inside the upper level of the skin; a *blood blister* goes down deeper and contains some blood released from broken capillaries. A normal amount of walking in shoes and hosiery that fit comfortably—neither too loose nor too tight—rarely results in blisters. When blisters do appear, it is best to protect them from further friction by the use of a sterile bandage strip.

Treatment: A blister that causes acute pain when walking can be treated as follows: after cleaning the area with soap and water, pat it dry and swab it with rubbing alcohol. Sterilize the tip of a needle in a flame, let it cool a little, and then puncture the edge of the blister, absorbing the liquid with a sterile gauze. The loose skin can be removed with manicure scissors that have been sterilized by boiling for ten minutes. The surface of raw skin should then be covered with an adhesive bandage. This procedure is best done before bedtime so that healing can begin before shoes are worn again.

If redness appears around the area of any blister and inflammation appears to be spreading, a doctor should be consulted promptly.

Bunions

A *bunion* is a deformation in the part of the foot that is joined by the big toe. The swelling and pain at the joint is caused by inflammation of the *bursa* (a fluid-filled sac) that lubricates the joint. Although bunions often develop because of wearing shoes that frequently accompany flat feet, they most don't fit correctly. Pain that is not too severe can be relieved by the application of heat; the condition may eventually be cured by doing foot exercises recommended by a physician, who will also help in the choice of correct footwear. A bunion that causes acute pain and limping can be treated by a simple surgical procedure.

Calluses

A *callus* is an area of the skin that has become hard and thick as a result of constant friction or pressure against it. Pain results when the callus is pressed against a nerve by poorly-fitting shoes. A painful callus can be partially removed by rubbing it—very cautiously—with a sandpaper file or a pumice stone sold for that purpose. The offending shoes should then be discarded for correctly fitted ones. Foot care by a podiatrist is recommended for anyone with recurring calluses and corns (see below), and especially for those people who have diabetes or any disorder of the arteries.

Corns

A *corn* is a form of callus that occurs on or between the toes. When the thickening occurs on the outside of the toe, it is called a *hard corn;* when it is located between the toes, it is called a *soft corn.* The pain in the affected area is caused by pressure of the hard inside core of the corn against the tissue beneath it. The most effective treatment for corns is to wear shoes that are the right size and fit. Corns can be removed by a podiatrist or chiropodist, but unless footwear fits properly, they are likely to return.

Treatment: To remove a corn at home, the toes should be soaked in warm water for about ten minutes and dried. The corn can be rubbed away with an emery file, or it can be treated with a few drops of ten percent salicylic acid in collodion, available from any druggist. Care should be exercised in applying the solution so that it doesn't reach surrounding tissue, since it is highly irritating to normal skin. The area can then be covered with a corn pad to relieve pressure. This treatment may have to be repeated several times before the corn becomes soft enough to lift out. Diabetics or those suffering from any circulatory disorder should never treat their own corns.

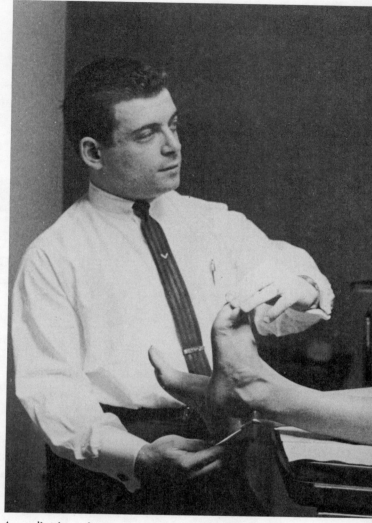

A podiatrist using a percussor to check reflexes.

Housemaid's Knee

Housemaid's knee is actually a form of *bursitis,* in which the fluid-filled bursa in front of the kneecap becomes inflamed by injury or excessive pressure, as because of constant kneeling. When the inflammation is mild, it can usually be corrected by rest. In the acute stage, the knee becomes swollen and painful, particularly when bent. It is especially prone to infection if scratched, bruised, or cut. Acute housemaid's knee is usually treated by anti-inflammatory type drugs, injections of cortisone, or by surgery under local anesthesia

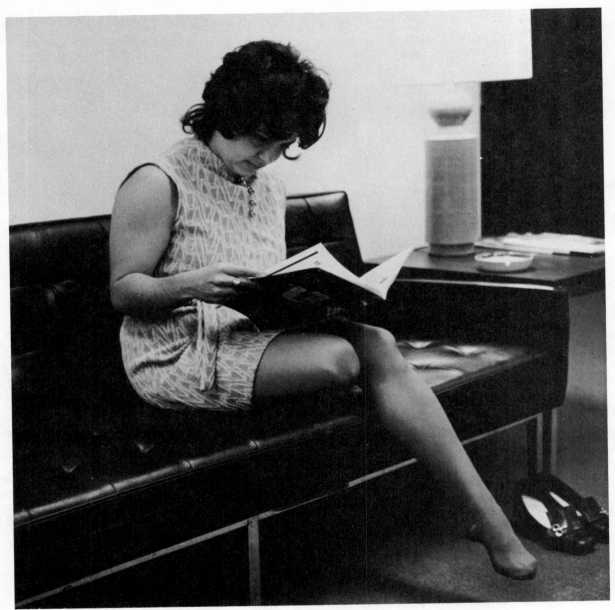

Sitting with a leg tucked under may feel comfortable for a while, but it is not recommended as a habit. It impedes circulation and may cause cramps.

in the doctor's office. Anyone whose daily activities involve a great deal of kneeling should make a habit of using a thick rubber mat.

Tennis Elbow

This disorder can affect not only tennis players but also people who have injured their elbow joint or subjected it to various stresses and strains. It may be a form of bursitis similar in nature to housemaid's knee, but it is more correctly called *tendonitis*, that is, an inflammation of the tendons which can affect any joint in the arms and legs. Rest and the application of heat usually relieve the painful symptoms. If the pain becomes acute, a doctor should be consulted.

Tenosynovitis

Tenosynovitis is an inflammation of a tendon sheath. One of the commoner sites of trouble is that of the wrist muscles. It can be caused by injury, infection, or constant use of the wrist muscles in piano-playing, typing, or some form of labor involving the wrist. The condition is usually treated by splinting the wrist and resting it for a while. Pain can be relieved with aspirin.

Writer's Cramp

Writer's cramp is a muscular pain caused by constant use of a set of muscles for a particular activity. The same set of muscles will function with no difficulty when the activity is changed. The best way to treat the discomfort is to give the muscles a rest from the habitual activity and to relieve the pain with heat and aspirin.

Other Muscle Cramps

A sharp cramp or pain in the leg muscles, and sometimes in the arm, can occur because blood circulation has been impaired, either by hardening of the arteries, or because of undue pressure, such as habitually sitting with one leg tucked under the upper thigh. The cramp is usually relieved by either changing the activity involved or by shifting the position of the affected limb. Constant or acute muscle cramps should be brought to the attention of a doctor.

The Exposed Integument

Common skin and scalp annoyances such as rashes, itches, dandruff, excessive perspiration, and infections of various kinds (such as athlete's foot and ringworm), as well as acne, wrinkles, and baldness, are discussed under *Skin and Hair,* p. 377.

Splinters

If lodged superficially in the hand, a splinter will usually work its own way out, but a splinter of no matter what size in the sole of the foot must be removed promptly to avoid its becoming further embedded by pressure and causing infection. The simplest method of removal is to pass a needle through a flame; let the needle cool; then after the skin surface has been washed with soap and water or swabbed with alcohol, press the point of the needle against the skin, scraping slightly until the tail of the splinter is visible and loosened. It can then be pulled out with tweezers that have been sterilized in boiling water or alcohol.

Hangnails

Hangnails are pieces of partly living skin torn from the base or side of the fingernail, thus opening a portion of the underskin to infection. A hangnail can cause considerable discomfort. It should not be pulled or bitten off; but the major part of it can be cut away with manicuring scissors. The painful and exposed area should then be washed with soap and water and covered with a sterile adhesive bandage. Hangnails are likely to occur when the skin is dry. They can therefore be prevented by the regular use of a hand cream or lotion containing lanolin.

"Normal" Disorders of the Blood and Circulation

Almost everybody is bothered occasionally by minor disturbances of the circulatory system. Most of the time these disturbances are temporary, and in many cases where they are chronic, they may be so mild as not to interfere with good health. Among the more common disturbances of this type are the following.

Anemia

Anemia is a condition in which there is a decrease in the number of red blood cells or in the hemoglobin content of the red blood cells. *Hemoglobin* is the compound that carries oxygen to the body tissues from the lungs. Anemia in itself is not a disease but rather a symptom of some other disorder, such as a deficiency of iron in the diet; excessive loss of blood due to injury or heavy menstrual flow; infection by industrial poisons; or kidney or bone marrow disease. A person may also develop anemia as a result of hypersensitivity (allergy) to various medicines.

In the simple form of anemia, caused by a deficiency of iron in the diet, the symptoms are rarely severe. There may be feelings of fatigue, a loss of energy, and a general lack of vitality. Deficiency anemia is especially common among children and pregnant women, and can be corrected by adding foods high in iron to the diet, such as liver, lean meat, leafy green vegetables, whole wheat bread, and dried peas and beans.

If the symptoms persist, a doctor should be consulted for diagnosis and treatment.

Varicose Veins

Varicose veins are veins that have become ropy and swollen, and are therefore visible in the leg, sometimes bulging on the surface of the skin. They are the result of a sluggish blood flow (poor circulation), often combined with weakened walls of the veins themselves. The condition is common in pregnancy and occurs frequently among people who find it necessary to sit or stand in the same position for extended periods of time. A tendency to develop varicose veins may be inherited.

Even before the veins begin to be visible, there may be such warning symptoms as leg cramps, feelings of fatigue, or a general achiness. Unless the symptoms are treated promptly, the condition may worsen, and if the blood flow becomes increasingly impeded, ulcers may develop on the lower area of the leg.

Treatment: Mild cases of varicose veins can be kept under control, or even corrected, by giving some help to circulation, as follows:

• Several times during the day, lie flat on your back for a few minutes, with the legs slightly raised.

• Soak the legs in warm water.

• Exercise.

• Wear lightly reinforced stockings or elastic stockings to support veins in the legs.

If varicose veins have become severe, a physician should be consulted. He may advise you to have injection treatment or surgery. See also p. 495.

Chronic Hypertension

Hypertension, commonly known as *high blood pressure,* is a condition that may be a warning of some other disease. In many cases, it is not in itself a serious problem and has no one underlying specific cause: this is called *functional, essential,* or *chronic hypertension.* The symptoms of breathing difficulty, headache, weakness, or dizziness that accompany high blood pressure can often be controlled by medicines that bring the pressure down, by sedatives or tranquilizers, and in cases where overweight is a contributing factor, by a change in diet, or by a combination of these.

More serious types of high blood pressure can be the result of kidney disease, glandular disturbances, or diseases of the circulatory system. Acute symptoms include chronic dizziness or blurred vision. Any symptoms of high blood pressure call for professional advice and treatment. A doctor should be consulted promptly.

Tachycardia

Tachycardia is the medical name for a condition that most of us have felt at one time or another—abnormally rapid heartbeat, or a feeling that the heart is fluttering, or pounding too quickly. The condition can be brought on by strong feelings of fear, excitement, or anxiety, or by overtaxing the heart temporarily with sudden exertion or

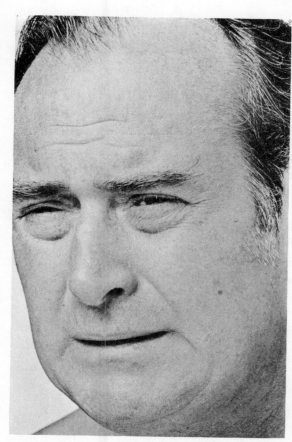

Symptoms of hypertension, or high blood pressure, include breathing difficulty, headache, and weakness. Medications can sometimes help control the condition.

too much exercise. It may also be the sign of heart disease, but in such cases, it is usually accompanied by other symptoms.

The most typical form of occasional rapid heartbeat is called *paroxysmal tachycardia*, during which the beat suddenly becomes twice or three times as fast as it is normally, and then just as suddenly returns to its usual tempo. When the paroxysms are frequent enough to be disturbing and can be traced to no specific source, they can be prevented by medicines prescribed by the doctor.

Nosebleed

Nosebleeds are usually the result of a ruptured blood vessel. They are especially common among children, and among adults

with high blood pressure. If the nosebleed doesn't taper off by itself, the following measures should be taken: the patient should be seated—he should not lie down—his clothing loosened, and a cold compress placed on the back of his neck and his nose. The soft portion of the nostril may be pressed gently against the bony cartilage of the nose for at least six minutes, or rolled wads of absorbent cotton may be placed inside each nostril, with part of the cotton sticking out to make its removal easier. The inserted cotton should be left in place for several hours and then gently withdrawn.

Fainting

Fainting is a sudden loss of consciousness, usually caused by an insufficient supply of blood and oxygen to the brain. Among the most common causes of fainting are fear, acute hunger, the sight of blood, and prolonged standing in a room with too little fresh air. Fainting should not be confused with a loss of consciousness resulting from excessive alcohol intake or insulin shock. A person about to faint usually feels dizzy, turns pale, and feels weak in the knees.

Treatment: If possible, the person should be made to lie down, or to sit with his head between his knees for several minutes. Should he lose consciousness, place him so that his legs are slightly higher than his head, loosen his clothing, and see that he gets plenty of fresh air. If smelling salts or aromatic spirits of ammonia are available, they can be held under his nose. With these procedures, he should revive in a few minutes. If he doesn't, a doctor should be called.

Troubles Along the Digestive Tract

From childhood on, most people are occasionally bothered by minor and temporary disturbances connected with digestion. Most of the disturbances listed below can

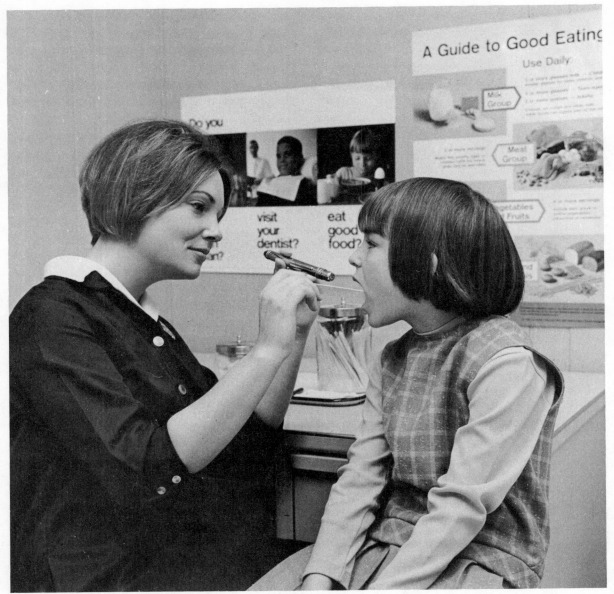

A school nurse examines a student's throat and mouth for inflammation or other symptoms of illness. Contrary to popular impression, a coated tongue is not necessarily a sign of illness.

be treated successfully with common sense and, if need be, a change in habits.

The Mouth

The digestive processes begin in the mouth, where the saliva begins chemically to break down some foods into simpler components, and the teeth and the tongue start the mechanical breakdown. Disorders of the teeth such as a malocclusion or poorly fitted dentures that interfere with proper chewing should be brought to the prompt attention of a dentist.

Inflammation of the gums: Also known as *gingivitis,* inflammation of the gums is caused by the bacteria that breed in food trapped in the spaces between the gums and the teeth. The gums become increasingly swollen, may bleed easily, and be sore enough to interfere with proper chewing.

The condition can be prevented by cleaning the teeth thoroughly and frequently, which includes the use of dental floss or the rubber tip on the toothbrush to remove any food particles lodged in the teeth after eating. Since gingivitis can develop into the more serious condition of *pyorrhea,* persistent gum bleeding or soreness should receive prompt professional treatment. See *Teeth and Gum Care,* p. 93.

Canker sores: Canker sores are small ulcers inside the lips, mouth, and cheeks. Their specific cause is unknown, but they seem to accompany or follow a virus infection, vitamin deficiency, or emotional stress. They may be additionally irritated by citrus fruit, chocolate, or nuts. A canker sore usually clears up in about a week without special treatment. A bland mouth rinse will relieve pain and, in some cases, speed the healing process.

Coated tongue: Although a coated tongue is commonly supposed to be a sure sign of illness, this is not the case. The condition may occur because of a temporary lack of saliva.

Glossitis: Glossitis, an inflammation of the tongue causing the tongue's surface to become bright red or, in some cases, glazed in appearance, may be a symptom of an infection elsewhere in the body. It may also be a symptom of anemia or a nutritional deficiency, or it may be an adverse reaction to certain forms of medication. If the inflammation persists and is accompanied by acute soreness, it should be called to a doctor's attention.

Halitosis or bad breath: Contrary to the millions of commercial messages on television and in print, bad breath cannot be cured by any mouthwash, lozenge, spray, or antiseptic gargle now on the market. These products can do no more than mask the odor until the basic cause is diagnosed and cured. Among the many conditions that may result in bad breath (leaving out such fleeting causes as garlic and onions) are

the following: an infection of the throat, nose, or mouth; a stomach or kidney disorder; pyorrhea; respiratory infection; tooth decay; improper mouth hygiene; and excessive drinking and smoking. Anyone who has been made self-conscious about the problem of bad breath should ask his doctor or dentist whether his breath is truly offensive and if it is, what to do about it.

Gastritis

Gastritis, one of the most common disorders of the digestive system, is an inflammation of the lining of the stomach which may occur in acute, chronic, or toxic form. Among the causes of *acute gastritis* are various bacterial or viral infections; overeating, especially heavy or rich foods; excessive drinking of alcoholic beverages; or food poisoning. An attack of acute gastritis may be severely painful, but the discomfort usually subsides with proper treatment. The first symptom is typically sharp stomach cramps, followed by a bloated feeling, loss of appetite, headache, and nausea. When vomiting occurs, it rids the stomach of the substance causing the attack but usually leaves the patient temporarily weak. If painful cramps persist and are accompanied by fever, a doctor should be consulted about the possibility of medication for bacterial infection. For a few days after an attack of acute gastritis, the patient should stay on a bland diet of easily digested foods, taken in small quantities.

Toxic gastritis: Toxic gastritis is usually the result of swallowing a poisonous substance, causing vomiting and possible collapse. It is an emergency condition requiring prompt first aid treatment and the attention of a doctor. See *Poisoning,* p. 686.

Chronic gastritis: Chronic gastritis is a recurrent or persisting inflammation of the stomach lining over a lengthy period. The condition has the symptoms associated with indigestion, especially pain after eating. It can be caused by excessive drinking of alcoholic beverages, constant tension or anxiety, or deficiencies in the diet. The most effective treatment for chronic gastritis is a bland diet from which caffeine and alcohol have been eliminated. Heavy meals should be avoided in favor of eating small amounts at frequent intervals. A tranquilizer or a mild sedative prescribed by a doctor may reduce the tensions that contribute to the condition. If the discomfort continues, a physician should be consulted about the possibility of ulcers. See under *Diseases of the Digestive System,* p. 522.

Gastroenteritis

Gastroenteritis is an inflammation of the lining of both the stomach and the intestines. Like gastritis, it can occur in acute or toxic forms as a result of food poisoning, excessive alcohol intake, viral or bacterial infections, or food allergies. Vomiting, diarrhea, and fever may be more pronounced and of longer duration. As long as nausea and vomiting persist, no food or fluid should be taken; when these symptoms cease, a bland, mainly fluid diet consisting of strained broth, thin cereals, boiled eggs, and tea is best. If fever continues and diarrhea doesn't taper off, a doctor should be called.

Diarrhea

Diarrhea is a condition in which bowel movements are abnormally frequent and liquid. It may be accompanied by cramps, vomiting, thirst, and a feeling of tenderness in the abdominal region. Diarrhea is always a symptom of some irritant in the intestinal tract; among possible causes are allergy, infection by virus or bacteria, accidentally swallowed poisonous substances, or excessive alcohol. Brief attacks are sometimes caused by emotions, such as overexcitement or anxiety.

Diarrhea that lasts for more than two days should be diagnosed by a physician to rule out a more serious infection, a glandular disturbance, or a tumor. Mild attacks

can be treated at home by giving the patient a light bland diet, plenty of fluids, and the prescribed dosage of a kaolin-pectin compound available at any drugstore.

Constipation

Many people have the mistaken notion that if they don't have a bowel movement every day, they must be constipated. This is not necessarily so. From a doctor's viewpoint, constipation is not determined by an arbitrary schedule of when the bowel should be evacuated, but by the individual's discomfort and other unpleasant symptoms. In too many instances, overconcern and anxiety about bowel movements may be the chief cause of constipation.

The watery waste that results from the digestion of food in the stomach and small intestine passes into the large intestine, or colon, where water is absorbed from the waste. If the waste stays in the large intestine for too long a time, so much water is removed that it becomes too solid and compressed to evacuate easily. The efficient removal of waste material from the large intestine depends on wavelike muscular contractions. When these waves are too weak to do their job properly, as often happens in the elderly or the excessively sedentary, a doctor may recommend a mild laxative or mineral oil.

Treatment: Constipation is rarely the result of an organic disorder. In most cases, it is caused by poor health habits; when these are corrected, the disorder corrects itself. Often, faulty diet is a major factor. Make sure that meals contain plenty of roughage in the form of whole-grain cereals, fruit, and leafy green vegetables. Figs, prunes, and dates should be included from time to time. Plenty of liquid intake is important, whether in the form of juices, soups, or large quantities of water. Scheduling a certain amount of exercise each day strengthens the abdominal muscles and stimulates muscle activity in the large intestine. Confronting the sources of worries and anxieties, if necessary with a trained therapist, may also be helpful.

An enema or a laxative should be considered only once in a while rather than as regular treatment. The colon should be given a chance to function properly without relying on artificial stimulation. If constipation resists these common-sense approaches, the problem should be talked over with a physician.

Hemorrhoids

Hemorrhoids, commonly called *piles,* are swollen veins in the mucous membrane inside or just outside the rectum. When the enlargement is slight, the only discomfort may be an itching sensation in the area. Acute cases are accompanied by pain and bleeding. Hemorrhoids are a very common complaint and occur in people of all ages. They are usually the result of straining to eliminate hard, dry stools. The extra pressure causes a fold of the membranous rectal lining to slip down, thus pinching the veins and irritating them.

Since hemorrhoids may be a symptom of a disorder other than constipation, they should be treated by a physician. If neglected, they may bleed frequently and profusely enough to cause anemia. Should a blood clot develop in an irritated vein, surgery may be necessary.

Treatment: Advertised cures should be avoided since they are not only ineffective but can cause additional irritation. Laxatives and cathartics, which may temporarily solve the problem of constipation, are likely to aggravate hemorrhoids.

If pain or bleeding becomes acute, a doctor should be consulted promptly. Treatment can be begun at home. Sitting for several minutes in a hot bath in the morning and again in the evening (more frequently if necessary) will provide temporary relief. Preventing constipation is of the utmost importance.

Anal Fissure

This is a condition in which a crack or split or ulcerated place develops in the area of the two anal sphincters, or muscle rings, that control the release of feces. Such breaks in the skin are generally caused by something sharp in the stool, or by the passage of an unusually hard and large stool. Although discomfort often accompanies a bowel movement when there is a fissure, the acute pain typically comes afterward. Healing is difficult because the injured tissue is constantly open to irritation. If the condition persists, it usually has to be treated by a minor surgical procedure. Intense itching in this area is called *anal pruritis.*

Minor Ailments in the Air Pipes

In addition to all the respiratory discomforts that go along with the common cold (see above, p. 410), there are various other ailments that affect breathing and normal voice production.

Bronchitis

Usually referred to as a chest cold, *bronchitis* is an inflammation of the bronchial tubes that connect the windpipe and the lungs. If bronchitis progresses down into the lungs, it can develop into pneumonia. Old people and children are especially susceptible to acute bronchitis. The symptoms include pain in the chest, a feeling of fatigue, and a nagging cough. If the infection is bacterial, it will respond to antibiotics. If it is viral, there are no specific medicines. The attack usually lasts for about ten days, although recovery may be speeded up with bed rest and large fluid intake.

Chronic bronchitis: Chronic bronchitis is a condition that may recur each winter, or may be present throughout the year in the form of a constant cough. The condition is aggravated by smoking and by irritants, such as airborne dust and smog. The swollen tissues and abnormally heavy discharge of mucus interfere with the flow of air from the lungs and cause shortness of breath. Medicines are available which lessen the bronchial phlegm and make breathing easier. People with chronic bronchitis often sleep better if they use more than one pillow and have a vaporizer going at night.

Coughing

Coughing is usually a reflex reaction to an obstruction or irritation in the trachea (windpipe), pharynx (back of mouth and throat), or the bronchial tubes. It can also be the symptom of a disease or a nervous habit. For a simple cough brought on by smoking too much or breathing bad air, medicines can be taken that act as sedatives to inhibit the reflex reaction. Inhaling steam can loosen the congestion (a combination of swollen membranes and thickened mucus) that causes some types of coughs, and hot drinks such as tea or lemonade help to soothe and relax the irritated area. Constant coughing, especially when accompanied by chest pains, should be brought to a doctor's attention. For a discussion of whooping

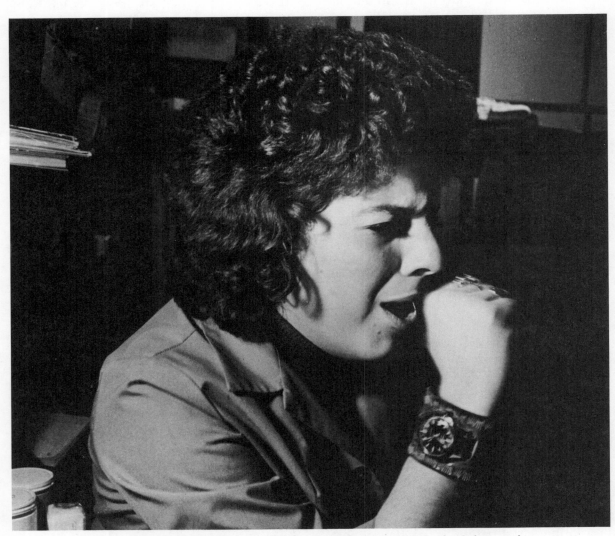

Irritation to the windpipe or to the soft, fleshy area at the back of the mouth induces coughing. Irritation is more likely to occur when throat tissues are dry.

cough and croup, see under *Birth, Infancy, and Maturation*, p. 99.

Laryngitis

Laryngitis is an inflammation of the mucous membrane of the larynx (voice box) that interferes with breathing and causes the voice to become hoarse or to disappear altogether. The condition may accompany a sore throat, measles, or whooping cough, or it may result from an allergy. Prolonged overuse of the voice, a common occupational hazard of singers and teachers, is also a cause. The best treatment for laryngitis is to go to bed, keep the room cool, and put moisture into the air from a vaporizer, humidifier, or boiling kettle. Don't attempt to talk, even in a whisper. Keep a writing pad within arm's reach and use it to spare your voice. Drinking warm liquids may help to relieve some of the discomfort.

Chronic laryngitis may result from too many acute laryngitis attacks, which can cause the mucous membrane to become so thick and tough that the voice remains permanently hoarse. The sudden onset of hoarseness that lasts for more than two weeks calls for a doctor's diagnosis.

Hiccups

Hiccups (also spelled *hiccoughs*) are contractions of the diaphragm, the great muscle responsible for forcing air in and out of our lungs. They may be brought on by an irritation of the diaphragm itself, of the respiratory or digestive system, or by eating or drinking too rapidly. Common remedies for hiccups include sipping water slowly, holding the breath, and putting something cold on the back of the neck. Breathing into a paper bag is usually effective because after a few breaths, the high carbon dioxide content in the bag will serve to make the diaphragm contractions more regular, rather than spasmodic. If none of these measures helps, it may be necessary to have a doctor prescribe a sedative or tranquilizer.

The Sensitive Eyes and Ears

Air pollution affects not only the lungs but the eyes as well. In addition to all the other hazards to which the eyes are exposed, airborne smoke, chemicals, and dust cause the eyes to burn, itch, and shed tears. Other common eye troubles are discussed below.

Sty

This pimplelike inflammation of the eyelid is caused by infection, which may be linked to the blocking of an eyelash root or an oil gland, or to general poor health. A sty can be treated at home by applying clean compresses of hot water to the area for about 15 minutes at a time every two hours. This procedure should cause the sty to open, drain, and heal. If sties are recurrent, a health checkup may be indicated.

Pinkeye

Pinkeye, an acute form of *conjunctivitis,* is an inflammation of the membrane that lines the eyelid and covers the eyeball, causing the eyes to become red and the lids to swell and stick together while sleeping. The condition may result from bacterial or viral infection—in which case it is extremely contagious—or from allergy or chemical irritation. A doctor should be consulted.

Conjunctivitis can be treated by washing the eyes with warm water, drying them with a disposable tissue to prevent the spread of infection, and applying a medicated yellow oxide of mercury ophthalmic ointment (as recommended by your physician) on the inner edges of the lids. This should be done upon rising in the morning and upon retiring at night. The eyes should then be closed until the ointment has spread. Apply compresses of hot water three or four times a day for five-minute periods.

Eyestrain

Eyestrain—with symptoms of fatigue, tearing, redness, and a scratchy feeling in

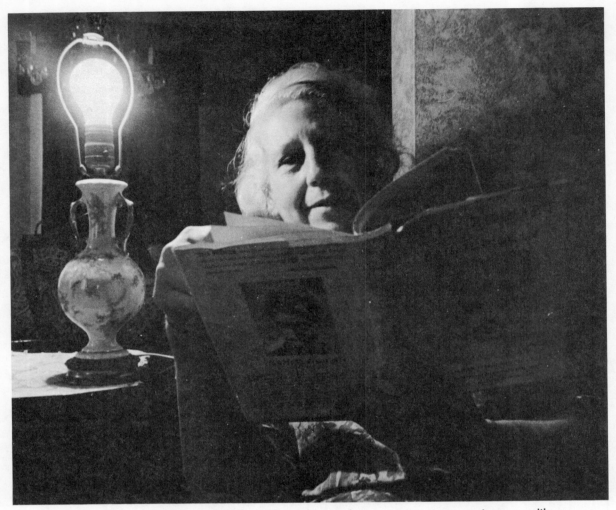

Reading with too dazzling a light, as this woman is doing, can cause eyestrain as readily as reading with too dim a light. The ideal reading environment is well-lighted but free of glare.

the eyelids—can be caused by a need for corrective glasses, by a disorder of the eye, or by overuse of the eyes that brings about fatigue. One of the most common causes of eyestrain, however, is improper lighting. Anyone engaged in close work, such as sewing or minature model building, and at all times when reading, should have light come from behind and from the side so that no shadow falls on the book or object being scrutinized. The light should be strong enough for comfort—not dazzling. Efforts should be made to avoid a shiny or highly polished work surface that produces a glare. To avoid eyestrain when watching tele-

vision, the picture must be in sharp focus; the viewer should sit at least six feet from the screen; and the room should not be in total darkness.

Ear Infections

Ear infections related to colds, sore throats, or tonsillitis can now be kept from spreading and entering the mastoid bone by the use of sulfa drugs and antibiotics. Any acute earache should therefore be called to a doctor's attention promptly. Aspirin can be taken for temporary relief from pain; holding a heating pad or a hot water bottle to the affected side of the face may also be helpful until proper medication can be prescribed.

Earwax

An excessive accumulation of earwax can sometimes cause pain as well as interfere with hearing. When the ear canal is blocked in this way, gently rotating a small wad of cotton may clean it. The ears should never be cleaned with sharp objects such as hairpins or matchsticks. If earwax has hardened too much to be removed with cotton, it can be softened by a few drops of hydrogen peroxide. When the wax is so deeply and firmly imbedded that it can't be removed at home, a physician may have to flush it out with a syringe.

Ear Blockage

A stopped-up feeling in the ear can be caused by a cold, and also by the change in air pressure experienced when a plane makes a rapid descent. The obstruction of the Eustachian tube can usually be opened by swallowing hard.

Ringing in the Ear

The general word for a large variety of noises in the ear is *tinnitus*. People who experience such noises describe the sounds in many ways: hissing, ringing, buzzing, roaring, whistling. When they are heard only occasionally for brief periods, without any other symptoms, they can be ignored. However, when they are constant, they should be considered a symptom of some disorder such as an infection, high blood pressure, allergy, or an improper bite (malocclusion). Sounds in the ears may also be caused by excessive smoking or drinking, or by large doses of aspirin or other medicines. In cases where the source of the ear disturbance can't be diagnosed and the noises become an unsettling nuisance, the doctor may recommend a sedative or tranquilizer.

The Path From the Kidneys

Cystitis

Cystitis is the general term for inflammation of the bladder caused by various types of infection. It is more common in women than in men. Infecting microbes may come from outside the body by way of the urethra, or from some other infected organ such as the kidney. When the bladder becomes inflamed, frequent and painful urination results.

Cystitis may also occur as a consequence of other disorders, such as enlargement of the prostate gland, a structural defect of the male urethra, or stones or a tumor in the bladder. Although there is no completely reliable way to prevent cystitis, some types of infection can be prevented by cleansing the genital region regularly so that the entrance of the urethra is protected against bacterial invasion. Cystitis is usually cured by medicines prescribed by a physician.

Prostatitis

Prostatitis is an inflammation of the prostate gland (present in males only), caused by an infection of the urinary tract or some other part of the body. It may occur as a result of venereal infection. The symptoms of painful and excessive urination generally respond favorably to antibiotics. *Acute prostatitis* is less common: the patient is likely to have a high fever as well as a discharge of pus from the penis. These symptoms should be brought to a doctor's attention without delay.

Excessive Urination

A need to empty the bladder with excessive frequency can be merely a nuisance caused by overexcitement or tension, or it can be the sign of a disorder of the urinogenital system. A doctor should be consulted if the problem persists.   EHH, Jr.

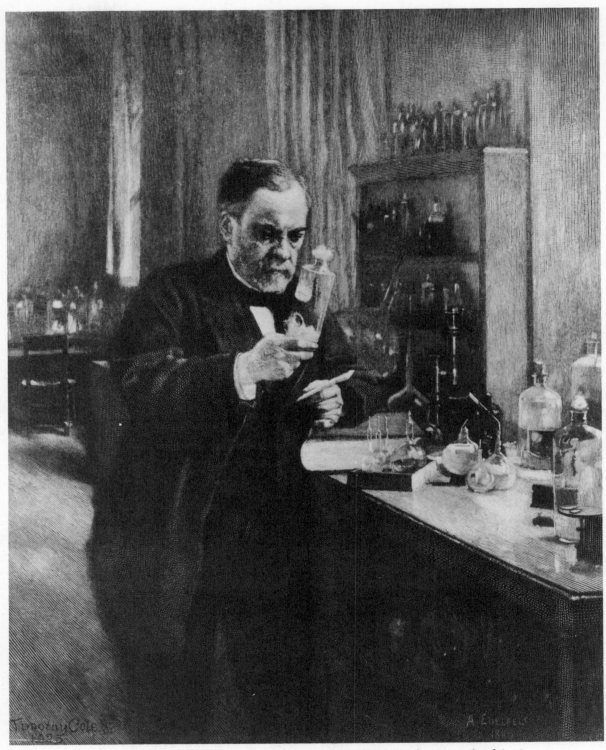

Much of our knowledge of bacteria comes originally from the research of Louis Pasteur (1822–1895). He proved that bacteria spread diseases, that the application of heat can kill germs (pasteurization), and that it is possible to immunize an animal against a disease by injecting it with weakened microbes (vaccination).

BIOLOGICAL CAUSES OF DISEASE

Cultivation

Bacteria are single-celled microscopic organisms that are shaped like rods, spheres, or spirals. Of the thousands of species and strains, only a small percentage cause disease. Most bacteria grow well in a dark, damp atmosphere at about the temperature of the human body. The bacteriologist cultivates them in test tubes (A) and glass Petri dishes (B) on special food called media. He watches for the formation of acid, alkali, or gas in the Smith fermentation tube (C). Bacteria enter the body through body openings such as the mouth and nose, and through wounds in the skin.

Bacteria

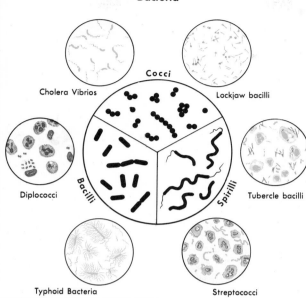

Cocci

Cholera Vibrios

Lockjaw bacilli

Diplococci

Bacilli

Spirilli

Tubercle bacilli

Typhoid Bacteria

Streptococci

Observation

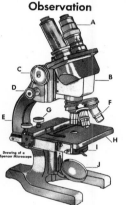

Drawing of a Spencer Microscope

THE MICROSCOPE

A. Eyepieces
B. Body
C. Coarse adjustment
D. Fine adjustment
E. Arm
F. Objectives
G. Mechanical stage
H. Stage
I. Condenser
J. Mirror

Transmission

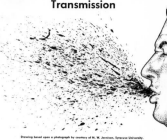

Drawing based upon a photograph by courtesy of M. W. Jennison, Syracuse University.

When a person talks, laughs, or sneezes, he expels droplets of saliva which carry great distances. These droplets carry germs, and if the person is sick, the germs may spread the sickness to other people when they are inhaled. Bacterial diseases are also spread by direct contact and by intermediate agents.

Infection

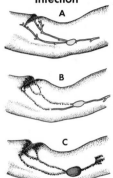

A

B

C

(A) represents an infected wound in which bacteria are growing. (B) shows the spread of infection through the lymph vessels. In (C) the bacteria have entered a lymph node (note swelling) and some have spread beyond toward a blood vessel. Infected wounds usually cause swelling, heat, redness, and pain.

Destruction

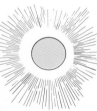
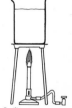

Boiling water (Also direct flame)

Germicides and Disinfectants

Sunlight (Ultraviolet)

Steam under pressure (Autoclave)

Worms

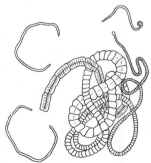

Worms, such as the tapeworm, hookworm, and round worm, are large enough to be seen without a microscope. They usually enter the body in food via the mouth and multiply in the intestines.

Protozoa

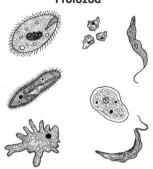

Protozoa are single-celled microscopic animals that enter the body through the mouth or insect bites. Malaria and amebic dysentery are caused by protozoa.

Fungi

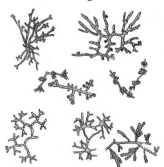

Fungi are many-celled microscopic plants larger than the bacteria. They cause many skin diseases, among the most widespread of which is ringworm (called "Athlete's foot" when on the feet).

Viruses

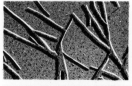
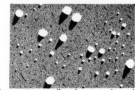

Viruses, too small to be seen through the ordinary microscope, may be seen and photographed by means of the electron microscope. They cause smallpox, rabies, and many other diseases.

Insect Carriers of Disease Germs

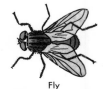

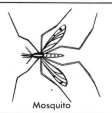

Fly

Flea

Tick

Louse

Mosquito

PHYSICAL AND CHEMICAL CAUSES OF DISEASE

(Typical Examples)

Physical

Mechanical Agents

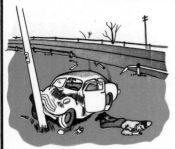 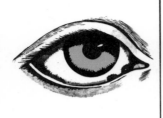

Disease can be caused by the widest variety of mechanical agents. At the left, the driver of an automobile involved in an accident has suffered concussion. Coal particles have lodged in the eye at the right and are causing irritation.

Motion

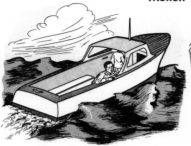 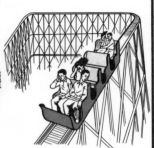

Uneven or unusual motion may cause disease in certain individuals. Motion sickness usually lasts only while the body is exposed to the motion. Seasickness and distress felt in a roller coaster are typical examples.

Temperature   Radiation   Electricity

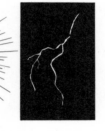

Diseases of various types may be caused by such physical agents as low temperature (freezing), high temperature (burning and scalding), radiation (sunstroke, X—ray burns), and electricity (shock and burns).

Pressure Changes

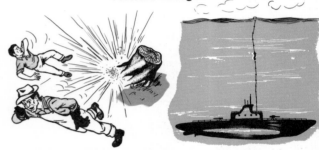

Life and health can be greatly endangered by pressure changes. At the left, two men are hit by the blast of an explosion. At the right, a man escapes from a sunken submarine but exposes his body to the direct and indirect danger of water pressure.

Chemical

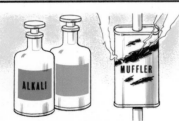

Inorganic Substances

Illness, injury or death may result from contacting, swallowing, or inhaling many chemical substances. Strong acids and alkalis are examples of such liquids. Carbon monoxide from internal combustion engines, such as in automobiles, represents one of the dangerous gases.

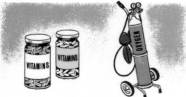

Deficiencies

Disease may be caused by the absence of or deficiency in certain essential substances. Numerous illnesses ranging from night blindness to rickets result from the lack of necessary vitamins in the diet. Likewise, an inadequate supply of oxygen will cause suffocation.

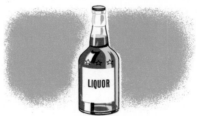

Alcohol

Alcohol is a habit-forming substance which in excessive amounts is harmful to health and shortens life. It depresses the nervous system, thus affecting mental functions, nerve control, and muscular coordination. Other effects may include lowered resistance to infection, diseases of the liver, kidneys, and heart.

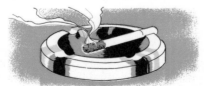

Tobacco

Persons who smoke excessively are not on the average as healthy as nonsmokers. Smokers have more heart and blood vessel disease as well as more cancer and other diseases of the lungs. From a health viewpoint, if you haven't started to smoke, don't—and if you have started, stop. Smoking definitely shortens life.

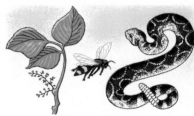

Organic Poisons

Many living plants and animals produce poisons which may cause serious illness and death in man. Among these are poison ivy and sumac and the venom of bees, snakes and lizards.

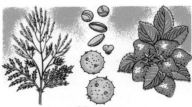

Allergens

Certain people react abnormally to foods and otherwise harmless materials. They are said to be allergic to these substances (allergens). Illustrated here are goldenrod, ragweed pollen and strawberries—common things to which many people are allergic.

FIRST AID
Control of Bleeding

Seriousness of Hemorrhage

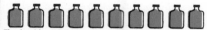

The healthy adult man has 1/13 of the weight of his body in pints of blood. Thus a man weighing 130 pounds would have 10 pints of blood.

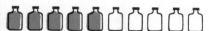

Loss of ½ or more of the blood is serious—often fatal. This amount can be lost in an incredibly short time (sometimes less than a minute) in severe bleeding. It is, therefore, clear that control of bleeding is one of the essentials of first aid. This chart illustrates the accepted methods for stopping external bleeding. In case of arterial bleeding, digital pressure should be used first, then direct pressure, and finally the tourniquet in case the others fail.

Internal bleeding, usually shown by bleeding from an orifice, such as an ear, cannot be controlled by any of these methods. A patient bleeding internally should be taken to a hospital immediately.

Kinds of Bleeding

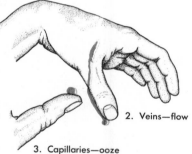

1. Arteries—spurt

2. Veins—flow

3. Capillaries—ooze

The type of blood vessel cut can be determined by the way in which blood is flowing from the wound. Arterial bleeding is much more serious than the others and must be stopped first.

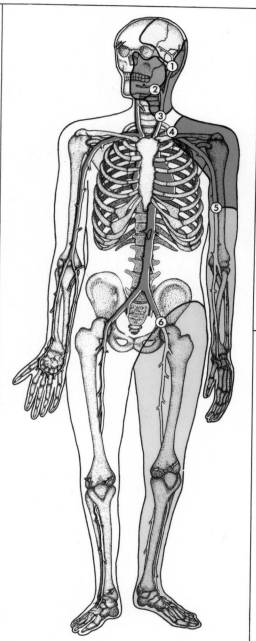

Direct Pressure

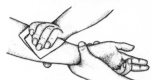

If digital pressure fails, or in case of venous bleeding, pressure should be applied directly to the wound, through a sterile gauze pad or a clean cloth. After the bleeding stops, a bandage may be applied.

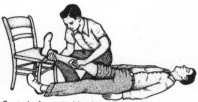

Control of venous bleeding may sometimes be brought about by elevation of the injured part.

A stimulant should never be given to an accident victim who is bleeding severely. It is also always necessary to watch for and prevent shock.

Using a Tourniquet

The tourniquet is a dangerous instrument and should be used only as a last resort to control arterial bleeding. These rules should be followed when using a tourniquet:
1. It should be at least 1½ inches wide.
2. It should be loosened for a few seconds at least every 20 minutes.
3. It should be placed one hand's breadth from the arm pit (arm) or the groin (leg).

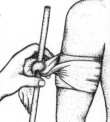

Arm

Leg

Digital Pressure
The Use of Pressure Points

Arterial bleeding may be controlled by applying pressure at certain points on the surface of the body where the main arteries are near the skin and lie close to a bone. These areas are known as pressure points. The six pressure points (duplicated on each side of the body) are illustrated in the central figure above and more complete description follows:

1.
Temporal is located in front of the ear on the cheek bone. It controls arterial bleeding above the eye and ear and halfway across the top of the head.
This area is shown in ☐ above.

2.
Facial is located on the jaw bone just in front of the curvature. It controls arterial bleeding halfway across the face below the level of the eye.
This area is shown in ☐ above.

3.
Carotid is located on the side of the neck just back of the windpipe. Compressing the carotid also shuts off the temporal and facial. It controls arterial bleeding in half of the entire head.
This area is shown in ☐ and , above.

4.
Subclavian is located in the hollow behind the collar bone. It controls arterial bleeding in the shoulder and arm. Compressing the subclavian also shuts off the axillary.
This area is shown in ☐ and ☐ above.

5.
Axillary is located on the inside of the upper arm about halfway between the shoulder and elbow. It controls arterial bleeding in the arm and hand.
This area is shown in ☐ above.

6.
Femoral is located in the middle of the groin. It controls arterial bleeding in the entire leg and foot.
This area is shown in ☐ above.

PREVENTION OF DISEASE

Natural Immunity and Resistance

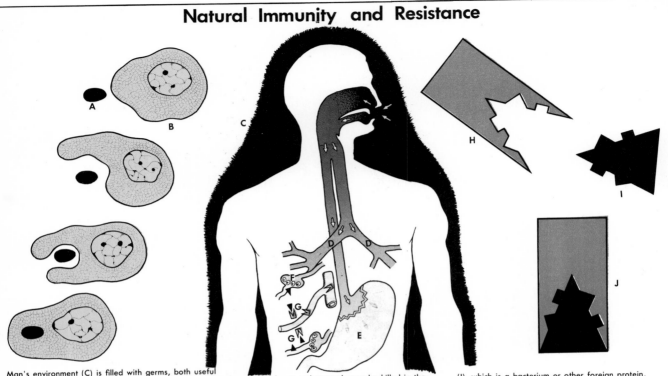

Man's environment (C) is filled with germs, both useful and harmful. The air he breathes and the food he eats bring them into his body. Many of the harmful germs are intercepted in the mouth and nose by mucous membranes extending into the lungs (D). Others are destroyed by acid in the stomach (E); those passing

beyond the lungs and stomach may be killed in the lymph nodes (F) or tissues (G) in either of two ways. In phagocytosis (left above), certain blood and tissue cells (B) engulf bacteria (A) and other foreign particles. In the antigen-antibody reaction (right above), an antigen

(I), which is a bacterium or other foreign protein, stimulates the body to produce a substance called an antibody (H). The antibody combines (J) with and neutralizes the antigen. An antibody can neutralize only that particular antigen which stimulated its production.

Passive Immunity

Active Immunity

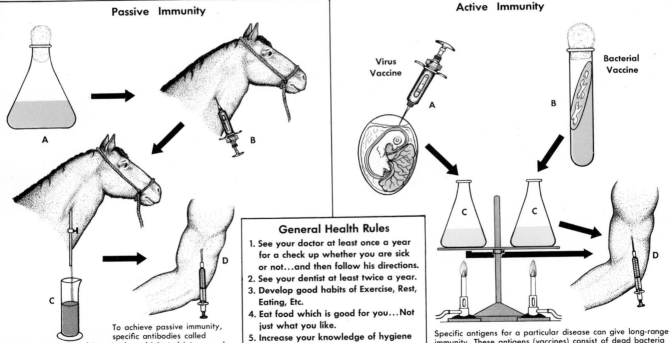

To achieve passive immunity, specific antibodies called antitoxins are produced in animals and injected into man. In (A) toxin-producing bacteria are grown in a flask. The toxin (an antigen) is separated from the bacteria and injected into horses (B). The horse builds up antitoxin in its blood. Blood is removed from the horse (C), the serum (containing antitoxin) is collected, purified, and injected into man (D) when needed. Immunity is temporary but is valuable in emergencies, such as after exposure to tetanus.

General Health Rules

1. See your doctor at least once a year for a check up whether you are sick or not...and then follow his directions.
2. See your dentist at least twice a year.
3. Develop good habits of Exercise, Rest, Eating, Etc.
4. Eat food which is good for you...Not just what you like.
5. Increase your knowledge of hygiene so you can help your doctor prevent disease.
6. Protect yourself from others who are sick.
7. Keep your body clean.
8. Take advantage of modern Medicines, Vaccines, Antitoxins, Etc.

Specific antigens for a particular disease can give long-range immunity. These antigens (vaccines) consist of dead bacteria or weakened viruses, and their injection is called vaccination. Immunity cased by vaccination is called active immunity. A virus is grown on living tissue such as a chicken embryo (A), then weakened with heat (C), chemicals, or exposure to ultraviolet light, and finally injected into man (D). Bacteria are grown (B), separated from the media, and killed by heat (C) or chemicals. The dead bacteria are injected into man (D)

CHAPTER 9

Disease

The Causes of Disease

When a person becomes sick, his life processes no longer function in a normal, balanced way. This malfunction, or disease, may involve the mind, the whole body, or just parts of the body.

Every illness is accompanied by the appearance of certain deviations from normal physical functions. These warning signals of disease have characteristic patterns referred to as symptoms and signs, and they aid doctors in *diagnosis*, the identification of disease. Once a person's illness is correctly diagnosed, doctors can foretell the probable course of the disease (*prognosis*) and prescribe the appropriate treatment (*therapy*). If the actual cause of the disease (*etiology*) is not known, doctors can still prescribe treatment to counter harmful body changes that may occur.

A *sporadic* disease is one that occasionally strikes a few persons in a community. An *epidemic* exists when a disease attacks a large segment of the population in a community within a short time. This is often the case with various types of influenza. Occasionally, the same disease spreads rapidly through several countries, an event described as a *pandemic*. Certain diseases, such as malaria, are always present in particular geographic areas, and these diseases are said to be *endemic* to that region. *Chronic* diseases are those that develop slowly and require long-term treatment, such as tuberculosis and psoriasis. *Acute* diseases are those that attack suddenly and progress rapidly, such as appendicitis. The period between the entry of a disease-causing organism in the body and the first onset of the symptoms of that disease is known as the *incubation period*.

A diseased portion of the body may influence the health of the rest of the body. Deterioration of the heart or arteries, for example, can reduce the blood flow to an arm or leg, which in turn reduces the supply of oxygen and nutrients to that limb. As a result, the afflicted limb will not heal easily if injured. Kidney or urethral stones can reduce the flow of urine to the bladder and thus increase the amount of urea in the blood, which results in uremic poisoning. Brain damage can affect all parts of the body.

Some diseases are the result of changes within the body itself, caused by aging, diet, physical damage, or other influences. Other

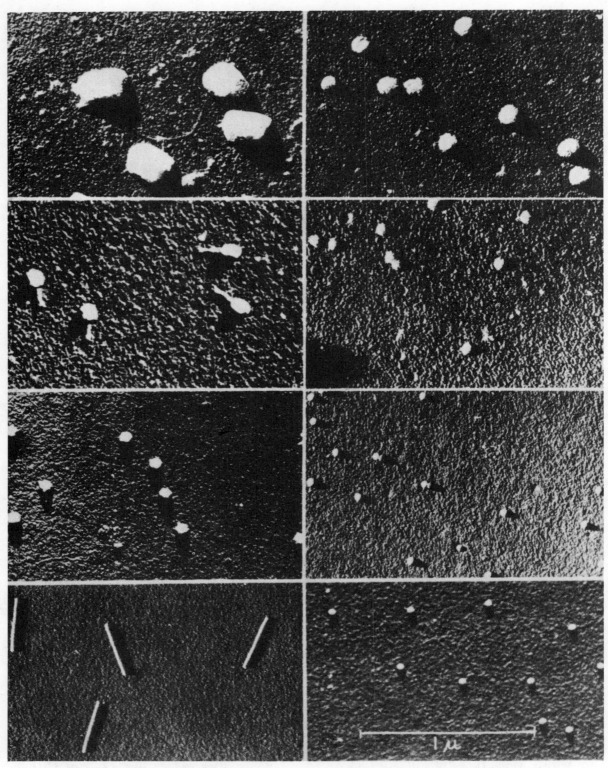

Micrographs (photographs of microscopic images) of viruses. The symbol μ in the lower right-hand box is the Greek letter mu, which stands for micron, 1/1000th of a millimeter, or less than 4/10,000ths of an inch. One can gauge from this how small are the viruses shown here.

diseases are the result of an invasion of the body by foreign life forms (*organisms*). These organisms may be large enough to be seen with the naked eye, as in the case of intestinal worms. They may be microscopic, as are bacteria, or so small they cannot be seen with a light microscope, as are the submicroscopic viruses. These disease-causing microorganisms have an intimate relationship with the body they inhabit, so that effective treatment is often a complex and difficult task.

Disease-causing organisms may be classified into the following several groups.

Viruses: These are the smallest known living organisms, and they are visible only under the electron microscope. Viruses cause a variety of infectious diseases, such as colds, mumps, and chicken pox. Their chief characteristic is that they multiply only in living tissue and thus cannot survive for long outside their host's body. The human body can be made immune to some viral diseases by the administration of *vaccines,* substances that trigger the body's virus-fighting mechanism before an infection actually occurs. Vaccination is a common practice in pediatric preventive medicine to protect children against smallpox, measles, and poliomyelitis.

Fungi: These are microscopic species of plant life, some of which can cause human diseases. *Histoplasmosis* is a chronic fungus disease of the lung, common in the southern United States. It may be mistaken for tuberculosis and is very difficult to treat. Another fungus disease, known as *ringworm* because of its red, circular ring of infection, may attack the scalp, skin, nails, or beard. The most common fungus disease in man is *athlete's foot* (ringworm of the foot), which attacks the sole of the foot and the area between the toes, causing reddening, cracking, scaling, and itching.

Parasites: These organisms thrive in the bloodstream or the digestive tract where they fulfill part of their normal life cycle.

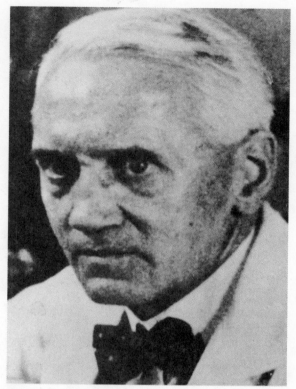

The bacteria-destroying capacity of the penicillin mold was discovered in 1929 by Sir Alexander Fleming (1881–1955). The subsequent development of penicillin to treat bacterial infections has saved an untold number of lives and must surely be considered one of the great medical achievements of this century.

Large wormlike parasites attach themselves to the digestive tract and drain away nutriments from the body. They vary in size from the two-millimeter long hookworm to the yard-long tapeworm. Other parasites, the malaria larvae, cause the typical chill and fever symptoms of that disease.

Cocci (singular *coccus*): These pus-forming organisms are responsible for a number of infectious diseases. Some examples are:

• *Staphylococcus,* which usually produces boils on the skin

• *Pneumococcus,* which is responsible for pneumonia

• *Gonococcus,* responsible for gonorrhea, the most common venereal disease

• *Streptococcus,* which causes such infections as strep throat and scarlet fever.

Bacilli: These microbes are large, elongated bacteria that may cause such diseases as diphtheria, dysentery, typhoid, and tuberculosis.

Spirochetes: These spiral-shaped organisms cause yaws and syphilis. They are identified by special blood tests and with the aid of a special microscope by which ultramicroscopic objects can be observed.

Rickettsiae: They resemble viruses in that they are very small, multiply only in living tissue, and are sometimes identified by means of an electron microscope. In North America, they are the cause of Rocky Mountain spotted fever, Q fever, and rickettsial pox.

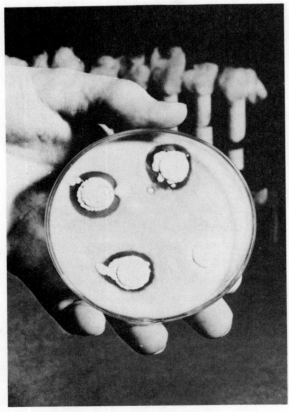

In screening for antibiotics, laboratory scientists use small disks of blotting paper saturated with experimental antibiotic solution. These disks are placed on the surface of "Petri" dishes seeded with bacteria. The potency of the antibiotic is detected by measuring the dark rings around the disks, which show that the antibiotic inhibited bacterial growth.

How Diseases Spread

Every infected person releases disease-causing organisms into the environment via the feces, saliva, blood, or discharges from the nose or mouth. The organisms enter a new victim primarily through the respiratory and urinogenital tracts, the mouth, or the skin. Infectious organisms may be acquired and carried from one person to another by blood-sucking insects, or they may be transmitted via blood donated for transfusions. In pregnant women, organisms can enter the unborn child via the placenta.

Food, water, and air are prime carriers of infectious diseases. Contaminated water, meat from diseased animals, and improperly cooked or preserved foods can introduce several deadly diseases into the body. Intestinal parasites in the muscle fibers of meat can remain viable if the meat is insufficiently cooked. One type of food poisoning caused by a species of the *salmonella* bacteria is often traced to improperly processed prepared foods.

Animals and human beings may spread diseases by direct contact with the source of infection, such as pets, rodents, insects, and food products. Some persons may carry a disease-causing microorganism (*pathogen*) without showing any symptoms or signs of the disease. Such human carriers can transmit diseases by direct physical contact or through the fine spray produced by coughing or sneezing.

Preventive Measures

Over the years, physicians have developed effective practices to prevent the transmission of disease from a sick person to a healthy one. Some of these techniques are discussed below under *Home Care of the Sick,* p. 446. However, both healthy and sick persons should take the following precautions to prevent the spread of disease and maintain good health:

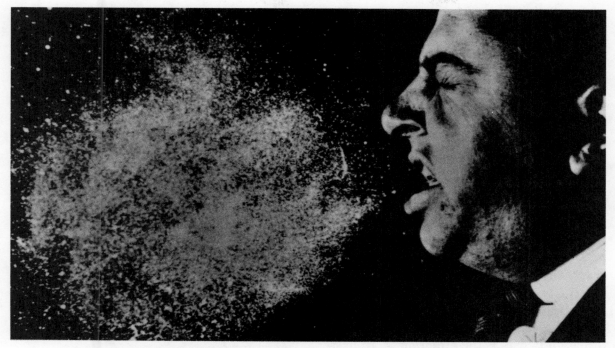

The fine spray of a sneeze disperses disease-causing microorganisms (pathogens) over a wide area. Insects, food, and direct contact are other ways in which disease is spread.

• Practice good personal hygiene habits, including brushing the teeth, bathing, cleaning hands and nails, and changing clothing regularly.

• Dispose of feces and urine in a flush toilet, chemical toilet, or at an isolated location sufficiently distant from water supplies. Using *germicides* (disinfectants) in toilet facilities reduces the germ population.

• Eat regular balanced meals to provide the body with the proper nutrition and the required amounts of vitamins, protein, and minerals.

• Avoid overindulgence in food, drink, and tobacco. Cirrhosis of the liver is associated with excessive drinking; cancer of the lung and heart disease have been linked to smoking; obesity has been associated with heart and circulatory diseases.

• Where possible, follow immunization schedules recommended by your physician and the United States Public Health Service.

• Have frequent medical and dental checkups even when you feel in perfect health. Your physician and dentist should be visited at least once a year.

• Avoid sexual promiscuity in order to reduce the possibility of acquiring and spreading venereal disease.

• Live in clean surroundings free of insects and rats.

• Maintain a regular schedule of moderate physical activity to preserve good circulation. Avoid excessive overwork and fatigue. Take time out for relaxation.

Recognizing Disease— Subjective Symptoms

When a person feels sick, he experiences changes in his normal state of well-being. These feelings are symptoms, called *subjective* because only the patient is aware of them. Almost all symptoms of disease fall into several broad categories.

Pain: This is the symptom that most often drives the patient to his doctor. Pain may be felt in various parts of the body and may vary in intensity and frequency. Chest pain is characteristic of some heart diseases. Abdominal pain may be an early warning sign of a serious gastrointestinal problem. Pain in the lower right abdomen may indicate acute appendicitis. Stones in the kidney or *ureter* produce flank pain.

Bleeding: Streaks of bright red or dark blood may appear in the stools or in the urine. Some women may bleed periodically between their menstrual cycles. A person may cough or vomit blood.

Gastrointestinal symptoms: Some digestive disorders lead to a loss of appetite (*anorexia*) followed by weight loss. Diarrhea, constipation, vomiting, and nausea are the most common symptoms of gastrointestinal disorders.

Urinogenital symptoms: Any difficulty in urination demands the attention of a physician. Typical symptoms include a burning sensation during urination, pus or blood in the urine, frequent urges to urinate, inability to empty the bladder, malodorous pus or bloody discharges, and small sores (*chancres*) at the external genitalia.

Miscellaneous symptoms: Among the other early warning signals of disease are dizziness (*vertigo*), general weakness, unsteady gait, tremors, abnormal increase in weight, fever or chills, constant sweating, discharges from ears and nostrils, swellings, boils, and abscesses. Lumps in the female breast may be indicative of benign or malignant tumors.

Diagnostic Procedures in Modern Medicine

Subjective symptoms are a valuable part of a patient's medical history, because they assist the physician in making an accurate diagnosis. It is advisable to make written notes of symptoms before visiting a physician. In making his diagnosis, the physician also relies on the clinical findings of a physical examination and on laboratory tests.

Methods of Clinical Diagnosis

In performing a physical examination, the physician looks for signs that provide objective evidence of disease, such as elevated temperature and high or low blood pressure. The four methods of clinical diagnosis are:

Visual inspection: With the help of special optical instruments the physician can examine the retina of the eye, the trachea, bronchi, urethra, stomach, and rectum. Every child knows the familiar command to say "Aaah," which permits a doctor to examine the throat for signs of reddening.

Feeling (palpation): By pressing and feeling the body, the physician is able to determine whether the shape, size, and lo-

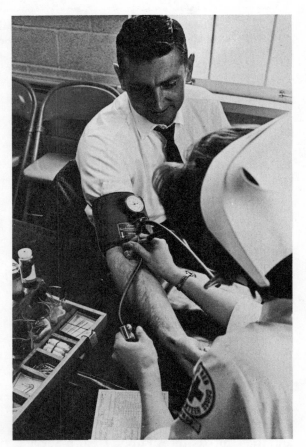

The taking of blood pressure depends upon listening to the sound of pumping blood—one illustration of listening (auscultation) used as a diagnostic tool.

cation of organs are normal or abnormal. He feels for glands and lymph nodes or for the enlargement of the prostate, uterus, spleen, or liver.

Listening (auscultation): The stethoscope is the basic instrument for studying the various sounds originating within the body. By listening to the sounds within the chest the physician can detect a normal or abnormal heartbeat. Rough breath sounds may indicate a respiratory tract infection. Multiple pregnancies are indicated when more than one fetal heartbeat is heard.

Striking (percussion): Parts of the body and body cavities resonate with a certain sound when tapped by special instruments or by the fingers. The sound of a chest or abdomen that contains fluid is different from the normal sound. The well-known test of the reflexes is performed by tapping the knee with a small rubber hammer.

Laboratory Tests

No matter how accurate a clinical diagnosis may be, a physician will still use laboratory tests to confirm his physical findings. He may call for one or more laboratory tests, which may be simple or quite complicated. Some of the diagnostic tests used in modern medicine are:

Blood analysis: Chemical analysis of the blood is used extensively to differentiate one disease from another. Blood chemistry will reveal higher than normal levels of blood sugar in diabetics. Anemia may be indicated by a decrease in red blood cells and hemoglobin. Leukemia may be suggested by an overproduction of white blood cells occurring with abnormal cell samples taken from blood-forming organs. The concentration of urea in the blood is an indication of kidney function and may be an early signal of gout. Blood-volume tests are used to determine the total amount of blood in the body. This test is important for patients who have lost blood during surgery or as the result of an accident.

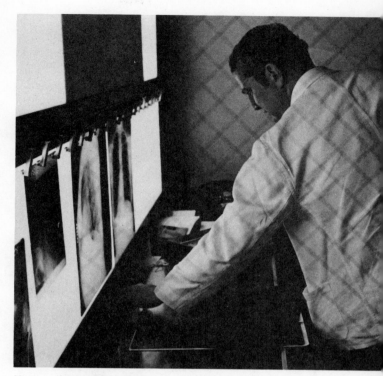

X rays, discovered in 1901 by Wilhelm Roentgen (or Röntgen, 1845–1923), have been increasingly diversified in use and are now indispensable in diagnosis.

A complete blood count (*CBC*) reveals the size, shape, and number of white cells, red cells, and platelets in a cubic millimeter of blood sample; a differential count determines the percentage of leukocytes and other cells. *Serological* studies are special blood serum tests of antigen-antibody reactions.

Urinalysis: Urine samples are tested for the presence of sugar and acetones, which may indicate a diabetic condition. Protein in the urine may signify kidney failure. Blood or pus in the urine are signs of other kidney or urinary diseases. The cloudy appearance of urine containing pus, the acidity of the urine, and its specific gravity all help the physician in making his diagnosis.

X-ray examination (radiology): This is the most useful tool for detecting abnormal anatomy and physiology. The X rays record the internal structure of the body on photographic film. The X-ray photograph, or

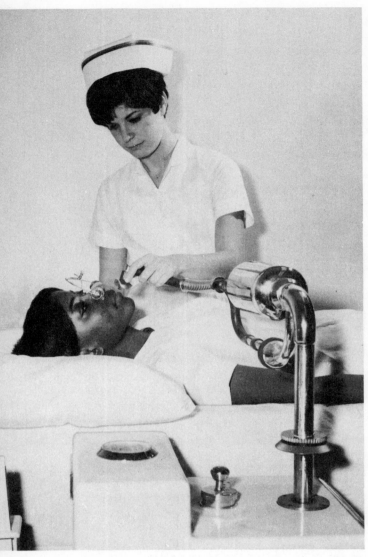

A student at a school for medical assistants administers a basal metabolic rate test to another student.

radiograph, is studied very carefully for any evidence of abnormality. Special techniques are used to X ray the circulatory system, the gastrointestinal system, and the spine. The diagnostician may also observe the X-ray image on a fluoroscope, a technique called *fluoroscopy.*

The nuclear age has added radioactive materials to the medical diagnostic tool kit. Some of these radioactive substances can be injected into the bloodstream to determine whether certain organs—such as the thyroid gland, liver, spleen, lungs, kidneys, and blood—are functioning properly. Such techniques permit doctors to study the structure and function of these organs in a way that would not be possible with conventional X rays.

Cerebrospinal fluid analysis: Samples of the clear colorless fluid that surrounds the brain and spinal cord can be withdrawn from the body by a spinal puncture and analyzed. Inflammatory conditions involving the central nervous system may be indicated by an increase in the cell count of the fluid. The presence of blood cells in the spinal fluid may signify damage to the brain or spinal cord, the result of certain types of strokes, or tumors. Bacteriological analysis may reveal infections. Chemical analysis is also usually performed.

Electrical activity: Electric impulses developed by the brain and by the heart muscle can be recorded graphically for analysis by specialists. *Electroencephalography (EEG)* records the electric signals given off by the brain. This technique involves placing electrodes on the scalp and recording the electric impulses, or brain waves, which are then interpreted by a neurologist. Graphic tracings of the currents developed by the heart muscle are recorded by a process known as *electrocardiography (EKG* or *ECG).* A graphic record, or *electrocardiogram,* is obtained through the use of metal electrodes attached to the chest wall and sometimes to the ankles. A cardiologist interprets the cardiogram to determine the functioning of the heart.

Hereditary and Congenital Diseases

Every person acquires certain characteristic traits from his parents—the color of skin, eyes, and hair, mental and emotional characteristics, blood grouping factors, and physique. The biological unit of inheritance

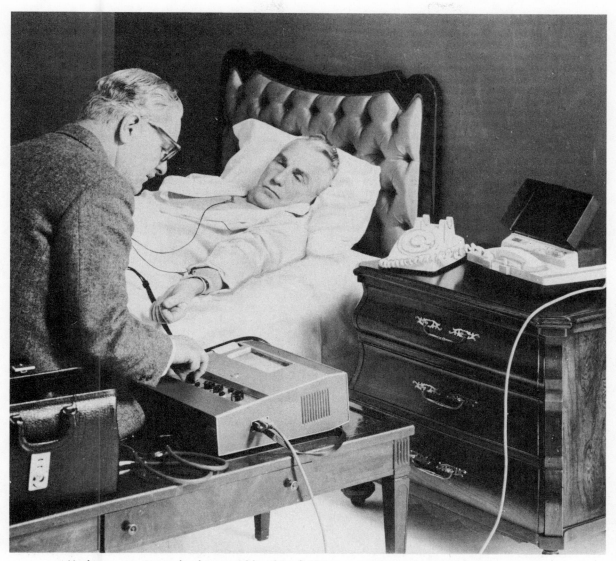

Modern computer technology enables this physician to send an electrocardiogram over an ordinary telephone line for analysis. Within minutes a report will be relayed to him.

(the *gene*) determines which of these characteristics are handed down from generation to generation.

An individual may also inherit certain illnesses from his parents, and these *hereditary* diseases may or may not manifest themselves early in life. Some hereditary diseases may skip one generation and show up in another. Among the more common hereditary diseases are sickle-cell anemia and hemophilia. Color blindness is also a common hereditary disorder.

Some birth abnormalities may originate during the development of the fetus, and these are classified as *congenital* abnormalities. Infectious diseases are the primary cause of congenital defects, venereal disease being one of the most significant. An infected mother may pass the disease to her unborn child via the placenta. German measles may cause congenital defects if the expectant mother contracts the disease during the first three or four months of pregnancy.

Home Care of the Sick

The physician must decide whether a patient can be treated at home or if his condition is serious enough to require hospitalization. For economic reasons some moderately serious diseases can be treated in the home, but regular visits by the family physician are necessary. A qualified nurse or nursing attendant can help to provide more effective home care.

Patients suffering from serious illnesses or from certain communicable diseases should be hospitalized. Home care facilities do not normally include the expensive and delicate medical equipment required for the complete care of these diseases. Communicable diseases require isolation and special disposal facilities to prevent the spread of the disease.

Home Care Supplies and Equipment

When caring for the sick in the home, certain supplies and items of equipment must be available in addition to a comfortable bed.

1. Disinfectants for soaking clothing and utensils used by the sick. Not all disinfectants are equally effective for every purpose. For clothing and food utensils, corrosive or poisonous disinfectants are to be avoided. Antiseptics do not kill bacteria; they only retard their growth. Among the common disinfectants that can be used in the home are:

• Alcohol, 75 percent by weight, used for disinfecting instruments and cleaning the skin

• Lysol for decontaminating clothing and utensils

• Soap with *hexachlorophene* (an antibacterial agent) for scrubbing the hands

• Carbolic acid (phenol) for disinfecting instruments and utensils. It is corrosive, poisonous, and very effective if used in 5 percent solution

• Cresol in 2.5 percent solution for disinfecting sputum and feces. It is less poisonous than phenol and can be obtained as an alkali solution in soap

• Boric acid, a weak antiseptic eyewash

• Phisoderm, a detergent cream, and Phisohex, a mixture of Phisoderm and 3 percent hexachlorophene. Both are proprietary products used to reduce skin bacteria.

2. Disposable rubber gloves, to be used when handling patients with open wounds or contagious diseases, as well as for cleaning feces.

3. Paper napkins and tissues for cleaning nasal and oral discharges.

4. Rectal and oral thermometers. The former is used primarily for infants, while the latter is used for adults and older children. Thermometers should always be thoroughly disinfected after use by soaking in isopropyl alcohol, and they should be washed prior to reuse.

5. Eating and drinking utensils to be used only by the patient. Disposable utensils are preferable.

6. Urinal, bedpan, and sputum cup for patients who cannot go to the toilet. After use, they should be thoroughly disinfected with cresol and washed with liquid soap containing hexachlorophene.

7. Personal toilet requisites: face cloths and towels, toilet soap, washbasin, toothbrush and toothpaste, comb, hairbrush, razor, and a water pitcher (if running water is not accessible to the patient).

8. Measuring glass graduated in teaspoon and tablespoon levels for liquid medication.

9. Plastic waste-disposal bags that can be closed and tied.

Nursing the Sick at Home

The sickroom should be one that is not used by other members of the family. Preferably, it should have its own toilet facilities. A cheerful decor and the sympathetic attitude of persons caring for the sick have a good psychological effect on the patient. Sickroom attendants should always wear clean clothing and scrub their hands before and after attending to the patient, so as to prevent cross-infection.

During the daily routine, the following written observations should be made:

1. The amount and kind of solids and liquids taken by the patient.

2. Bowel movement—frequency, consistency of stools, presence of blood.

3. Urination—frequency, amount, presence of burning sensation, color.

4. Morning, noon, and evening body temperature. The body temperature of a healthy adult varies within one or two degrees of 98.6° Fahrenheit (37° Centigrade). Normal rectal temperature for most people is ½ to 1 degree higher than the oral temperature. For infants a 100° temperature may be considered normal.

5. General mental and physical condition of the patient—subjective symptoms, irritability, cheerfulness, attitude.

6. Hours of sleep.

7. Medications administered. Medications should be given only on the instructions of the physician.

Disposal of body refuse from the sick should include disinfecting the utensils with a 2.5 percent solution of cresol and washing them very thoroughly with liquid soap containing hexachlorophene. The toilet bowl and seat should also be washed daily and rinsed with cresol or Lysol after each use by the patient. Eating and drinking utensils can be washed with liquid soap containing hexachlorophene and boiled for 30 minutes. Using disposable utensils eliminates the necessity for this procedure. Clothing and linens should be soaked in a disinfectant before being stored for separate laundering. All disposable items should be placed in a plastic bag which should be sealed before being thrown away or incinerated.

Daily sickroom duties should include changing bed clothing, which may require rolling the patient to one side of the bed to

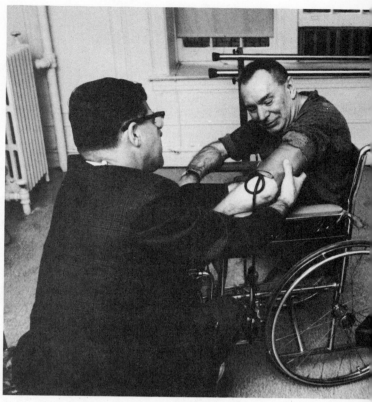

Many chronic diseases can be treated in the home. Some hospitals have a department of home care for this purpose, scheduling regular visits by physicians.

remove half of the linens, then rolling him to the other side to complete the operation. Daily attention to personal hygiene—washing, toothbrushing, hair combing, and shaving are important to the health and well-being of the patient. These personal attentions should be followed by rubbing the elbows, shoulders, back, and heels with alcohol or soothing lotion. The floor, furniture, windows, and walls should be cleaned and dusted frequently.

Sickroom personnel should not attempt to diagnose the patient's illness and should refrain from discussing the illness with the patient himself. By observing the directives of the physician with special reference to diet and medication, home care of the sick may follow the hospital pattern in helping the patient along the road to recovery and good health.   AAD

DISEASES OF
THE SKELETAL SYSTEM

Birth Defects

As the fetus develops in the womb, its bony skeleton first appears as soft cartilage, which hardens into bone before birth. The calcium content of the mother's diet aids the fetus in bone formation and in the development of the normal human skeleton. Thus the basic skeletal structure of an individual is formed before his birth. In some instances, the bones of the fetus develop abnormally, and such defects are usually noticeable soon after delivery.

The causes of skeletal birth defects are not always known. Some may be due to hereditary factors; others have been traced to the mother's exposure to X rays, atomic radiation, chemicals, drugs, or to disease during pregnancy. Among the more common birth defects are extra fingers, toes, or ribs, or missing fingers, hands, toes, feet, or limbs. Sections of the spine may be fused together, often without causing serious problems later in life, although some fused joints can hinder the motion of limbs. The sections of the skull may unite prematurely, retarding the growth of the brain.

Bone Disorders and
Dietary Problems

Since bone consists of living cells, it is constantly changing as old cells die and new cells take their places. Any systemic disease during the growing period may temporarily halt the growth of long bones. As the aging process continues, dead bone cells are not replaced as consistently as in earlier life. The bony skeleton thus loses some of its calcium content, a process known as *decalcification* or *bone atrophy,* and the bones become fragile.

Osteoporosis: This metabolic disorder is marked by porousness and fragility of the bones. When the condition is associated with old age, it is referred to as senile *osteoporosis.* Its exact cause is not known, but protein deficiency, lack of gonadal hormones, or inadequate diet may be contributing factors.

Osteoporosis can originate in youth from improper metabolism of calcium or phosphorus, elements necessary for healthy bones. It can also result from a deficiency in the sex hormones, androgen and estrogen—which is why it often appears after menopause. Another cause is atrophy due to disuse and lack of stress and strain on the bones.

Osteogenesis imperfecta: During the formation and development of bones, a process called *osteogenesis,* the bones may grow long and thin but not to the required width, becoming brittle so that they fracture easily. This condition is known as *osteogenesis imperfecta.* The individual may grow out of the condition in the middle twenties after suffering numerous fractures while growing up. A child thus afflicted cannot participate in games or other strenuous physical activities.

Paget's disease: Paget's disease is characterized by a softening of the bones followed by an abnormal thickening of the bones. Its cause is unknown, and it manifests itself after the age of 30. It may cause pain at the thighs, knees, or legs, as well as backache, headache, and general fatigue. Symptoms include deafness, deformity of the pelvis, spine, and skull, and bowed legs. Although there is no known cure, Paget's disease is not usually fatal, but is eventually disabling.

Osteomyelitis: Osteomyelitis is an inflammation of the bone caused by fever-inducing (*pyrogenic*) microorganisms. The microbes reach the bone from infected tissues through the bloodstream. The infection can originate from wounds, compound fractures, or respiratory infections.

Diet

A proper diet is necessary to maintain the health of the skeletal system. The body's retention of the bone-building minerals, phosphorus and calcium, depends on vitamin D, which is manufactured in the human skin through the action of the sun's ultraviolet radiation.

Rickets: An insufficient supply of vitamin D and a lack of exposure to sunlight leads to a vitamin-deficiency disease known as *rickets.* It can occur in infants and small children who live in northern latitudes and thus are not exposed to sufficient sunlight to permit their body to manufacture vitamin D. Rickets slows growth and causes bent and distorted bones and bandy legs. Symptoms first appear between the age of six months and the end of the first year. If rickets is recognized in time, it can be cured by a diet containing adequate vitamin D and by exposure to sunlight. If the disease is unchecked, the bones may develop permanent curves.

Joint Diseases

Arthritis

Many types of *arthritis* and related disorders give rise to painful inflammation of the joints. The most common is *rheumatoid arthritis,* which involves spontaneous changes in the musculoskeletal system. Arthritic symptoms can also result from infectious diseases such as gonorrhea and tuberculosis, or diseases such as gout, psoriasis, and rheumatic fever.

Rheumatoid arthritis: This is a chronic disease, the most prominent symptoms of which are usually pain and swelling of the joints of the fingers, wrists, knees, and feet. Other symptoms may include fatigue, weakness, fever, and warm, red, or swollen joints.

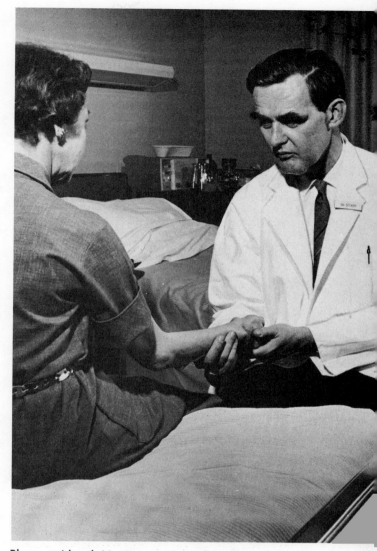

Rheumatoid arthritis causes pain and swelling of the joints. Here a patient's wrist and hand, typical sites of the disease, are examined by a physician. Rheumatoid arthritis is more common in women than in men.

Pain in the joints leads to spasms of adjacent muscles and the characteristic feeling of stiffness. Physical activity reduces the feeling of stiffness, while lack of exercise tends to increase stiffness and pain.

The cause of the disease is unknown, and it usually develops slowly over a period of months or years. Its onset may be triggered by physical or emotional stress. The disease is much more frequent among women than men. The symptoms may increase or de-

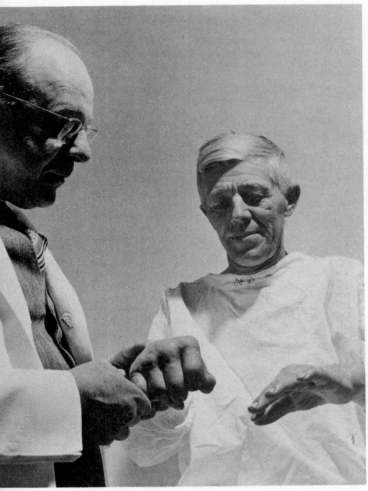

Because arthritic joints become painful and stiff, many patients tend to avoid movement and exercise, causing adjoining muscles to stiffen. Exercise of affected joints is beneficial, and arthritis patients must overcome their reluctance to move these joints.

crease spontaneously and unpredictably. There is even a chance that the disease will disappear completely during the first year after its onset.

The available methods of treatment do not cure the disease but relieve the symptoms so that the pain is reduced and normal movement is facilitated. Proper nutrition, heat, rest, and exercise are also helpful. A number of drugs can reduce the inflammation of the joints, but they may have undesirable toxic side effects. Accordingly, before any drug therapy is embarked upon, the patient should seek the advice of a physician specializing in arthritic disorders.

The most common drug used to treat arthritis is aspirin, which may have to be taken in high doses. Occasional side effects include gastrointestinal bleeding and buzzing in the ears. The cortisone-type (steroid) drugs have proven effective in controlling severe cases of the disease. They can be given orally or injected directly into the joints. However, these drugs generate a number of undesirable side effects, and withdrawal often results in a severe recurrence of the original symptoms. Thus, steroid drug therapy is a long-term process that can make the patient totally dependent on the medication.

Steroids are more useful in treating arthritic children, who have a better tolerance for them. About three-fourths of the cases of juvenile rheumatoid arthritis disappear spontaneously. If the disease persists, it tends to retard the child's growth and development.

Exercise of the arthritic joint helps prevent the adjoining muscles from shrinking and weakening. Patients tend to avoid moving the arthritic joint because of pain and stiffness, but this reluctance should be overcome, and the joint should be exercised within the tolerable limits of pain. A program of physiotherapy—including hot packs and exercise—can be extremely helpful.

Osteoarthritis: Osteoarthritis, arthritis of the bone, is a degenerative joint disease found in middle-aged persons, usually over age 40. Wear and tear on joints is the chief cause, and as one ages, tissue-repair capacity lessens. Thus joint damage from a torn ligament or rheumatoid arthritis may eventually lead to osteoarthritis.

The symptoms come on gradually over a period of many months, with pain and limitation of joint movement. Mild attacks usually require no treatment. Severe cases require aspirin, pain-killing drugs, physiotherapy, and weight loss to reduce the load on the affected joints. Joint destruction, especially in the hip, may require prosthetic replacement.

Pyrogenic arthritis: This fever-inducing condition is a result of microbial infection. The arthritic-causing organisms infect the joints and induce fever and pain with limitation of joint movement by muscle spasm and swelling. As in most infections, the treatment includes bed rest and antibiotics. If untreated, joint destruction is possible.

Gout

Gout is a metabolic disease common in men over age 40; it may also occur in women after menopause. The disease is con-

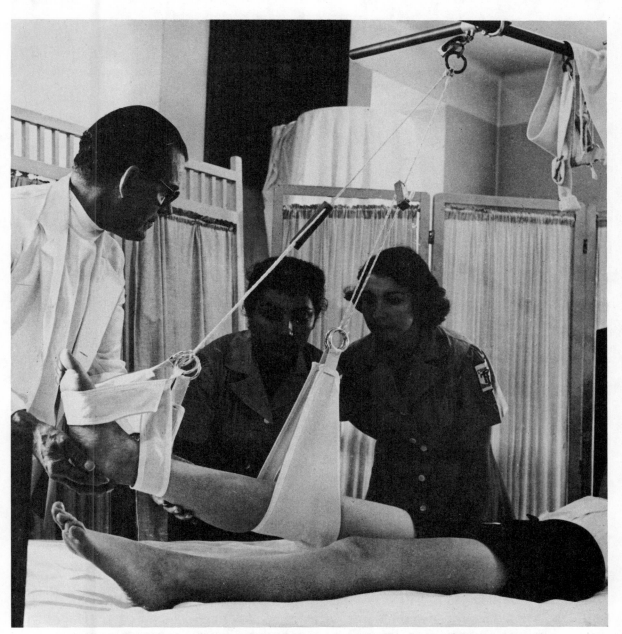

Physical therapy can often bring about significant improvement in arthritis patients. Here a physical therapist demonstrates the use of a pulley device in a program of exercises.

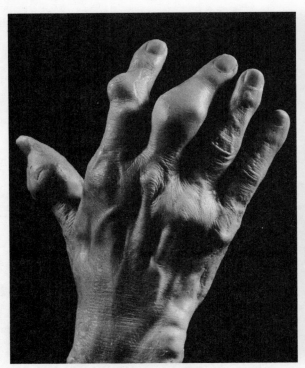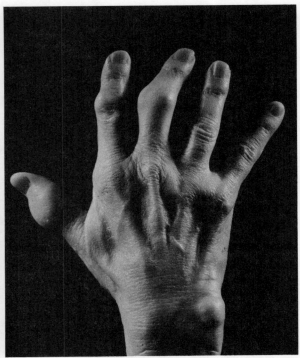

The hand of a gout patient (*left*). Excess uric acid causes crystals to form around the joints, producing the swellings characteristic of this disease. At right, the same hand after treatment.

sidered hereditary, and is associated with an excess of uric acid in the blood from abnormal metabolism of urea. An excess of vitamin D contributes to the development of gout.

Urea deposits in the joints, kidneys, and external ear herald the onset of the disease. The early symptoms, which may disappear and reappear, include pain at night and swollen joints, especially in the big toe. Certain drugs, such as Colchicine, Benamid, Alopurinal, or a combination of them, may be useful in controlling gout over a period of time. They should be taken, of course, under a physician's supervision. Untreated gout may lead to severe joint destruction.

Bursitis

The *bursa* is a fluid-filled sac located in the muscle near most joints. The fluid lubricates the joint, thereby providing smooth joint movement. Infection or injury may cause inflammation of the bursa. This con-

dition is known as *bursitis* and can be very painful. Most commonly affected are the shoulder, knee, and hip.

Calcium deposits in the shoulder tendon or calcification of the bursa (*calcific bursitis*) leads to more painful shoulder problems. This may be similar to *interstitial calcinosis,* a condition in which calcium deposits are found in the skin and subcutaneous tissues of children. Recovery from calcific bursitis is achieved by medical care, minor surgery, and resting the inflamed joint. Radiation treatments can sometimes speed the recovery process.

Injury to Joints

Injury (*trauma*) to joints should not be taken lightly, especially if pain persists. Youngsters very often indulge in rough play —tackling on the football field, hockey, tree climbing—which may result in injury. Broken bones (*fractures*) and displaced joints (*dislocations*) may remain undiagnosed and untreated even in adults, who may not consider the injury serious enough to obtain medical advice.

Untreated joint injuries can mean that fractures and dislocations heal with the bones out of alignment. Permanent deformity and *traumatic arthritis* are two possible complications.

Fractures and Dislocations

A fracture is a break in a bone as a result of injury or pathological weakness. Tumors, for example, can destroy bones to such an extent that a spontaneous fracture occurs due to pathological weakness. Osteoporosis (see above) can also cause such fractures.

Kinds of Fractures

Incomplete fractures are those which do not destroy the continuity of the bone. In a *complete fracture,* the bone is completely broken across. A *simple* or *closed fracture* is one in which the fragments are held together under the surface of the skin by the muscles and soft tissues. In a *compound* or *open fracture* one or both fragments pierce the skin, resulting in an open wound. In some cases the bony fragments can be seen protruding through the skin.

Comminuted fractures are the result of crushed bones. Several fragments appear at the trauma site. *Greenstick fractures* occur when one side of the bone is broken and the other bent. This type of fracture is more common in long bones, especially the forearms, clavicle, and legs of young children.

Dislocations

A dislocation is a displacement of any part, especially a bone. During this process the joint-capsule ligaments and muscle may be torn. The displaced bones must be reset by a bone specialist in their original position and immobilized until healing is complete. If this is not done, there is every possibility that the unhealed muscles will

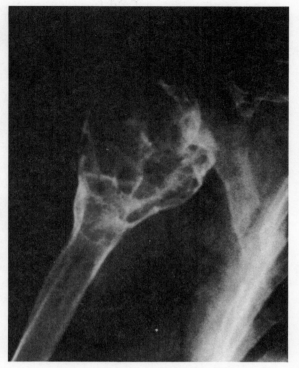

A bone tumor of the upper humerus (bone leading from elbow to shoulder). Tumors can destroy bones so extensively that a spontaneous fracture results.

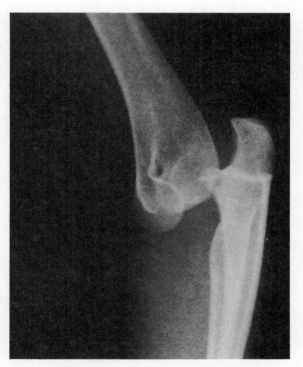

A dislocation at the elbow joint. Dislocated bones must be reset by a bone specialist and immobilized.

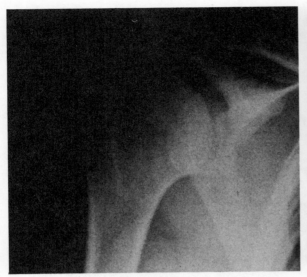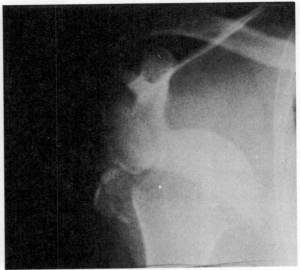

A normal shoulder (*left*) and a fracture/dislocation of the shoulder joint (*right*). Injuries in contact sports can be minimized if players wear the proper protective equipment at all times.

not provide the necessary support, thereby causing chronic spontaneous dislocation.

Athletic Injuries

Anyone involved in strenuous sports can suffer fractures, dislocations, torn cartilage, and other injuries. These injuries are not confined to the professional athlete; in fact, amateur athletes often lack the body conditioning and equipment that save professional players from injury. Knee fractures and torn knee cartilage are common injuries. These injuries can be serious in view of such possible complications as osteoarthritis.

Medical care should always be sought following a serious accident at play or on the athletic field. Children sometimes conceal injury for fear of parental punishment. A babysitter may be reluctant to report a child's accident or fall. Children should always inform their parents of falls and spills. This will permit early treatment of fractures and dislocations and avoid permanent deformity and traumatic arthritis.

Healing of Fractures

When a bone breaks, new bone cells called *callus* are laid down at the ends of the fracture to unite the fragments. This is the beginning of the healing process, the speed of which is dependent on the nature of the fracture.

Simple, incomplete, and greenstick fractures heal readily. However, compound fractures have wounds and fragments to complicate the healing process. Cleaning and suturing the wound and administering antibiotics reduce the chance of infection and promote healing.

Comminuted fractures may have to be disimpacted and all fragments reset, usually by an orthopedic or general surgeon. Some very serious fractures of the extremities may require surgical insertion of metallic pins, nails, plates, wires, or screws to hold the fragments in proper position, thereby promoting rapid healing with minimal deformity. Such devices must be made from corrosion-free and rustproof metals since they may remain in the body for a few months or throughout the person's lifetime.

Age and the healing process: The age of the fracture victim determines the speed of healing. In healthy, normal children, broken bones mend quickly because a rapid bone-cell manufacturing process is constantly in progress during the growth of the child. This is further advanced by proper diet, including daily intake of milk and milk products to provide the calcium required to build healthy bones.

In younger adults, new bone cells do not develop as rapidly as in the growing child, but under normal circumstances, this will not present problems with the healing of fractures. Fractures in the aged heal slowly or not at all, depending on the age and health of the individual.

Treatment of fractures: Correction of a fracture or dislocation is called *reduction* and is usually performed by an orthopedic surgeon. Bones that are merely cracked do not require reduction; they heal with the aid of immobilization. More serious fractures require manipulation, pressure, and sometimes, as mentioned above, wires, pins, nails, and screws, to bring the fragments together so that they can unite.

Healing of fractures and dislocations following reduction requires proper immobilization, which also reduces pain by preventing movement of the fragments. Immobilization is usually accomplished by the use of splints or plaster casts, or by applying *traction*. Traction subjects the fractured member to a pulling force by means of a special apparatus, such as a system of weights and pulleys.

After a fracture or dislocation is reduced and immobilized in a cast, the injury is X-rayed to insure that the immobilized reduction will heal without deformity. If the reduction is not satisfactory, the cast is removed, the fragments are remanipulated to provide better reduction, and a new cast or bandage is applied. Periodic X-ray rechecks help the doctor ascertain the degree of new bone formation as the healing continues. Casts are also checked to make sure there is not excess swelling of tissues and compression of blood vessels in the area.

How long a cast remains on depends on the extent of the injury and the rapidity of healing. A broken wrist may heal in four to

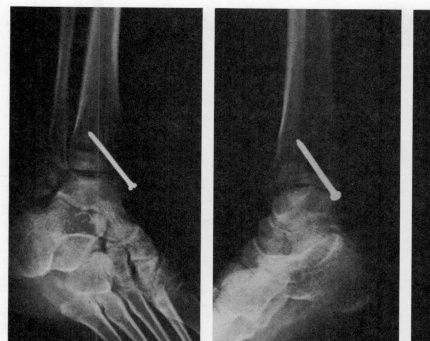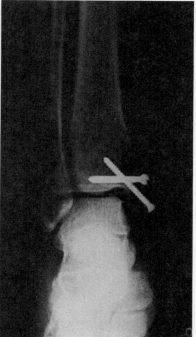

Surgical insertion of screws may be required in certain serious fractures to hold fragments in proper position. Shown here are X rays of ankle fractures reset and secured by screws.

six weeks while a fractured tibia may require four months of immobilization in a plaster cast.

Amputation

Clogging or blockage of blood vessels reduces or cuts off the supply of blood to an extremity. When this happens, tissues below the blockage may die, and wounds will not heal due to lack of oxygenated blood and nutrition. Industrial and automobile accidents, frostbite, and crush injuries may make healing impossible. *Gangrene,* or the death of soft tissues, can sometimes result from injury, infection, or severe circulatory disturbance.

In all these instances, in order to save the person's life, the surgeon may have to *amputate* the extremity just above the site of trauma or blockage and at a location that will make the healing process possible. Following some amputations the patient may be fitted with a *prosthetic* device, an artificial limb. For below-the-knee amputations, artificial legs and feet are commonly used.

Pelvis and Hip Disorders

The hip joint presents most of the problems in the pelvic area. Symptoms may appear in early infancy in the form of congenital hip dislocation, in older children as tuberculous and transient arthritis, as slipped epiphysis in young adults, and as osteoarthritis in adults and the aged. Early diagnosis of these conditions is very important in reducing the possibility of permanent deformity.

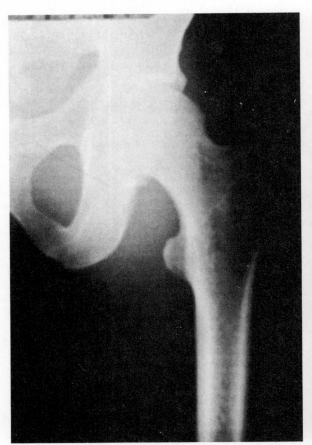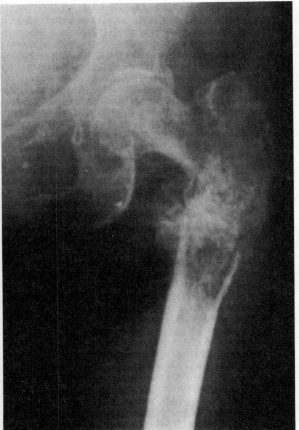

The normal hip (*left*) and a hip showing involvement of bone disease (*right*). Osteoarthritis is a chronic disorder, found especially in older people, that may result in bone degeneration.

Diagnosis is achieved by physical examinations for signs of abnormal joint stability and mobility, postural changes, unstable and painful hip movement, fixed joint deformity, and pain in the lower back. Measurement of both lower limbs may indicate the presence of abnormal hip structure. X-ray examination of the pelvic area and both hips aids in diagnosis, as does blood analysis, which may yield evidence of early signs of gouty or arthritic conditions.

Congenital Dislocation of the Hip

Dislocation of the hip is the most common congenital problem of the pelvic area. It is found more in girls than in boys in a five to one ratio. Babies born from a breech presentation, buttocks first, are more likely to develop this abnormality than those delivered headfirst. The condition may be the result of inherited characteristics.

Clinical examination of infants, especially breech-born girls, may reveal early signs of congenital hip dislocation, with the affected hip appearing shorter than the normal side. If the condition is not diagnosed before the infant is ready to walk, the child may begin walking later than is normal. The child may develop a limp and an unsteady gait, with one leg shorter than the other.

Early diagnosis of this condition is important, followed by immediate reduction and immobilization by means of a plaster cast or by applying traction. Permanent deformity, dislocation, uneven pelvis, retarded walking, limping, and unsteady gait are possible complications if this condition remains untreated. Surgery is sometimes required.

Other Diseases Affecting the Hip

Arthritis: Joint disease or hip injury may result in osteoarthritis in the hip, one of the most prominent causes of disability in older persons. It produces pain in the hips, inner thigh, the groin, and very often in the knee. Walking, climbing steps, sitting, and bending become very painful, since the joint is destroyed due to the degeneration of bone and cartilage. Stress and strain on the hip joint further aggravates the condition, which becomes worse with advancing age. See also *Arthritis,* p. 449.

Small children sometimes suffer from transient arthritis of the hip, of unknown cause, manifested by pain, limitation of hip movement, and impeded walking. Since the condition usually disappears within six weeks, the only treatment is bed rest. Transient arthritis must not be mistaken for the more serious pyrogenic hip arthritis of children and adults, marked by high fever.

Slipped epiphysis: This occurs in late childhood, between the ages of 9 and 18. The head of the *femur,* or thighbone, slips from its normal position, affecting one or both hips. The individual feels pain in the hip and knee, has limitation in joint movement, and walks with a limp. Usually there is evidence of endocrine disturbances.

Legg-Perthes' disease: This is an inflammatory condition of unknown origin involving the bone and cartilage of the femoral head. It is found mostly in children between 4 and 12 years old and usually affects one hip. The symptoms are thigh and groin pain, joint movement limitation, and a walking impediment.

Successful treatment requires extended hospitalization with weight traction applied to the diseased hip, and limitation of body weight on the affected side. Untreated Legg-Perthes' disease leads to permanent hip joint deformity and possible osteoarthritis around middle age.

Coxa vara: This hip deformity is due to a misshapen femur and causes shortening of the leg on the affected side; as a result, the person walks with a limp. The condition may be related to bone softening due to rickets, poorly joined fractures of the hip, or congenital malformation of the hip joint. Some cases may require surgical correction.

Any attack of persistent unexplained hip pains, limitation of movement, and walking impediments should be referred to the family doctor for further investigation. Early diagnosis is crucial in controlling and eradicating many of the crippling diseases of the pelvic area.

Injury to the Pelvis

Pelvic injuries are most often caused by falls in the home or on slippery streets, and by industrial or automobile accidents.

The pelvis bears the entire weight of the body from the waist up and must bear the stress of general body motion during daily activity. The bony architecture of the pelvis does not readily permit the use of a plaster cast to immobilize a fracture. Consequently, fractures of the pelvis require bed rest for at least three weeks, depending on the nature of the injury and the age of the patient.

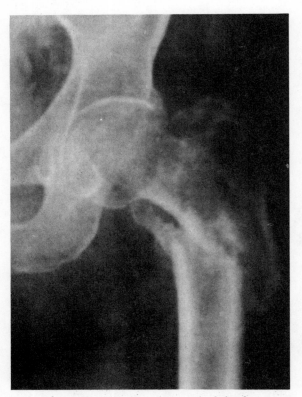

A healing fracture of the upper end of the femur, or thigh bone. Hip fractures require hospitalization.

Simple fractures in children and young adults heal readily with complete bed rest and proper home care. Among the aged, the creation of new bone cells occurs more slowly, and this complicates the management of serious pelvic fractures in people over 65. Prolonged inactivity from extensive bed rest presents other health hazards for the aged, such as sluggish digestion and respiratory or vascular complications.

Treatment of hip fractures: Falls cause a variety of hip fractures—the most common type of pelvic injury. Intense pain with limitation of hip movement and external rotation of the lower leg are indications of a hip fracture. When this occurs, a doctor should be contacted immediately. The patient should be placed flat in bed until medical advice has been obtained. Proper diagnosis requires X-ray examinations.

Patients with hip fractures must be hospitalized. Although a hip fracture may be treated with traction, this method requires months of bed rest and is rarely used. The best method for treating such fractures is to nail the hip together with a metallic pin. The operation is performed by a surgeon, usually an orthopedist, who uses X-ray examinations during surgery to ascertain that the pin is in the correct position. Some hip fractures may also require a metallic plate screwed to the bone to help immobilize the fracture.

After plates and pins have been inserted, the patient can be out of bed within a day. This speeds recovery and prevents the complications of prolonged bed rest. Hip nails are usually left in the patient, depending on the nature of the fracture and the patient's age. Recuperation includes periodic medical checkups and X-ray examinations.

Pubic fractures can cause ruptures of the bladder with urine leaking into the pelvic cavity. Routine urinalysis for the presence of blood cells is always necessary in cases of pelvic fractures. Surgical repair of the bladder may be required.

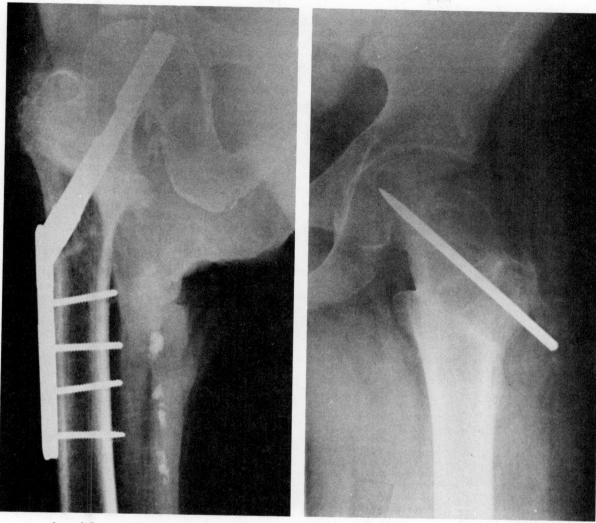

Immobilizing a fractured hip with metallic pins (as shown here) or with plates screwed to the bone enables the patient to avoid the months of bed rest that would otherwise be necessary.

Back Pain and Its Causes

Most adults have experienced some form of back pain. Back pain is a serious physical impairment in persons of all ages, but it occurs more frequently in older persons.

Lumbago and Sciatica

Lumbago refers to general pain in the lower back. Technically, it is not a disease but a symptom that is accentuated by bending, lifting, turning, coughing, or stooping. Pain from neuritis of the sciatic nerve adds to one's misery, with the pain shooting down the legs. This form of back pain is commonly known as *sciatica*, and, like lumbago, can be considered a symptom of some other condition. Treatment depends on the underlying cause of both.

Rheumatoid Spondylitis

Rheumatoid or *ankylosing spondylitis* is a chronic inflammatory condition of unknown origin involving the joints of the spinal column. It becomes progressively worse and produces an abnormal fusion (or *ankylosing*) of the joints. The symptoms are generally found in males in their twenties and thirties and start with severe low back pain. The symptoms migrate to the upper spinal column and produce agonizing generalized back pain with stiffness and limitation of movement. Treatment includes physical exercise to maintain spinal flexibility, radiation therapy, analgesics to relieve the pain, and anti-inflammatory agents.

Slipped and Herniating Disks

Between each vertebra is a fibro-cartilaginous disk that acts as a cushion. These disks are subjected to strain with every movement of the body, especially in the erect position. Increased pressure may cause a disk to protrude or herniate into the vertebral canal, causing what is referred to as a *slipped disk*. This condition can also be brought on by injury, age degeneration, unaccustomed physical activity, or heavy lifting.

The herniating disk presses against nerves in the area, resulting in low back pain, sciatica, and in some instances, disabling muscle spasm. Back rest and a surgical corset may help milder forms of slipped disk by allowing natural healing to take place. Treatment may also include bed rest with intermittent traction to the legs for several weeks. Spinal fusion may be required in severe cases.

Spondylolisthesis

A forward displacement of one vertebral body over another results in a very painful condition known as *spondylolisthesis*. In mild cases there may be no symptoms at all. But in more advanced forms, there is severe low back pain when in the erect position and on bending, with the pain radiating to the legs. The displaced vertebra interferes with nerve roots in that area.

Mild cases require no treatment. Severe cases may require fusion of the vertebral segments with bone grafting; less severe symptoms can be relieved by a specially fitted corset.

Muscle Spasms and Strained Ligaments

Lack of physical exercise and unaccustomed bending can cause acute backache from undue muscle strain. Backache from strain on the ligaments is not uncommon in women following childbirth. The symptoms are similar to general low back pain. Physiotherapy with moist heat and massage helps restore muscular tone and relieve the pain. Muscle-relaxing drugs are sometimes prescribed.

Sacroiliac Pain

The *sacroiliac* joints, in the lower back where the *iliac* (hipbone) joins the sacrum, are a common location for osteoarthritic changes, rheumatoid arthritis, tuberculosis, and ankylosing spondylitis. The most common site of pain is in the lower lumbar region, radiating to the thighs and legs. X-ray diagnosis helps to pinpoint the cause of this particular form of back pain.

Defects and Diseases of the Spine

The normal human spine follows a shallow S-shaped curve. If the curve is greater than normal, that condition is described as a *lordosis*. This type of spinal curvature is uncommon except in late pregnancy, and is caused by hip deformity or a defect in posture.

Other Spinal-Curve Deformities

Scoliosis: This is a lateral curvature of the central part of the spine and appears mostly in children from birth and young adults up to age 15. Early diagnosis and proper orthopedic care are important. If scoliosis appears in early adulthood, the prognosis is better than if the disease starts in infancy. Growth of the curvature ends when the individual's skeletal development ceases.

Scoliosis creates an ugly spinal deformity, and this is usually the only symptom. Some-

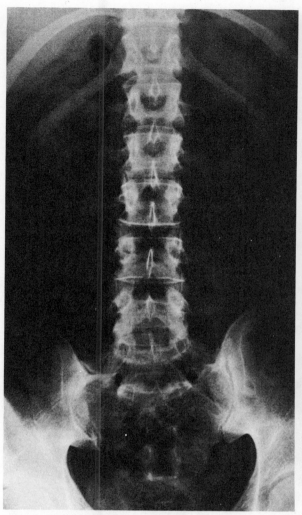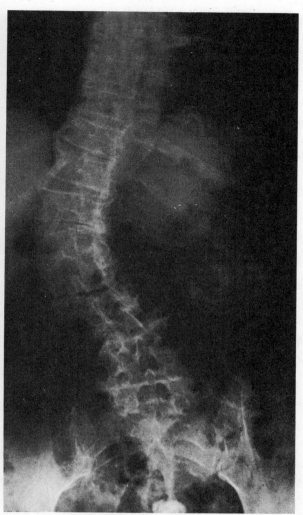

Normal lumbar spine (*left*); lateral curvature (scoliosis) of the lumbar spine (*right*). This deformity of the central part of the spine may appear in children from birth to the age of 15.

times there may be an acute attack of sciatica. Treatment of scoliotic children requires hospitalization. In simple cases, a cast is applied from the chest to the waist to reduce the curvature. Fusion of the vertebral bodies with bone grafting to maintain the fusion may be necessary.

Kyphosis: This is a dorsal spinal curvature characterized by a humpback appearance. A person with this disorder develops an abnormal-looking thorax (or chest) due to the hump in the back, and may sometimes find it difficult to lie on his back. The condition is brought on by untreated fractures of a vertebral body, a spinal tumor, osteoporosis, or spinal tuberculosis. If the principal cause is diagnosed and treated, recovery is possible.

Spinal Arthritis

The aging process is the principal cause of spinal arthritis. Other contributing factors are disk lesions and injury. Spinal arthritis causes pronounced bone degeneration and disability. The sufferer experiences severe back pain radiating to the thighs as a result of interference of the nerve roots from *osteophytes,* or spurs, formed in the joints. In mild cases, physical therapy may be the only treatment required. See *Arthritis,* p. 449.

Spinal Tuberculosis

Chronic pulmonary tuberculosis can spread to the skeletal system, including the vertebral column. Spinal tuberculosis, also known as *Pott's disease,* affects one or more vertebrae in children and young adults. It is currently a relatively rare disease.

The diseased vertebrae may collapse due to pressure from the vertebrae above, resulting in a humpback deformity and possible paralysis of the lower limbs. The usual symptoms are back pain, stiffness, and limited movement. Antibiotics are administered to combat and cure the infection.

Spinal Infections

Fever-inducing microorganisms may reach the spine via the blood and lymph

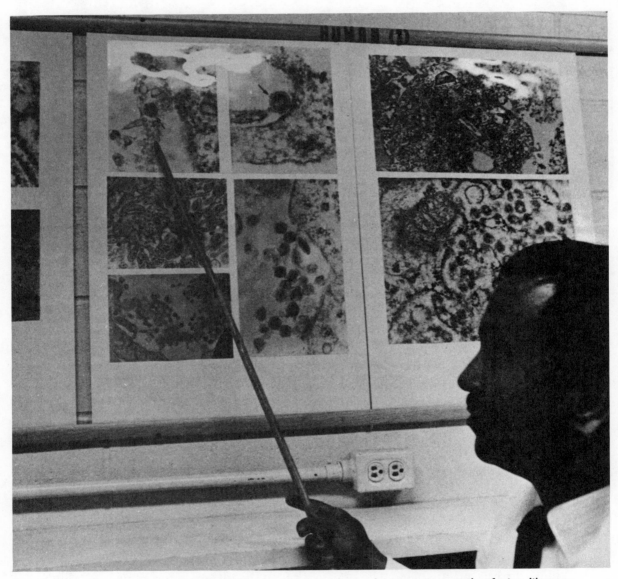

A scientist in a cancer research laboratory points to an electron micrograph of virus-like particles in human tissue. Viruses are suspected of being causative agents of some forms of cancer.

channels, resulting in spinal osteomyelitis or a general inflammation of the vertebrae. This results in bone destruction, pressure on the spinal cord, and paralysis of the legs. Successful treatment includes bed rest, drug therapy, and sometimes a body jacket (for immobilization) made from plaster of paris.

Tumors

The spinal column is affected by both malignant and benign tumors. They can either destroy the bony makeup of the affected vertebra, apply pressure to the spinal cord with resultant paralysis, or interfere with the nerve roots.

Spinal tumors are generally destructive. Some, like *meningiomas* and *neurofibromas*, result in lack of control over bowel and bladder function in addition to the loss of functioning of the lower extremities. Malignant tumors of the spinal column may originate from cancer of the prostate, uterus, bladder, lungs, or breast.

The symptoms of spinal tumors are pain, deformity, weakness, and lower limb paralysis. Diagnosis requires careful study of the subjective symptoms, as well as special tests and radiological examinations. Treatment may involve radiation therapy and chemotherapy; some tumors can be surgically removed. In many instances, the patient may be given analgesics to relieve the pain.

Spinal Injuries

Most spinal injuries originate from automobile accidents, industrial mishaps, falls, athletics, or from fights and beatings. Spinal injuries can create fractures that compress or sever the spinal cord, with resultant paralysis. A diving accident or headlong fall may cause a concussion and possible fractures of the cervical spine. Head-on collisions in the sports arena and automobile accidents are the chief causes of cervical spine fractures.

An individual who jumps from a considerable height and lands on his feet, especially on his heels, may easily fracture his spine. Sudden pain in the thoracic spine following a jump should receive immediate medical attention and investigation.

Victims of spinal injuries should be moved as little as possible. While waiting for professional help, the patient should be placed on his back and made as comfortable as possible. If an accident or explosion victim is wedged between debris, attempts should be made to free him, but his body should be kept flat with as little movement as possible. No attempt should be made to have the person sit up or stand before he has been examined by a physician. Unnecessary movement of victims of spinal injury can damage the spinal cord and cause permanent paralysis.

Whiplash injuries, the most common form of injury to the spine, occur most often during head-on and rear-end automobile accidents which suddenly jerk the neck and injure the cervical vertebrae. Accident victims thus injured may undergo months of agonizing headaches and pain in the neck. Immobilization of the neck by a surgical collar will reduce some of the pain and aid the healing process.

Diagnosis and Treatment of Spinal Problems

The following are a few of the more common methods of diagnosing and treating spinal disorders.

Spinal Tap

The removal of *cerebrospinal fluid* for laboratory investigation is a diagnostic procedure commonly known as a *spinal tap*. This fluid, which surrounds the brain and spinal cord, can indicate abnormal conditions of the spine and the central nervous system. The withdrawal of cerebrospinal fluid requires puncturing the spinal canal with a needle under sterile conditions. Samples of fluid withdrawn are sent to the diagnostic laboratory for analysis. The patient is usually confined to bed on his back for at least 12 hours afterwards.

Removal of Disks and Spinal Fusion

A severely herniated disk can be surgically removed to relieve pain and other symptoms. Disk removal is followed by fusion of the vertebral bodies on both sides of the removed disk. Fusion is accomplished by bridging the vertebral space with a bone graft.

Decompression of Fractures

Anyone with a spinal injury should be taken to the emergency ward of the nearest hospital for X-ray examinations that will reveal possible fractures. If the fracture compresses against the spinal cord, the extremities may be paralyzed. In such cases, a neurosurgeon or an orthopedist may perform a delicate operation, lifting the fracture fragments away from the spinal cord, thereby relieving the pressure and reestablishing control and movement of the paralyzed extremities.

Fractures of the cervical spine can be decompressed by applying traction to the neck. Frequent X-ray rechecks are required to assess the degree of healing and new bone formation. Patients with fractured vertebrae undergo a lengthy rehabilitation with frequent medical rechecks and physical therapy. In some severe cases of spinal fractures that result in paralysis, the individual is never able to walk again.

Radiology

X-ray examination of the skeletal system involves plain film studies or a special examination called *myelography*. Air or an oily iodine compound is injected into the spinal canal before taking X-ray pictures. The air or iodine outlines the spinal canal in contrast to the surrounding body tissues.

The Rib Cage

Every normal human being has 12 pairs of ribs attached to the spine, but some people are born with extra ribs on one or both sides.

Congenital Anomalies

Although extra ribs are usually harmless, an extra rib projecting into the neck can damage nerves and the artery located in that area. In adults extra neck ribs may cause shooting pains down the arms, general periodic numbness in the arms and hands, weak wrist pulse, and possible diminished blood supply to the forearm. Surgery may be required to remove the rib and thereby relieve the pressure on the nerves or artery. Minor symptoms are treated by physiotherapy.

Congenital absence of one or more ribs is not uncommon. An individual may be born with some ribs fused together. Neither condition creates any serious threat to health.

Bone Lesions

Cancerous tumors of the bony thorax result in the destruction of ribs, clavicles, and sternum. Since the bone marrow of the sternum plays an important role in the manufacture of new blood cells, it can act as a vehicle for the spread of cancer cells to other parts of the body.

Injury to the Rib Cage

Accidents, athletic injuries, and fights account for most injuries to the rib cage. Any blow to the chest can cause rib fractures, which hurt when one coughs or inhales. Hairline and incomplete fractures are less serious than complete fractures, where the fragments are usually sharp and pointed. Such fractured ribs can tear the lungs, causing air to leak into the pleural space, with possibly serious results. The lung can collapse as a result of being punctured. Punctured blood vessels can hemorrhage into the pleural space. The accumulated blood may have to be withdrawn before it reduces the capacity of the lungs to carry out their normal function.

Severe chest injuries—crush injuries with multiple fractures—require hospitalization. The patient must be confined to bed and kept under constant medical observation and treatment. If the lung has collapsed, it has to be reinflated. In simple rib fractures the chest may be strapped to immobilize the fragments and promote rapid healing. Generally, analgesics alone are enough.

Fractures of the sternum are caused by direct blows to the sternal area, as is usually the case with automobile accidents when the steering wheel hits the driver's chest. This injury can be avoided if the driver wears a shoulder-restraining belt, and if his car is equipped with a collapsible steering column.

Chest pains following a blow to the area of the sternum should be medically investigated by means of X-ray diagnosis for possible fracture. The fracture fragments may have to be wired together and remain in place until the injury has healed. For simple fractures, rest may be the only treatment required. The serious complication of a fractured sternum in a steering wheel accident is contusion of the heart; it should be evaluated by means of an electrocardiogram.

The Skull, Face, and Jaw

Birth Defects

Various malformations of the skull, face, and jaw can appear at birth or soon after. They include *macrocephaly* (enlarged head) and *microcephaly* (very small head). Microcephaly is caused by the premature fusion of the cranial sutures in early childhood. If brain growth increases very rapidly during the first six months of life in infants whose skulls have fused prematurely, the brain cannot expand sufficiently within the rigid skull, and mental retardation results. Surgery is used to widen the sutures to permit normal brain development.

Cleft lip and *cleft palate* are common facial deformities and are visible at birth. These are longitudinal openings in the upper lip and palate. They result from failure of the area to unite in the normal manner during embryonic stages of pregnancy. They should be corrected at an early age. If surgery is performed in infancy there is a good chance that the child will mature with little or no physical evidence of the affliction and with no psychological damage as a result of it. See *Cleft Palate and Cleft Lip,* p. 403, for further information.

Skull Injuries

Although the skull is very thick, it is not invulnerable. Head injuries can result from sports or playground accidents, falls, automobile or industrial accidents, or sharp blows to the head. Head injuries can cause linear or hairline skull fractures, depressed skull fractures (dents), brain injury due to fracture fragments or foreign bodies piercing the brain (as in the case of a bullet wound), or *concussion* with or without bone damage. The effects of concussion can show up as dizziness, nausea, loss of consciousness, weak pulse, and slowed respiration.

Any of these injuries can cause blood vessels to rupture and bleed. The resulting blood clots form what is known as a *subdural hematoma*, which may cause increased pressure on the brain. Patients with a subdural hematoma feel dizzy, slip slowly into unconsciousness, and may die unless immediate hospital care is available. Usually half of the body on the opposite side of the clot becomes paralyzed.

A depressed fracture can also apply pressure on the brain at the area of the depression. Surgery is required to relieve the pressure.

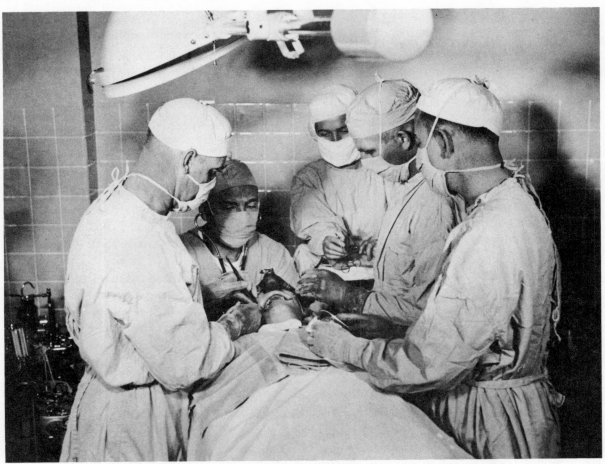

An oral surgeon and his staff operate on a patient under general anesthesia.

No skull injury should be treated lightly. A child may hit his head in a playground or in the backyard and conceal this from his parents, or a babysitter may be afraid of losing her job if she reports such a fall. An alcoholic may slip on the street and strike his head on the sidewalk. Anyone who suffers a blow to the head or who falls on his head should be observed carefully for possible later complications. If such incidents are followed by vomiting, drowsiness, and headaches, immediate medical attention should be sought.

Facial Injuries

A blow to the eye may fracture the upper or lower borders of the eye socket. It can also cause what is commonly known as a black eye, the blue-black appearance of which is due to bleeding under the skin. The swelling can be reduced by applying an ice pack to the area.

Fractures of the facial bones, jaw, and nose result from a direct blow to these areas. The impact may rupture blood vessels and cause bleeding in the sinuses. Fractures of the nose and jawbone may be severe enough to cause facial deformity. Dislocation of the jaw is a common problem caused by trauma. It may also occur spontaneously in certain individuals by an unusually wide-mouthed yawn or laugh. It is an uncomfortable rather than painful experience.

Serious facial injury requires hospitalization and surgical restoration. Skin lacerations may have to be sutured and the scars removed by plastic surgery; fractures of the jaw and mouth may require surgical wiring for stabilization and immobilization before healing can take place. In some instances both jaws may be wired together until healing takes place.

The Mouth and the Teeth

Pathological conditions in the mouth include abscesses and tumors that are very often located in the gums. On occasion, diseases such as leukemia, infectious mononucleosis, or lymphomas can manifest themselves with lesions in the mouth; these may even be the first manifestations of the disease. Periodontal disease (pyorrhea) be-

gins as an inflammatory condition of the membrane surrounding each tooth and is characterized by pockets of infection around the tooth. If untreated, it can cause extreme discomfort and eventual tooth loss.

Tooth Decay and Treatment

The most common teeth problem is *dental caries,* commonly called cavities. The decay process first affects the *dentin,* the bony interior of the tooth, finally exposes the *pulp* and destroys the tooth. The typical symptoms are toothache, face ache if the nerves are exposed, and painful reaction to hot and cold liquids or foods.

Treatment of teeth varies from filling cavities, extracting dead and badly decay-

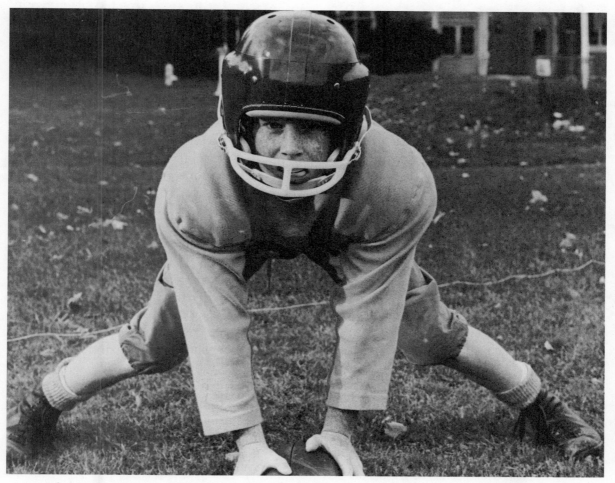

A helmet can prevent a skull fracture or concussion; it should always be worn in contact sports.

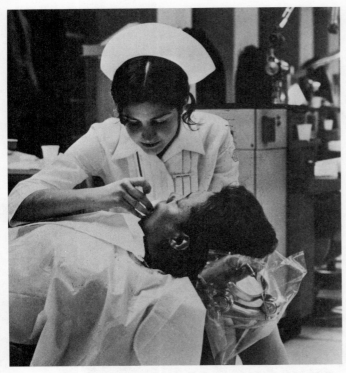

Teeth should be cleaned regularly by a dentist or hygienist to prevent decay and serious gum disease.

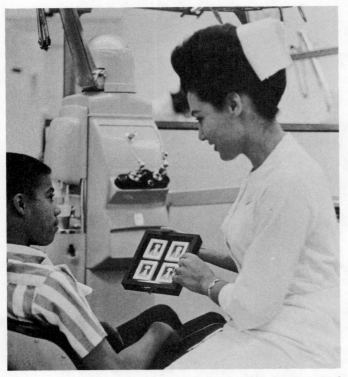

Regular visits to the dentist permit early diagnosis and treatment of tooth decay and diseases of the gums.

ing teeth, incising and draining abscesses, employing root canal procedures to save a dead tooth, and cleaning the teeth.

When oral surgery is being performed, the dental surgeon injects a local anesthetic into the gums and nerve endings. The effect of the anesthetic disappears about four hours after the operation. Sometimes a general anesthetic is used to put the patient to sleep during the operation.

Simple procedures such as filling cavities require only a local anesthetic or none at all. The dentist drills the cavity to remove the decaying portion and fills the cavity with *amalgam,* a mixture of silver, tin, and mercury with small amounts of copper and zinc. The filling replaces the original tooth material and prevents further decay.

When teeth are extracted, the empty spaces are filled by a partial dental plate or a complete set of upper and lower teeth if all must be removed. Some artificial teeth are removable; others may be permanently anchored between existing teeth.

Decay Prevention

The following precautions will help maintain healthy teeth:

• Eat a proper diet containing a daily supply of milk and milk products to provide the body with enough calcium to build strong teeth. Adequate calcium intake is important during pregnancy since the fetal bone and tooth formation starts at that time.

• Brush teeth after every meal to free the teeth of food particles which, when left in the mouth, promote tooth decay.

• Visit the dentist once or twice a year so that he can diagnose and treat tooth problems in their early stages.

• Avoid excessive eating of candy and other sweets in order to reduce the amount of sugar around the teeth, thereby reducing tooth decay.

• Have children drink fluoridated water to help promote healthy teeth and prevent decay.   AAD

DISEASES OF THE MUSCLES AND NERVOUS SYSTEM

We have the capacity to perceive our environment by receiving sensory messages—sound, light, touch and pain, an awareness of our position in space—to associate these with other sensory messages, to store the information, and then to call it back to our consciousness as needed. The control of our body parts is also a function of the nervous system, and movement may range from gross to the most delicate. Further, many aspects of our behavior are not at all mysterious and can be explained in terms of a series of neuro-electrochemical events. In short, our human existence is a reflection of the state of our nervous system, the normal function of which can be disturbed in many ways.

For example, if any part of the brain has developed abnormally, the usual function of that structure would be expected to be altered. Abnormalities present at birth are called *congenital* defects. If the nervous system does not receive a normal blood supply because of the obstruction of a blood vessel, or if there is a tear in the vessel with subsequent hemorrhage, the cells are deprived of blood and will die. These lesions are *vascular* or *cerebrovascular* accidents. Cerebral injury, or *trauma*, can destroy brain tissue, with subsequent loss of normal function; infection of the nervous system may also permanently injure tissue. Finally, changes in normal body chemistry can alter brain function and are considered *metabolic, toxic,* or *degenerative* diseases. It is not surprising, then, that such a beautifully organized nervous system is vulnerable to the hazards of living.

Nervous Diseases

A patient referred to a *neurologist,* a physician who specializes in diseases of the nervous system, will be asked to tell the history of the problem in great detail, for that history will describe the nature of the disorder; the neurological examination will help to localize the problem. After the neurological examination is completed, the physician may order radiographs (X rays) of the skull and spinal column and an electroencephalogram. The *electroencephalogram (EEG)* or brain wave test, assists in localizing a brain abnormality or describing the nature of a convulsive disorder. A specific diagnosis is not based upon the EEG alone, but rather the EEG is used to corroborate the doctor's clinical impression of the disease process.

It may also be necessary to perform a *lumbar puncture (spinal tap)* in order to obtain a specimen of the *cerebrospinal fluid (CSF),* the fluid that circulates within the brain structures. This laboratory test is a benign, relatively painless procedure when performed by a skilled physician and is extremely useful in making a diagnosis. It entails a needle puncture under sterile conditions in the midline of the lower spine as the patient lies on his side or sits upright.

Occasionally, other more specialized diagnostic tests are used to better enable the physician to visualize the structure of the brain and the spinal cord. Air can be introduced directly into the cavities (*ventricles*) within the brain in a process called *ventriculography,* or through a needle similar to that used in a lumbar puncture, (*pneumoencephalography*) and the darkness of shadows on the X rays will outline the brain structure.

Another specialized neuroradiological test is the *angiogram.* A radio-opaque material that can been seen on X ray is injected into the blood vessels that supply the brain. Since the vessels can be plainly seen on the X-ray film, any displacement of those vessels from the normal position is evident.

A third type of contrast study is called a *myelogram*. A similar radio-opaque liquid is introduced through a spinal needle into the sac-enclosed space around the spinal cord. Any obstructive or compressive lesion of the spinal cord is thus seen on the radiogram and helps to confirm the diagnosis.

Each of these contrast studies helps the physician better understand the structures of the brain or spinal cord and may be essential in order for him to make a correct diagnosis.

Cerebral Palsy

The term *cerebral palsy* is not a diagnosis but a label applied to a child who has a problem in locomotion. Interpretations of what cerebral palsy is are many and varied, but in general refer to nonprogressive abnormalities of the brain that have occurred early in life from many causes. The label implies that there is no active disease process but rather a static or nonprogressive lesion that may affect the growth and development of the child.

Symptoms: Included under the category of cerebral palsy are such problems as limpness (flaccidity), *spasticity* of one or all limbs, or incoordination or some other disorder of movement. In some patients, quick jerks affect different parts of the body at different times (*chorea*); in others, slow writhing, incoordinated movements (*athetosis*) are most pronounced in the hands and arms. Incoordination of movement may also be seen in muscles used for speaking and eating, so that speech becomes slurred, interrupted, or jerky; the patient may drool because of the incoordinated muscle action that prevents efficient swallowing of saliva. This does little to improve the physical appearance of the child and, unfortunately, he may look mentally subnormal.

The fact that a patient has an abnormality that is responsible for difficulty in locomotion does not mean that he will be mentally retarded. There is a greater likelihood that he will be mentally slow, but patients in this group of disease states range from normal to superior in intelligence, a fact that emphasizes that each child must be assessed individually.

A complete physical examination must be completed, and to determine the patient's functional status complete psychological testing should be performed by a skilled psychologist.

Treatment: Treatment for cerebral palsy is a continuing process involving a careful surveillance of the patient's physical and psychological status. A physical therapist, under the doctor's guidance, will help to mobilize and maintain the function of the neuromuscular system. Occasionally, an orthopedic surgeon may surgically lengthen a tendon or in some way make a limb more functional. A speech therapist can provide additional speech training, and a vocational therapist is helpful in assisting the patient to find appropriate life's work. The key position in the patient's care is the primary physician, usually the pediatrician, who with care and understanding guides the patient through the years.

Bell's Palsy

Bell's palsy (named after Sir Charles Bell) is a paralysis of the facial nerve that may affect men and women at any age, though it occurs most commonly between the ages of 30 and 50. The onset of the facial paralysis may be abrupt: the patient can awaken one morning unable to move one side of his face. He can't wrinkle one side of his forehead or raise the eyebrow; the eye will not close on the affected side, and when attempting to smile, the face is pulled to the opposite side. Occasionally the patient may experience discomfort about the ear on the involved side. There is no difficulty in swallowing, but since the muscles about the corner of the mouth are weak,

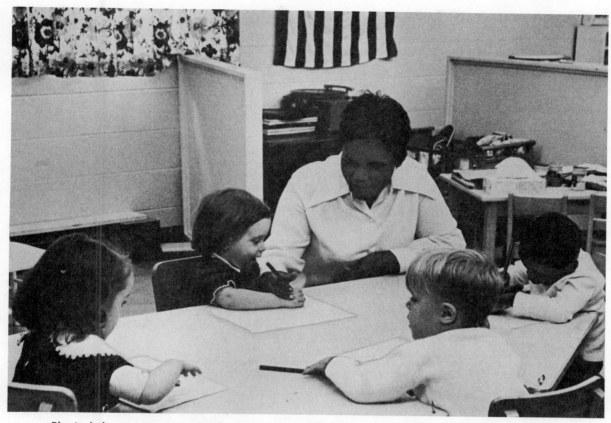

Physical therapy is essential for cerebral palsy patients. Here a therapist works with children in manipulating pencils—a means of improving hand-eye coordination and finger dexterity.

drooling is not uncommon, and food may accumulate in the gutter between the gum and the lip.

Bell's palsy can affect the branch of the facial nerve that supplies taste sensation to the anterior part of the tongue, and the branch that supplies a small muscle in the middle ear (the *stapedius*) whose function is to dampen loud sounds. Depending on the extent that the facial nerve is affected, the patient may be unable to perceive taste on the side of the paralysis, or he may complain of loudness of sound (*hyperacusis*).

The most probable cause of Bell's palsy is an inflammation of the nerve as it passes through a bony canal within the skull (the Fallopian canal) or inflammation of that bony canal with subsequent swelling and compression of the nerve. It is not uncommon that the patient has a history of preceding exposure to a cold breeze, such as sleeping in a draft or riding in an open car. Any patient who has a facial weakness should be carefully evaluated by a physician, preferably a neurologist, to be quite certain that there is no other neurologic abnormality. When the diagnosis of Bell's palsy is certain, some therapeutic measures can be taken.

Treatment: There is no specific treatment for Bell's palsy, but many physicians recommend massage, application of heat, and passive or active exercise of the weak muscles. These therapeutic measures do not specifically influence the course of the facial nerve paralysis, but they are thought to be useful in maintaining tone of the facial muscles and preventing permanent deformity. Occasionally a V-shaped adhesive tape splint can be applied to the affected side of the face, from the corner of the mouth to the temple. Some physicians treat the condition with steroids such as cortisone, which may hasten recovery if begun at the onset of the illness.

In treating Bell's palsy, it is important to remember that when the eyelid does not close normally, the conjunctiva and cornea are not fully lubricated, and corneal lesions may develop from excessive dryness or exposure to the air. For this reason, some ophthalmic lubrication may be recommended by the attending doctor.

About 80 percent of the patients with Bell's palsy recover completely in a few days to weeks, and 10 to 15 percent recover more slowly, over a period of three to six months. The remaining 5 to 10 percent will have some residual facial deformity.

Epilepsy

Since convulsions are usually such dramatic episodes, there is little wonder that they have been recorded in earliest medical writings. Even today, fear is associated with convulsions, and many patients with seizures suffer needlessly because of incorrect and incomplete information passed down through the years. The term needs some clarification; one should know that a *seizure* means the same as a *convulsion* or a fit, and that *epilepsy* is a condition that is manifested by convulsions. It is a common malady of mankind, occurring in both sexes in about 0.5 percent of the population of the United States. Although one cannot be specific about the inheritance of epilepsy, more family members of epileptics have had

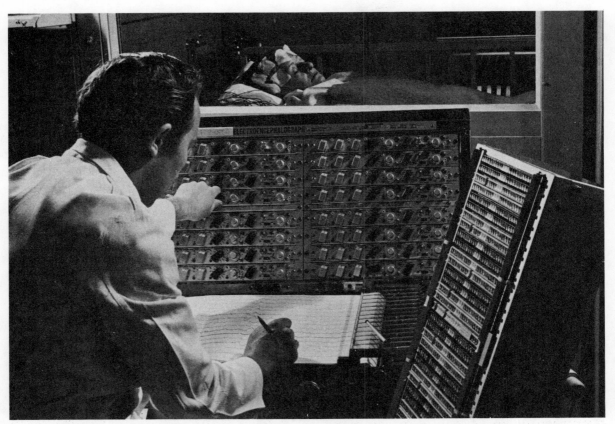

Electroencephalography, the measurement of electric impulses in the brain, is useful in the diagnosis of epilepsy. An EEG taken during a seizure is likely to show exceptionally high bursts of energy. Even between seizures, the EEG of most epileptics shows some irregularities.

seizures than have the family members of nonepileptics, a situation that suggests a constitutional or predispositional basis of inheritance.

The fit is a sign of an underlying brain abnormality that can be structural, chemical, or electrical. It is not unusual that a specific cause is not found to explain its occurrence, in which case the disorder is usually called *idiopathic epilepsy*. A convulsive state can be defined as a recurring, paroxysmal alteration in brain function that begins and ends spontaneously. About one-half of the patients experience an *aura*, a momentary sensory perception of an unusual nature, just before they lose consciousness. The aura may be an unpleasant or unusual smell, an odd feeling, numbness, or a strange fear. Some patients cannot describe the sensation; others may feel strange or a little confused for hours or even days before the seizure. Such early warnings are known as *prodromes*. Following the attack, patients often complain of a headache or confusion or may fall into a deep sleep for minutes or hours.

Grand Mal Convulsions

The *grand mal* is a generalized convulsion during which the patient may initially look strange or bewildered, suddenly groan or scream, lose consciousness and become stiff (*tonic phase*), stop breathing, fall to the ground unless supported, and then begin to jerk the arms and legs (*clonic phase*). Occasionally, there is a loss of bowel and bladder control. The duration of the entire seizure, both the tonic and clonic phases, is less than two minutes—frequently less than one minute—followed by postconvulsive confusion, headache, or deep sleep that may last from minutes to hours.

Focal Convulsion

When the convulsion is limited to one part of the body, the disorder is focal, and is considered to be a *focal convulsion*. Com-

monly, one side of the face, the thumb and fingers of the same side, or one entire side of the body is involved. The patient does not always lose consciousness during the focal spell and may be aware of his surroundings and circumstances, although unable to speak clearly. Focal convulsions in adults commonly indicate some focal brain abnormality, but this is less true in a child, who may have a focal seizure without evidence of a focal brain lesion.

Temporal Lobe (Psychomotor) Convulsions

Psychomotor convulsions are characterized by stereotyped muscle movements: a smacking of the lips, a seemingly purposeful movement or activity such as rising from a chair and walking about, the repetition of words or a phrase, or incoherent speech. Some patients, if physically restrained during the episode, may appear belligerent and obstreperous. The entire episode usually lasts less than several minutes and the patient often "awakes" confused and unable to recall what has happened.

Petit Mal Convulsions

Petit mal seizures are characterized by momentary staring spells, as if the patient were suspended in the middle of his activity. The patient does not fall down. These spells usually begin in childhood or at adolescence and have been called lapses or absences. They may occur many times throughout the day. It is very common that the lapses go unnoticed for weeks or months because the patient appears to be daydreaming.

Since the patient usually has no clear recollection of what happens during any of the epileptic convulsions, it is wise to have someone who has seen the attack accompany him to the doctor. Usually the physician does not see the patient during the seizure and must rely on the description to make the correct diagnosis. Then the doctor begins the detective work to find the cause of the fit. He will examine the patient completely, obtain blood tests, an EEG, and a lumbar puncture, if indicated. However, even after all these studies, he often can find no specific cause.

Treatment of Epilepsy

The treatment of epilepsy consists primarily of medication for prevention of the seizures and is very effective. About one-half of all patients are completely controlled and another quarter have a significant reduction in frequency and severity of the attacks. The medication must be taken regularly according to the physician's instructions. However, medicine is not the only treatment. The patient should have adequate rest, good nutrition, and an understanding family. Vigorous body-contact sports and solitary swimming should be avoided.

Because of ignorance and misinformation, some people regard epileptics as frightening or mysterious, and patients may suffer unnecessarily and unjustly. In fact, behavioral abnormalities in patients with seizures are commonly the reflection of how they are viewed by others. The patient should be carefully observed by an understanding physician who watches not only for medical but for psychological problems.

Further information about epilepsy can be obtained from the Epilepsy Foundation of America, 1419 H Street, N.W., Washington, D.C. 20005; or from the U.S. Department of Health, Education and Welfare, Public Health Services, National Institutes of Health, Bethesda, Md. 20014.

Parkinson's Disease

Patients with *Parkinson's disease* are easily recognized because they have similar characteristics of tremor, muscle stiffness, and a decrease of movement. This combination of symptoms is caused by degeneration of the nerve cells deep within the brain (*basal ganglia*) and the brain surface (*cerebral cortex*) and can follow encephalitis, a brain injury, or exposure to toxic substances; it may also occur without any known injury to the brain.

The tremor, or shaking, usually involves the fingers and the wrist, but sometimes the arms, legs, or head are involved to the extent that the entire body shakes. Characteristically, the tremor occurs when the patient is at rest. It stops or is much less marked during a voluntary muscle movement, only to start once again when that movement has been stopped. There is no tremor when the patient is asleep.

Early in the disease, the patient is aware that one leg seems a bit stiff; later, the arm does not swing normally at his side when he is walking. He moves about more slowly with stooped-over head and shoulders. Often he has difficulty in starting to walk, but once started he cannot stop unless he grabs onto the wall or some other object. The face appears expressionless, the speech is slurred, and written figures are small and uneven (*micrographia*) because of the ri-

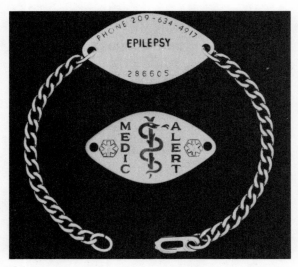

In order to avoid having an epileptic convulsion mistaken for some other disorder and treated improperly, some epileptics wear a bracelet or necklace that identifies their disease. These emblems are available for a slight charge from the Medic Alert Foundation, Turlock, California 95380, a nonprofit organization.

gidity and the tremor. Mental faculties are usually not impaired, but as might be expected in such a chronic disease in which the patient cannot move or communicate normally, mood disturbances are common.

Treatment: For many years *Parkinsonism* was treated with drugs derived from *belladonna,* but the results were less than gratifying and the side effects were sometimes as unpleasant as the disease. Synthetic compounds with fewer side effects were introduced, but there was still need for better therapy. Neurosurgical procedures were then devised by which very small destructive lesions were produced in the brain, with subsequent lessening of the symptoms. The most gratifying improvements following neurosurgery are usually seen in patients under the age of 60 whose symptoms are confined primarily to one side of the body.

More recently, there has been increasing evidence that the symptoms of Parkinson's disease are related to a decreased concentration of *dopamine,* a neurochemical substance in the structures of the brain. A neurochemical substance called *levodopa,* very closely allied to dopamine, has been found to alleviate effectively the symptoms of Parkinsonism. It is thought that this substance is converted into dopamine within the neurostructures of the brain. At this time, levodopa is the most effective control for the symptoms of Parkinson's disease.

Infections of the Nervous System

Like any other organ system, the brain and its associated structures may be host to infection. These infections are usually serious because of the significantly high death rate and incidence of residual defects. If the brain is involved in the inflammation, it is known as *encephalitis;* inflammation of the brain coverings, or *meninges,* is called *meningitis.*

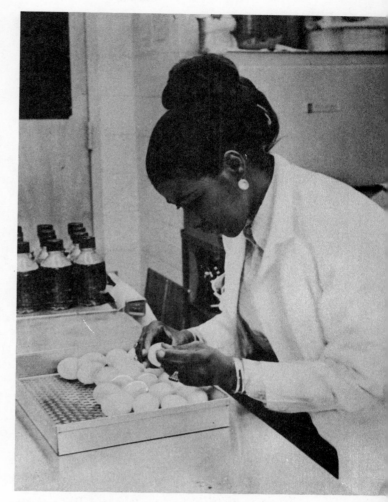

A research technician injects sterile chicken eggs with influenza virus in a Parkinson's-disease study.

Encephalitis

Encephalitis is usually caused by a virus, and, since the symptoms are not specific, the diagnosis is usually made by special viral immunologic tests. Both sexes of all age groups can be afflicted. Most patients complain of fever, headache, nausea or vomiting, and a general feeling of malaise. The mental state varies from one of mild irritability to lethargy or coma, and some patients may have convulsions. The physician becomes suspicious after completing the history and the physical examination, but the diagnosis is usually established by laboratory tests that include examination of the CSF (cerebrospinal fluid), the EEG, and viral studies of the blood, CSF, or stool. Since there is no specific treatment for viral encephalitis at the present time, particular attention is paid to general supportive care.

Meningitis

Meningitis is an inflammation of the coverings (*meninges*) of the brain and spinal cord and may occur in both sexes at any time of life. The patient often has a preceding mild respiratory infection and later complains of headache, nausea, and vomiting. Fever and neck stiffness are usually present early in the course of the disease, at which time the patient is commonly brought to the physician for examination. If there is any question of meningitis, a lumbar puncture is performed and the CSF examined. It is not possible to make a specific clinical diagnosis of meningitis without examination of the cerebrospinal fluid.

Meningitis is usually caused by bacteria or a virus. It is important to learn what the infectious agent is in order to begin appropriate therapy. Bacterial infections can be treated by antibiotics, but there is no known specific treatment for viral (*aseptic*) meningitis. Meningitis is a life-threatening disease, and despite modern antibiotic therapy, the mortality rate varies from 10 to 20 percent.

Poliomyelitis

Poliomyelitis is an acute viral illness affecting males and females at any time of life, though most commonly before the age of ten. It may also be called *polio, infantile paralysis*, or *Heine-Medin disease.*

Polio is caused by a virus that probably moves from the gastrointestinal tract via nerve trunks to the central nervous system, where it may affect any part of the nervous system. However, the disease most often involves the larger motor neurons (*anterior horn cells*) in the brain stem and spinal cord, with subsequent loss of nerve supply to the muscle. The neuron may be partially or completely damaged; clinical recovery is, therefore, dependent on whether those partially damaged nerves can regain normal function.

Patients with polio can be considered in one of two categories: asymptomatic and symptomatic. Those persons who have had no observed symptoms of the disease, but in whom antibodies to polio can be demonstrated, belong in the *asymptomatic* group. The *symptomatic* group, on the other hand, is comprised of patients who have the clinical disease, with either residual paralysis (paralytic polio) or no residual paralysis (nonparalytic polio).

Symptoms: The symptoms of poliomyelitis are similar to other acute infectious processes. The patient may complain of headache, fever, or *coryza* (head cold or runny nose), or he may have loose stools and malaise. One-fourth to one-third of patients improve for several days only to have a recurrence of fever with neck stiffness. Most patients, however, do not improve, but rather have a progression of their symptoms, marked by neck stiffness and muscle aching. They are often irritable and apprehensive, and some are rather lethargic.

The important question is whether or not the patient will have muscle paralysis, and this should be evident within the first few weeks. Some have muscle paralysis at the onset of their symptoms, others will be aware of loss of muscle function several weeks after the onset, but in about one-half of patients, the paralysis occurs during the second to the fifth day of the disease. Patients experience a muscle spasm or stiffness, and may complain of muscle pain, particularly if the muscle is stretched.

The extent of the muscle paralysis is variable, ranging from mild localized weakness to a state where most of the skeletal muscles are paralyzed. Proximal muscles (for example, those about the shoulder-arm, or hip-thigh) are involved more often than distal

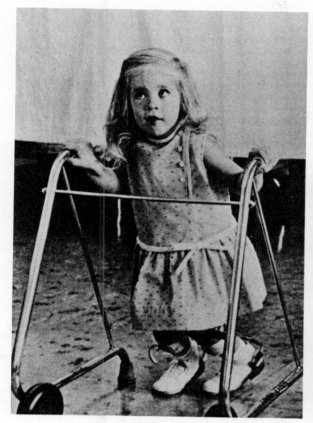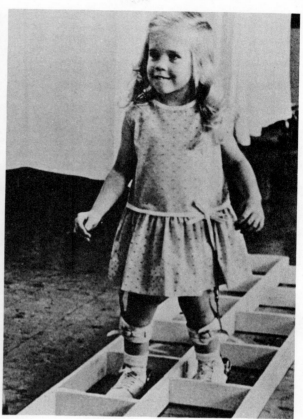

Physical therapy for poliomyelitis patients can increase strength and range of motion. This little girl is using a walker and step-box as part of her gait training.

muscles (for example, of the extremities), and the legs are affected more often than the arms. When the neurons of the lower brain stem, cervical and thoracic spinal cord are affected, the patient may have a paralysis of the muscles used in swallowing and breathing. This circumstance, obviously, is life-threatening, and particular attention must be paid to the patient's ability to handle secretions and to his respiration. If independent, spontaneous respiration is not possible, patients must be given respiratory assistance with mechanical respirators.

Treatment: There is no specific treatment for acute poliomyelitis. The patient should be kept at complete bed rest, and attention given to general supportive care, assuring adequate nutrition and fluid intake. Muscle spasm has been treated with hot as well as cold compresses, and no one method has

been universally beneficial. Careful positioning of the patient with the musculature supported in a position midway between relaxation and contraction is probably of benefit, and skilled physical therapy is of great importance.

Immunization. Since the early 1900s, attempts had been made to produce an effective vaccine against poliomyelitis, with success crowning the efforts of Dr. Jonas Salk in 1953. Today vaccination is accomplished with either the Salk vaccine (killed virus) that is given intramuscularly, or the Sabin (live attenuated virus) given orally. There is little question that immunization with poliomyelitis vaccine has proven to be highly effective in eradicating the clinical disease within the community, and it is now a part of routine immunization for all children.

Dementia

Dementia is a term used to describe the patient who has suffered mental deterioration, with particular regard to memory and thought processes. Such deterioration can be seen in many diseases affecting the brain: infection, brain injury, such toxic states as alcoholism, brain tumors, or cerebral arteriosclerosis.

The presenile dementias (*Alzheimer's disease*) represent a group of brain degenerative diseases in which the mental deterioration first becomes apparent in middle age. Commonly, the first clue may be demonstrations of unusual unreasonableness and impairment of judgment. The patient can no longer grasp the content of a situation at hand and reacts inappropriately. Memory gradually fades and recent events are no longer remembered, but events that occurred early in life can be recalled. The patient may wander aimlessly or get lost in his own house. There is progressive deterioration of physical appearance and personal hygiene, and, finally, the command of language deteriorates. Unfortunately, there is a relentless progression of the process, and the patient becomes confined to bed and quite helpless.

Whether or not the mental deterioration seen in the aged, senile dementia, is a specific brain degeneration or is secondary to cerebral arteriosclerosis is not yet settled. It does appear, however, that senile dementia is probably secondary to a degenerative process similar to that of Alzheimer's disease but occurring late in life.

Whether or not dementia can be halted depends upon its cause. If, for example, the dementia is secondary to brain infection or exposure to toxic material, eradication of the infectious agent or removal of the toxin may be of distinct benefit in arresting the dementing process. Unfortunately, there is no specific treatment for the brain degenerative processes.

Muscle Diseases

When one hears the words muscle disease, one thinks only of muscular dystrophy and pictures a small child confined to a wheelchair. But there are many diseases other than muscular dystrophy in which muscle is either primarily or secondarily involved, and many of these diseases do not have a particularly bad prognosis. Muscle diseases may make their presence known at any time, from early infancy to old age; no age group or sex is exempt.

The hallmark of muscle disease is weakness, or loss of muscle power. This may be recognized in the infant who seems unusually limp or *hypotonic*. Often the first clue to the presence of muscle weakness is a child's failure to achieve the developmental milestones within a normal range of time. He may be unusually clumsy or have difficulty in running, climbing stairs, or even walking. Occasionally a teacher is the first one to be aware that the child cannot keep up with classmates and will report this fact to the parents. The onset of the muscle weakness can be so insidious that it may go unnoticed or be misinterpreted as laziness until there is an obvious and striking loss of muscle power.

This is true in the adult as well who at first may feel tired or worn out and then realize that he cannot keep up his previous pace. Often his feet and legs are involved in the beginning. He may wear out the toes of his shoes and may then recognize that he must raise his legs higher to avoid tripping or dragging the toes, or must expend more energy to raise the legs in climbing stairs, or even to climb one step at a time. Getting out of bed in the morning may be a chore, and rising from a seated position in a low chair or from the floor may be difficult or impossible. Those with arm involvement may recognize that the hands are weak; if the shoulder muscles are involved, there is often difficulty in raising the arms over the head. The patient may take a long time in recognizing the loss of muscle power because the human body can so well compensate or use other muscles to perform the same motor tasks. If the weakness is present for a considerable length of time, there may be a wasting, or a loss of muscle bulk.

Diagnostic Evaluation of Muscle Disease

In evaluating patients with motor weakness, the physician must have a complete history of the present complaints, past history of the patient, and details of the family history. A general physical and neurological examination is required, with particular reference to the motor, or musculoskeletal system. In most cases, the physician will be able to make a clinical diagnosis of the disease process, but occasionally the examination does not reveal whether the nerve, the muscle, or both are involved. In order to clarify the diagnosis, some additional examinations may be required, mainly determination of serum enzymes (a good indicator of loss of muscle substance), a muscle biopsy, and an electromyogram.

Enzymes are essential for the activity of normal body chemistry. Since the normal blood concentration of some enzymes specifically related to muscle chemistry is known, the determination of blood concentrations of these enzymes can provide additional evidence that muscle chemistry is either normal or abnormal.

A muscle *biopsy* is the surgical removal of a small segment of muscle, which is then prepared for examination under the microscope. The examination of the biopsy specimen enables the physician to visualize any abnormality in the appearance of the muscle fibers, supporting tissue, small nerve twigs, and blood vessels. The muscle biopsy can be of great value in making a correct diagnosis, but occasionally, even in good hands, there is not sufficient pathological change from the normal state to identify the disease process.

Electromyography (EMG) is a technique used to study electrical activity of muscle.

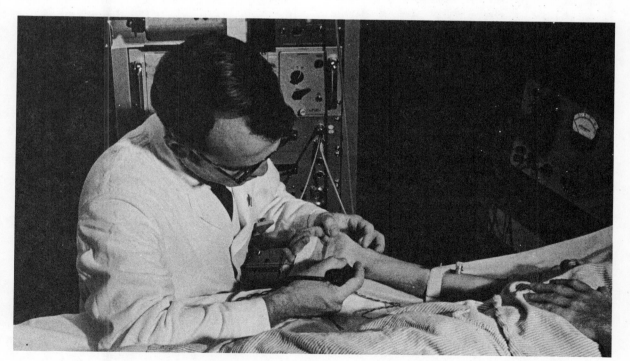

A physician measures the electrical activity of an arm muscle by electromyography (EMG).

Fine needles attached to electronic equipment are inserted into the muscle to measure the electrical activity, which is recorded on an *oscilloscope,* a special electronic device. It is not a particularly painful process when performed by a skilled physician, and the information gained may be important in establishing a diagnosis.

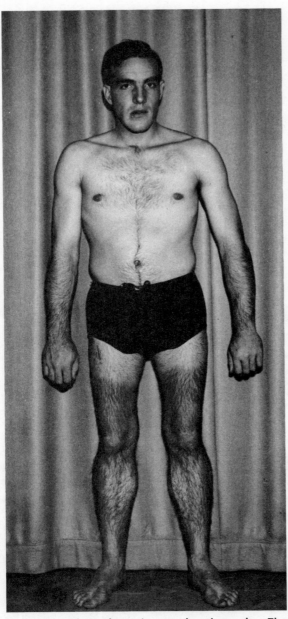

A patient with Duchenne's muscular dystrophy. The muscular appearance is typical, but in spite of muscle enlargement, muscular weakness is usually present

Muscular Dystrophy

In 1886, Dr. Guillaume Duchenne described a muscle disease characterized by weakness and an increase in muscle size and the supporting connective tissue of those muscles. He named the disease *pseudohypertrophic* (false enlargement) muscular paralysis, but it is now known as *Duchenne's muscular dystrophy.*

Subsequently other varieties of muscular dystrophy (MD) have been described and have been classified according to the muscles involved and inheritance. By definition, MD is an inherited, degenerative disease of the muscles. Any abnormality of muscle, whether pathologic, biochemical, or electrical, but without nerve involvement, is called a *myopathy.*

Duchenne's MD is observed almost entirely in males. However, its inheritance through the maternal side of the family means that the mother can pass the clinical disease to her son; her daughters will not demonstrate the disease but are potential carriers to their sons. The mother receives the ability to transmit the disease from her mother. More than one-quarter of the cases of Duchenne's MD are sporadic, that is, without any known family history of the disease. There are rare cases of Duchenne's MD in females who have *ovarian dysgenesis,* a condition in which normal female chromosomal makeup is lacking.

The disease process in Duchenne's MD may be apparent during the first few years of life when the child has difficulty in walking or appears clumsy. The muscles of the pelvis and legs are usually affected first, but the shoulders and the arms soon become involved. About 90 percent of the patients have some enlargement of a muscle or group of muscles and appear to be rather muscular and strong; however, as the disease progresses, the muscular enlargement disappears. Most patients progressively deteriorate and at the age of about 10 to 15 are unable to walk. Once the child is confined to a wheelchair or bed, there is a progressive deformity with muscle contracture and with death coming usually toward the end of the second decade. A small percentage of patients appear to have an arrest of the disease process and survive until the fourth or fifth decade. Despite herculean attempts to unravel the riddle of muscular dystrophy, the problem is yet unsolved.

A benign variety of MD, *Becker type,* begins at 5 to 25 years of age and progresses slowly. Most of the reported patients with Becker type are still able to walk 20 to 30 years after the onset of the disease.

Facio-scapulo-humoral MD: This type of MD affects males and females equally and is thought to be inherited as a dominant trait. The onset may be at any age from childhood to adult life, but is commonly first seen in adolescence. The muscles affected, as indicated by the name of the disease, are those of the face and shoulders, usually with abnormal winging of the *scapula* (either of the large, flat bones at the backs of the shoulders). There is also a characteristic appearance of lip prominence, as if the patient were pouting. Occasionally there is an involvement of the anterior leg muscles, and weakness in raising the foot. The disease progresses more slowly than Duchenne's type, and some patients can remain active for a normal life span.

Limb-girdle MD: This type of MD is less clearly delineated than the others. Males and females are equally affected and the onset is usually in the second or third decade, but the process may start later. It is probably inherited as a recessive trait, but many cases are sporadic. It may first affect the muscles of the pelvis or the shoulder, but in 10 to 15 years both pelvis and shoulder girdles are usually involved. The disease varies considerably from patient to patient; sometimes the disease process appears to be arrested after involvement of either

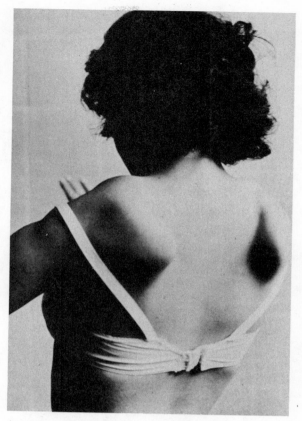

A patient with facio-scapulo-humoral muscular dystrophy. Muscles of the face and shoulders are wasted. Note the protruding scapulae (shoulder blades).

the pelvis or the shoulder, and the patient may then have a benign course. Most, however, have significant difficulty in walking by middle age.

Other varieties of MD: These include ocular, oculopharyngeal, and a distal form (farthest away, as in small muscles of the hands or feet). *Ocular MD* involves the muscles that move the eye as well as the eyelids; occasionally, the small muscles of the face and the shoulder girdle are affected. *Oculopharyngeal MD* involves not only the muscles that move the eye and the eyelids but may also affect the throat muscles, so that patients have difficulty in swallowing food (*dysphagia*). *Distal MD* is rare in the United States but has been reported in Scandinavia. Both sexes can be affected. Usually after the fifth decade, the patient recognizes weakness of the small muscles of the hands and the anterior leg muscles that assist in raising the toes. The disease is relatively benign and progresses slowly.

Treatment: There is no specific treatment for any form of MD, but the patient's life can be made more pleasant and probably prolonged if careful attention is paid to good nutrition, activity without overfatigue, and avoidance of infection. Physical therapists can be helpful in instructing the pa-tient or the parents in an exercise program that relieves joint and muscle stiffness. Sound, prudent, psychological support and guidance cannot be overemphasized.

The Myotonias

This is a group of muscle diseases charac-terized by *myotonia,* a continuation of the muscle contraction after the patient has vol-untarily tried to relax that contraction. It is best observed in the patient who holds an object firmly in his hand and then tries to release his grasp suddenly, only to realize that he cannot let go quickly. There are two major members of this group of diseases and several other less common variants.

Myotonia congenita: This condition is usually present at birth, but is recognized later in the first or second decade of life when the child complains of stiffness or when clumsiness is noted. A child with this condition appears very muscular and has been called the "infant Hercules." The unu-sual muscular development persists through-out life, but the myotonia tends to improve with age.

Myotonic dystrophy: The other major variety of myotonia, *myotonic dystrophy,* is a disease in which many organ systems in addition to muscle are involved. Both males and females are affected equally, and the onset may occur at any time from birth to the fifth decade. It is not unusual for a patient to recognize some clumsiness, but he may not be aware that he has a muscle disease. The myotonia may range from mild to severe. There is a striking similarity in the physical appearance of patients with myotonic dystrophy, the features of which include frontal baldness in the male, wast-ing and weakness of temporal muscles, muscles of the forearm, hands, and anterior leg muscles. Other physical abnormalities include cataracts in about 90 percent of the patients, small testicles, and abnormality of the heart muscle. Thickening and other bony abnormalities have been seen in the

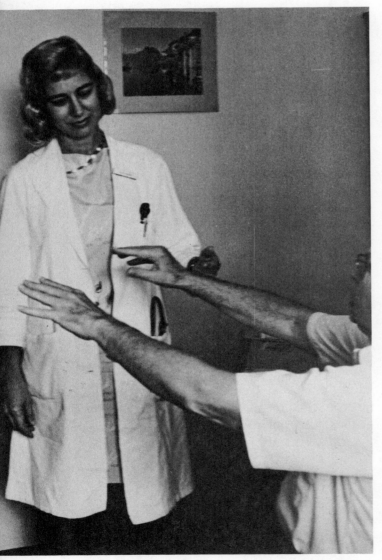

A physician indicates the level at which she wants the patient to hold his arms in a neurological test.

skull radiogram and, with time, many patients become demented.

Treatment: As in the case of muscular dystrophy, there is no specific treatment for myotonia. Some drugs, such as quinine, have limited value in decreasing the abnormally prolonged muscular contractions, but as yet no treatment has been completely effective.

Polymyositis

Polymyositis is a disorder of muscular and connective tissues affecting both sexes, males more commonly than females. It can occur at any age, although usually after the fourth decade. It is characterized by muscle weakness with associated muscle wasting; about half of the patients complain of muscle pain or tenderness. The disease may begin suddenly, but often follows an earlier mild, febrile illness. Changes in the skin are common, including a faint red-violet discoloration particularly about the eyelids, and these changes are often associated with mild swelling. There may be a scaly rash. Some patients have ulcerations over the bony prominences. About one-quarter of the patients with polymyositis complain of joint stiffness and tenderness and an unusual phenomenon in which the nailbeds become blue (*cyanotic*) after minor exposure to cold.

Treatment: The treatment involves the administration of cortisone preparations, which may be required for many years. General supportive care, including appropriate physical therapy, is recommended.

Myasthenia Gravis

Myasthenia gravis is characterized by muscle weakness and an abnormal muscle fatigability (pathologic fatigue); patients are abnormally weak after exercise or at the end of the day. The disease affects males and females from infancy to old age, but it is most common during the second to the fourth decades. There is no complete ex-

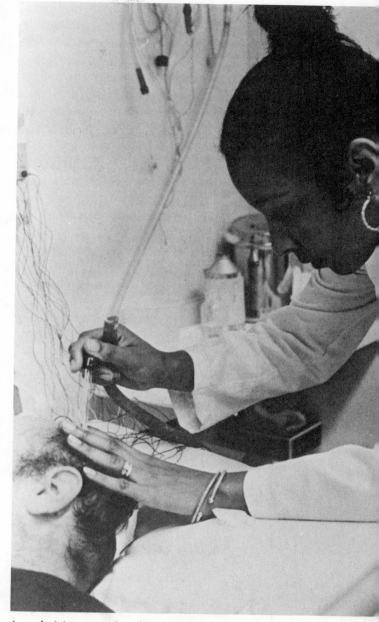

A technician attaches leads to a patient's scalp in preparation for an electroencephalogram.

planation for myasthenia gravis, but it is believed that there is some defect in the transmission of a nerve impulse to the muscle (*myoneural junction defect*). The disease may occur spontaneously, during pregnancy, or following an acute infection, and there appears to be a curious association with diseases in which there is an immunologic abnormality, such as tumors of the thymus gland, increased or decreased activity of the thyroid gland, or rheumatoid arthritis.

Usually there is an insidious onset of generalized weakness, or weakness confined to small groups of muscles. Normal muscle power may be present early in the day, but as the hours pass the patient notices that one or both eyelids droop (*ptosis*) or he may see double images (*diplopia*). If he rests and closes his eyes for a short time, the ptosis and the diplopia clear up, only to return after further muscle activity. The weakness can also be seen in the trunk or the limbs, and some patients have involvement of the muscles used in speaking, chewing, or swallowing (*bulbar* muscles). Some are weak all the time and have an increase in that weakness the longer they use their muscles. The muscles used in respiration may be affected in patients with severe myasthenia, and these patients must be maintained on a respirator for varying periods of time.

Treatment: Myasthenia gravis is treated with drugs that assist in the transmission of the nerve impulse to the muscle. Medication is very effective, but the patient should be carefully observed by the physician to determine that the drug dose and the time of administration are right, so that the patient may have the benefit of maximal muscle power. Surgical removal of the thymus gland, *thymectomy,* may prove of benefit to some patients in lessening the symptoms of muscle weakness; however, not all patients have clinical improvement of the disease after thymectomy, and patients must be selected very carefully by the physician. Myasthenia gravis is another chronic disease in which long-term careful observation by the physician is most important in obtaining an optimal medical and psychological outcome.   BOB

DISEASES OF
THE CIRCULATORY SYSTEM

It's called the river of life, the vital fluid, the five or six quarts of blood that stream through the 60,000 tortuous miles of arteries, veins, and capillaries.

Blood contains many elements with specific functions—red cells to transport oxygen from the lungs to body tissues, white cells to fight off disease, and tiny elements called *platelets* to help form clots and repair tears in the blood vessel wall. All float freely in an intricate complex of liquid proteins and metals known as *plasma.*

Because of the blood's extreme importance to life, any injury to it—or to the grand network of channels through which it flows—may have the most serious consequences. The troubles that beset the circulation may be grouped into two categories: diseases of the blood and diseases of the blood vessels.

Diseases of the Blood

Diseases of the blood include disorders that affect the blood elements directly (as in the case of *hemophilia,* where a deficiency in clotting proteins is at fault) as well as abnormalities in the various organs involved in maintaining proper blood balance (i.e., spleen, liver and bone marrow). The various ills designated and described below are arranged according to the blood component most affected (i.e., clotting proteins, red blood cells, and white blood cells).

Hemorrhagic or Clotting-Deficiency Diseases

The blood has the ability to change from a fluid to a solid and back to a fluid again. The change to a solid is called *clotting*. There are mechanisms not only for sealing off breaks in the circulatory system when serious blood loss is threatened, but also for breaking down the seals, or clots, once the damage has been repaired and the danger of blood loss is eliminated. Both mechanisms are in continuous, dynamic equilibrium, a delicate balance between tissue repair and clot dissolution to keep us from bleeding or literally clogging to death.

Clotting involves a very complex chain of chemical events. The key is the conversion of an inactive blood protein, *fibrinogen*, into a threadlike sealant known as *fibrin*. Stimulus for this conversion is an enzyme called *thrombin*, which normally also circulates in an inactive state as *prothrombin* (formed from vitamin K in the daily diet).

For a clot to form, however, inactive prothrombin must undergo a chemical transformation into thrombin, a step requiring still another chemical—*thromboplastin*. This agent comes into play only when a tissue or vessel has been injured so as to require clot protection. There are two ways for thromboplastin to enter the bloodstream to spark the chain of events. One involves the release by the injured tissue of a substance that reacts with plasma proteins to produce thromboplastin. The other requires the presence of blood platelets (small particles that travel in the blood) and several plasma proteins, including the so-called antihemophilic factor. Platelets tend to clump at the site of vessel injury, where they disintegrate and ultimately release thromboplastin, which, in the presence of blood calcium, triggers the prothrombin-thrombin conversion.

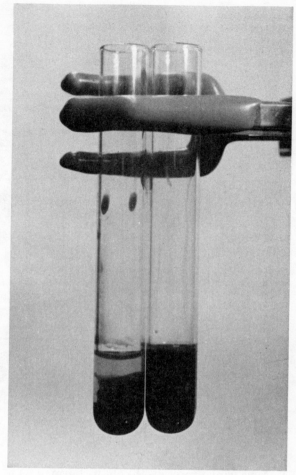

Chemicals called anticoagulants are used to retard clotting. Left standing for two hours, the blood in the left test-tube has formed a clot, but that of the right, treated with an anticoagulant, remains unchanged.

The clot-destroying sequence is very similar to that involved in clot formation, with the key enzyme, *fibrinolysin*, existing normally in an inactive state (*profibrinolysin*). There are also other agents (e.g. *heparin*) in the blood ready to retard or prevent the clotting sequence, so that it doesn't spread to other parts of the body.

Naturally, grave dangers arise should these complex mechanisms fail. For the moment, we shall concern ourselves with hemorrhagic disorders arising from a failure of the blood to clot properly. Disorders stemming from excessive clotting are discussed below under *Diseases of the Blood*

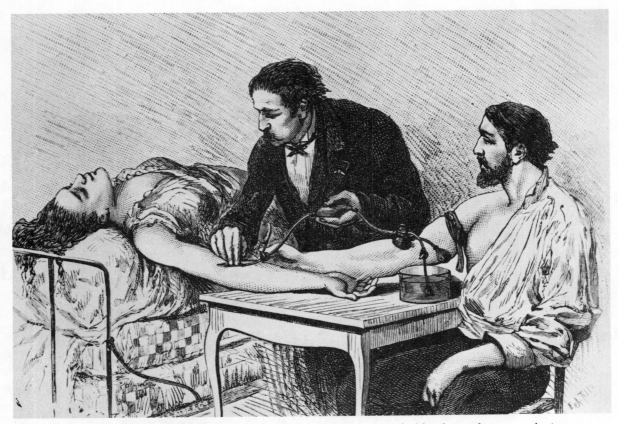

This illustration from a 19th-century medical book shows an early blood transfusion employing the direct method, in which the donor's blood flows directly into the patient's bloodstream.

Vessels, since they are likely to happen as a consequence of pre-existing problems in the vessel walls.

Hemophilia: Hemophilia is probably the best known (although relatively rare) of the hemorrhagic disorders, because of its prevalence among the royal families of Europe. In hemophilia the blood does not clot properly and bleeding persists. Those who have this condition are called *hemophiliacs* or bleeders. The disease is inherited, and is transmitted by the mother, but except in very rare cases only the male offspring are affected. Hemophilia stems from a lack of one of the plasma proteins associated with clotting, *antihemophilic factor (AHF).*

The presence of hemophilia is generally discovered during early childhood. It is readily recognized by the fact that even small wounds bleed profusely and can trigger an emergency. Laboratory tests for clotting speed are used to confirm the diagnosis. Further investigation may occasionally turn up the condition in other members of the family.

In advanced stages, hemophilia may lead to anemia as a result of excessive and continuous blood loss. Bleeding in the joints causes painful swelling, which over a long period of time can lead to permanent deformity and hemophilic arthritis. Hemophiliacs must be under constant medical care in order to receive quick treatment in case of emergencies.

Treating bleeding episodes may involve the administration of AHF alone so as to speed up the clotting sequence. If too much blood is lost a complete transfusion may be necessary. Thanks to modern blood bank techniques, large quantities of whole blood can be made readily available. Bed rest and hospitalization may also be required. For bleeding in the joints, an ice pack is usually applied.

Proper dental hygiene is a must for all hemophiliacs. Every effort should be made to prevent tooth decay. Parents of children with the disease should inform the dentist so that all necessary precautions can be taken. Even the most common procedures, such as an extraction, can pose a serious hazard. Only absolutely essential surgery should be performed on hemophiliacs, with the assurance that large amounts of plasma are on hand.

Purpura: Purpura refers to spontaneous hemorrhaging over large areas of the skin and in mucous membranes. It results from a deficiency in blood platelets, elements essential to clotting. Purpura is usually triggered by other conditions: certain anemias, leukemia, sensitivity to drugs, or exposure to ionizing radiation. In newborns it may be linked to the prenatal transfer from the maternal circulation of substances that depress platelet levels. Symptoms of purpura include the presence of blood in the urine, bleeding from the mucous membranes of the mouth, nose, intestines and uterus. Some forms of the disease cause arthritic changes in joints, abdominal pains, diarrhea and vomiting—and even gangrene of the skin, when certain infectious organisms become involved.

To treat purpura in newborns, physicians may exchange the infant's blood with platelet-packed blood. Sometimes drug therapy with *steroids* (i.e., cortisone) is prescribed. In adults with chronic purpura it may be necessary to remove the spleen, which plays an important role in eliminating worn-out blood components, including platelets, from the circulation. Most physicians prescribe large doses of steroids coupled with blood transfusions. Purpura associated with infection and gangrene also requires appropriate antibiotic therapy.

Red Cell Diseases

Half the blood is plasma; the other half is made up of many tiny blood cells. The biggest group in number is the red blood cells. These cells contain a complicated chemical called *hemoglobin,* which brings oxygen from the lungs to body cells and picks up waste carbon dioxide for expiration. Hemoglobin is rich in iron, which is what imparts the characteristic red color to blood.

Red blood cells are manufactured by bones all over the body—in the sternum, ribs, skull, arms, spine and pelvis. The actual factory is the red bone marrow, located at bone ends. As red cells mature and are ready to enter the blood stream, they lose

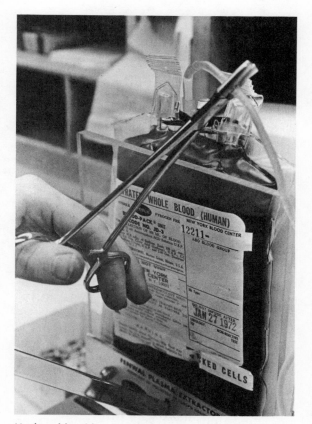

Modern blood bank techniques can make large quantities of whole blood available to hemophiliacs. Blood can also be fractionated (separated into components) for use of the antihemophilic factor (AHF) of plasma.

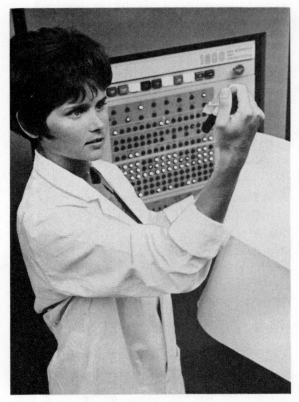

A computer linked to automated testing instruments provides blood test results quickly and accurately.

Abnormalities in the size, shape, or hemoglobin content of the erythrocytes may also account for anemic states. Any such irregularity interferes with the red cell's ability to carry its full share of oxygen to body tissues. It also tends to weaken the red cells so that they are more likely to be destroyed under the stresses of the circulation.

Anemia may result from:

• Nutritional deficiencies which deprive the body of elements vital to the production of healthy cells

• Diseases or injuries to organs associated with either blood cell formation (bone marrow) or blood cell destruction (spleen and liver)

• Excessive loss of blood, the consequences of surgery, hemorrhage, or a bleeding ulcer

• Heredity, as in the case of *sickle cell anemia* (where the red cells are misshapen).

their nuclei to become what are called *red corpuscles* or *erythrocytes*. With no nucleus, a red corpuscle is relatively short-lived (120 days). Thus, the red cell supply must be constantly replenished by bone marrow. And busy factories they are, since 20 to 25 trillion red corpuscles normally travel in the circulation. The spleen is responsible for ridding the body of the aged corpuscles, but it is not an indiscriminate sanitizer, inasmuch as it salvages the hemoglobin for reuse by the body.

To measure levels of red cells, physicians make a blood count by taking a smidgen of blood from a patient's fingertip. The average number of red cells in healthy blood is about five million per cubic millimeter for men, and four and one-half million for women.

Anemia: Anemia exists when the red cell count stays persistently below four million.

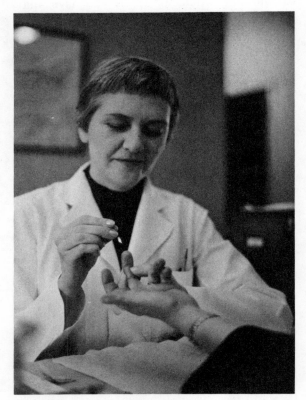

A pricked finger yields enough blood to determine the proportion of red blood cells in a blood count.

Hemolytic anemia: There are also several kinds of disorders known as *hemolytic anemias* that are linked to the direct destruction of red cells. Poisons such as snake venom, arsenic, and lead can cause hemolytic anemia. So can toxins produced by certain bacteria as well as by other organisms, such as the parasites that cause malaria, hookworm, and tapeworm. Destruction of red cells may also stem from allergic reactions to certain drugs or transfusions with incompatible blood.

The various anemias range from ailments mild enough to go undetected to disorders which prove inevitably fatal. Many are rare; among the more common are:

Pernicious anemia: Pernicious anemia, or *Addison's anemia,* is associated with a lack of hydrochloric acid in the gastric juices, a defect which interferes with the body's ability to absorb vitamin B_{12} from the intestine. Since the vitamin acts as an essential stimulus to the production of mature red blood cells by the bone marrow, its lack leads to a reduced output. Moreover, the cells tend to be larger than normal, with only half the life-span of the normal erythrocyte.

The symptoms are characteristic of most anemias: pale complexion, numbness or a feeling of "pins and needles" in the arms and legs, shortness of breath (from a lack of oxygen), loss of appetite, nausea, and diarrhea (often accompanied by significant weight loss). One specific feature is a sore mouth with a smooth, glazed tongue. Advanced stages of the disease may be marked by an unsteady gait and other nervous disorders, owing to degeneration of the spinal cord. Red cell count may drop as low as 1,000,000. Several kinds of tests may be necessary to differentiate pernicious anemia from other blood diseases—a test for hydrochloric acid levels, for example.

Pernicious anemia, however, is no longer so pernicious, or deadly, as it once was—not since its cause was identified. Large, in-

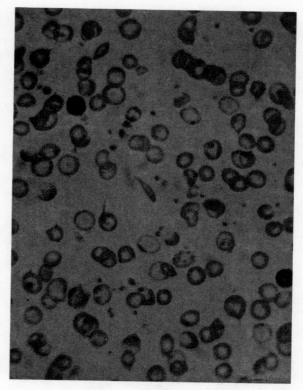

A photomicrograph of a blood smear showing sickle cells amidst the normal red cells. The solid dark circles are white cells. The very small dark spots are platelets, which are abnormally numerous here.

jected doses of vitamin B_{12} usually restore normal blood cell production.

Sickle-cell anemia: Sickle-cell anemia, an inherited abnormality, occurs almost exclusively among black people. Widespread in tropical Africa and Asia, sickle-cell anemia is also found in this country, affecting perhaps 1 in 500 American blacks. The blood cells are sickle-shaped rather than round, a structural aberration arising from a defect in the manufacture of hemoglobin, the oxygen-carrying component.

A differentiation should be made between sickle-cell anemia, the full-blown disease, and sickle cell trait. Anemia occurs when the offspring inherits the sickle-cell gene from both parents. For these people life stretches out in endless bouts of fatigue punctuated by a series of crises of excruciating pain lasting days or

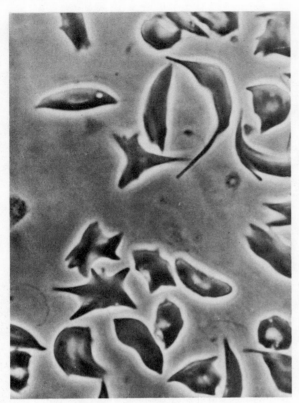

Sickle cells magnified 1000 times. Inherited sickle-cell anemia affects about one black American in 500.

even weeks. In some cases there is permanent paralysis. The crises often require long-term hospitalization. The misshapen cells increase the patient's susceptibility to blood clots, pneumonia, kidney and heart failure, strokes, general systemic poisoning due to bacterial invasions, and, in the case of pregnant women, spontaneous abortion. Ninety percent of the patients die before age 40, with most dead by age 30. Half are dead by age 20, with a number also suffering from poor physical and mental development.

Those with only one gene for the disease have sickle cell trait. They are not likely to have too much trouble except in circumstances where they are exposed to low oxygen levels (the result, say, of poor oxygenation in a high-altitude plane). Administration of anesthesia or too much physical activity may also bring on some feverish attacks. Those with the trait are also carriers of the disease, since they can pass it on to the next generation. Two out of every 25 black Americans are said to be carrying the trait.

Iron-deficiency anemia: Iron-deficiency anemia is a common complication of pregnancy, during which time the fetus may rob the maternal blood of much of its iron content. Iron is essential to the formation of hemoglobin. The deficiency can be further aggravated by digestive disturbances (i.e. a lack of hydrochloric acid) which may hinder the absorption of dietary iron from the intestines. Some women may not observe proper dietary habits, thereby aggravating the anemic state. Successful treatment involves increasing iron intake, with iron supplements and an emphasis on iron-rich foods, including eggs, cereals, green vegetables, and meat, especially liver.

Polycythemia: Polycythemia is the opposite of anemia; the blood has too many red corpuscles. The most common form of the disease is *polycythemia vera* (or *erythremia*). In addition to the rise in corpuscle count, there is a corresponding rise—as much as three-fold—in blood volume to accommodate the high cell count, and increased blood viscosity. Symptoms include an enlarged spleen, blood-shot eyes, red mouth and red mucous membranes—all due to excess red cells. Other common characteristics are weakness, fatigue, irritability, dizziness, swelling in the ankles, choking sensations, viselike chest pains (angina pectoris), rapid heart beat, and sometimes severe headaches. There is also an increased tendency toward both clotting and hemorrhaging.

The disease occurs primarily in the middle and late years and is twice as prevalent in males than females. The cause is unknown, but polycythemia is characterized by stepped-up bone marrow production activity.

Radiation therapy is one method for controlling this hyperactivity. Low iron diets and several forms of drug therapy have been tried with varying degrees of effectiveness. A one-time panacea, blood-letting—to drain off excess blood—appears to be of considerable value. Many patients survive for years with the disease. Premature death is usually the result of vascular thrombosis (clotting), massive hemorrhage, or leukemia.

The Rh factor: Rh disease might also be considered a form of anemia—in newborns. The disorder involves destruction of the red blood cells of an as-yet unborn or newborn infant. It is brought about by an incom-

patability between the maternal blood and fetal blood of one specific factor—the so-called *Rh* factor. (*Rh* stands for *rhesus* monkey, the species in which it was first identified.) Most of us are *Rh* positive, which is to say that we have the *Rh* protein substance on the surface of our red cells. The *Rh* factor is, in fact, present in 83 percent of the white population and 93 percent of the black. Those lacking it are classified as *Rh* negative.

A potentially dangerous situation exists when an *Rh* negative mother is carrying an

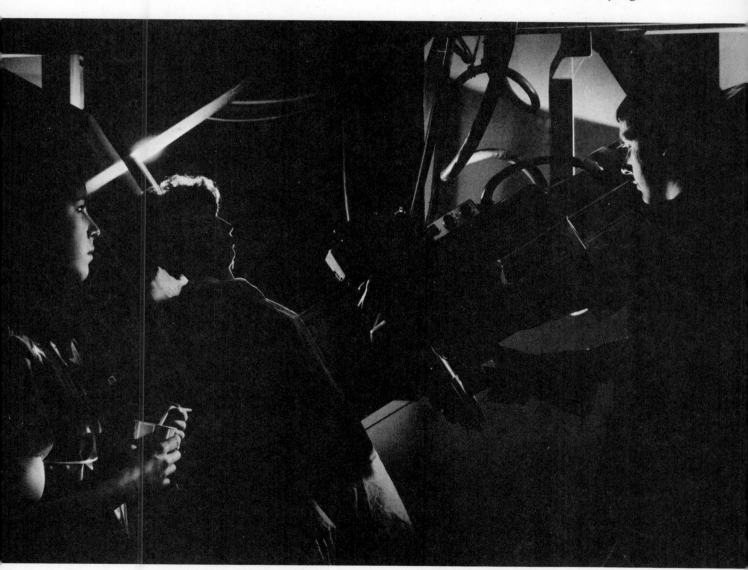

Radiation therapy being administered in the treatment of blood disease.

Rh positive baby in her uterus. Although the mother and unborn baby have separate circulatory systems, some leakage does occur. When *Rh* positive cells from the fetus leak across the placenta into the mother's blood, her system recognizes them as foreign and makes antibodies against them. If these antibodies then slip across into the fetal circulation, damage is inevitable.

The first baby, however, is rarely affected because it takes time for the mother's body to become sensitized to the *Rh* positive cells. But should she become pregnant with another child, the now-sensitized mother's blood produces a large quantity of destructive antibodies that could result in stillbirth, death of the infant shortly after birth or, if the child survives, jaundice and anemia.

Modern medicine has reduced the fatality rate and considerably improved the prognosis. Severely affected newborns are being treated by complete blood transfusions— even while still in the womb—to draw off all the *Rh* positive cells. After birth and as it grows older, the child will once again produce *Rh* positive cells in its bone marrow— but by that time the danger from the mother's antibodies is past. Recently an *Rh* vaccine to prevent the problem from ever occurring was developed. After *Rh* negative women give birth to their first *Rh* positive baby, they are immunized with the anti-*Rh* serum to prevent them from manufacturing these dangerous antibodies.

White Blood Cell Diseases

For every 600–700 or more red corpuscles, there is one white blood cell, or *leukocyte*. White cells, unlike red corpuscles, have nuclei; they are also larger and rounder. About 70 percent of the white cell population have irregularly-shaped centers, and these are called *polymorphonuclear leukocytes* or *neutrophils*. The other 30 percent are made up of a variety of cells with round nuclei called *lymphocytes*. A cubic millimeter of blood normally contains anywhere from 5,000 to 9,000 white cells (as compared with the 4–5 million red cells).

White cells defend against disease, which explains why their number increases in the bloodstream when the body is under infectious assault. There are some diseases of the blood and blood-forming organs themselves that can increase the white count. Disorders of the spleen, for example, can produce white cell abnormalities, because this organ is a major source of lymphocytes (cells responsible for making protective antibodies). Diseases of the bone marrow are likely to affect neutrophil production.

Leukemia: Leukemia, characterized by an abnormal increase in the number of white cells, is one of the most dangerous of blood disorders. The cancerlike disease results from a severe disturbance in the functioning of the bone marrow. Chronic leukemia, which strikes mainly in middle age, produces an enormous increase in neutrophils, which tend to rush into the bloodstream at every stage of their development, whether mature or not. Patients with the chronic disease may survive for several years, with appropriate treatment.

In acute leukemia, more common among children than adults, the marrow produces monster-sized, cancerous-looking white cells. These cells not only crowd out other blood components from the circulation, they also leave little space for the marrow to produce the other elements, especially the red cells and platelets. Acute leukemias run their fatal course in a matter of weeks or months—although there have been dramatic instances of sudden remission. The cause is unknown, but recent evidence strongly suggests that a virus may be responsible for at least some forms of the disease.

Modern treatment—radiation and drugs —is aimed at wiping out all of the malignant cells. A critical stage follows treatment, however. For with the disappearance of these abnormal cells and the temporary disruption of marrow function, the patient is

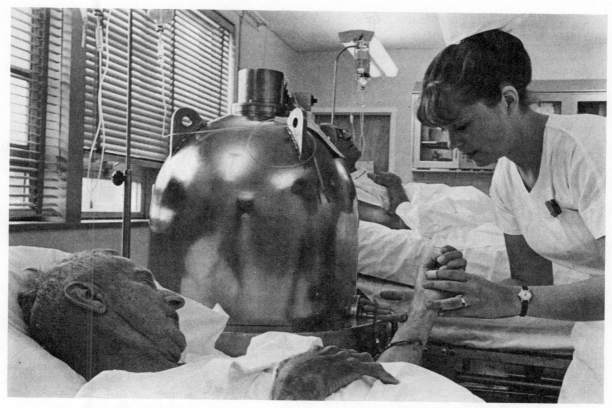

Because red blood cells are much more resistant to radiation damage than leukemic white cells, irradiation of the blood is one way to destroy diseased cells without injuring other cells. Arterial blood is propelled by the heart action of these patients through plastic tubing into the shielded container, past an intense source of gamma rays, and back into each patient's arm.

left with his defenses against infection down. He also runs a great risk of hemorrhage. Therefore, he is usually kept in isolation to ward off infections. In addition he may be given white cell and platelet transfusions along with antibiotic therapy. Eventually—and hopefully—the marrow will revert to normal function, freed of leukemic cell production.

Agranulocytosis: Agranulocytosis is a disease brought on by the direct destruction of neutrophils (also called *granulocytes*). Taken over a long period of time, certain types of drugs may bring about large-scale destruction of the neutrophil supply. Symptoms include general debilitation, fatigue, sleeplessness, restlessness, headache, chills, high fever (often up to 105°), sore mouth and throat, along with psychologically aber-

rant behavior and mental confusion. White cell count may fall as low as 500 to 2000. Sometimes agranulocytosis is confused with leukemia.

Treatment involves antibiotic therapy to ward off bacterial invasion, a likelihood that is increased owing to the lowered body resistance. In advanced cases, hospitalization and transfusions with fresh blood are necessary. Injections of fresh bone marrow may also be prescribed.

Leukopenia: Leukopenia is less severe than agranulocytosis. It too involves a reduction of circulating white cells to counts of less than 5000. It is usually the result of allergic reactions to some chemical or drug.

Infectious mononucleosis: Infectious mononucleosis, also known as *glandular fever* or *kissing disease,* is characterized by the presence in the bloodstream of a large number of lymphocytes, many of which are abnormally formed. The disease is mildly contagious—kissing is thought to be one popular source of transmission—and occurs chiefly among children and adolescents. The transmitting agent, however, has yet to be discovered, though some as yet unidentified organism is strongly suspected.

The disease is not always easy to diagnose. It can incubate anywhere from four days to four weeks, at which point the patient may experience fever, headache, sore throat, swollen lymph nodes, loss of appetite, and a general feeling of weakness.

The disease runs its course in a matter of a week or two, although complete recovery may take a while longer. Bed rest and

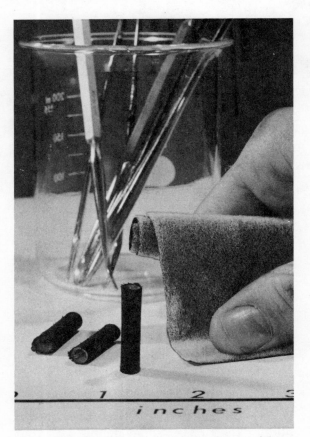

Man-made blood vessels fashioned from polyester velour fabric (right) simulate functions of veins and arteries. Still in the experimental stage, they may soon aid people suffering from vascular diseases.

conservative medical management is often enough for complete patient recovery. A few severe cases may require hospitalization because of occasional complications, such as rupture of the spleen, skin lesions, some minor liver malfunctions, and occasionally hemolytic anemia or purpura.

Diseases of the Blood Vessels

Diseases of the blood vessels deal with problems arising primarily from adverse changes in the vessel walls, such as hardening of the arteries, stroke, varicose veins, and other disorders.

A healthy circulation depends to a large extent not only on the condition of the blood-forming organs but on the pipelines through which this life-sustaining fluid flows. The arteries, which carry blood away from the heart, and the veins, which bring it back, are subject to a wide range of maladies. They may become inflamed, as in the case of arteritis, phlebitis, and varicose veins; or they may become clogged—especially the arteries—as a result of atherosclerosis (hardening of the arteries) or blood clots (thrombosis and embolism).

The Inflammatory Disorders

Arteritis: Arteritis, or inflammation of the arterial wall, usually results from infections (e.g. syphilis) or allergic reactions in which the body's protective agents against invading organisms, the antibodies, attack the vessel walls themselves. In these instances, the prime source of inflammation must be treated before the arterial condition can heal.

Phlebitis: Phlebitis is an inflammation of the veins, a condition that may stem from an injury or may be associated with such conditions as varicose veins, malignancies, and infection. The extremities, especially the legs, are vulnerable to the disorder. The symptoms are stiffness and hot and painful swelling of the involved region. Phlebitis brings with it the tendency of blood to form blood clots (*thrombophlebitis*) at the site of inflammation. The danger is that one of these clots may break away and enter the bloodstream. Such a clot, on the move, called an *embolus,* may catch and become lodged in a smaller vessel serving a vital organ, causing a serious blockage in the blood supply.

Physicians are likely to prescribe various drugs for phlebitis—agents to deal with the suspected cause of the disorder as well as *anticoagulants* (anti-clotting compounds) to ward off possible thromboembolic complications.

Varicose veins: Varicose veins, which are veins that are enlarged and distorted, primarily affect the leg vessels, and are often troublesome to people who are on their feet for many hours. Varicose veins develop because either the walls or the valves of veins are weakened. Some people may be born with weakened veins or valves. In others, the damage may develop from injury or disease, such as phlebitis. More women than men seem to have this condition, but it is common among both sexes. In women, the enlarged veins sometimes occur during pregnancy, but these may well diminish and disappear after delivery. Some elderly people are prone to this condition because the blood vessels lose their elasticity with aging, with the muscles that support the vein growing less sturdy.

In most instances, the surface veins lying just beneath the skin are involved. If there are no other complications, these cases are seldom serious, although they may be disturbing because of unsightliness. Doctors have remedies, including surgery, for making varicosed veins less prominent.

When varicose veins become severe, it is usually because the vessels deeper in the leg are weak. Unchecked, this situation can lead to serious complications, including swelling (*edema*) around the ankles and lower legs. The skin in the lower leg may

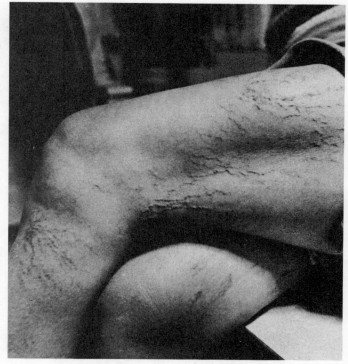

Weakened walls or valves of the veins can lead to varicose veins, where the veins become enlarged and distorted. Tiny hemorrhages may discolor the skin.

become thin and fragile and easily irritated. Tiny hemorrhages may discolor the skin. In advanced stages, hard-to-treat leg ulcers and sores may erupt.

Most of the complicating problems can be averted with early care and treatment. Doctors generally prescribe elastic stockings even in the mildest of cases and sometimes elastic bandages to lend support to the veins. They may recommend some newer techniques for injecting certain solutions that close off the affected portion of the vein. On the other hand, surgery may be indicated, especially for the surface veins, in which the varicose section is either tied off or stripped, with the blood being rerouted to the deeper vein channels.

While long periods of standing may be hard on varicosed legs, so are uninterrupted stretches of sitting, which may cause blood to collect in the lower leg and further distend the veins. Patients are advised to get

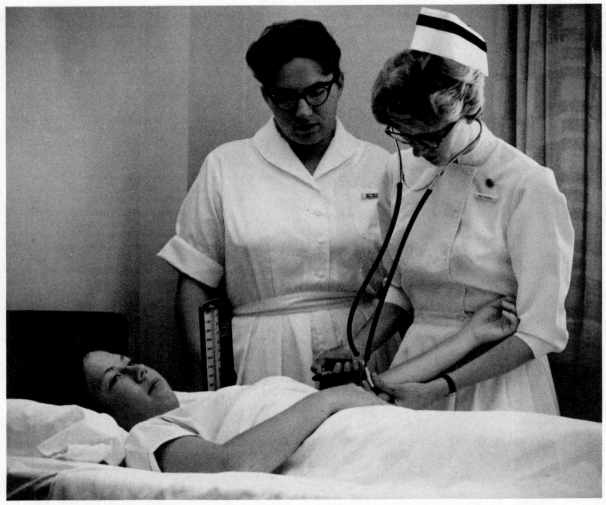

Atherosclerosis refers to the thickening of the interior walls of the blood vessels by deposits of fat. Blood pressure readings can help in assessing the condition of blood vessel walls.

up and walk about every half hour or so during any extended period of sitting. A good idea, too, is to sit with the feet raised, whenever possible, to keep blood from collecting in the lower legs.

The Vessel-Clogging Disorders

Atherosclerosis: Atherosclerosis (hardening of the arteries) is the nation's most serious health problem, the underlying cause of a million or more deaths each year from heart attack and stroke. It is the process whereby fats carried in the bloodstream gradually pile up on the walls of arteries, like rust in a pipe. The vessels become brittle and roughened; the channel through which blood flows grows narrower. Eventually the organs and tissues supplied by the diseased arteries may be sufficiently deprived of their normal oxygen delivery so as to interfere with proper function. Such a cutback in the pipeline supply is called *ischemia*. This fat deposit poses its greatest hazard when it occurs in the vessels serving the heart, brain and, sometimes, the lower extremities.

In the last case, for instance, a reduced supply of blood may cause irreversible damage and ultimately lead to death of the leg tissues unless proper circulation is restored.

Bacterial invasion may follow; the area may swell, blacken, and emit the distinctly offensive smell of the deadly infection. Such a condition is known as *gangrene,* a severe disorder that may require amputation above the site of blockage if other measures, including antibiotic therapy, fail. Diabetics more commonly than others may develop atherosclerotic obstructions in leg arteries. Such persons must take care to avoid leg injuries, since the further loss of blood, as from a cut, in an already poorly served tissue area can bring on what is termed *diabetic gangrene.*

When the coronary arteries nourishing the heart are involved, even a moderate reduction in blood delivery to the heart muscle may be enough to cause angina pectoris, with its intense, suffocating chest pains.

Thrombosis: Thrombosis, a blood clot that forms within the vessels, is a great, everpresent threat that accompanies atherosclerosis. The narrowed arteries seem to make it easier for normal blood substances to adhere to the roughened wall surfaces, forming clots. If the clot blocks the coronary arteries, it may produce a heart attack— damage to that part of the heart deprived by vessel obstruction. For a detailed account of atherosclerosis and heart attack, see under *Heart Disease,* p. 500.

Stroke: Stroke, like heart attack, is a disorder usually due to blockage brought on by the atheroslerotic process in vessels supplying the brain. This sets the stage for a *thrombus,* or blood clot fixed within a vessel, which would not be likely to occur in arteries clear of these fatty deposits. A stroke may be a result of an interruption of blood flow through arteries in the brain or in neck vessels leading to the brain.

Sometimes the shutoff of blood flow, or *embolism,* may be triggered by a wandering blood clot that has become wedged in cerebral vessels. This kind of clot, known as an *embolus,* is a thrombus that has broken free into the circulation.

A stroke may also stem from hemorrhaging, where a diseased artery in the brain bursts. A cerebral hemorrhage is most likely to occur when a patient has atherosclerosis in combination with hypertension (high blood pressure). (For a discussion of hyper-

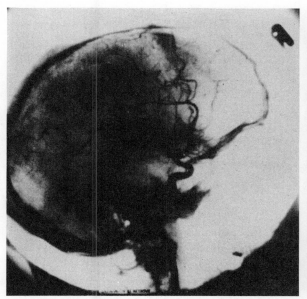
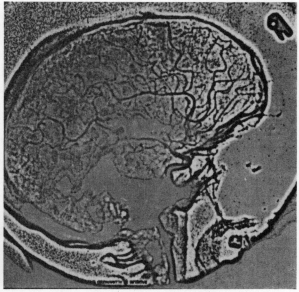

Digital computer techniques can be used to clarify X rays. The computer-enhanced X ray of a human skull (*right*) shows the frontal blood vessels more clearly than an ordinary X ray (*left*).

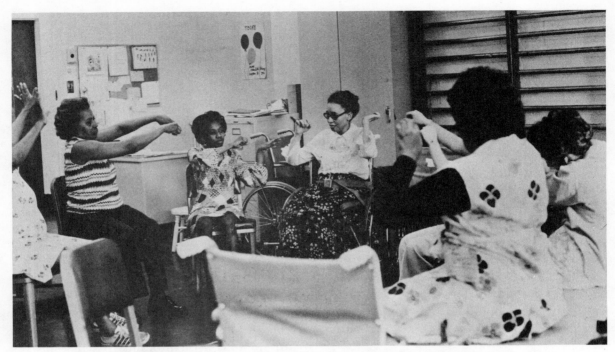

Intensive rehabilitation is most important in the treatment of stroke patients. These women are learning to regain control of their bodies through dance therapy.

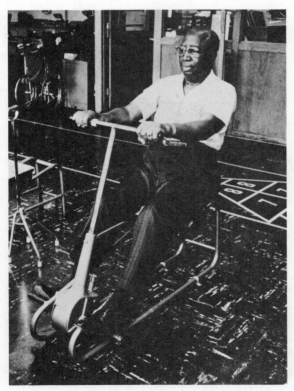

Daily sessions on a bicycle exerciser are part of the physical therapy prescribed for many stroke patients.

tension, see *Hypertensive Heart Disease*, p. 512.) Hemorrhage is also a danger when an aneurysm forms in a blood vessel. An *aneurysm* is a blood-filled pouch that balloons out from a weak spot in the artery wall. Sometimes, too, pressure from a mass of tissue—a tumor, for example—can produce a stroke by squeezing a nearby brain vessel shut.

When the blood supply is cut off, injury to certain brain cells follow. Cells thus damaged cannot function; neither, then, can the parts of the body controlled by these nerve centers. The damage to the brain cells may produce paralysis of a leg or arm; it may interfere with the ability to speak or with a person's memory. The affected function and the extent of disability depend on which brain region has been struck, how widespread the damage is, how effectively the body can repair its supply system to this damaged area, and how rapidly other areas of brain tissue can take over the work of the out-of-commission nerve cells.

Frequently there are symptoms of impending stroke: headaches, numbness in the limbs, faintness, momentary lapses in memory, slurring of speech, or sudden clumsiness. The presence of these symptoms does not always mean a stroke is brewing; sometimes they are quite harmless. But should they be stroke warning signals, the physician can take some preventive action. He may recommend anticoagulant therapy as well as drugs to bring down elevated blood pressure. In some cases, he might decide to call for surgical replacement of diseased or weakened sections of arteries leading to the brain.

Once a stroke has occurred, the most important step is intensive rehabilitation. Not everyone needs such a program, inasmuch as some people are only slightly affected by a stroke. Others may recover quickly from what seems like a severe stroke. But still others may suffer such serious damage that it may take a long time to regain even partial use of the faculty involved. A great deal, however, can be done to help, especially for patients who are partially paralyzed and those with *aphasia*—the inability to deal with language properly because of damage to the brain's speech center. For rehabilitation to be most effective, it should be started as soon as possible after the stroke.

Embolus and thrombus: An embolus, or thrombus that has broken away into the bloodstream, is, as we have seen, sometimes the direct cause of a stroke. A heart attack may also cause a stroke. Bacterial action may soften a thrombus so that it separates into fragments and breaks free from its wall anchorage. Thrombi are not the only source of emboli; any free-floating mass in the bloodstream, be it an air bubble, clumps of fat, knots of cancer cells, or bacteria, can prove dangerous.

Usually, however, emboli originate as thrombi in the veins, especially the leg veins. Breaking free, the clump of clot material wanders into the bloodstream to be car-

ried towards the right chamber of the heart and then onward into the lungs, unless dissolved before that. Once in the pulmonary arteries there is a growing threat that the moving mass will catch in one of the smaller branches of the lung circulation. This life-threatening blockage is called a *pulmonary embolism.*

This disorder takes at least 50,000 lives a year; most occur during or following prolonged periods of hospitalization and bed rest. The lack of activity slows the blood

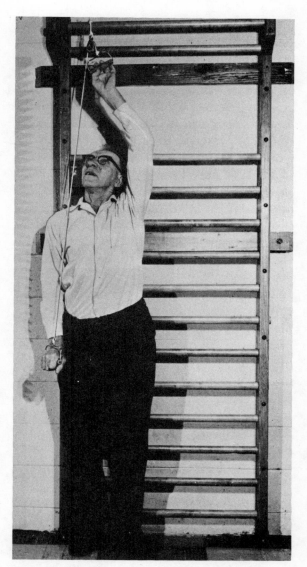

Physical therapy for stroke should begin as soon as possible. This patient is strengthening arm muscles.

flow and increases the danger of thrombi —and ultimately emboli. Prevention requires getting the patient out of bed as soon and as often as possible to stimulate leg circulation. The nonambulatory patient, meanwhile, is encouraged to move his legs by raising them, or changing position so as to step-up blood flow.

The detection of a large embolus—symptoms include shortness of breath and chest pains—may require emergency surgery for removal. In most instances, however, treatment usually means administering anticoagulants to prevent new clots from emerging while allowing the body to rid itself of the existing embolus.   BP, AAD

HEART DISEASE

Heart disease is the commonly used, catch-all phrase for a number of disorders affecting both the heart and blood vessels. A more apt term is cardiovascular disease, which represents America's worst health scourge. More than 27,000,000 Americans of all ages are afflicted with some kind of cardiovascular ailment. When considered together, heart and circulatory system diseases, including stroke, account for more than one-half of all deaths each year in the United States, a total of over 1,000,000 people.

The most frequent cause of death from cardiovascular disease is *coronary artery disease,* brought on by obstructions that develop in the coronary vessels nourishing the heart muscle. These fatty blockages impair adequate delivery of oxygen-laden blood to the heart muscle cells. The result may be *angina pectoris:* short episodes of viselike chest pains that strike when the heart fails to get enough blood; or it may be a full-blown heart attack, where blood-starved heart tissue dies.

One out of every five American males will have a heart attack before the age of 60. Heart attacks strike about 1.6 million annually, killing over 600,000. Overall, more than 6 million adults either definitely have or are suspected of having some degree of

coronary disease; for this reason it has been labeled the "20th century epidemic," or the "black plague of affluence."

Hypertensive heart disease is an impairment of heart-pumping function stemming from persistent *hypertension* (high blood pressure). Untreated, elevated pressure makes the heart work harder, causing it to enlarge and sometimes, to fail. It can also lead to serious damage to the kidneys and acceleration of the vessel-clogging process responsible for most heart attacks and strokes. Hypertension is the most common of the cardiovascular diseases, affecting about 22 million Americans, with more than half having some degree of heart involvement. A little more than 60,000 deaths are directly attributable to hypertension and hypertensive heart disease.

Rheumatic heart disease, the leftover scars of a rheumatic fever attack, claims the lives of 14,000 annually. It generally strikes children between the ages of 5 and 15. All told, 1,600,000 persons are suffering from rheumatic heart disease, with about 100,000 new cases reported each year.

Congenital heart disease includes that collection of heart and major blood vessel deformities that exist at birth and appear in 8 out of every 1,000 live births, or 25,000 cases yearly, Nine thousand deaths annu-

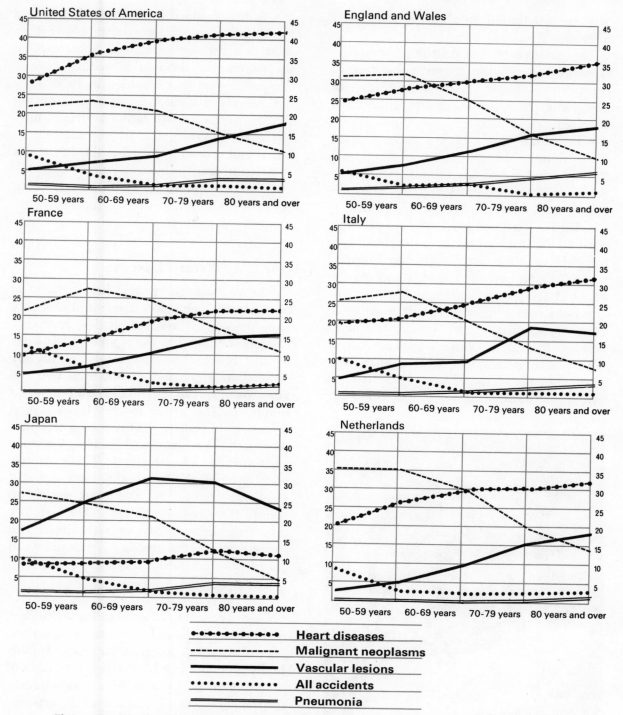

United States of America

England and Wales

50-59 years 60-69 years 70-79 years 80 years and over

France

Italy

50-59 years 60-69 years 70-79 years 80 years and over

Japan

Netherlands

50-59 years 60-69 years 70-79 years 80 years and over

●—●—●—●—●—●—● **Heart diseases**
- - - - - - - - - - **Malignant neoplasms**
━━━━━━━ **Vascular lesions**
• • • • • • • • • • **All accidents**
═══════ **Pneumonia**

These graphs illustrate the relative frequency of the five major causes of death among people aged 50 or over in six different countries. The horizontal lines represent the percentage of deaths from all causes attributed to the particular disease. Note that in these graphs, which are based upon recent figures compiled by the World Health Organization (WHO), vascular lesions, which include strokes, are considered separately from heart diseases. The percentage of deaths resulting from cardiovascular diseases, therefore, can be arrived at by adding together the figures for heart diseases and vascular lesions.

ally are attributed to these inborn heart abnormalities.

This grim portrait of death and disability is improving rapidly, however, because of research uncovering new knowledge for protecting the heart and its pipelines. For example:

• Rheumatic fever, once a major menace of childhood, has been subdued effectively through the use of antibiotics, which can eradicate streptococcal infections, the precursor of rheumatic disease; theoretically, the disease has been made wholly preventable. In the last two decades the death rate from rheumatic heart disease has dropped more than 85 percent within the 5- to 24-year-old age group.

• Bold new surgery makes it possible to cure or alleviate most congenital heart defects, to replace defective heart valves with plastic substitutes, and to open new sources of blood to a heart with diseased coronary arteries.

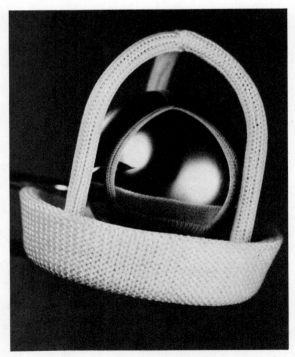

This artificial aortic valve prosthesis consists of a metal frame and seating ring completely covered with a synthetic fabric, and a hollow ball of stellite.

• A broad arsenal of drugs that makes almost all cases of hypertension—whether mild or severe—controllable, helps explain the 63 percent drop in the death rate as compared with that recorded in 1950.

• Advances in coronary care are lowering the heart attack death rate. Physicians, having learned to recognize the coronary-prone individual, are able to prescribe life styles to forestall heart attack.

• Out-of-kilter heart rhythms are being restored to normal with permanently implanted pacemakers.

Coronary Artery Disease

To keep itself going, the heart relies on two pencil-thick main arteries. Branching from the aorta, these vessels deliver freshly oxygenated blood to the right and left sides of the heart. The left artery is usually somewhat larger and divides into two sizable vessels, the circumflex and anterior branches. The latter is sometimes called the artery of sudden death, since a clot near its mouth is common and leads to a serious and often fatal heart attack. These arteries wind around the heart and send out still smaller branches into the heart muscle to supply the needs of all cells. The network of vessels arches down over the heart like a crown—in Latin, *corona*—hence the word *coronary*.

Atherosclerosis

Coronary artery disease exists when flow of blood is impaired because of narrowed and obstructed coronary arteries. In virtually all cases, this blockade is the result of atherosclerosis, a form of *arteriosclerosis*, the thickening and hardening of the arteries. *Atherosclerosis*, from the Greek for porridge or mush, refers to the process by which fat carried in the bloodstream piles up on the inner wall of the arteries like rust in a pipe. As more and more fatty substances, including cholesterol, accumulate,

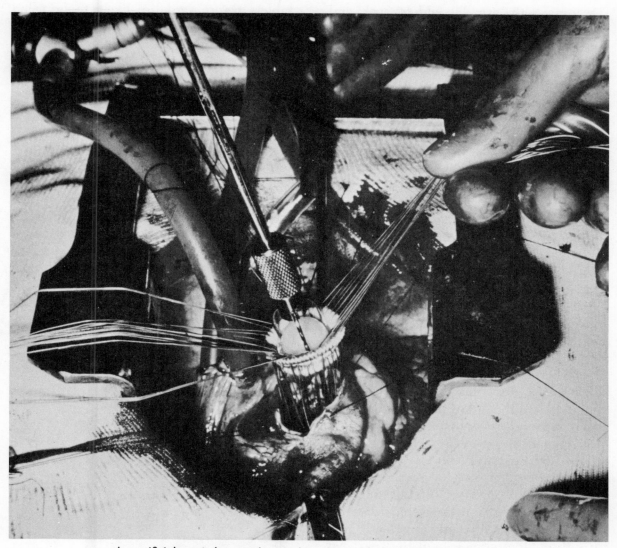

An artificial aortic heart valve, replacing a defective valve, is being inserted into a human heart. Its padded ring will be stitched to the human tissues.

the once smooth wall gets thicker, rougher, and harder, and the blood passageway becomes narrower.

This fatty clogging goes on imperceptibly, a process that often begins early in life. Eventually, blood flow may be obstructed sufficiently to cause the heart muscle cells to send out distress signals. The brief, episodic chest pains of angina pectoris announce that these cells are starving and suffering for lack of blood and oxygen. Flow may be so severely diminished or

totally plugged up that a region of the heart muscle dies. The heart has been damaged; the person has had a heart attack.

Angina

Angina pectoris means chest pain. Usually the pain is distinctive and feels like a vest being drawn too tightly across the chest. Sometimes it eludes easy identification. As a rule, however, the discomfort is felt behind the breastbone, occasionally spreading to the arms, shoulders, neck, and jaw. Not all chest pain indicates angina; in most cases it may simply be gas in the stomach.

Symptoms

Angina attacks are likely to appear when sudden strenuous demands are placed on the heart. They may come from physical exertion—walking uphill, running, sexual activity, or the effort involved in eating and digesting a heavy meal. Watching an exciting movie or sporting event can trigger it; so might cold weather. An attack can occur even when the individual is lying still or asleep—perhaps the result of tension or dreams.

Whatever the trigger, the heart is called upon to pump more blood to meet the body's stepped-up needs. To do so means working harder and faster. If one or more of the heart's supply lines is narrowed by disease, the extra blood and oxygen required to fuel the pump cannot get through to a region of the heart muscle. Anginal pain is a signal that muscle cells are being strained by an insufficiency of oxygen; they are, as it were, gasping for air.

The attacks usually are brief, lasting only a matter of minutes. Attacks stop when the person rests. Some people, apparently, can walk through an attack, as if the heart has gotten a second wind, and the pain subsides.

Treatment

Treatment may involve merely rearranging activity to avoid overly taxing physical labors or emotional situations likely to induce discomfort. A major medication used for angina is *nitroglycerine*. It dilates small coronary blood vessels, allowing more blood to get through. Nitroglycerine pellets are not swallowed but are placed under the tongue, where they are quickly absorbed by blood vessels there and sped to the heart; discomfort passes in minutes. Often anginal attacks can be headed off by taking the tablets before activities likely to bring on an attack.

Another anginal drug coming into widespread use is *propranolol*. There is some evidence that propranolol and nitroglycerine taken together may compound the effectiveness of therapy.

Angina does not mean a heart attack is inevitable. Many angina patients never have one, probably because their hearts have developed collateral circulation. Fortunately, an auxiliary system of very tiny pipelines lacing the heart exists in a dormant state as a potential escape hatch for the diseased heart. As the coronary arteries narrow, the collateral vessels gradually grow larger and wider, switched on, presumably, by the oxygen shortage. Thus, they may provide an

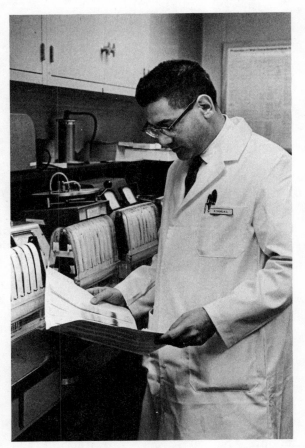

This endocrinologist is engaged in research on the effects of cholesterol-reducing drugs in helping to protect coronary patients against recurrent attacks.

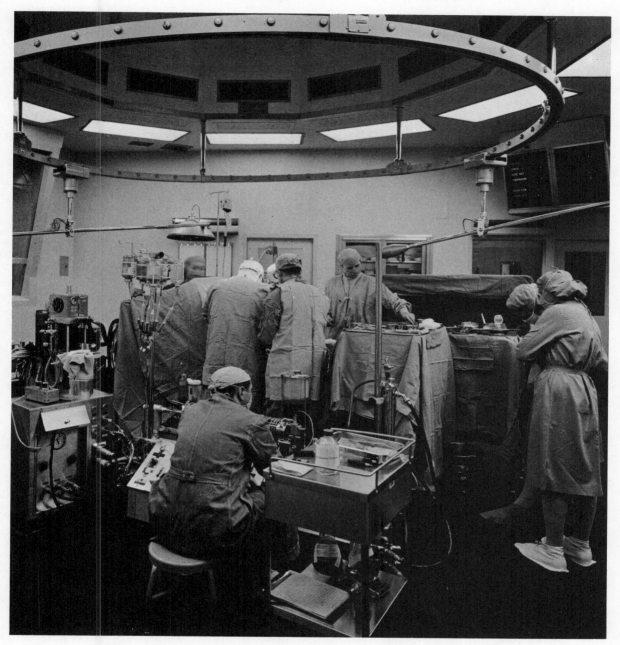

Open-heart surgery has been made possible by the heart-lung machine (*foreground*), which gives surgeons time to work on a relatively bloodless heart.

alternate route for blood to the afflicted area of the heart muscle. As the collateral system continues to develop, it may cause anginal symptoms to lessen. Although this may not prevent a heart attack, these newly activated pathways might make the attack less severe.

Coronary Artery Surgery

In general, surgery for angina is reserved for the severely restricted, incapacitated patient for whom medical treatment has been a failure. A procedure devised recently in Canada for bringing new sources of blood to the heart with clogged arteries may be of value in some cases. It involves implanting into the wall of the left ventricle an artery that normally supplies blood to the chest. One drawback is the time it takes —often a matter of months—for the implanted artery to develop the necessary collateral linkages to be of help to the heart.

Ideally, surgeons would like to operate directly on the coronary arteries, especially when the obstructing atherosclerotic deposits are confined to short, accessible vessel segments. Early attempts to do this, however, have brought high mortality and a low percentage of cures.

Endarterectomy, which means reaming out the trouble-making blockage, is still in the experimental stage. Carbon dioxide, forced in under high pressure to blow the deposits loose, has been used as a reaming tool in experiments. The diseased core is then cut free and pulled out through an incision in the coronary artery. Still another direct technique involves bypassing the diseased portion of the artery with a synthetic blood vessel graft taken from the patient's leg artery.

Heart Surgery

Direct surgery on the heart is possible because of the development of the heart-lung machine, which takes over the job of oxygenating and pumping blood into circulation, thus giving surgeons time to work directly on a relatively bloodless heart.

To choose patients appropriate for surgery, physicians use a reviewing system called *arteriography,* which allows them to watch blood flowing through the coronary artery system and to evaluate with accuracy the degree and location of obstruction. A substance opaque to X rays is injected into the coronary arteries and then followed by X ray as it runs its course through the vessels supplying the heart muscle.

Despite the newspaper headlines and dramatic history-making operations of re-

cent years, heart transplants must still be considered experimental. One reason is the logistics problem: getting and storing enough donor hearts to meet the demand. More important, however, is the immunological barrier. The body's defense against disease regards the new heart as foreign and attacks it, just as it would bacteria and viruses. Until scientists have learned how to thwart rejection consistently, heart transplants will have to be performed only on a limited, highly selective basis.

Heart Attack

Physicians have other names for heart attack: coronary occlusion, coronary thrombosis, myocardial infarction. *Coronary occlusion* means total closure of the coronary artery. This may be caused by fatty deposits that have piled up high enough to dam the flow channel.

Or it may be that a blood clot, or *thrombus,* forming in the coronary artery, has suddenly caught on the roughened, fat-clogged area and plugged up the vessel. In this case the occlusion is called a *coronary thrombosis. Myocardial infarction* refers to the actual damage or death of heart muscle (*myocardium*) resulting from the occlusion.

Heart attack hits males hardest. The frequency of heart attacks begins to build rapidly among men between the ages of 30 and 40 but is almost unknown in women of the same age group. The odds begin evening out as women approach and pass menopause. Despite this, during the same 40 to 44 age period, the ratio of male to female heart attacks may be as high as 24 to one.

The incidence of heart attacks increases with age. The peak years for male heart attacks are in the 55 to 59 age bracket. The percentage of deaths from first heart attacks is highest among men, say, in their forties, as compared with those in their sixties,

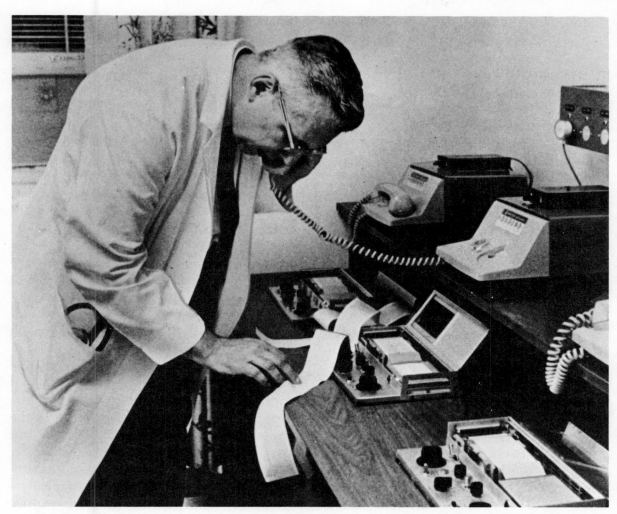

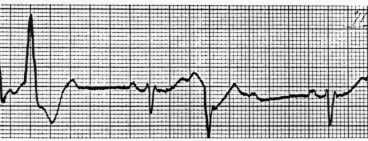

The electrocardiogram at the right was transmitted via Data-Phone—through telephone lines—from a distant hospital. It shows that the patient is suffering from a severe heart disturbance. The cardiac specialist above can confer with the patient's private doctor immediately after interpreting the electrocardiogram, thus facilitating diagnosis and insuring prompt and accurate treatment.

presumably because they do not have as well-developed collateral circulation to protect them.

Symptoms

Sometimes heart attacks are so vague or indistinct that the victim may not know he has had one. Often a routine electro-cardiogram—the squiggly-lined record of the heart's activity—turns up an abnormality indicative of an *infarct,* or injured area. This is another instance of the importance of periodic check-ups. Special blood tests can also detect substances which may leak out into the circulation when heart muscle cells are injured.

Most heart attacks, however, do not sneak by. There are well-recognized symptoms. The most common are:

• A feeling of strangulation

• A prolonged, oppressive pain or unusual discomfort in the center of the chest that may radiate to the left shoulder and down the left arm

• Abnormal perspiring

• Sudden, intense shortness of breath

• Nausea or vomiting (Because of these symptoms, an attack is sometimes taken for indigestion; usually, coronary pains are more severe.)

• Occasionally, loss of consciousness.

Treatment

Knowing these warning signals and taking proper steps may make the difference between life and death. Call a physician or get to a hospital as soon as possible. Time is crucial. Most deaths occur in the initial hours after attack. About 25 percent, for example, die within three hours after onset of their first heart attack.

Often, death is not due to any widespread damage to the heart muscle, but rather to a disruption in the electric spark initiating heart muscle contraction—the same spark measured by the electrocardiogram. These out-of-kilter rhythms, including complete heart stoppage or cardiac arrest, are often reversible with prompt treatment.

Coronary care units: For this reason special hospital centers called coronary care units have been created. Here, around-the-clock electronic sentries keep watch over the patient's vital functions, particularly the heart's electrical activity. The critical period is 72 hours, during which time as many as 90 percent of heart attack patients experience some type of electrical disturbance or *arrhythmia* (rhythmic irregularity). Not all are dangerous in themselves, but they may be the forerunner of chaotic rhythms that are dangerous indeed. The onset of any irregular beat alerts a member of the 24-hour-a-day, specially-trained nursing staff to initiate the appropriate countermeasures while a physician is being summoned.

Fibrillation

The most dangerous rhythmic disorder is ventricular *fibrillation,* in which the lower chambers of the heart contract in an uncoordinated manner, causing blood-pumping to cease completely. Treated within one minute, the patient has a 90 percent or better chance of surviving. A delay of three minutes means a survival rate of less than 10 percent because of extensive and irreversible brain and heart damage.

Treatment involves use of an instrument called a *defibrillator.* Through plates applied to the chest, the device sends a massive jolt of electricity into the heart muscle to get the heart back on the right tempo.

More signficantly, it is now also possible to head off ventricular fibrillation, so that the already compromised heart will not have to tolerate even brief episodes of the arrhythmia. Ventricular fibrillation is invariably heralded by an earlier, identifiable disturbance in the heart beat. Most frequently, the warning signal is a skipped or premature ventricular beat. Picked up by the coronary care monitoring equipment, the signal alerts the unit staff to administer heart-calming medicaments that can ward off the danger. One such drug is *lidocaine,* a long-used dental anesthetic found to have the power to restore an irritated heart to electrical tranquility.

The advent of coronary care has produced striking results. Where in use, these units have reduced heart attack deaths among hospitalized patients up to 30 percent. If all heart victims surviving at least a few hours received such care, more than 50,000 lives could be saved annually.

Failure of Heart Muscle

Most deaths in coronary care units, however, result not from electrical failure but power failure—the result of massive injury to the heart muscle. So large an area of the muscle is put out of commission, at least temporarily, that the still healthy portion is unable to cope with the body's ceaseless blood needs.

Success in treating failures of the heart muscle has not been great. Various devices for assisting the weakened heart with its pumping burden are still in the experimental stage. The problem is to create a device that will do most, if not all, of the work for the struggling left ventricle over a period of days or weeks to give the heart muscle a chance to rest and recover.

Emergency Care

Most heart attack victims never reach the hospital. About 400,000 die before getting there, as many as 60 percent in the first hour. Evidence suggests that many of these sudden deaths result from ventricular fibrillation or cardiac arrest—reversible disturbances when treated immediately.

These considerations led to the concept of mobile coronary care units—of bringing

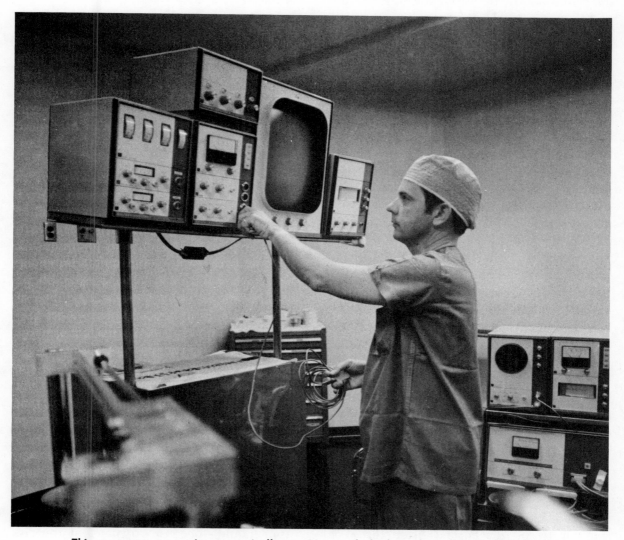

This coronary care unit automatically monitors and displays the patient's vital functions, including body temperature, blood pressure, and heartbeat rate and rhythm. It can also pace the heart by electrical stimulation to restore and maintain a normal heartbeat.

the advanced techniques of heart resuscitation to the victims. Originated in 1966 in Belfast, North Ireland, the practice of having a flying squad of specially equipped ambulances ready to race with on-the-spot aid to heart attack patients has been spreading to more U.S. communities, successfully reducing mortality.

Recently developed *external cardiopulmonary resuscitation* (*ECPR*), more popularly known as *closed-chest massage,* has also reduced out-of-hospital heart attack mortality figures. Used in conjunction with mouth-to-mouth breathing, ECPR is an emergency procedure for treating cardiac arrest. The lower part of the breastbone is compressed rhythmically to keep oxygenated blood flowing to the brain until appropriate medical treatment can be applied to restore normal heart action; often ECPR alone is enough to restart the heart. The technique should be performed only by trained personnel, however, because it involves risks, such as the danger of fracturing a rib or rupturing a weakened heart muscle if too much pressure is applied.

Recuperation

Beyond the 72-hour crisis period, the patient will still require hospitalization for three to six weeks to give the heart time to heal. During the first two weeks or so, the patient is made to remain completely at rest. In this period, the dead muscle cells are being cleared away and gradually replaced by scar tissue. Until this happens, the damaged area represents a dangerous weak spot. By the end of the second week, the patient may be allowed to sit in a chair and then to walk about the room. Recently, some physicians have been experimenting with getting patients up and about earlier, sometimes within a few days after their attack. Although most patients are well enough to be discharged after three or four weeks, not everyone mends at the same rate, which is why doctors hesitate to pre-

dict exactly when the patient will be released or when he will be well enough to resume normal activity.

About 15 percent of in-hospital heart attack deaths come in the post-acute phase owing to an *aneurysm,* or ballooning-out, of the area where the left ventricle is healing. This is most likely to develop before the scar has toughened enough to withstand blood pressures generated by the heart's contractions. The aneurysm may kill either by rupturing or by so impairing pumping efficiency that the heart fails and the circulation deteriorates.

Most heart attack patients are able to return to their precoronary jobs eventually. Some, left with anginal pain, may have to make adjustments in their jobs and living habits. What kind of activity the patient can ultimately resume is an individual matter to be worked out by the patient with his physician. The prescription usually involves keeping weight down and avoiding undue emotional stress or physical exertion; moderate exercise along with plenty of rest is encouraged.

Prevention

Scientists do not have all the answers to atherosclerosis as yet. What is apparent, though, is that not one but a mosaic of factors are involved.

Long-term population studies have helped to point up individual characteristics and living habits that raise heart attack risk. These include such factors as sex, heredity, overweight, high blood pressure, lack of exercise, cigarette smoking, high blood levels of cholesterol and other fatty substances, and the presence of diabetes.

The identification of these risk factors has given the physician an important new weapon: a way to spot coronary-prone individuals years before any overt symptoms appear and—because so many of the risk factors are controllable—a promising program for reducing this risk.

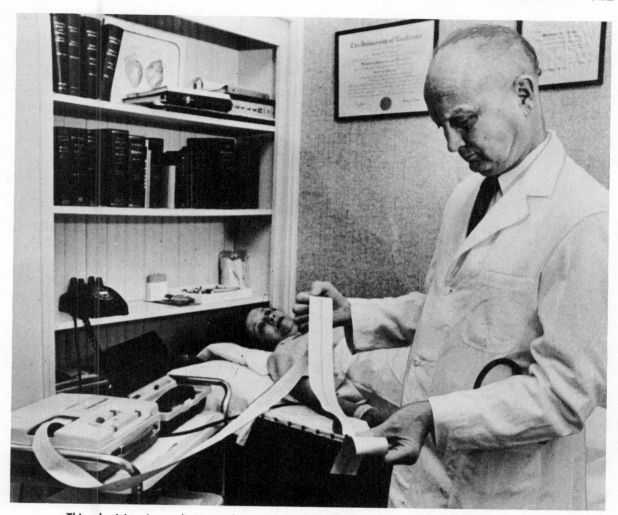

This physician is reading an electrocardiogram while it is being sent simultaneously via Data-Phone—a system utilizing telephone lines—to a cardiac laboratory for interpretation.

These are some of the recommendations:

• Eat less saturated fat and cholesterol. Egg yolks are rich in cholesterol. Saturated animal fats—as in butter, cheese, cream and whole milk—help to raise cholesterol levels. Use skimmed (fat free) milk. Substitute polyunsaturated vegetable fats for saturated fats as often as possible. This means, for example, cooking with vegetable oils and eating poultry and fish. Polyunsaturates tend to lower blood cholesterol. The more cholesterol in the circulation, presumably, the more material is available to build up the blood-blocking atherosclerotic deposits.

• Control high blood pressure. Hypertension sharply increases the chances of heart attack. A man whose blood pressure at *systole* (the moment the heart contracts) is higher than 160 has four times the risk of an individual with a systolic blood pressure under 120. In almost all cases, elevated blood pressure can be brought under control.

• Don't smoke. The heart attack death rate is 50 to 200 percent higher, depending on age and number of cigarettes consumed, among men who smoke as compared with nonsmokers. Giving up the habit can decrease the coronary risk to that of the non-

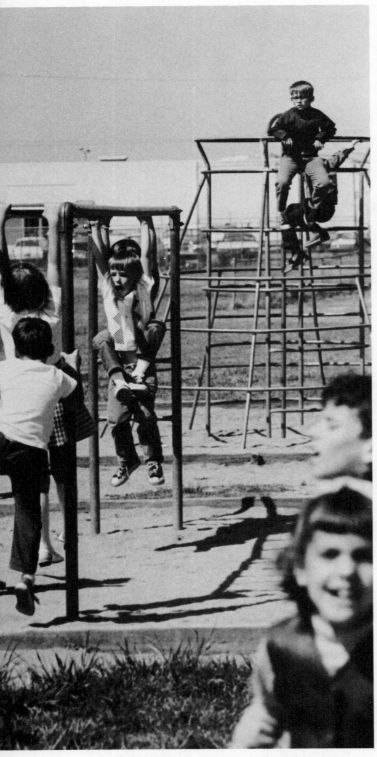

A lifelong habit of exercise is believed to be important in improving blood circulation. Studies indicate that people who are active have a better chance to survive heart attacks than people who are inactive.

smoker; the danger from smoking appears to be reversible. A combination of two or more risk factors not only increases the risk, it compounds it. A male cigarette smoker with high cholesterol and high blood pressure may have a risk ten times higher than the man with none.

• Count calories. Get down to your proper weight and stay there. Excess weight taxes the heart, makes it work harder. Middle-aged men who are 20 percent overweight run as much as two to three times the risk of a fatal heart attack than their trimmer counterparts.

• Exercise regularly. Your physician can tell you what the best exercise program is for your age and physical condition. Studies show active men to be better able to survive a heart attack than sedentary individuals. The belief is that exercise promotes the development of collateral circulation.

Children can benefit most of all, perhaps, if they are trained from the start in this life-long prescription.

Hypertensive Heart Disease

Hypertension, or elevated blood pressure, results from a persistent tightening or constriction of the body's very small arterial branches, the *arterioles*. This clenching increases the resistance to blood flow and sends the blood pressure up, just as screwing down the nozzle on a hose builds up pressure in the line. The heart must now work harder to force blood through. Over a period of time, the stepped-up pumping effort may cause the heart muscle to thicken and enlarge, much as the arm muscles do on a weight lifter. Eventually, the overworked circulatory system may break down, with resultant failure of the heart or kidneys, or the onset of stroke. The constant hammering of blood under high pressure on the walls of the arteries also accelerates the development of atherosclerosis and heart attacks.

How Blood Pressure Is Measured

Blood pressure is measured in millimeters of mercury with an instrument called a *sphygmomanometer*. The device consists of an inflatable cuff attached to a mercury meter. The physician wraps the cuff around the arm and inflates it with air from a squeeze-bulb. This drives the mercury column up towards the top of the gauge while shutting off blood flow through the brachial artery in the arm. With a stethoscope placed just below the cuff, the physician releases the air and listens for the first thudding sounds that signal the return of blood flow as the blood pressure on the wall of the artery equals the air pressure in the cuff. He records this mercury meter reading. This number represents the systolic pressure, the force developed by the heart when it contracts.

By continuing to let air out, the physician reaches a point where he can no longer hear the pulsing sounds of flowing blood. He marks the gauge reading as the *diastolic* pressure, the pressure on the artery when the heart is relaxing between beats. Thus, two numbers are used to record blood pressure, the systolic followed by the diastolic.

Recorded when the patient is relaxed, normal systolic pressure for most adults is between 100 and 140, and diastolic between 60 and 90. Many factors, such as age and sex, account for the wide variations in normal readings from individual to individual. Systolic blood pressure, for example, tends to increase with age.

Normally, blood pressure goes up during periods of excitement and physical labor. Hypertension is the diagnosis when repeated measurements show a persistent elevated pressure—160 or higher for systolic and 95 or more for diastolic.

In addition to the sphygmomanometer reading in the examination for high blood pressure, the physician shines a bright light in the patient's eyes so that he can look at

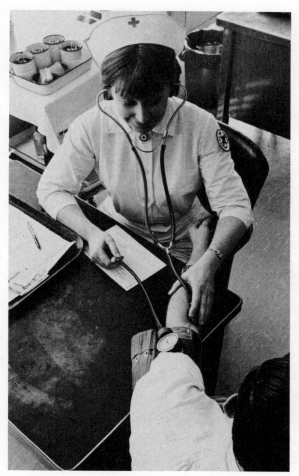

The cuff of the sphygmomanometer is inflated, thus shutting off blood flow and driving up a column of mercury. Air is then released from the cuff, and as blood flow returns, the systolic pressure is recorded. Diastole occurs when pulsing sounds cease.

the blood vessels in the retina, the only blood vessels that are readily observable. Any damage there due to hypertension is usually a good index of the severity of the disease and its effects elsewhere in the body.

An electrocardiogram and X ray may be in order to determine if and how much the heart has been damaged. The physician may also perform some tests of kidney function to ascertain whether hypertension, if detected, is of the essential or secondary kind, and if there has been damage to the kidneys as well.

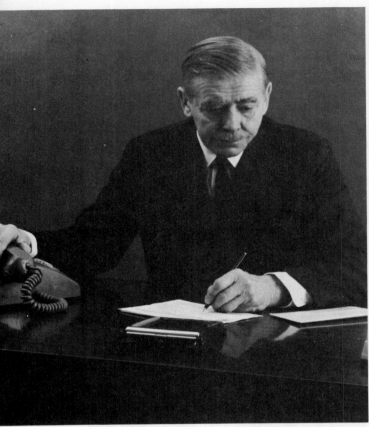

Being subjected to the constant stress of a high-pressure job is one suspected cause of hypertension.

Causes

About 85 percent of all hypertension cases are classified as *essential*. This simply means that no single cause can be defined. Rather, pressure is up because a number of factors—none of which has yet been firmly implicated—are operating in some complex interplay.

One theory holds that hypertension arises from excessive activity of the sympathetic nervous system, which helps regulate blood vessel response. This notion could help explain why tense individuals are susceptible to hypertension. Emotional reactions to unpleasant events or other mental stresses prompt the cardiovascular system to react as it might to exercise, including widespread constriction of small blood vessels and increased heart rate.

The theory suggests that repeated episodes of stress may ultimately affect pressure-sensitive cells called *baroreceptors*. Situated in strategic places in the arterial system, these sensing centers are thought to be preset to help maintain normal blood pressure, just as a thermostat works to keep a house at a preset temperature. Exposure to regularly recurrent elevated blood pressure episodes may bring about a resetting of the baroreceptors—or *barostats*—to a new, higher normal. Once reset, the barostats operate to sustain hypertension.

Symptoms

Essential hypertension usually first occurs when a person is in his thirties. In the early stages, one may pass through a transitional or prehypertensive phase lasting a few years in which blood pressure rises above normal only occasionally, and then more and more often until finally it remains at these elevated levels.

Symptoms, if they exist at all, are likely to be something as nonspecific as headaches, dizziness, or nausea. As a result, without a physical examination to reveal its presence, a person may have the disease for years without being aware of it. That can be dangerous, since the longer hypertension is left untreated, the greater the likelihood that the heart will be affected.

About 15 percent of cases fall under the *secondary hypertension* classification, because they arise as a consequence of another known disorder. Curing the underlying disorder also cures the hypertension. Usually it is brought on by an obstruction of normal blood flow to the kidney because of atherosclerotic deposits in one or both of its major supply lines, the renal arteries. Many patients can be cured or substantially improved through surgery.

Treatment

The outlook is good for almost all patients with essential hypertension, whether mild or severe, because of the large arsenal of antihypertensive drugs now at the physician's disposal. Not all drugs will benefit all patients, but where one fails another or several in combination will almost invariably succeed. Even the usually lethal and hard-to-treat form of essential hypertension described as malignant is beginning to respond to new medications. *Malignant hypertension,* which may strike as many as five percent of hypertensive victims, does not refer to cancer, but rather describes the rapid, galloping way blood pressure rises.

Mild hypertension often may be readily treated with tranquilizers and mild sedatives, particularly if the patient is tense, or with one of a broad family of agents known as *diuretics.* These drugs flush the body of excess salt, which appears to have some direct though poorly-understood role in hypertension.

Against more severe forms, there are a large number of drugs which work in a variety of ways to offset or curb the activity of the sympathetic nervous system so that it relaxes its hold on the constricted arterioles.

Rheumatic Fever and Rheumatic Heart Disease

Rheumatic heart disease is the possible sequel of rheumatic fever. Triggered by streptococcal attacks in childhood and adolescence, rheumatic fever may leave permanent heart scars. The heart structures most often affected are the valves.

Causes

The cause of rheumatic fever is still not entirely understood. It is known that rheumatic fever is always preceded by an invasion of bacteria belonging to the group A beta hemolytic streptococcus family. Sooner or later, everybody has a strep infection, such as a strep throat or scarlet fever. Most of us get over it without any complications. But in 1 out of every 100 children the strep infection produces rheumatic fever a few weeks later, even after the strep attack has long since subsided. The figure may rise to 3 per 100 during epidemics in closed communities, such as a children's camp.

The invasion of strep sparks the production of protective agents called antibodies. For some reason, in a kind of biological double-cross, the antibodies attack not only the strep but also make war on the body's own tissues—the very tissues they are called upon to protect.

Researchers are now suggesting the possible reason, although all the evidence is not yet in. According to a widely-held theory, the strep germ possesses constituents (*antigens*) which are similar in structure to components of normal, healthy cartilage and connective tissue—found abundantly in joints, tendons, and heart valves—in susceptible individuals. Failing to distinguish between them, the antibodies attack both. The result: rheumatic fever, involving joint and valve inflammation and, perhaps, permanent scarring.

Prevention

The development of antibiotics has made rheumatic fever preventable. These drugs can knock out the strep before the germs get a chance to set off the inflammatory defense network sequences, but early detection is necessary. Among the symptoms of strep are a sore throat that comes on suddenly, with redness and swelling; rapidly acquired high fever; nausea and headaches. The only sure way to tell, however, is to have a throat swab taken by passing a sterile piece of cotton over the inflamed area. This culture is then exposed for 24 hours to a laboratory dish containing a substance that enhances strep growth. A positive identification calls for prompt treatment to kill the germs before the complica-

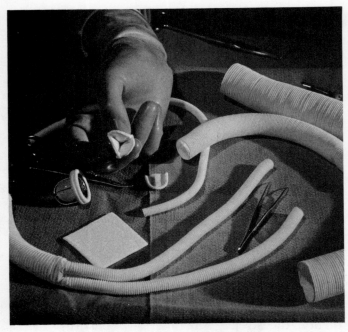

Shown here are artificial blood vessels, a patch, and heart valves: from left, a mitral ball valve, an aortic valve (held in hand), and an aortic valve leaflet.

tions of rheumatic fever have a chance to set in.

Unfortunately, many strep infections may be mild enough to escape detection. The child may recover so quickly that the parents neglect to take the necessary precautions, but the insidious processes may still be going on in the apparently healthy child. This is a major reason why rheumatic fever is still with us, though in severe decline.

Symptoms

Rheumatic fever itself is not always easy to diagnose. The physician must detect at least one of five symptoms, derived by the American Heart Association from the work of the late Dr. T. Duckett Jones. The so-called Jones criteria include:

• Swelling or tenderness in one or more joints. Usually, several joints are involved, not simultaneously but one after the other in migratory fashion.

• Carditis or heart inflammation

• Heart murmur (see p. 517)

• An unusual skin rash, which often disappears in 24 to 48 hours

• Chorea, or St. Vitus's dance, so-called because of the uncoordinated, jerky and involuntary motions of the arms, legs, or face, which result from rheumatic inflammation of brain tissue. It may last six to eight weeks and even longer, but when symptoms disappear there is never any permanent damage and the brain and nervous system return to normal.

• Hard lumps under the skin and over the inflamed joints, usually indicating severe heart inflammation.

Confirmation of rheumatic fever also requires other clinical and laboratory tests, to determine, for example, the presence of strep antibodies in the patient's blood. Rheumatic fever does not always involve the heart; even when it does, permanent damage is not inevitable. Nor does the severity of the attack have any relationship to the development of rheumatic heart disease.

The real danger arises when heart valve tissue becomes inflamed. When the acute attack has passed and the inflammation finally subsides, the valves begin to heal, with scar tissue forming.

Scar tissue may cause portions of the affected valve leaflets to fuse together. (*Leaflets* are the flaps of the heart valves.) This restricts leaflet motion, impeding the full swing action and thereby blood flow through the valve. This condition is called valvular *stenosis*. The leaflets may become shrunken or deformed by healing tissue, causing *regurgitation* or backspill because the valve fails to close completely.

Both stenosis and regurgitation are often present. Most susceptible are the *mitral valve*, which regulates flow from the upper to the lower left chambers of the heart, and the *aortic valve*, the gateway between the left ventricle and the general circulation. Rarely attacked are the two valves in the right chambers.

Treatment

During the acute stages of rheumatic fever, the patient is given heavy doses of antibiotics to rid the body of all strep traces, aspirin to control swelling and fever, and sometimes such hormones as ACTH and cortisone to reduce inflammation.

In the past, rheumatic fever spelled mandatory bed rest for months. Now the routine is to get the patient up and about as soon as the acute episode is over to avert the problem of psychological invalidism. The biggest restriction, especially for young people, is that no participation in competitive sports or other severely taxing exercises is allowed for two to three months while a close watch is kept on cardiac status.

The patient with valve damage can in many cases be treated medically, without the need for surgical intervention. He may, of course, have to desist from certain strenuous activities, but in all other ways he can lead a relatively normal life. Surgical relief or cure is available, however, for patients with severe damage or those who may, with age, develop progressive narrowing or leakage of the valves.

Surgery: Stenotic valves can be scraped clear of excess scar tissue, thereby returning the leaflets to more normal operation. In some cases individually scarred leaflets are replaced with synthetic substitutes. The correction of severe valvular regurgitation requires replacement of the entire valve with an artificial substitute, or, as some surgeons prefer, with a healthy valve taken from a human donor dying of other causes.

Heart Murmurs and Recurrences of Rheumatic Fever

The prime sign that rheumatic heart disease has developed is a heart murmur—although a heart murmur does not always mean heart disease. The murmur may be only temporary, ceasing once the rheumatic fever attack subsides and the stretched and

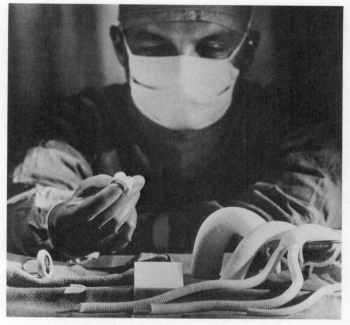

Research continues to develop better ways to repair damaged hearts. Shown here are valves, patching material, and artificial blood vessels.

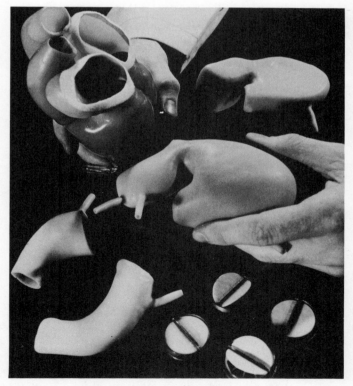

Heart parts made of rubber. Beginning at the upper left and moving clockwise: outer heart, atrial ventricular halves, valves, pulmonary artery, aorta.

swollen valves return to normal. To complicate matters more, many heart murmurs are harmless. Such functional murmurs may appear in 30 to 50 percent of normal children at one time or another.

As many as three in five patients with rheumatic fever may develop murmurs characteristic of scarred valves—sounds of blood flowing through ailing valves that fail to open and close normally.

Anyone who has had an attack of rheumatic fever has about a 50–50 chance of having one again unless safeguards are taken. As a result, all patients are placed on a daily or monthly regimen of antibiotics. The preventive dose, although smaller than that given to quell an in-progress infection, is enough to sabotage any attempts on the part of the strep germs to mount an attack.

There is some encouraging evidence that rheumatic fever patients who escape heart damage the first time around will do so again should a repeat attack occur. On the other hand, those with damaged valves will probably sustain more damage with subsequent strep-initiated attacks.

Endocarditis

One of the additional bonuses of antibiotic therapy is that it has all but eliminated an invariably fatal complication to which rheumatic patients were especially vulnerable—an infection of the heart's outside lining, or *endocardium*, called *subacute bacterial endocarditis*. The scar tissue provides an excellent nesting site for bacteria to grow.

The responsible germs are found in almost everyone's mouth and usually invade the bloodstream after dental surgery. Fortunately, it is easy to prevent or cure because the germs offer little resistance to antibiotics. As a precaution, dentists are usually advised to give rheumatic fever patients large doses of penicillin (or other antibiotics to those allergic to penicillin) before, during, and after dental work.

Congenital Heart Disease

There are some 35 recognized types of congenital heart malformations. Most—including all of the 15 most common types—can be either corrected or alleviated by surgery. The defects result from a failure of the infant's heart or of the major blood vessels near the heart to mature normally during development in the womb.

The term *blue baby* refers to the infant born with a heart impairment that prevents blood from getting enough oxygen. Since blood low in oxygen is dark bluish red, it imparts a blue tinge to the skin and lips.

The cause of inborn heart abnormalities is not known in most cases. Some defects can be traced to maternal virus infection, such as German measles (rubella), during the first three months of pregnancy when the fetus' heart is growing rapidly. Certain drugs, vitamin deficiencies, or excessive exposure to radiation are among other environmental factors known to be associated with such defects.

Heart abnormalities may come singly or in combination. There may be, for example, a hole in the walls separating the right and left heart chambers, or a narrowing of a valve or blood vessel which obstructs blood flow, or a mixup in major blood vessel connections—or a combination of all of these.

Diagnosis

A skilled cardiologist often can make a reasonably complete diagnosis on the basis of a conventional physical examination, including visual inspection of the infant's general condition, blood pressure reading, X ray, blood tests, and electrocardiogram. For more complex diagnosis, the physician may call for either *angiography* or *cardiac catheterization*. The former, a variation of coronary arteriography, allows direct X-ray visualization of the heart chambers and major blood vessels. In cardiac catheterization, a thin plastic tube or catheter is in-

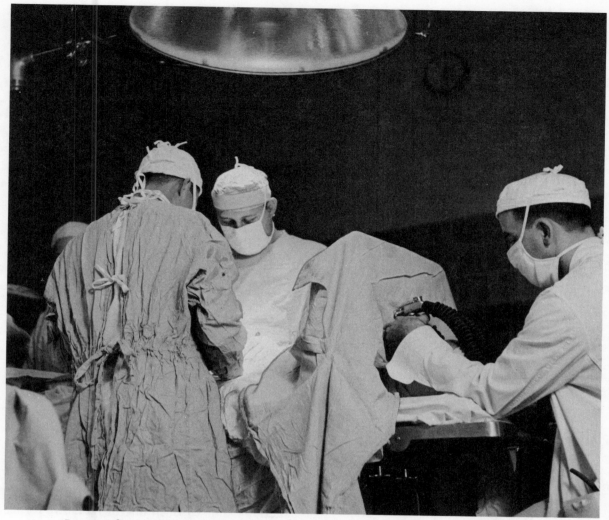

Recent refinements in surgical methods and post-operative care have enabled surgeons to perform life-saving heart surgery even on newborn infants with remarkable success.

serted into an arm or leg vein. While the physician watches with special X-ray equipment, the tube is advanced carefully through the vein until it reaches the heart chambers, there to provide information about the nature of the defect.

Treatment

From these tests, the cardiologist together with a surgeon can decide for or against surgery. Depending on the severity of the disease, some conditions may require an immediate operation, even on days-old infants. In other conditions, the specialists may instead recommend waiting until the infant is older and stronger before surgery is undertaken. In a number of instances, the defect may not require surgery at all.

Open-heart surgery in infants with inborn heart defects carries a higher risk than does the same surgery in older children. Risks must be taken often, however, since about one-third will die in the first month if untreated, and more than half within the first year.

Refinements in surgical techniques and post-operative care have given surgeons the confidence to operate on infants who are merely hours old with remarkable success. Specially adapted miniature heart-lung machines may also chill the blood to produce *hypothermia,* or body cooling. This slows metabolism and reduces tissue oxygen needs so that the heart and brain can withstand short periods of interrupted blood flow.

A good deal has been learned, too, about the delicate medical management required by infants during the surgical recovery period. All of this accounts for the admirable record of salvage among infants who would have been given up for lost only a few years ago.

Congestive Heart Failure

Heart failure may be found in conjunction with any disease of the heart—coronary artery disease, hypertension, rheumatic heart disease, or congenital defects. It occurs when the heart's ability to pump blood

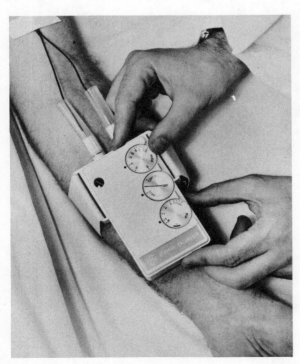

This cardiac pacemaker is designed to provide temporary external stimulation of the heart through internal electrodes. It may be used during heart surgery or before an internal pacemaker can be implanted.

has been weakened by disease. To say the heart has failed, however, does not mean it has stopped beating. The heart muscle continues to contract, but it lacks the strength to keep blood circulating normally throughout the body. Doctors sometimes refer to the condition as cardiac insufficiency or *dropsy,* although the latter term is seldom heard anymore.

When the heart fails to pump efficiently, the flow slows down, causing blood returning to the heart through the veins to back up. Some of the fluid in the blood is forced out through the thin walls of smaller blood vessels into surrounding tissues. Here the fluid piles up, or congests.

The result may be swelling, or *edema,* which can occur in many parts of the body but is most commonly seen in the legs and ankles. Fluids sometimes collect in the lungs, interfering with breathing and making the person short of breath. Heart failure also affects the ability of the kidneys to rid the body of sodium and water. Fluid retained in this way adds to the edema.

Treatment

Treatment usually includes a combination of rest, drugs, diet, and restricted daily activity. *Digitalis,* in one of its many forms, is usually given to strengthen the action of the heart muscle. It also slows a rapid heart beat, helps decrease heart enlargement, and promotes secretion of excess fluids. Care must be taken to find the right dose, since this will vary from person to person. When edema is present, diuretics are prescribed to speed up the elimination of excess salt and water. Many improved diuretics are available today. A sodium-restricted diet is generally necessary to reduce or prevent edema. Patients will also probably need bed rest for a while, with a gradual return to slower-paced activity.

Most important, however, is the adequate treatment of the underlying disease that led to heart failure in the first place.

(*Below*) An implantable cardiac pacemaker suitable for patients with heart block or for those with normal heart rhythm who require occasional stimulus. It is powered by six silver mercury cells designed to last up to five years. (*Right*) Electronic components of an experimental nuclear pacemaker, shown in relation to a dime. (*Below, right*) A nuclear-powered pacemaker and electrode (heart lead), which is normally placed in contact with the left ventricle of the heart. The device is about two-thirds the size of a package of cigarettes and weighs only three ounces. It is hoped that longer-lived nuclear power units of this type will eventually reduce the frequency of surgical replacement of the batteries to about once every ten years.

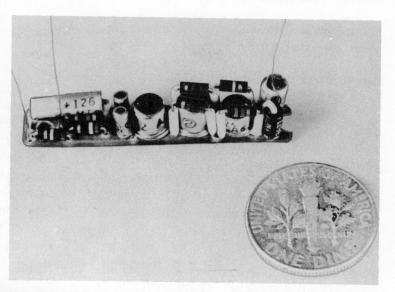

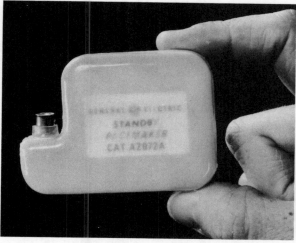

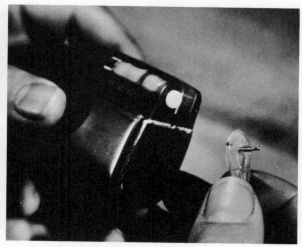

Heart Block

Sometimes the scars resulting from rheumatic fever, heart attack, or surgical repair of the heart may damage the electrical network in a way that blocks normal transmission of the signal between the upper and lower chambers. The disruption, called *atrio-ventricular block*, may so severely slow down the rate at which the ventricles beat that blood flow is seriously affected, especially to the brain. Blackouts and convulsions may ensue.

For less serious slowdowns, there are nervous system stimulants to keep the heart from lagging. In the case of *Stokes-Adams syndrome*—where the ventricles may not beat from four to ten seconds—drugs are not enough. An artificial electronic pacemaker, implanted in the body and connected to the heart by wires, has been successfully applied to more than 20,000 Americans. This pacemaker fires electrical shocks into the ventricle wall to make it beat at the proper rate. Currently, the devices are powered by tiny batteries which must be replaced surgically every 18 months or so. Longer lasting fuel sources, including nuclear power in miniature, are on the horizon.   BP

DISEASES OF THE DIGESTIVE SYSTEM

Digestive Functions and Organs

The function of the digestive system is to accept food and water through the mouth, to break down the food's chemical structure so that its nutrients can be absorbed into the body, a process called *digestion,* and to expel undigested particles. This process takes place as the food passes through the entire *alimentary tract.* This tract, also called the *gastrointestinal tract,* is a long, hollow passageway that begins at the mouth and continues on through the esophagus, the stomach, the small intestine, the large intestine, the rectum, and the anus. The salivary glands, the stomach glands, the liver, the gallbladder, and the pancreas release substances into the gastrointestinal tract that help the digestion of various food substances.

Digestion

Digestion begins in the mouth where food is shredded by chewing and mixed with saliva, which helps break down starch into sugars and lubricates the food so that it can be swallowed easily. The food then enters the *esophagus,* a muscular tube that forcibly squeezes the food down toward the stomach, past the *cardiac sphincter,* a ring of muscle at the entrance of the stomach that opens to allow food into the stomach.

The stomach acts as a reservoir for food, churns the food, mixes it with gastric juices, and gradually releases the food into the small intestine. Some water, alcohol, and glucose are absorbed directly through the stomach into the bloodstream. Enzymes secreted by the stomach help break down proteins and fats into simpler substances. Hydrochloric acid secreted by the stomach kills bacteria and prepares some minerals for absorption in the small intestine. Some food may leave the stomach one minute after it enters, while other parts of a meal may remain in the stomach for as long as five hours.

The food passes from the stomach to the first section of the small intestine, the *duodenum,* where it is acted on by pancreatic enzymes that help break down fats, starches, proteins, and other substances. While the food is in the duodenum it is also digested by *bile,* which is produced by the liver and stored in the gallbladder. During a meal, the gallbladder discharges its bile into the duodenum. The bile promotes the absorption of fats and some vitamins.

The semidigested food is squeezed down the entire length of the intestines by a wavelike motion of the intestinal muscles called *peristalsis.* Digestion is largely completed as the food passes through 20 feet of small intestine, which absorbs the digested food substances and water and passes them into the bloodstream. The food nutrients are distributed by the bloodstream throughout the body and used by the body cells.

Those parts of the food that are indigestible, such as the skins of fruits, pass into the large intestine, or *colon,* along with bacteria, bile, some minerals, various cells, and mucus. This combination of substances makes up the *feces,* which are stored in the colon until *defecation.* Some water and salts in the feces are absorbed through the walls of the colon into the bloodstream. This conserves the body's fluids and dries the feces. The formation of a semisolid fecal mass helps precipitate defecation.

The Oral Cavity

The Salivary Glands

The smell of food triggers the salivary glands to pour saliva into the mouth; that is what is meant by "mouth-watering" odors.

THE DIGESTIVE SYSTEM

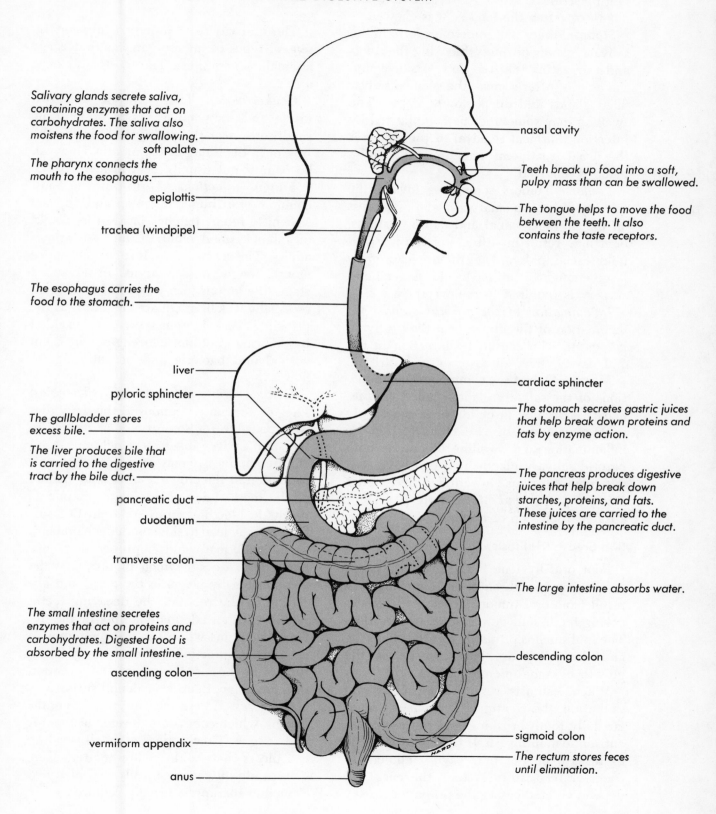

Salivary glands secrete saliva, containing enzymes that act on carbohydrates. The saliva also moistens the food for swallowing.

soft palate

The pharynx connects the mouth to the esophagus.

epiglottis

trachea (windpipe)

nasal cavity

Teeth break up food into a soft, pulpy mass than can be swallowed.

The tongue helps to move the food between the teeth. It also contains the taste receptors.

The esophagus carries the food to the stomach.

liver

pyloric sphincter

The gallbladder stores excess bile.

The liver produces bile that is carried to the digestive tract by the bile duct.

pancreatic duct

duodenum

transverse colon

cardiac sphincter

The stomach secretes gastric juices that help break down proteins and fats by enzyme action.

The pancreas produces digestive juices that help break down starches, proteins, and fats. These juices are carried to the intestine by the pancreatic duct.

The large intestine absorbs water.

The small intestine secretes enzymes that act on proteins and carbohydrates. Digested food is absorbed by the small intestine.

ascending colon

vermiform appendix

anus

descending colon

sigmoid colon

The rectum stores feces until elimination.

HARDY

During a meal, saliva is released into the mouth to soften the food as it is chewed.

Stones: Stones will sometimes form in the salivary glands or ducts, blocking the ducts and preventing the free flow of saliva into the mouth. After a meal, the swollen saliva-filled glands and ducts slowly empty. The swelling may sometimes be complicated by infection. Surgical removal of the stones is the usual treatment; sometimes the entire gland is removed.

Tumors: Tumors sometimes invade the salivary gland. An enlarged gland may press on the auditory canal and cause deafness, or it may result in stiffness of the jaw and mild facial palsy. The tumors can grow large enough to be felt by the fingers, and surgery is required to remove them.

Inflammation of the parotid glands: Inflammation of the upper (*parotid*) salivary glands may be caused by infection in the oral cavity, liver disease, or malnutrition.

Mumps: One of the commonest inflammations of the salivary glands, called *mumps,* occurs especially in children. It is a highly contagious virus disease characterized by inflammation and swelling of one or both parotid salivary glands, and can have serious complications in adults. See under *Birth, Infancy, and Maturation,* p. 99, for a fuller discussion of mumps.

Bad Breath (Halitosis)

Poor oral hygiene is the principal cause of offensive mouth odor, or *halitosis.* It can result from oral tumors, abscesses from decaying teeth, and gum disease or infection. The foul smell is primarily due to cell decay, and the odors are characteristic of the growth of some microorganisms.

When halitosis results from poor oral sanitation, the treatment is obvious—regular daily tooth brushing and the use of an antiseptic mouthwash. If the halitosis is due to disease of the oral cavity, alimentary tract, or respiratory system, the cure will depend on eradicating the primary cause.

Nonmalignant Lesions

The oral cavity is prone to invasion by several types of microorganisms that cause nonmalignant lesions. The most prominent are:

Canker sores: These are of unknown origin and show up as single or multiple small sores near the molar teeth, inside the lips, or in the lining of the mouth. They can be painful but usually heal in a few days.

Fungus infections: Thrush is the most common oral fungus infection and appears as white, round patches inside the cheeks of infants, small children, and sometimes adults. The lesions may involve the entire mouth, tongue, and pharynx. In advanced stages the lesions turn yellow. Malnutrition, especially lack of adequate vitamin B, is the principal cause. Fungus growth is also aided by the use of antibiotic lozenges, which kill normal oral bacteria and permit fungi to flourish.

Dental caries and vitamin deficiencies: Lack of adequate vitamins in the daily diet is responsible for some types of lesions in the oral cavity. Insufficient vitamin A in children under five may be the cause of malformation in the crown, dentin, and enamel of the teeth. Lack of adequate vitamin C results in bleeding gums. Vitamin D insufficiency may lead to slow tooth development.

An inadequate and improper diet supports tooth decay, which in turn may be complicated by ulcers in the gums and abscesses in the roots of the decaying teeth. A diet with an adequate supply of the deficient vitamins will cause the symptoms to disappear. Infections, abscesses, cysts, or tumors in the mouth require the attention of a physician, dentist, or dental surgeon.

Chancres: These are primary syphilis lesions, which commonly develop at the lips and tongue. They appear as small, eroding red ulcers that exude yellow matter. They can invade the mouth, tonsils, and pharynx. Penicillin therapy is usually required.

The Esophagus

Varices

Varices (singular: *varix*) are enlarged and congested veins that appear in the esophagus due to increased blood pressure to the liver in patients with liver cirrhosis. This disease is most common in chronic alcoholics. Esophageal varices can be complicated by erosion of the mucous lining of the esophagus due to inflammation or vomiting. This causes hemorrhaging of the thin-walled veins, which can be fatal.

Bleeding esophageal varices may require hospitalization, immediate blood transfusions, and surgery.

Hiatus Hernia

The lower end of the esophagus or part of the stomach can sometimes protrude through the diaphragm. This *hiatus hernia*, sometimes referred to as a *diaphragmatic hernia*, can be due to congenital malformation; in adults, the principal cause is weakness of the muscles around the opening of the esophagus leading into the stomach.

In individuals who are obese and who have large stomachs, the stomach contents may be forced back into the lower esophagus, causing this area to herniate. Other causes include stooping, bending, or kneeling, which increases pressure in the stomach. Pregnancy may increase abdominal pressure in the same manner as obesity.

Typical symptoms are vomiting when the stomach is full, heartburn with pain spreading to the ears, neck, and arms, swallowing difficulty with the food sometimes sticking in the esophagus, and a swollen abdomen. The vomiting may occur at night, with relief obtained by getting up and walking about for a few minutes. Belching will relieve the distension and *antacids* (acid neutralizers) may be prescribed to counter gastric hyperacidity.

Conservative treatment involves eating small portions at frequent intervals. Dieting and a reduction in weight cause the symptoms to disappear. When the symptoms are due to pregnancy, they disappear after delivery. When medical management is not successful, surgical repair of the hernia is necessary. See also *Hernias*, p. 531.

Achalasia

Achalasia is abnormal dilation of the lower esophagus caused by failure of the cardiac sphincter to relax and allow food to

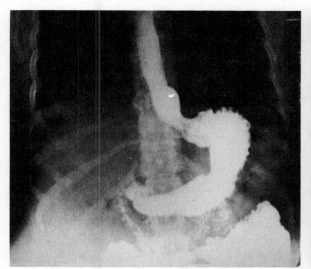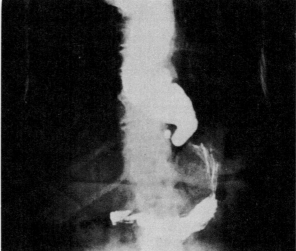

(*Left*) A normal esophagus. (*Right*) An esophagus abnormally distended with food (achalasia) because of the failure of the cardiac sphincter to relax and allow food to enter the stomach.

enter the stomach. Food collects in the esophagus and does not flow into the stomach. The patient feels as though the food is sticking in the middle of his chest wall. Small amounts of food may eventually pass into the stomach, and the mild pain or discomfort disappears.

If the condition persists, the pain may increase to become a continuous burning sensation at each meal, due to inflammation of the esophagus by accumulated food. If the patient lies down, some of this esophageal content will regurgitate and enter the pharynx. If the vomitus gets into the lungs, the end result may be *aspiration pneumonia,* a form of pneumonia caused by inhaling particles of foreign matter.

The disease is difficult to control, and the condition tends to return, so that surgery is often used to create a permanent opening between the esophagus and stomach.

Swallowing Difficulty

Difficulty in swallowing is called *dysphagia,* which should not be confused with *dysphasia,* a speech impairment. Dysphagia may be caused by lesions in the mouth and tongue, acute inflammatory conditions in the oral cavity and pharynx (mumps, tonsillitis, laryngitis, pharyngitis), lesions, cancers, or foreign bodies in the esophagus. Strictures in the esophagus—from esophageal ulcers or from swallowing corrosive liquids—will also impair swallowing.

Stomach and Intestines

Indigestion (Dyspepsia)

There are times when the gastrointestinal tract fails to carry out its normal digestive function. The resulting indigestion, or *dyspepsia,* generates a variety of symptoms, such as heartburn, nausea, pain in the upper abdomen, gases in the stomach (*flatulence*), belching, and feeling of fullness after eating.

Indigestion can be caused by ulcers of the stomach or duodenum and by excessive or too rapid eating or drinking. It may also be caused by emotional disturbance.

Constipation

Constipation is the difficult or infrequent evacuation of feces. The urge to defecate is normally triggered by the pressure of feces on the rectum and by the intake of food into the stomach. On the toilet, the anal sphincter is relaxed voluntarily, and the fecal material is expelled. The feeling to defecate should be attended to as soon as possible. Habitual disregard of the desire to empty the bowels reduces intestinal motion and leads to constipation.

Daily or regular bowel movements are not necessary for good health. Normal bowel movements may occur at irregular intervals due to variations in diet, mental stress, and physical activity. For some individuals, normal defecation may take place as infrequently as once every four days.

Simple constipation: In simple constipation, the patient may have to practice good bowel movement habits, which include a trip to the toilet once daily, preferably after breakfast. Adequate fluid intake and proper diet, including fresh fruits and green vegetables, can help restore regular bowel movement. Laxatives can provide temporary relief, but they inhibit normal bowel function and lead to dependence. When toilet-training young children, parents should encourage but never force them to have regular bowel movements, preferably after breakfast.

Chronic constipation: Chronic constipation can cause feces to accumulate in the rectum and *sigmoid,* the terminal section of the colon. The colonic fluid is absorbed and a mass of hard fecal material remains. Such impacted feces often prevent further passage of bowel contents. The individual suffers from abdominal pain with distension and sometimes vomiting. A cleansing enema will relieve the fecal impaction and related symptoms.

In the overall treatment of constipation, the principal cause must be identified and corrected so that normal evacuation can return.

Intestinal Obstructions

Obstruction to the free flow of digestive products may exist either in the stomach or in the small and large intestines. The typical symptoms of intestinal obstruction are constipation, painful abdominal distension, and vomiting. Intestinal obstruction can be caused by the bowel's looping or twisting around itself, forming what is known as a *volvulus*. Malignant tumors can either block the intestine or press it closed.

In infants, especially boys, a common form of intestinal obstruction occurs when a segment of the intestine folds into the section below it. This condition is known as *intussusception,* and can significantly reduce the blood supply to the lower bowel segment. The cause may be traced to viral infection, injury to the abdomen, hard food, or a foreign body in the gastrointestinal tract.

The presence of intestinal obstructions is generally determined by consideration of the clinical symptoms, as well as X-ray examinations of the abdomen. Hospitalization is required, since intestinal obstruction has a high fatality rate if proper medical care is not administered. Surgery may be needed to remove the obstruction.

Diarrhea

Diarrhea is the frequent and repeated passage of liquid stools. It is usually accompanied by intestinal inflammation, and sometimes by the passing of mucus or blood.

The principal cause of diarrhea is infection in the intestinal tract by microorganisms. Chemical and food poisoning also brings on spasms of diarrhea. Long-standing episodes of diarrhea have been

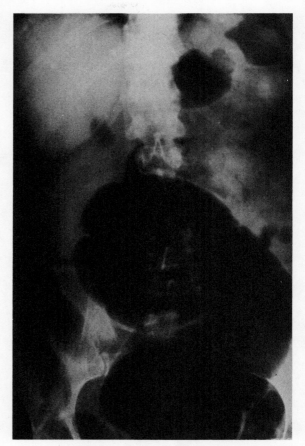

This X ray reveals volvulus of the colon, a looping of the bowel around itself, causing an obstruction.

traced to inflammation of the intestinal mucosa, tumors, ulcers, allergies, vitamin deficiency, and in some cases emotional stress.

Patients with diarrhea commonly suffer abdominal cramps, lose weight from chronic attacks, or have vomiting spells. A physician must always be consulted for proper diagnosis and treatment; this is especially important if the attacks continue for more than two or three days. Untreated diarrhea can lead to dehydration and malnutrition; it may be fatal, especially in infants.

Dysentery

Dysentery is caused by microorganisms that thrive in the intestines of infected individuals. Most common are *amoebic dysentery,* caused by amoeba, and *bacillary dys-*

entery, caused by bacteria. The symptoms are diarrhea with blood and pus in the stools, cramps, and fever. The infection is spread from person to person through infected excrement that contaminates food or water. The bacteria and amoeba responsible can also be spread by houseflies which feed on feces as well as on human foods. It is a common tropical disease and can occur wherever human excrement is not disposed of in a sanitary manner.

Dysentery must be treated early to avoid erosion of the intestinal wall. In bacillary dysentery, bed rest and hospitalization are recommended, especially for infants and the aged. Antibiotic drugs may be administered.

In most cases the disease can be spread by healthy human carriers who must be treated to check further spread.

Typhoid

Enteric fever or *typhoid* is an acute, highly communicable disease caused by the

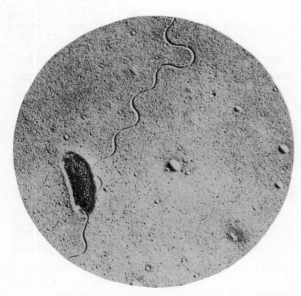

A microphotograph of bacilli of cholera, a disease marked by diarrhea and vomiting that is often fatal due to dehydration. Cholera, an epidemic disease, is generally confined to those countries having primitive sanitary facilities, since it is spread by food and water contaminated by infected fecal matter.

organism *Salmonella typhosa.* It is sometimes regarded as a tropical disease because epidemic outbreaks are common in tropical areas where careless disposal of feces and urine contaminates food, milk, and water supplies. In any location, tropical or temperate, where unsanitary living predominates, there is always the possibility that the disease can occur. Flies can transmit the disease, as can shellfish that live in typhoid-infested waters.

The typhoid bacilli do their damage to the mucosa of the small intestines. They enter via the oral cavity and stomach and finally reach the lymph nodes and blood vessels in the small bowel.

Symptoms: Following an incubation period of about ten days, general bodily discomfort, fever, headache, nausea, and vomiting are experienced. Other clinical manifestations include abdominal pain with tenderness, greenish diarrhea (or constipation), bloody stools, and mental confusion. It is not unusual for red spots to appear on the body.

If untreated, typhoid victims die within 21 days of the onset of the disease. The cause of death may be perforation of the small bowel, abdominal hemorrhage, toxemia, or other complications such as intestinal inflammation and pneumonia.

Treatment and prevention: A person can best recover from typhoid if he receives diligent medical and nursing care. He should be isolated in a hospital on complete bed rest. Diet should be restricted to highly nutritious liquids or preferably intravenous feeding. Destruction of the bacilli is achieved by antibiotic therapy, usually with Chloromycetin.

The best way to prevent the spread of typhoid is to disinfect all body refuse, clothing, and utensils of the infected. Isolation techniques practiced in hospitals prevent local spread. Milk and milk products should be pasteurized; drinking water should be chlorinated.

Human beings can carry the disease and infect others without themselves becoming ill; they are usually not aware that they are carriers. Within recent years, a vaccination effective for a year has been developed. People traveling to areas where sanitation practices may be conducive to typhoid should receive this vaccination. In such areas, it is usually a good practice to boil drinking water as well.

Foreign Bodies in the Alimentary Tract

Anyone who accidentally swallows a foreign body should seek immediate medical aid, preferably in a hospital. Foreign bodies that enter the gastrointestinal tract may cause obstruction anywhere along the tract, including the esophagus. For proper emergency procedures, see *Obstruction in the Windpipe,* p. 676.

Dental plates and large chunks of meat have been known to cause fatal choking. A foreign body in the esophagus may set off a reflex mechanism that causes the trachea to close. The windpipe may have to be opened by means of a *tracheostomy* (incision in the windpipe) to restore breathing. If the object swallowed is long and sharp-pointed, it may perforate the tract.

Foreign bodies in the esophagus are usually the most troublesome. Small fish bones may stick to the walls of the esophagus; large pieces of meat may block the tract. X-ray studies aid the doctor in locating the swallowed object and in determining how best to deal with it.

Small objects like coins and paper clips may pass through the digestive tract without causing serious problems. Their progress may be checked by X rays of the abdomen. Examination of stools will indicate whether or not the entire object has been expelled. With larger objects, the problem of blockage must be considered. It is sometimes necessary for a surgeon to open the stomach in a hospital operating room and remove the foreign object.

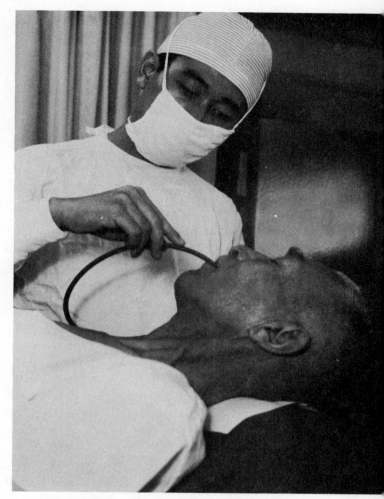

A gastrocamera is introduced into the patient's stomach, where it takes color photographs of the interior walls as an aid in the diagnosis of disorders.

Ulcers

A *peptic ulcer* is an eroded area of the mucous membrane of the digestive tract. The most common gastrointestinal ulcers are found in the lower end of the esophagus, stomach, or duodenum and are caused by the excessive secretion of gastric acid which erodes the lining membrane in these areas.

The cause of ulcers is obscure, but any factor that increases gastric acidity may contribute to the condition. Mental stress or conflict, excessive food intake, alcohol, and caffeine all cause the stomach to increase its output of hydrochloric acid.

The disease is sometimes considered to be hereditary, especially among persons with type O blood. Symptoms usually appear in individuals of the 20 to 40 age group, with the highest incidence in persons over age 45. Peptic ulcers of the stomach (*gastric ulcers*) and duodenal ulcers occur more frequently in men than in women. Ulcers are common in patients with arthritis and chronic lung disease.

Symptoms: Early ulcer symptoms are gastric hyperacidity and burning abdominal pain which is relieved by eating, vomiting, or the use of antacids. The pain may occur as a dull ache, especially when one's stomach is empty, or it may be sharp and knifelike.

Other manifestations of a peptic ulcer are nausea, which is associated with heartburn and regurgitation of gastric juice into the esophagus and mouth; excessive gas; poor appetite with undernourishment and weakness in older victims; black stools due to a bleeding ulcer.

The immediate goal of ulcer therapy is to heal the ulcer; the long-term goal is to prevent its recurrence. An ulcer normally heals through the formation of scar tissue in the ulcer crater. The healing process, under proper medical care, may take several weeks. The disappearance of pain does not necessarily indicate that the ulcer has healed completely, or even partially. The pain and the ulcerative process may recur at regular intervals over periods of weeks or months.

Although treatment can result in complete healing and recovery, some victims of chronic peptic ulcers have a 20 to 30 year history of periodic recurrences. For such patients, ulcer therapy may have to be extended indefinitely to avoid serious complications. If a recurrent ulcer perforates the stomach or intestine, or if it bleeds excessively, it can be quickly fatal. Emergency surgery is always required when perforation and persistent bleeding occur.

Treatment: The basic principles of ulcer therapy are diet, rest, and the suppression of stomach acidity. A patient with an active gastric ulcer is generally hospitalized for three weeks to make certain that he receives the proper diet and to remove him from sources of emotional stress, such as business or family problems. During hospitalization the healing process is monitored by X-ray examination. If there is no evidence of healing within three to four weeks, surgery may be advisable. For patients with duodenal ulcers, a week or two of rest at home with proper diet may be sufficient.

Ulcer diets consist of low-residue bland foods taken in small amounts at frequent intervals, as often as once an hour when pain is severe. The preferred foods are milk, soft eggs, jellies, custards, creams, and cooked cereals. Since ulcer diets often lack some essential nutrients, prolonged dietary treatment may have to be augmented with daily vitamin capsules. Antispasmodic medication may be prescribed to reduce contractions of the stomach, decrease the stomach's production of acid, and slow down digestion. Antacids, such as the combination of aluminum hydroxide and magnesium trisilicate, may be required after meals and between feedings. Spicy foods, alcohol, coffee, cola and other caffeine-containing drinks, large meals, and smoking should be strictly avoided.

If the ulcer does not respond to medical therapy, or if pain persists, surgery may be the preferred treatment. Such surgery is elective surgery, a matter of choice, as opposed to the emergency surgery required by large, bleeding, or perforated ulcers. After the removal of the acid-producing section of the stomach, some patients may develop weakness and nausea as their digestive system adjusts to the reduced size of their stomach. A proper diet of special foods and fluids, plus sedatives, can alleviate the condition. The chances for complete recovery are good.

Diverticula

A *diverticulum* is an abnormal pouch caused by herniation of the mucous membrane of the digestive tract. The pouch has a narrow neck and a bulging round end. Diverticula are found in the esophagus, stomach, duodenum, colon, and other parts of the digestive tract.

The presence of diverticula in any segment of the digestive tract is referred to as *diverticulosis*. When diverticula become inflamed the condition is known as *diverticulitis*. The latter is a common form of disease of the sigmoid colon and is found in persons past the age of 45.

In mild cases, there may be no symptoms. On the other hand, a diverticulum may sometimes rupture and produce the same symptoms as an acute attack of appendicitis—vomiting and pain with tenderness in the right lower portion of the abdomen. Other symptoms are intermittent constipation and diarrhea, and abdominal pain.

Diverticulosis is treated by bed rest, restriction of solid food and increase of fluid intake, and administration of antibiotics. Surgery is recommended when diverticulosis causes obstruction of the colon or creates an opening between the colon and the bladder, or when one or more diverticula rupture and perforate the colon. The outlook for recovery following surgery is good.

Hemorrhoids (Piles)

Hemorrhoids or *piles* are round, purplish protuberances at the anus. They are the results of rectal veins that become dilated and rupture. Hemorrhoids are very common and are often caused by straining due to constipation, pregnancy, or diarrhea.

Hemorrhoids may appear on the external side of the anus or on the internal side; they may or may not be painful. Rectal bleeding and tenderness are common. It is important to emphasize, however, that not all rectal

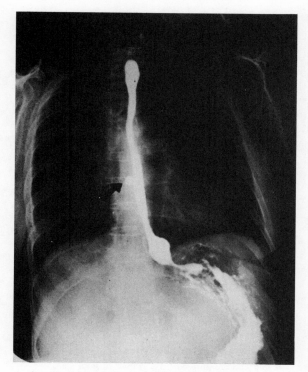

A diverticulum of the esophagus, shown by arrow, is a pouch caused by herniation of mucous membranes.

bleeding is due to hemorrhoids. Small hemorrhoids are best left untreated; large painful ones may be surgically reduced or removed. *Prolapsed* piles—those that have slipped forward—are treated by gentle pressure to return the hemorrhoidal mass into the rectum. The rectal and anal opening must be lubricated to keep the area soft. Other conditions in the large bowel can simulate hemorrhoids and need to be adequately investigated.

Hernias

Hernias in the digestive tract occur when there is muscular weakness in surrounding body structures. Pressure from the gastrointestinal tract may cause a protrusion or *herniation* of the gut through the weakened wall. Such hernias exist in the diaphragmatic area (*hiatus hernias,* discussed above on p. 525), in the anterior abdomen (*ventral hernias*), or in the region of the groin (*inguinal hernias*). Apart from hiatus her-

INGUINAL HERNIA

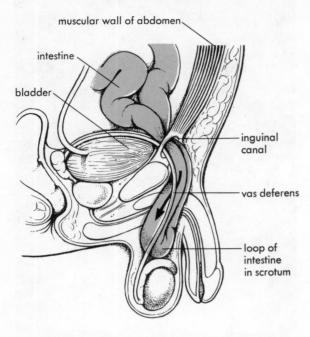

muscular wall of abdomen

intestine

bladder

inguinal canal

vas deferens

loop of intestine in scrotum

In this type of indirect hernia, a loop of small intestine has pushed through the weakened inguinal canal in the abdominal wall and descended into the scrotal sac.

nias, inguinal hernias are by far the most common.

One of the prevalent causes of intestinal obstruction is a *strangulated hernia.* A loop of herniated bowel becomes tightly constricted, blood supply is cut off, and the loop becomes gangrenous. Immediate surgery is required since life is threatened from further complications.

Except for hiatus hernias, diagnosis is usually made simple by the plainly visible herniated part. In men, an enlarged scrotum may be present in untreated inguinal hernias. The herniating bowel can be reduced, that is, manipulated back into position, and a truss worn to support the reduced hernia and provide temporary relief. In all hernias, however, surgical repair is the usual treatment.

Gastritis

Gastritis is inflammation of the mucosa of the stomach. The patient complains of *epigastric* pain—in the middle of the upper abdomen—with distension of the stomach, loss of appetite, nausea, and vomiting.

Attacks of acute gastritis can be traced to bacterial action, food poisoning, peptic ulcer, the presence of alcohol in the stomach, the ingestion of highly spiced foods, or overeating and drinking. Occasional gastritis, though painful, is not serious and may disappear spontaneously. The general treatment for gastritis is similar to the treatment of a gastric ulcer.

Enteritis

Enteritis, sometimes referred to as *regional entertitis,* is a chronic inflammatory condition of unknown origin that affects the small intestine. It is called regional because the disease most often involves the terminal ileum, even though any segment of the digestive tract can be involved. The diseased bowel becomes involved with multiple ulcer craters and ultimately stiffens because of fibrous healing of the ulcers.

Regional entertitis occurs most often in males from adolescence to middle age. The symptoms may exist for a long period before the disease is recognized. Intermittent bloody diarrhea, general weakness, and lassitude are the early manifestations. Later stages of the disease are marked by fever, increased bouts of diarrhea with resultant weight loss, and sharp lower abdominal pain on the right side. This last symptom sometimes causes the disease to be confused with appendicitis, since in both conditions there is nausea and vomiting. Occasionally in women there may be episodes of painful menstruation.

Treatment involves either surgical removal of the diseased bowel or conservative medical management and drug therapy. In acute attacks of enteritis, bed rest and intravenous fluids are two important aspects of treatment. Medical management in less severe occurrences includes a daily diet rich in proteins and vitamins, excluding harder foods such as fresh fruits and vegetables. Antibiotics are prescribed to combat bacterial invasion.

Colitis

Colitis is an inflammatory condition of the colon, of uncertain origin, and often chronic. It may result from a nervous predisposition which leads to bacterial or viral infection. The inflammation can cause spasms that damage the colon, or can lead to bleeding ulcers that may be fatal.

In milder forms, colitis first appears with diarrhea in which red bloody streaks can be observed. The symptoms may come and go for weeks before the effects become very significant. As the disease process advances, the diarrhea episodes become more frequent; more blood and mucus are present in the feces. These are combined with abdominal pain, nausea, and vomiting. Due to loss of blood the patient often becomes anemic and thin. If there are ulcer craters in the mucosa, the disease is called *ulcerative colitis*.

Hospitalization is necessary in order to provide proper treatment that will have a long-term effect. Surgery is sometimes necessary if an acute attack has been complicated by perforation of the intestines or if chronic colitis fails to respond to medical management.

Nonoperative treatment includes control of diarrhea and vomiting by drug therapy. Antibiotics are given to control infection and reduce fever, which always accompanies infection. A high protein and vitamin diet is necessary. But if the diarrhea and vomiting persist, intravenous feeding becomes a must. Blood transfusions may be required for individuals who have had severe rectal bleeding. Since there is no absolute cure, the disease may recur.

Appendicitis

The *vermiform appendix* is a narrow tubular attachment to the colon. It can become obstructed by the presence of undigested food such as small seeds from fruits, or by hard bits of feces. This irritates the appendix and causes inflammation to set in. If it is obstructed, pressure builds within the appendix due to increasing secretions, a situation that can result in rupture of the appendix. A ruptured appendix can be rapidly fatal if *peritonitis,* inflammation of the peritoneal cavity, sets in.

In most cases the onset of appendicitis is heralded by an acute attack of pain in the center of the abdomen. The pain intensity increases, shifts to the right lower abdomen with nausea, vomiting, and fever as added symptoms. Some individuals, however, suffer from recurrent attacks of dull pain without other signs of gastrointestinal disease, and these may not be significant enough to warrant immediate hospitalization.

Diagnosis of appendicitis is usually dependent on the above symptoms, along with tenderness in the appendix area, increased pulse rate, and decreasing blood pressure. The last two are very significant if the appendix ruptures and peritonitis sets in. Whenever these symptoms are observed, the patient should be rushed to the nearest hospital.

Immediate surgical removal of the diseased appendix by means of a small incision is necessary in all nonperforated acute cases. This type of operation (*appendectomy*) is no longer considered major surgery. If the appendix ruptures and peritonitis is evident, emergency major surgery is necessary to drain the infection and remove the appendix. In the absence of postoperative complications, the patient recovers completely. One of the major problems of appendicitis is early diagnosis to prevent dangerous complications.

Intestinal Parasites

Not all the diseases of man are caused by microscopic organisms. Some are caused by parasitic worms, *helminths,* which invade the digestive tract, most often via food and water. In recent years government health agencies have largely eliminated the prime sources of worm infection: unwholesome meat or untreated sewage that finds its way into drinking water. Nevertheless, helminths still exist. Drugs used to expel worms are called *vermifuges* or *anthelmintics.*

The following are among the major intestinal parasites:

Tapeworms (*cestodes*)*:* These ribbon-shaped flat worms are found primarily in beef, fish, and pork that have not been thoroughly cooked. There are several species ranging from inch-long worms to tapeworms that grow to about 30 feet and live for as long as 16 years.

Tapeworms attach themselves to intestinal mucosa and periodically expel their eggs in excreta. If such feces are carelessly disposed of, the eggs can reach drinking water and be taken in by fish or ingested by grazing cattle. The eggs hatch in the animal's large bowel and find their way into the bloodstream by boring through the intestinal wall. Once in the blood they eventually adhere to muscles and live a dormant life in a capsule.

People who eat raw or partially cooked meat and fish that are infested with tapeworms become infected. The worms enter the bowel, where they feed, grow, and produce eggs. When the egg-filled segments are excreted, the cycle begins anew. Tapeworm infection is usually asymptomatic. They are discovered when egg-laden segments in feces are recognized as such.

Medication must be given on an empty stomach, followed later by a laxative. This will dislodge the worms and enable the body to purge itself of them. A weekly check of stools for segments of the worms may be necessary to confirm that the host is free of the parasites.

Hookworms: There are many species of these tiny, threadlike worms which are usually less than one centimeter long. They are found principally in tropical and subtropical areas of China, North Africa, Europe, Central America, and the West Indies, but they are by no means extinct in the United States.

The eggs are excreted in the feces of infected individuals, and if fecal materials are not well disposed of, the eggs may be found on the ground of unsanitary areas. In warm, moist, conditions they hatch into larvae that penetrate the skin, especially the feet of people who walk around barefooted. The larvae can also be swallowed in impure water.

Hookworm-infected individuals, most often children, may experience an inflammatory itch in the area where the larvae entered. The host becomes anemic from blood loss, due to parasitic feeding of the worms, develops a cough, and experiences abdominal pain with diarrhea. Sometimes there is nausea or distended abdomen. Diagnosis is confirmed by laboratory analysis of feces for the presence of eggs.

Successful treatment requires administration of anthelmintic drugs, preferably be-

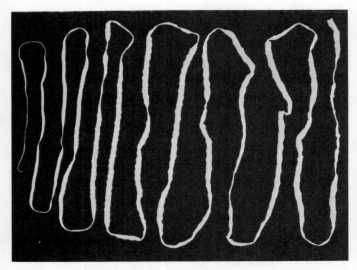

Tapeworm eggs are usually taken into the body via improperly cooked food. Some adults, such as this specimen of the genus *Taenia,* can grow to 30 feet.

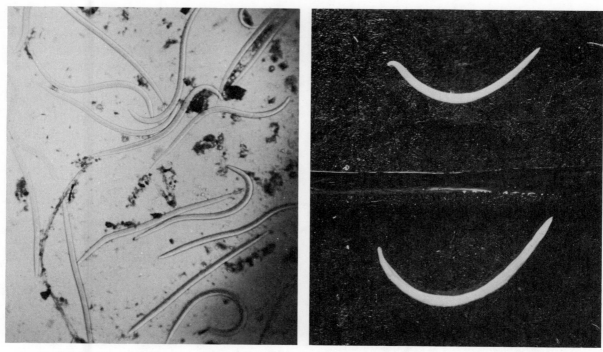

Hookworm eggs hatch into larvae (*left,* greatly enlarged) that can penetrate the skin of a bare foot. (*Right,* also much enlarged) Two adult hookworms: one (*top*) a variety with teeth resembling flat plates (genus *Necator*), the other (*bottom*) having hook-shaped teeth (genus *Ancylostoma*).

fore breakfast, to destroy the worms. Weekly laboratory examination of the feces for evidence of hookworm eggs is a necessary precaution in ascertaining that the disease has been eradicated. Untreated hookworm infestation very often leads to small bowel obstruction.

Trichinosis: This sometimes fatal disease is caused by a tiny worm, *Trichinella spiralis,* which is spread to man by eating improperly cooked pork containing the tiny worms in a capsulated form. After they are ingested the worms are set free to attach themselves to the mucosa of the small intestines. Here they mature in a few days and mate, the male dies and the female lays eggs that reach the muscles via the vascular system.

Trichinella organisms cause irritation of the intestinal mucosa. The infected individual suffers from abdominal pains with diarrhea, nausea, and vomiting. Later stages of the disease are marked by stiffness, pain, and swelling in the muscles, fever with sweating, respiratory distress, insomnia, and swelling of the face and eyelids. Death may result from complications such as pneumonia, heart damage, or respiratory failure. Despite government inspection of meats, all pork should be well-cooked before eating.

Threadworms (nematodes): These worms, also called pinworms, infect children more often than adults. Infection occurs by way of the mouth. The worms live in the bowel and sometimes journey through the anus, where they cause intense itching. The eggs are laid at the anal opening, and can be blown about in the air and spread in that manner. The entire family must be medically treated to kill the egg-laying females, and soothing ointment should be applied at the rectal area to relieve the itching. Good personal hygiene, especially hand washing after toilet use, is an essential part of the treatment.

Round worms (ascaris): These intestinal parasites closely resemble earthworms. The eggs enter the digestive tract and hatch in the small bowel. The young parasites then penetrate the walls of the bowel, enter the bloodstream and find their way to the liver, heart, and lungs.

Untreated roundworm infestation leads to intestinal obstruction or blockage of pancreatic and bile ducts caused by the masses of roundworms, which usually exist in the hundreds. Ingestion of vermifuge drugs is the required treatment.

Food Poisoning

Acute gastrointestinal illnesses may result from eating food that is itself poisonous, from ingesting chemical poisons, or from bacterial sources. The bacteria can either manufacture *toxins* (poisonous substances) or cause infection. Improperly canned fish, meats, and green vegetables may encourage the growth of certain toxin-manufacturing organisms that resist the action of gastric juice when ingested. A person who eats such foods may contract a type of food poisoning known as *botulism.* The symptoms include indigestion and abdominal pain, nausea and vomiting, blurred vision, dryness in the mouth and throat, and poor muscular coordination.

If the toxins become fixed in the central nervous system, they may cause death. Emergency hospitalization is required, where antitoxins are administered intravenously and other measures are taken to combat the effects of botulism.

Salmonella food poisoning is caused by a species of bacteria by that name and is spread by eating contaminated meat, or by eating fish, egg, and milk products that have not been properly cooked or stored or inadequately refrigerated. The organisms are also transmitted by individuals who handle well-prepared food with dirty hands. Victims suffer from vomiting, diarrhea, abdominal pain, and fever. This type of food poisoning can be fatal in children and the aged, especially if the latter are ailing. Medical treatment with hospitalization, administration of broad-spectrum antibiotics, and intravenous fluids (to replace body loss due to vomiting) is required.

Some people develop allergic reactions to certain foods and break out in severe rashes after a meal containing any of these foods. Among such foods are fruits, eggs, and milk or milk products. Vomiting or diarrhea may also occur. The best treatment is to avoid eating such foods and, when necessary, supplement the diet with manufactured protein and vitamins.

Liver Disease

Cirrhosis

Chronic disease of the liver with the destruction of liver cells is known as *cirrhosis.* A common cause is excessive intake of alcoholic beverages along with malnutrition. However, there are other predisposing factors, such as inflammation of the liver (*hepatitis*), syphilis, intestinal worms, jaundice or biliary tract inflammation, and disorders in blood circulation to the liver.

Victims of cirrhosis are usually anemic and have an elevated temperature, around 100 degrees Fahrenheit. Alcoholics very often lose weight, suffer from indigestion, and have distended abdomens.

Accurate diagnosis of cirrhosis depends on complex laboratory tests of liver function, urine, and blood. If liver damage is not too far advanced, treatment of the complications and underlying causes can aid the liver cells in the process of regeneration. In long-standing chronic disease, liver damage may be irreversible. Alcoholics who forgo alcohol may be restored to health, depending on the extent of liver damage, with a proper diet rich in proteins and vitamins.

Successful treatment of liver cirrhosis may require long hospitalization with drug therapy and blood transfusions. During alcoholic withdrawal, the patient may require close medical observation and psychiatric help. If the patient's jaundice improves and his appetite returns, recovery in milder cirrhosis cases is possible.

Jaundice

In diseases of the liver and biliary tract, excessive bile pigment (*bilirubin*) is recirculated into the bloodstream. It enters the mucous membranes and skin, giving them the characteristic yellow pigmentation of the disease.

Gallstones or tumors that obstruct the free flow of bile are one cause of jaundice. Other causes include hepatitis, overproduction of bile pigments with resultant accumulation of bile within the liver, cirrhosis, and congenital closure of the bile ducts, the last a common cause of jaundice in infancy.

Apart from the typical yellow appearance of the skin, jaundice generates such symptoms as body itching, vomiting with bile (indicated by the green appearance and bitter taste of vomit), diarrhea with undigested fats present in the stools, and enlargement of the liver with pain and tenderness in the right upper abdomen.

Treatment of jaundice requires continued medical care with hospitalization. Surgery may be necessary to remove stones in the biliary tract or other obstructions. If there is bacterial infection, antibiotic therapy is necessary.

Hepatitis

Inflammation of the liver results in the disease known as *hepatitis*. The most common cause is an infectious process brought on by viruses, jaundice, or high fevers. Other causes of hepatitis include intestinal parasites, circulatory disturbances (such as congestive heart failure), hypersensitivity to drugs, damage to the liver or kidneys, or bacterial infection elsewhere in the body.

One common form of this disease is *infectious hepatitis,* a highly contagious viral infection that often attacks children and young adults, especially those who congregate in large groups. Infectious hepatitis has been known to break out as an epidemic in schools, summer camps, music festivals, and military installations.

The virus is spread by food and water contaminated by feces from infected individuals; good sanitation thus becomes a vital preventive factor. Whole blood used in transfusions can transmit the organisms if the donor is infected. This form of the disease is known as *serum hepatitis*. With the great increase in the use of blood transfusions in recent years in complex surgery, the danger of transmitting serum hepatitis by infected blood or infected syringes has become correspondingly greater. Drug addicts are particularly vulnerable to serum hepatitis from the use of shared, infected needles.

Symptoms: The incubation period of infectious hepatitis lasts from one to six weeks —that of serum hepatitis is longer—followed by fever with headache, loss of appetite (especially for fatty foods), and gastrointestinal distress (nausea, vomiting, diarrhea, or constipation). As the disease progresses, the liver becomes enlarged and the patient jaundiced. There may be some pain in the right upper abdomen.

Treatment: Bed rest, preferably hospital isolation, is a necessary step in the initial treatment stages. Drug therapy with steroids may hasten the recovery process, which may take three to four weeks. When discharged from the hospital, the patient is usually very weak.

Untreated hepatitis causes severe liver damage and may result in coma due to liver failure. Sometimes death occurs. Several assaults on the liver reduce the regeneration process and promote cirrhosis. Persons who

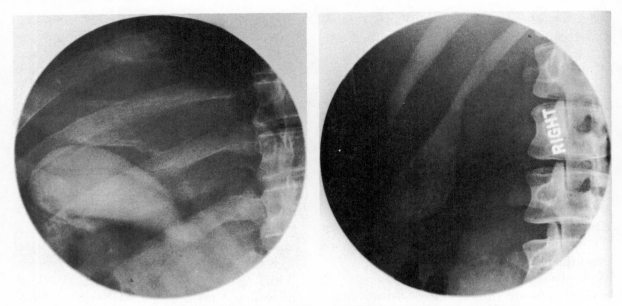

The normal gallbladder (*left*), and a diseased gallbladder (*right*) filled with stones. The small stones are comprised of calcium carbonate, cholesterol, and bile salts.

may have been exposed to the causative virus can receive temporary immunity if they are given an injection of gamma globulin, especially if there is an epidemic. Recent research directed toward the development of a vaccine against serum hepatitis has been very encouraging, and gives rise to the hope that some day wide-scale outbreaks of this disease may become a thing of the past.

Gallbladder Disease

The biliary tract is very often plagued by the presence of stones, either in the gallbladder or in one of the bile ducts. Gallstones are mostly a mixture of calcium carbonate, cholesterol, and bile salts, and can occur either as one large stone, a few smaller ones, or several very small stones.

When fats from the daily diet enter the small intestines, the concentrated bile from the gallbladder is poured into the duodenum via the bile ducts. Bile is necessary if fats are to be digested and absorbed. If stones are present in the biliary tract, the gallbladder will contract, but little or no bile will reach the fats in the small bowel.

A sharp pain to the right of the stomach is usually the first warning sign of gallstones, especially if the pain is felt soon after a meal of fatty foods—eggs, pork, mayonnaise, or fried foods. The presence of stones very often causes inflammation of the gallbladder and such symptoms as occasional diarrhea and nausea with vomiting and belching. The abdominal area near the gallbladder is usually very tender.

Untreated gallbladder disease leads to several possible complications. The obstructed bile pigments may be recirculated in the bloodstream, causing jaundice. Obstruction of the ducts causes increased pressure and may also result in perforation of the gallbladder or ducts. Acute inflammation of the biliary tract is always a possibility due to the irritation caused by the concentrated bile.

A gallbladder that is full of stones or badly diseased must be surgically removed for the patient's health to improve. In milder cases, other treatment and special diet can prevent attacks.

Treatment and Diagnosis of Gastrointestinal Disorders

Some medications used in treating gastrointestinal disorders, such as antacids and laxatives, can be purchased without prescription. Such medications should be taken only upon a physician's advice.

Treatment of gastrointestinal diseases may require low-residue diets—that is, a diet of foods that pass through the digestive tract very readily without a large amount of solid fecal residue. Included are low-fat meals, liquids, and finely crushed foods. Diagnostic tests may require overnight fasting, fat-free meals, or eating specific foods. Bland meals are vital in the treatment of peptic ulcers and should consist of unspiced soft foods and milk. Raw fruits and vegetables, salads, alcohol, and coffee do not belong in a bland diet. See under *Nutrition and Weight Control*, p. 295, for further information on special diets.

X-ray examinations play an important role in diagnosis of gastrointestinal disorders, such as ulcers, diverticuli, foreign bodies, malignant lesions, obstruction, achalasia of the esophagus, and varices.

Plain film radiographs are used in initial studies in cases where intestinal obstruction or perforation is suspected. Metallic foreign bodies are easily demonstrated on plain X rays of the digestive tract.

GI Series

By filling the digestive tract with *barium sulfate*, a substance opaque to X rays, a radiologist can locate areas of abnormality. Barium sulfate can be mixed as a thin liquid or paste and be swallowed by the patient during studies of the esophagus, stomach, and small intestines. The type of radiological examination which utilizes such a barium meal is known as a *GI* (gastrointestinal) *series*. The large bowel is examined with the barium mixture administered through the rectum like a standard enema, and is known as a *barium enema*. This makes it possible to visualize the inner walls of the colon.   AAD

DISEASES OF THE RESPIRATORY SYSTEM

The human body cannot survive for more than a very few minutes in an environment that lacks oxygen. Oxygen is required for the normal functioning of all living body cells. This vital gas reaches the body cells via the bloodstream; each red blood cell transports oxygen molecules to the body tissues. The oxygen comes from the atmosphere one breathes, and it enters the bloodstream through the very thin membrane walls of the lung tissue, a fresh supply of oxygen entering the bloodstream each time a person inhales. As the red blood cells circulating through the walls of the lung tissue pick up their fresh supply of oxygen, they release molecules of carbon dioxide given off by the body cells as a waste product of metabolism. When a person exhales, the lungs are squeezed somewhat like a bellows, and the carbon dioxide is expelled from the lungs.

The automatic action of breathing in and out is caused by the alternate contraction and relaxation of several muscle groups. The main muscle of breathing is the *diaphragm*, a layer of muscle fibers that separates the organs of the chest from the organs of the abdomen. Other muscles of respiration are located between the ribs, in the neck, and in the abdomen. As the diaphragm contracts to let the lungs expand, the other muscles increase the capacity of the *thorax,* or chest cavity, when one inhales. The muscles literally squeeze the lungs and chest when an individual exhales.

Any disease of the muscles and bones of the chest wall or of the passages leading from the nose to the lung tissue—containing the small air sacs where the gases are actually exchanged—will interfere to some extent with normal function. As with any organ of the body, there is a great reserve built into the lungs that assures that small to even moderate amounts of diseased tissue can exist without compromising their ability to sustain life. However, when disease of the lungs, air passages, *thoracic* (rib) *cage,* or any combination of these parts decreases the capacity of the reserve areas, then the oxygen supply to all the organs

and tissues of the body becomes deficient, and they become incapable of performing their vital functions.

Diseases of the thoracic cage are relatively uncommon. Certain forms of arthritis cause fixation of the bony cage and limit expansion when breathing. Various muscle and nervous system diseases weaken the muscles used to expand the chest for breathing.

Diseases of the *bronchi* or air passages tend to narrow those tubes and thereby limit the amount of air that can pass through to the tiny *alveoli* or air sacs. Other conditions affect the alveoli themselves, and, if widespread enough, allow no place for the oxygen and carbon dioxide to be exchanged.

The most common forms of lung disease are infections caused by viruses, bacteria,

THE ACTION OF THE DIAPHRAGM

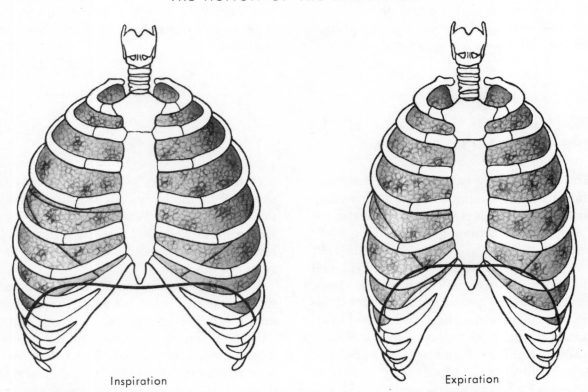

Inspiration

Expiration

The thorax, or chest cavity, is enlarged when air is drawn into the lungs (inspiration), and the diaphragm is accordingly stretched. The diaphragm contracts to squeeze together the lungs and expel breath during expiration, and the volume of the thorax is thereby reduced.

or fungi. Infection is always a potential threat to the lung, since this organ is in constant contact with the outside air and therefore constantly exposed to infectious agents. It is only through elaborate defenses that the body is able to maintain normal functions without interference by these agents.

The major defenses are simply mechanical and consist mainly of the hairs in the nose and a mucous blanket coating the inside of the bronchi. The very small hairs (called *cilia*) in the breathing passage act as a filtering system; mucous membranes of the bronchi help to intercept small particles as they are swept along by the action of the cilia. Whenever these structures are diseased, as in chronic bronchitis, there is a much greater likelihood of acquiring infection.

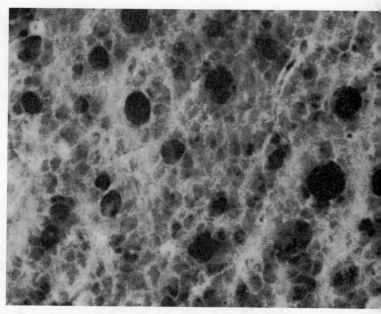

Normal lung tissue, greatly enlarged, of a man in his late sixties. The larger spaces are bronchioles.

The Common Cold, Influenza, and Other Viral Infections

The Common Cold

The common cold is the most prevalent illness known to mankind. It accounts for more time lost from work than any other single condition. The infection rate varies from one individual to another.

Surveys indicate that about 25 percent of the population experiences four or more infections a year, 50 percent experience two or three a year, and the remaining 25 percent have one or no infections in a year. There is also some variation from year to year for each person, explained often by the amount of exposure to young children, frequent extreme changes in weather, fatigue, and other factors.

For years it has been felt that chilling plays a role in causing the common cold, and, although difficult to prove, there is almost certainly some truth to the idea. By some as yet unclear process, chilling probably causes certain changes in our respiratory passages that make them susceptible to viruses that otherwise would be harmless.

The common cold affects only the upper respiratory passages: the nose, sinuses, and throat. It sometimes is associated with fever. Several viruses have been implicated as the cause for the common cold. But in the study centers that investigate this illness, isolation of a cold virus is only achieved in about one half of the cases. These viruses are not known to produce any other significant illnesses. Most likely they inhabit the nose and throat, often without producing any illness at all.

Symptoms: The major part of the illness consists of about three days of nasal congestion, possibly a mild sore throat, some sneezing and irritation of the eyes (though not as severe as in hay fever), and a general feeling of ill health often associated with some muscle fatigue and aching. After three days the symptoms abate, but there is usually some degree of nasal congestion for another ten days.

Prevention is difficult, and there is no specific treatment. The natural defenses of

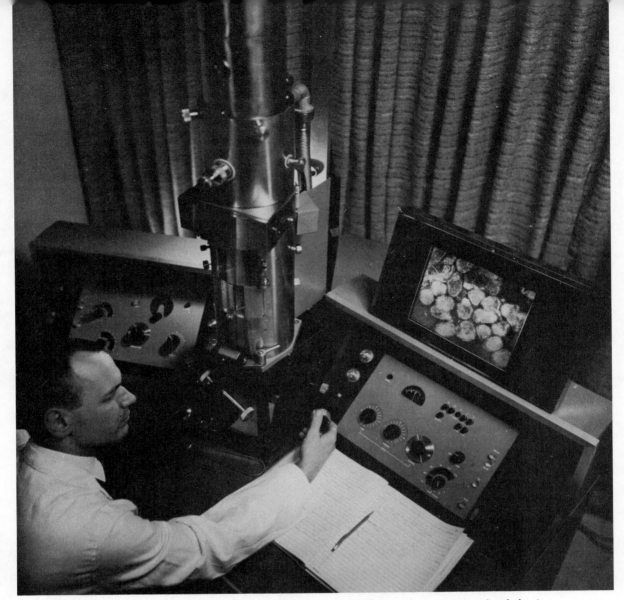

Displayed on the light box of an electron microscope is a photomicrograph of the influenza virus. Electron microscopy gave scientists their first clear look at this virus in 1960.

the body usually are capable of resolving the infection. Attention should be paid to avoiding further chilling of the body, exhausting activity, and late hours that can further lower the defenses and lead to complications.

Complications: Ear infection may develop due to blockage of the *eustachian tube,* which leads from the back of the throat to the inner part of the ear. That complication is heralded by pain in the ear. Bronchitis and pneumonia may be recognized early by the development of cough and production of *sputum* (phlegm). *Sinu-*

sitis develops when the sinus passages are obstructed so that the infected mucus cannot drain into the pharynx (as in postnasal drip). The pain develops near the sinus cavity involved. These complications can and should be treated with specific drugs, and, if they develop, a physician should be consulted.

Influenza

A number of other viruses cause respiratory illness similar to the common cold, but are much more severe in intensity and with frequently serious, and even fatal, complications. The best known member of the group is the *influenza* (flu) virus. It can cause mild symptoms that are indistinguishable from those of the common cold, but in the more easily recognizable form it is ushered in by fever, cough, and what doctors refer to as *malaise*—chills, muscle ache, and fatigue.

The symptoms of influenza appear quickly; they develop within hours and generally last in severe form from four to seven days. The disease gradually recedes over the following week. The severity of the local respiratory and generalized symptoms usually forces the influenza patient to stay in bed.

Not only is the individual case often severe, but an outbreak of influenza can easily spread to epidemic proportions in whole population groups, closing factories, schools, and hospitals in its wake. There have been 31 very severe *pandemics* (epidemics that sweep many countries) that have occurred since 1510. The most devastating of these pandemics occurred in 1918; it led to the death of twenty million people around the world. Rarely is death directly attributable to the influenza virus itself, but rather to complicating bacterial pneumonia or to the failure of vital organs previously weakened by chronic disease.

Flu shots: Inoculation is fairly effective in preventing influenza, but is not long lasting and has to be renewed each year. Unfortunately, there are several different types of influenza virus, and a slightly different vaccine is needed to provide immunity to each type of infection. Each recent epidemic in the United States has been the result of a different strain, and although there have been several months' warning before the epidemics started, it has been difficult to mass-produce a vaccine in time to use it before the epidemic developed.

Treatment: Once acquired, there is no cure for influenza, but the body defenses are usually capable of destroying the virus if given the necessary time and if the de-

fenses are not depressed by other illness. Fluids, aspirin, and bed rest help relieve the symptoms. Special attention should be paid to sudden worsening of fever after seeming recovery, or the onset of sputum production. In elderly people more intensive medical care is often necessary, including hospitalization for some.

Pneumonia

Pneumonia might be defined as any inflammation of the lung tissue itself, but the term is generally applied only to infections of an acute or rapidly developing nature caused by certain bacteria or viruses. The term is generally not used for tuberculous or fungal infections. The most common severe pneumonia is that caused by the *pneumococcus bacterium*.

Pneumonia develops from inhaling infected mucus into the lower respiratory passages. The pneumococcus is often present in the nasal or throat secretions of healthy people, and it tends to be present

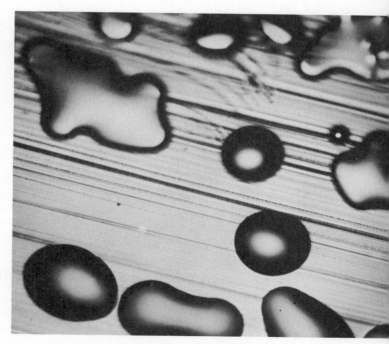

A photomicrograph of colonies of the pneumococcus bacteria, which cause a severe form of pneumonia.

even more often in the same secretions of an individual with a cold. Under certain conditions these secretions may be *aspirated,* or inhaled, into the lung. There the bacteria rapidly multiply and spread within hours to infect a sizable area. As with the common cold, chilling and fatigue often play a role in making this sequence possible. Any chronic debilitating illness also makes one very susceptible to pneumonia.

Pneumonia develops very suddenly with the onset of high fever, shaking chills, chest pain, and a very definite feeling of total sickness or malaise. Within hours enough pus is produced within the lung for the patient to start coughing up thick yellow or greenish sputum which often may be tinged or streaked with blood. The patient has no problem in recognizing that he has suddenly become extremely ill.

Prior to penicillin the illness tended to last about seven days, at which time it would often suddenly resolve almost as quickly as it started, leaving a healthy but exhausted patient. But it also could frequently lead to death or to serious complications, such as abscess formation within the chest wall, meningitis, or abscess of the brain. Since penicillin is so very effective in curing this illness today, doctors rarely see those complications.

The response of pneumococcal pneumonia to penicillin is at times one of the most dramatic therapeutic events in medicine. After only several hours of illness the patient presents himself to the hospital with a fever of 104 degrees, feeling so miserable that he does not want to eat, talk, or do anything but lie still in bed. Within four to six hours after being given penicillin he may have lost his fever and be sitting up in bed eating a meal. Not everyone responds this dramatically, but when someone does, it is striking.

There is no guaranteed way to prevent pneumonia. The advice to avoid chilling temperatures, overexertion, and fatigue when one has a cold is directed principally toward avoiding pneumonia. Anybody exposed to the elements, especially when fatigued and wearing damp clothing, is particularly susceptible to pneumonia; this explains its frequent occurrence among army recruits and combat troops. The elderly and debilitated become more susceptible when exposed to extremes of temperature and dampness.

Pneumonia is not really a contagious illness except in very special circumstances, so that isolation of patients is not necessary. In fact, all of us carry the pneumococcus in our noses and throats, but we rarely have the constellation of circumstances that lead to infection. It is the added physical insults that allow pneumonia to take hold.

Other Kinds of Pneumonia

All bacteria are capable of causing pneumonia and they do so in the same manner, via the inhalation of infected upper airway secretions. Some diseases, such as alcoholism, tend to predispose to certain bacterial pneumonias. Usually these are not as dramatic as those caused by the pneumococcus, but they may be much more difficult to treat and thereby can often be more serious.

Far less severe are the pneumonias caused by certain viruses or a recently discovered organism that seems to be intermediate between a virus and bacterium. The term *walking pneumonia* is often applied to this type, because the patient is often so little incapacitated that he is walking about and not in bed. These apparently occur in the same way as the bacterial pneumonias, but the difference is that the infecting agent is not capable of producing such severe destruction. These pneumonias are usually associated with only mild temperature elevation, scant amount of sputum production, and fewer general body symptoms. They should be suspected when coughing dominates the symptoms of a cold, especially if it turns from a dry or nonproductive cough to one that produces sputum. Antibiotic therapy tends to hasten recovery and prevent the complication of bacterial pneumonia.

Pleurisy

No discussion of pneumonia is complete without mention of *pleurisy*. This term refers to any inflammation of the lining between the chest wall and the lung. Infection is only one of the causes, but probably the most common, of inflammation of the *pleura*. Pleurisy is almost always painful, the pain being felt on inhaling and exhaling but not when the breath is quietly held for a brief period. It is a symptom that always deserves the attention of a physician and investigation of its cause. The same type of pain on breathing can often be mimicked by a strain of the chest wall muscles, but the difference can usually be determined by a physician's examination. If not, a chest X ray will help to reveal the cause of the pain.

Tuberculosis

At the turn of the century *tuberculosis* was the leading cause of death in the world; now it is eighteenth. The change in status is due both to the discovery of antibiotics and to modern preventive measures. In this century most other infectious diseases have likewise decreased in incidence and severity for similar reasons. The general decline leaves tuberculosis still at the top of the list as the leading cause of death among infectious diseases. And tuberculosis remains a very serious health problem, accounting for 40,000 new illnesses every year in the United States. In contrast to a disease like influenza, doctors already have the tools with which to eliminate tuberculosis. But many factors, primarily social, make that a very distant possibility.

Tuberculosis is caused by one specific type of bacterium. Certain ethnic groups seem particularly susceptible to the disease,

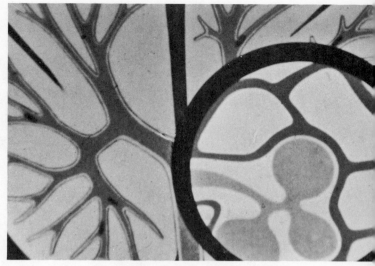

These photographs illustrate how tubercle bacilli infiltrate the air sacs of the lungs. Bacilli (dark, rod-like spots) have been breathed into the lungs.

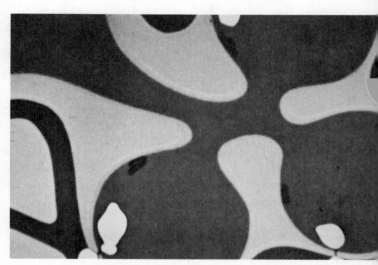

The tubercle bacilli have settled on the walls of air sacs of the lung. White cells from a nearby capillary move through the capillary wall into the air sacs.

but the reasons are unclear. The American Indian and the Eskimo are two susceptible groups. However, there is no recognized hereditary factor. The disease is different from many commonly known infections in several ways. Unlike pneumonia, tuberculosis is a chronic and painless infection, measured more in months than in days. Because of this pattern, it not only takes a long

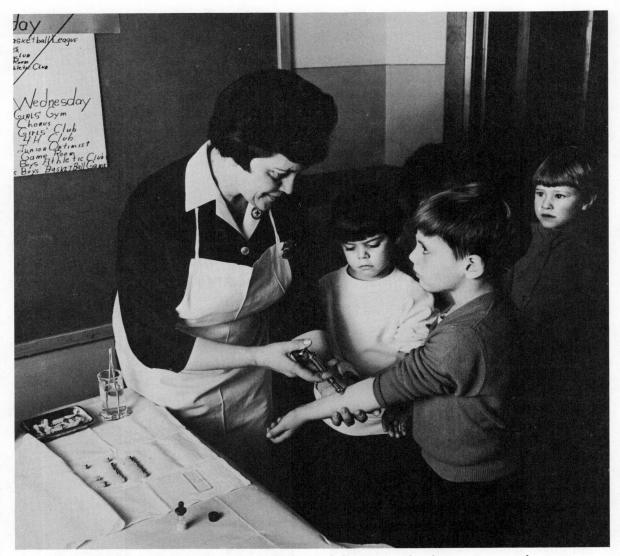

Mass tuberculosis testing programs in schools can help uncover the disease at an early stage.

time to develop serious disease, but it also takes a long time to effect a cure.

Another very important difference between tuberculosis and many other infections is its ability to infect individuals without causing symptoms of illness, but then lie dormant as a potential threat to that person for the rest of his life. The early stages of the disease do not produce any symptoms. Consequently a patient develops large areas of diseased tissue before he begins to feel sick. Screening procedures, therefore, are very important in detecting early disease in patients who feel perfectly healthy. Another is the skin testing of schoolchildren, which is carried out routinely in many communities today.

How Tuberculosis Spreads

Tuberculosis is contracted by inhaling into the lungs bacteria that have been coughed into the air by a person with advanced disease. It is, therefore, contagious, but not as contagious as measles, mumps, or chickenpox. Unlike those illnesses, it usually requires fairly close and prolonged contact with a tuberculous patient before the infection is passed on. Once the bacteria are inhaled, the body defenses are usually capable of isolating them into small areas within the tissues, thereby preventing any significant destruction or disease. However, though defenses are able to isolate the bacteria, they are not able to destroy all of them. Some bacteria persist in a state in which they are unable to break out and destroy tissue, but they always maintain the potential to do so at a time when the body defenses are impaired.

In about 20 percent of individuals the body defenses are not initially capable of isolating the tubercle bacilli. These individuals, mostly children, develop progressive tuberculosis directly following their initial contact. Others are successful in preventing actual disease at the time of initial contact, but they join a large group with the potential for active disease at some time in the future. Most of the new cases of active tuberculosis come from this second group; their defenses break down years after the initial contact and resultant infection.

Weight loss, malnutrition, alcoholism, diabetes, and certain other chronic illnesses are particularly likely to lead to deterioration of the defense mechanisms holding the tuberculosis organisms in check. Still other individuals develop active disease with no recognizable condition to account for the loss of defenses. In fact, the most likely age group to develop active disease as a result of breakdown of past infection is the 20 to 30-year-old group.

Once active disease has appeared it usually involves the chest, although it can develop anywhere in the body. There is gradual spread of inflammation within lung tissue until large areas are involved. Holes, or cavities, are formed as a result of tissue destruction. These contain large numbers of tuberculosis organisms and continue to enlarge as new tissue is destroyed at the edges. At any stage of this development

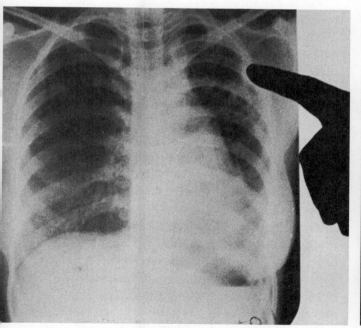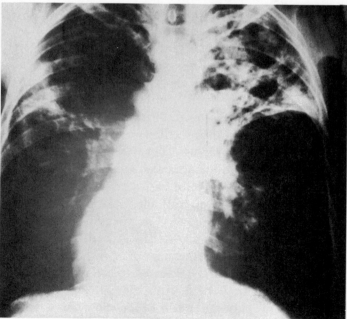

Tissue destruction in the lungs caused by tuberculosis results in cavities that show up as shadows on X-ray film. (*Left*) A physician points to such a shadow. (*Right*) The shadows on this X ray reveal far advanced cavitary tuberculosis.

organisms may find their way into the bloodstream and new foci of disease can spring up throughout the body. The sputum becomes loaded with organisms that are coughed into the air and go on to infect other individuals. The infected sputum from one area of the lung may gain access to other areas and cause development of diseased tissue there as well.

Treatment

Before the modern era of drug treatment all these events followed an inexorable course to death in 85 percent of people with active tuberculosis. Only a lucky few were able to survive as cured, usually because their disease was found at an early stage. That survival was often at the expense of years confined to a sanatorium. Because of its almost uniform outcome and the required separation from family and home, tuberculosis was formerly looked upon with quite as much dread as cancer is today.

The sanatorium rest cure of tuberculosis was first developed in the mid-nineteenth century at a time when the cause of the disease was unknown. In 1882, Robert Koch first demonstrated the tuberculosis organism, thereby proving the disease was an infection. As the twentieth century progressed general public health measures helped limit the number of new cases, and new surgical procedures were developed to treat the disease. These measures were effective enough to arrest tuberculosis in another 25 percent of cases, brightening somewhat the dismal outlook of the past century.

But the discovery of specific antibiotics in the 1940s made the real difference in tuberculosis. Because of drug treatment, surgery is rarely resorted to today, although it still may be helpful in certain patients. Now patients with tuberculosis can face a relatively bright future without having to be hospitalized for prolonged periods or enduring periods of endless disability.

Tuberculosis Control

People still contract tuberculosis, and people still die from it. Two of the principal causes of death are delayed therapy and interruptions in therapy, the latter leading to the development of tuberculosis organisms that are unaffected by drugs. Both of these causes are often under the control of the patient. The first can be avoided by seeing a physician whenever one develops a cough that lasts more than two weeks, especially when it is not associated with the typical symptoms of a cold at the outset. The other symptoms of developing tuberculosis are also seen in other illnesses, and should always lead one to recognize that he is sick and needs to consult his physician. These symptoms are weight loss, loss of appetite, fever, and night sweats. When tuberculosis is diagnosed, the patient must follow carefully the directions regarding medication, which is always continued for a long time after the patient has regained his feeling of well-being.

There are other ways, however, to attack tuberculosis, even before one becomes sick. Once a person has had contact with tuberculosis, even though he usually does not develop active disease, he produces antibodies against the bacteria. A person with such antibodies can be recognized by injecting under the skin specially prepared material from dead tuberculosis bacteria which gives rise to a reaction within the skin after two days. This material is called *tuberculin* and the test is known as the *tuberculin test*.

There are now many mass screening programs of tuberculin testing for schoolchildren, hospital personnel, and industrial groups. Those with positive skin test reactions are screened further for the presence of active disease. If they are found to be active cases, they are treated during what is usually an early and not very severe stage of the disease. The other people with positive tuberculin tests, without any evidence of active disease, are candidates for *prophylactic* (preventive) *therapy*. This therapy employs *isoniazid* (*INH*), the most effective of many drugs for the treatment of tuberculosis and one that has virtually no side effects. Treatment for one year has been shown to reduce greatly the chance of future progress from the merely infected state to the state of active disease.

The goal of prophylactic therapy is chiefly to prevent the far more serious development of active disease. But, in addition, by preventing disease before it develops physicians can prevent the infection of others, since the typical patient with tuberculosis has already infected some of those living with him before he becomes ill and seeks medical attention. The surface has just been scratched in this regard, however, as there are estimated to be 25 million people in the United States who would demonstrate reactions to tuberculin tests. Many of these people have never been tested and are not aware of the potential threat within them.

In most foreign countries the tuberculosis problem is much more serious. An estimated 80 percent of the populations of the countries of Asia, Africa, and South America would show positive tuberculin skin tests, with the number of active cases and deaths being proportionately high.

Respiratory Diseases Caused by Fungi

Two fungal diseases affecting respiration are of great importance in particular regions of the United States. They are both caused by types of fungi capable of growing within mammalian tissue, thereby infecting and destroying it. Both cause chronic diseases very similar to tuberculosis and may lead to death, though that is a far less common outcome—even when untreated—than in tuberculosis.

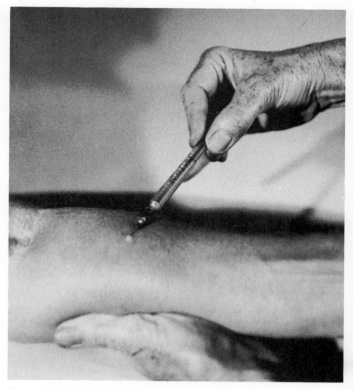

The tuberculin test is given to determine if antibodies are being produced against the tubercle bacilli, which may be present without active disease.

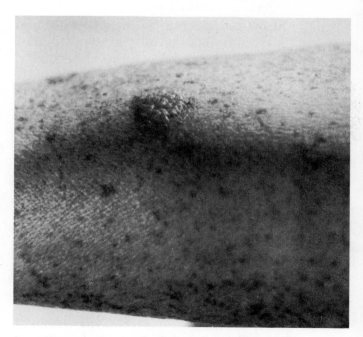

A positive reaction to the tuberculin test demands further screening for the presence of active disease. If none is found, preventive therapy is indicated.

The spores of the fungi are inhaled from the air, and the response of the body is similar to that in tuberculosis in that most people become merely infected (the spores being contained by body defenses) while a few develop progressive disease. The body also produces antibodies, and consequently skin tests similar to the tuberculin test can identify infected individuals.

Histoplasmosis (named for a fungus called *histoplasma*) organisms are prevalent in the Midwest, generally in the areas of the Ohio, Mississippi, and Missouri Rivers. Largely unknown prior to World War II, histoplasmosis has been studied extensively since. Local epidemics have brought it to public attention on several occasions. The fungus grows readily in soil containing large amounts of bird (chickens, pigeons, starlings) or bat excrement. One of the better ways to assure exposure is to clean out an old chicken coop. The concentration of organisms may reach such high levels in bat caves that entry by spelunkers may prove fatal. In contrast to tuberculosis, the amount of exposure seems to play a very important role in determining the extent of disease. There also seem to be few cases of late breakdown (the rule in tuberculosis). Most people develop the active disease, if at all, at the time of their initial exposure.

Coccidioidomycosis (for *coccidioides* fungus) also generates in the soil, in this case in California, the southwest United States, and Mexico. It grows best in hot, dry soil. The common names for this disease are *desert rheumatism* or *valley fever*. Infection and disease occur in a similar pattern to that of histoplasmosis. Skin testing of large population groups for both these fungi in the appropriate geographical areas indicates that the majority of exposed individuals quite adequately contain the initial infection and never develop any illness or active disease.

Because Americans travel into infected regions, these diseases are being seen more frequently in people who do not live where the fungi are found. Both conditions, fortunately, are often self-limited, even when active disease develops. For more severe cases there is a drug, *Amphotericin-B*, which is quite effective; however, since it is also quite toxic to the patient, it must be given in progressive doses starting with a small initial dose, to permit the body's tolerance to build up. It is hoped that less toxic agents will be found in the future that will be just as effective against the fungus.

Allergic Respiratory Diseases

Hay fever (*allergic rhinitis*) and *asthma* are two very common allergic diseases of the respiratory tract. The two have much in common as to age at onset, seasonal manifestations, and causation. Hay fever involves the *mucosa,* or lining, of the upper respiratory tract only, whereas asthma is confined to the bronchial tubes of the lower respiratory tract. Physicians usually distinguish two main types of asthma, allergic and infectious. The infectious type of asthma resembles bronchitis, with cough and much wheezing as well. The discussion here will be confined to the allergic form of asthma.

In hay fever and asthma the allergenic substance causing the reaction is usually airborne, though it can be a food. In most cases the offender is pollen from a plant. The pollen is inhaled into the nostrils and alights upon the lining of the respiratory passages. In the allergic individual, antibodies react with the proteins in the pollen and cause various substances to be released from the tissue and blood cells in the immediate area. These substances, in turn, produce vessel engorgement in the area and an outpouring of mucus, plus certain irritating symptoms that result in a stuffy or runny nose and itchy eyes. The same reactions occur in the bronchial lining in asthma, but the substances released there also cause constriction of the bronchial

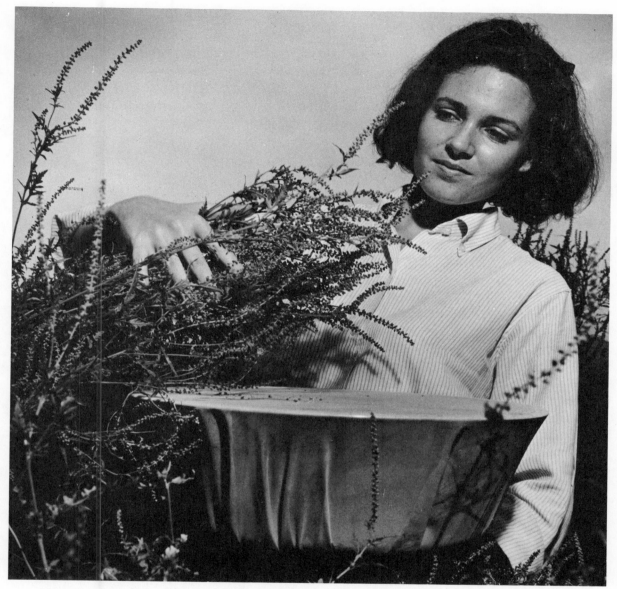

Ragweed pollen, the most common airborne allergen, is collected so that extracts may be used in desensitizing injections that help the body develop immunity against future allergy attacks.

muscle and consequent narrowing of the passages. This muscular effect and the narrowing caused by greatly increased amounts of mucus in the passages are both responsible for the wheezing in asthma.

Hay Fever

Hay fever is never a threat to life, but in severe cases it can upset one's life patterns immensely. For unknown reasons it is more common in childhood, where it is often seen in conjunction with eczema or asthma. The tendency to develop hay fever, eczema, and asthma is hereditary. The transmission of the hereditary factors is complex, so that within a family group any number of individuals or none at all may exhibit the trait.

Most people with hay fever have their only or greatest difficulty in the summer months because of the airborne pollens from

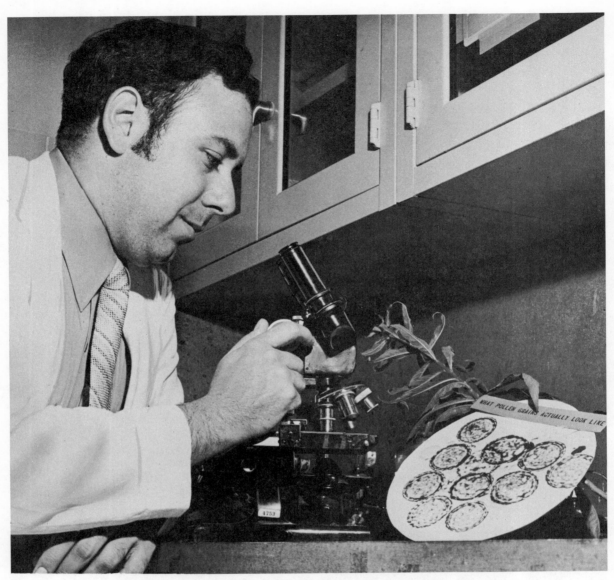

Ragweed pollen is monitored and reported on daily during the hay-fever season from this control center for the New York City metropolitan area.

trees, grasses, flowers, and molds that are prevalent then. The most notorious of all pollens is the ragweed pollen. This weed pollinates around August 15 and continues to fill the air until late September. In many cities an official pollen count is issued every day, and those with severe difficulty can avoid some trouble by staying outside as little as possible on high-count days. *Antihistamine* drugs are used to counteract the nasal engorgement in hay fever. These drugs counteract the effects of *histamine*, which is one of the major substances released by the allergic reaction.

Allergic Asthma

Allergic asthma is the result of the allergic reaction taking place in the bronchial mucosal lining rather than in the nasal lining. A person may suffer from both asthma and hay fever. The common inciting factors are pollens, hair from pets (especially cats), house dust, molds, and certain foods (especially shellfish). When foods are responsible, the reaction initially occurs within the bloodstream, but the major effect is felt within the lung, which is spoken of as the target organ.

Most allergic asthma is seen in children. For unclear reasons it usually disappears spontaneously at puberty. In those who continue to have difficulty after puberty, the role of infection as a cause for the asthma usually becomes more prominent. Allergic

asthma attacks start abruptly and can usually be aborted rather easily with medication.

People with asthma are symptom-free much of the time. When exposed to high concentrations of pollen they begin wheezing and producing sputum. Wheezing refers to the high-pitched squeaking sound that is made by people exhaling through narrowed bronchi. Associated with the wheezing and sputum is a distinct sensation of shortness of breath that varies in severity

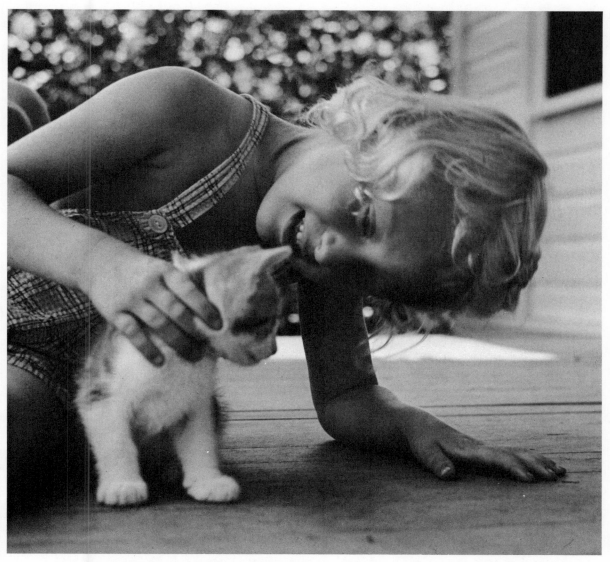

Allergic asthma is often caused by a reaction to pets, especially cats, or to pollens, dust, molds, or certain foods. Swollen mucous membranes of the bronchi interfere with normal breathing.

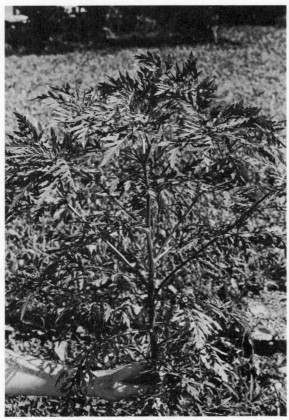

Hay fever affects the lining of the upper respiratory tract—the nasal passages and throat. Pictured here is the ragweed plant, whose pollen is one of the chief causes of hay fever and allergic asthma.

according to the nature of the attack. Milder attacks of asthma often subside spontaneously, merely with relaxation. This is especially true when the wheezing is induced by nonspecific factors, such as a cloud of dust, cold air, or exercise. Asthmatic individuals have more sensitive air passages and they are more easily bothered by these nonspecific irritants.

Treatment: For more severe attacks of asthma there are several types of treatment. There are oral medications that dilate the bronchi and offset the effects of the allergic reaction. Antihistamines, however, exert no effect on asthma and may even worsen the condition. Also available are injectable medications, such as adrenaline, and sprays, that contain substances similar to adrena-

line and that can be inhaled. Any or all of these methods may be employed by the physician. During times of high exposure it is often helpful to take one of the oral medications on a regular basis, thereby avoiding minor episodes of wheezing.

The best therapy for asthma and hay fever is avoidance of the allergen responsible for attacks. Obviously, cats and certain foods can be avoided more readily than pollens and other airborne substances. The first requisite, however, is to identify the offender. The most important method of identification is the patient's medical history. Sometimes the problem is easy, as when the patient states that he only has trouble during the ragweed season. At other times a great amount of detective work may be required. Skin testing is used to complement the history. The skin test merely involves the introduction under the skin (usually within a tiny scratch) of various materials suspected of being allergens. If the individual has antibodies to these substances he will form a hive at the site of introduction. That he reacts does not necessarily mean that his asthma is due to that test substance, because many people have reactions but no hay fever or asthma. The skin test results need to be interpreted in the light of the history of exposure.

If the substance so identified cannot be avoided, then hyposensitization may prove useful. This form of treatment is based on the useful fact that the human body varies its ability to react depending upon the degree and the frequency of exposure. In a hyposensitizing program, small amounts of pollen or other extract are injected frequently. Gradually the dose of extract is increased. By this technique many allergic individuals become able to tolerate moderate exposure to their offending material with little or no symptoms. Hyposensitization does not succeed in everyone, but it is usually worth attempting if other approaches are unsuccessful.   PBB

LUNG DISEASE

Two present-day problems of major proportions are not diseases in themselves, but both are detrimental to health. These are smoking and air pollution. The former is a habit that, in some users, can produce as serious results as narcotics or alcohol addiction. Knowledge of air pollution has grown with the increased public awareness of our environment. It is quite clear that there are many serious consequences produced by the products with which we foul our air. Both tobacco and air pollution are controllable: one by individual will, the other by public effort.

Smoking

Eighty-five million Americans smoke, and the vast majority of these people smoke cigarettes. This discussion will therefore center on cigarettes. The number of new smokers is increasing, which offsets the number of quitters, thereby producing a new gain in smokers each year. There was a temporary absolute decline in 1964 when the first U.S. Surgeon General's report on smoking outlined the many hazards, but that trend quickly reversed itself. The tobacco industry spends $280 million per year to promote smoking. The U.S. Public Health Service and several volunteer agencies spend $8 million in a contrary campaign to discourage smoking.

Dangers of Smoking

There is still great discussion about how cigarettes adversely affect human beings. There is no question that smokers are prone to many diseases only rarely seen in nonsmokers. It is very likely that no specific factor in cigarette smoke causes disease all by itself, but that multiple factors pro-

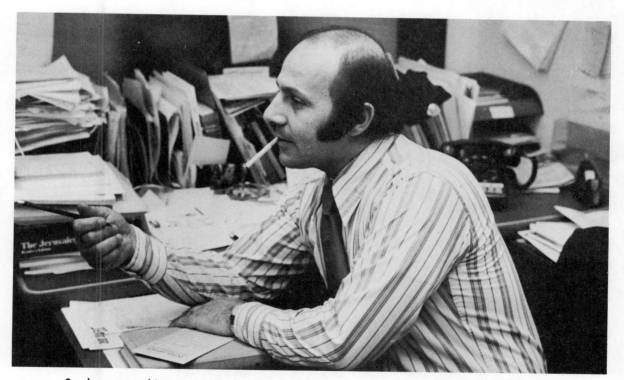

Smokers are subject to many diseases only rarely seen in nonsmokers. Studies both here and abroad have shown a clear relationship between cigarette smoking and lung disease.

duce the conditions under which disease can begin. Smoking has been strongly implicated in bronchitis and emphysema, lung cancer, oral and laryngeal cancer, heart disease, and peripheral vascular disease. All of these conditions are seen in nonsmokers, but large population studies demonstrate a much higher incidence in smokers.

In addition to the circumstantial evidence correlating a greater incidence of many diseases with smoking, there has been varied research on the biological effects of tobacco smoke on animals and humans. Some of these direct effects of tobacco smoke suggest its capacity for producing disease in the smoker. Smoking lowers skin temperature, often by several degrees, principally through the constricting effect of nicotine on blood vessels. Carbon monoxide levels rise in the blood when a person is smoking. The ability to expel air rapidly from the lungs is somewhat impaired even by a single cigarette. Adverse changes in the activity of several important chemicals in the body can be demonstrated after smoking. All of these effects of smoking, and the many others known, are difficult to interpret as conclusive evidence that disease results as a direct consequence. But the changes are certainly disturbing.

The principle arguments of the tobacco manufacturers and cigarette supporters have been that the population studies produce only circumstantial evidence and that the demonstrable biological effects do not necessarily produce disease. They also point out that no single ingredient in tobacco smoke can be shown to produce cancer, despite many attempts. But the thousands of physicians who have quit smoking in the

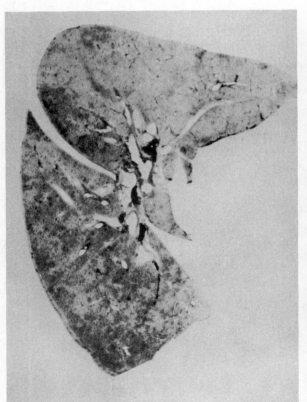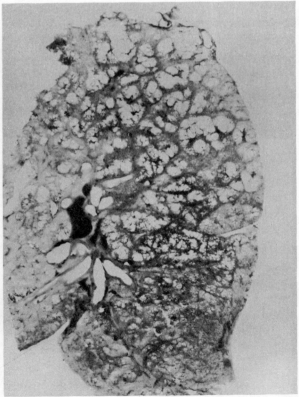

One of the effects of cigarette smoking is illustrated by these photographs. (*Left*) Normal lung tissue, with air sacs too fine to be visible. (*Right*) Lung tissue of a heavy smoker, showing numerous enlarged air sacs.

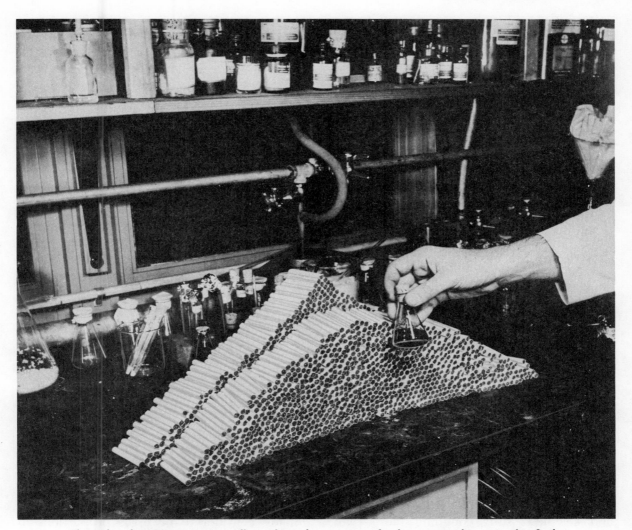

This pile of 2000 cigarettes will produce the amount of tobacco tar shown in the flask.

last few years do not need absolute cause-and-effect proof. Nor are they blind to the fact that tobacco smoke may create conditions under which these diseases are more readily apt to develop.

The number of cigarettes an individual smokes is one of the determinants of eventual damage, although individual susceptibility is also important. If a person smokes one pack a day for one year he has smoked one pack-year; if he smokes one pack a day for two years or two packs a day for one year, he has smoked two pack-years, and so on. Calculating by pack-years, it appears that 40 pack-years is a crucial time period

above which the incidence of cancer of the lung, emphysema, and other serious consequences rises rapidly. Smoking three packs a day, it takes only about 13 years to reach this critical level.

Breaking The Smoking Habit

Obviously, the best way not to smoke is never to start. Unfortunately, young people are continuing to join the smoking ranks at a rapid rate. The teen-ager often is one of the hardest persons to convince of the hazards of smoking. He is healthy, suffers less from the fatigue, headaches, breathlessness, and other immediate effects of smoking, and he often feels the need to smoke to keep up with his peers. Once he starts, it is not long before he becomes addicted. The addiction to cigarettes is very real. It is more psychological dependency than the physical addiction associated with narcotics, but there are definite physical addiction aspects to smoking that are mostly noted when one stops.

For most people it is quite a challenge to stop smoking. There are many avenues to travel and many sources now available to aid one on the way. They include smoking clinics that offer group support and medical guidance to those anxious to quit. The clinics vary in their format but basically depend on the support given the smoker by finding other individuals with the same problems and overcoming the problems as a group. The medical guidance helps people recognize and deal with withdrawal symptoms as well as helping them with weight control.

Withdrawal Symptoms

Withdrawal symptoms vary from person to person and include many symptoms other than just a craving for a cigarette. Many people who stop smoking become jittery and sleepless, start coughing more than usual, and often develop an increased appetite. This last withdrawal effect is especially disturbing to women, and the need to prevent weight gain is all too often used as a simple excuse to avoid stopping the cigarette habit or to start smoking again. The weight gained is usually not too great, and one generally stops gaining after a few weeks. Once the cigarette smoking problem is controlled, then efforts can be turned to weight reduction. Being overweight is also a threat to health, but ten extra pounds, even if maintained, do not represent nearly the threat that confirmed smoking does.

Despite all efforts, many individuals who would like to stop smoking fail in their attempts. The best advice for them is to keep trying. Continued effort will at least tend to decrease the amount of smoking and often leads to eventual abstinence, even after years of trying. If a three-pack-per-day smoker can decrease to one pack a day or less, he has helped himself even though he is still doing some damage. For prospective quitters it is important to remember that cigarette smoking is an acquired habit, and that the learning process can be reversed. The problem most people have is too little knowledge of the dangers and too much willingness to believe that disease and disability cannot strike them, just the other fellow.

Air Pollution

While 85 million Americans pollute the air they breathe individually with cigarettes, all 200 million of us collectively pollute the atmosphere we all breathe. Some people are obviously more responsible than others, but air, water, and land pollution is a disease of society and can only be solved through a concerted effort by the whole society. Pollution has always been a problem to man. As we have become more urbanized the problem has grown. It has now reached what many consider to be crisis proportions in our large cities and even in some of our smaller ones.

We have had ample warning. In 1948 a killer smog engulfed Donora, Pennsylvania, killing 20 persons and producing serious illness in 6,000 more. In 1952 a lingering smog over London was blamed for 4,000 deaths in a few weeks. New York City has had several serious encounters with critical smog conditions that have accounted for many illnesses and deaths. The exteriors of many buildings in our cities are showing signs of vastly increased rates of decay due to the noxious substances in the air. It is estimated that air pollution costs the United States $11 billion a year in damage, illness, and in other ways. Even if all this loss of

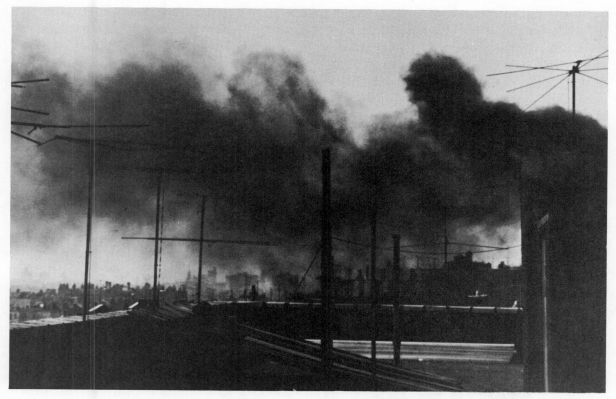

As society has become more urbanized and technology has increased, pollution problems have grown accordingly. This smoking apartment-house chimney is a symptom of the problem.

life and property were not a result it would clearly be more pleasant to live in a clean atmosphere than in a foul one.

Air pollution in any one area varies greatly from day to day and even from hour to hour. The amount of air pollution depends mainly on the production of smoke and gases and the prevailing weather conditions. Pollutants include *particulate matter* in smoke that is first dispersed by the wind and then removed from the atmosphere by falling back to earth. Other major pollutants are organic gases and vapors, most of which are very toxic to humans in substantial concentrations. These include sulfur dioxide, nitrogen dioxide, carbon monoxide, ozone, and many others. These substances depend upon dilution in clean air to keep them from reaching toxic concentrations. That dilution depends principally upon the wind. When the air is stagnant these prod-

ucts do not disperse adequately in the atmosphere, and at these times many people suffer from burning eyes, increased cough, breathlessness, sore throat, and similar symptoms. To correct conditions at that point the only solution is to reduce emission of pollutants. Many large cities have developed staged plans for reducing emissions in a crisis.

Pollution and Disease

The diseases caused by air pollution are subtle and elusive. When pollution levels are significantly increased most people with moderate to severe chronic lung disease notice more symptoms, and some become quite ill. People with mild lung disease but severe heart disease may find their heart problem to be much more bothersome. Studies show that many more persons die or are hospitalized for lung and related disorders during periods of high pollution than at other times. Evidence suggests that more lung cancer develops in and around large cities, but it is difficult to prove that this is solely due to air pollution. There even appear to be more common colds in high-pollution areas than in low ones.

For those people with lung disease who live in high-pollution areas there are several ways to reduce the irritation on particularly bad days. Staying indoors and exerting oneself as little as possible are two basic precepts. If one has an air conditioner or air filter system, he does even better by staying inside. These measures are aimed at reducing pollutant exposure and reducing the oxygen requirements of the body.

In the past decade efforts at controlling air pollution have increased greatly. But

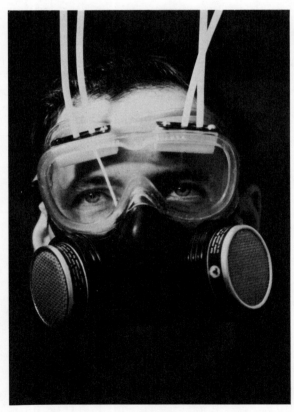

A volunteer undergoes tests to determine the effects of auto exhaust, irradiated by sunlight, on the human eye. Pollution-free air is released through one set of tubes, irradiated exhaust through the other.

the increased control is not yet keeping pace with the new production each year, which amounts to an added 12 million tons of pollutants. See also *Air Pollution*, p. 357, under *The Environment and Health*.

Emphysema and Bronchitis

Emphysema and chronic bronchitis are diseases that involve the whole lung. They can be of varying severity, and both are characterized by the gradual progression of breathlessness.

Because chronic bronchitis is almost invariably associated with pulmonary emphysema, the combined disorder frequently is called *obstructive-airway disease*. The disease involves damage to the lung tissue, with a loss of normal elasticity of the air sacs (*emphysema*), as well as damage to the *bronchi*, the main air passages to the lungs. In addition, chronic bronchitis is marked by a thickening of the walls of the bronchi with increased mucus production and difficulty in expelling these secretions. This results in coughing and sputum production.

The condition known as *acute bronchitis* is an acute process generally caused by a sudden infection, such as a cold, with an exaggeration of bronchitis symptoms. If a spasm of the bronchi occurs, accompanied by wheezing, the ailment is called infectious or nonallergic asthma.

Obstructive-airway disease is very insidious, and characteristically people do not, or will not, notice that they are sick until they suddenly are very sick. This is partly due to chronic denial of the morning cough and breathlessness, but also to the fact that we are fashioned in such a way as to have great reserve strength in our organs. As the disease progresses one starts using up his reserve for exertion. Since most people's life styles allow them to avoid exertion easily, the victim of this disease may have only rare chances to notice his

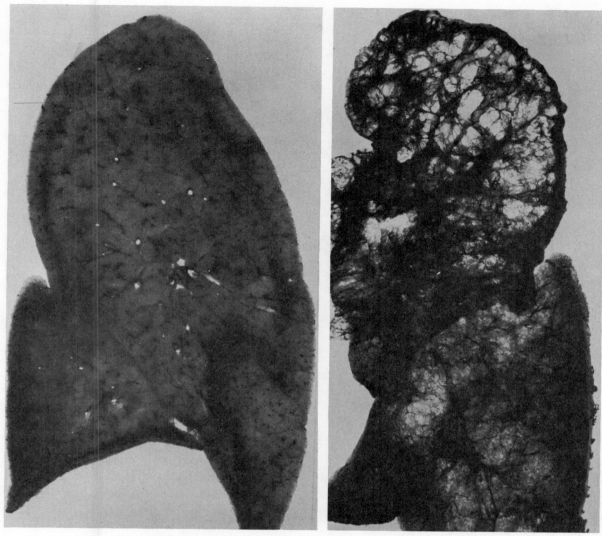

Inflated lung slices of (*left*) person with normal lungs and (*right*) person suffering from emphysema, a disease characterized by a loss of normal elasticity of the air sacs.

breathlessness. Then, suddenly, within a period of a few months he becomes breathless with ordinary activity because he has used up and surpassed all his reserve. He goes to a doctor thinking he has just become sick. Usually this event occurs when the patient is in his fifties or sixties and little can be done to correct the damage. The time for prevention was in the previous 30 years when elimination of smoking could have prevented much or all of the illness.

Chronic cough and breathlessness are the two earliest signs of chronic bronchitis and emphysema. A smoker's cough is not an insignificant symptom. It indicates that very definite irritation of the bronchi has developed and it should be respected early. Along with the cough there is often production of phlegm or sputum, especially in the morning, due to less effective emptying of the bronchial tree during the relatively motionless period of sleep. Another early manifestation of disease is the tendency to develop chest infections along with what would otherwise be simple head colds. With these chest infections there is often

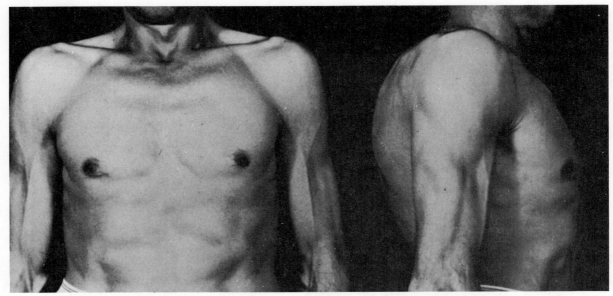

Two views of an emphysematic. Note the barrel chest due to stretched air sacs in the lungs. Such lung-tissue damage is irreversible, but smoking aggravates the problem considerably. Stopping smoking will slow the progression of the disease, and the patient will feel noticeably better.

a tightness or dull pain in the middle chest region, production of sputum, and sometimes wheezing.

Treatment

Once emphysema or bronchitis are diagnosed there are many forms of therapy that can help. Stopping smoking is the most important measure, and will in itself often produce dramatic effects. The more bronchitis the patient has the more noticeable the effect, as the bronchial irritation and mucous production decrease, cough lessens, and a greater sense of well-being ensues. The emphysema component does not change, as the damage to the air sacs is irreversible, but the progression may be greatly slowed. When chest infections develop they can be treated with antibiotics.

For more severe disease a program of breathing exercises and graded exertion may be beneficial. When these people develop heart trouble as a result of the strain on the heart, treatment to strengthen the heart is rewarding. For those with the most advanced stage of the disease new methods

of treatment have been devised in recent years. One of the most encouraging is the use of controlled oxygen administration, a treatment that can sometimes allow a patient to return to an active working life from an otherwise helpless bed-and-chair existence. But it must be remembered that all these measures produce little effect if the patient continues to smoke.

The problems encountered by patients with obstructive disease do not encompass merely that disease alone. Because of their smoking history these patients are also prone to develop lung cancer. All too often a person with a potentially curable form of lung cancer is unable to undergo surgery because his lungs will not tolerate the added strain of surgery. Patients with obstructive disease are also more prone to pneumonia and other infectious pulmonary conditions. When these develop in the already compromised lung, it may be impossible for the patient to maintain adequate oxygen supply to his vital tissues. If severe and prolonged enough, the patient dies from pulmonary failure.

Despite the emphasis placed on smoking as the predominant factor for the development of obstructive disease, there are people with the disease who have never smoked. For many of these individuals there is no known cause for their disease. However, a group of younger people with obstructive disease have been found to be deficient in a particular enzyme. (*Enzymes* are agents that are necessary for certain chemical reactions.) Individuals with this deficiency develop a particularly severe form of emphysema, become symptomatic in their third or fourth decade, and die at a young age. They may not smoke, but if they do, the disease is much more severe. Just how the enzyme deficiency leads to emphysema is not clear, but a great amount of research is being conducted on this new link to try to learn more about the causes of emphysema.

The Pneumoconioses

Pneumoconiosis is a chronic reaction of the lung to any of several types of inhaled dust particles. The reaction varies somewhat but generally consists of initial inflammation about the inhaled particle followed by the development of scar tissue. The pneumoconioses develop predominantly from various occupational exposures to high concentrations of certain inorganic compounds that cannot be broken down by the cells of the body. The severity of the disease is proportional to the amount of dust retained in the lung.

Silica is the most notorious of these substances. People who work in mining, steel production, and any occupation involved with chipping stone, such as manufacturing monuments, are exposed to silica dust. Many of the practices associated with these occupations have been altered over the years because of the recognition of the hazard to workers. Other important pneumoconioses involve talc and asbestos particles, cotton fibers, and coal dust. Coal dust has gained wide attention in recent years with the heightened awareness of *black lung,* a condition seen in varying degrees in coal miners. The attention has resulted in a federal black lung disease law under which more than 135,000 miners have filed for compensation.

Although there are individual differences in reaction to the varied forms of pneumoconiosis, the ultimate hazard is the loss of functioning lung tissue. When enough tissue becomes scarred, there is interference with oxygenation. Those people with pneumoconiosis who smoke are in great danger of compounding their problem by adding obstructive disease as well.

Prevention

Once the scarring has taken place there is no way to reverse the process. Therefore, the answer to the pneumoconioses is to

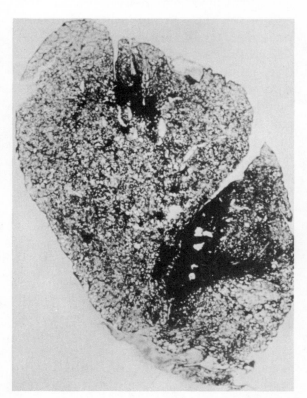

Lung tissue of a coal miner afflicted with pneumoconiosis (black lung), caused by inhaling coal dust.

prevent the exposure. Attention to occupational diseases in the United States has lagged about 30 years behind Europe, so that we are just now beginning to show concern about certain industrial practices condemned as hazardous in many European countries in the 1940s. New lung diseases caused by inhaled substances are discovered every year, and more will undoubtedly be found in the future. People in industries in which there is exposure to industrial dust should be aware of the potential danger and should be prepared to promote the maintenance of protective practices and the investigation of new ideas and devices. In those jobs where masks have already been supplied, the workers should wear them, a practice too often neglected.

Pulmonary Embolism

Pulmonary embolism is a condition in which a part of a blood clot in a vein breaks away and travels through the heart and into the pulmonary circulatory system. Here the vessels leading from the heart branch like a tree, gradually becoming smaller until finally they form *capillaries*, the smallest blood vessels. Depending on its size, the clot will at some point reach a vessel through which it cannot pass, and there will lodge itself. The clot disrupts the blood supply to the area supplied by that vessel. The larger the clot, the greater is the area of lung that loses its blood supply, and the more drastic the results to the patient.

This condition develops most commonly in association with inflammation of the veins of the legs (*thrombophlebitis*). People with varicose veins are particularly susceptible to thrombophlebitis. Because of constrictions produced by garters or rolled stockings, or just sitting with crossed legs for a long time, the sluggish blood flow already present is aggravated, and a clot may form in a vessel. Some people without varicose veins can also develop clots under the same conditions. The body often responds to the clot with the reaction of inflammation, which is painful. However, when there is no inflammatory response, there is no warning to tell that a clot has formed. In either situation there is always a chance that a piece may break off the main clot and travel to the lung. Of recent concern in this regard are studies that appear to link oral contraceptives with the incidence of clotting, thereby leading to pulmonary embolism. The number of women affected in this way by the Pill is small, but enough to be of concern.

The symptoms of pulmonary embolism are varied and may be minor or major. Most common are pleurisy—marked by chest pain during breathing—shortness of breath, and cough with the production of blood. Once the pulmonary embolism is diagnosed the treatment is simple in the less severe cases, which are the majority. But in cases of large clots and great areas of lung deprived of blood supply there may be catastrophic effects on the heart and general circulation.

Prevention

Certain preventive measures are worthwhile for all people. Stockings should not be rolled, because that produces a constricting band about the leg that impairs blood flow and predisposes to clot formation. Especially when taking long automobile or airplane rides one should be sure to stretch the legs periodically. Individuals with varicose veins or a history of thrombophlebitis should take these precautions more seriously. People who stand still for long periods during the day should wear elastic support stockings regularly and elevate their feet part of the day and at night.

When considering the use of oral contraceptives the physician must weigh the risks of developing clots from the drug against the psychological, social, and physical risks of pregnancy. The risk from oral

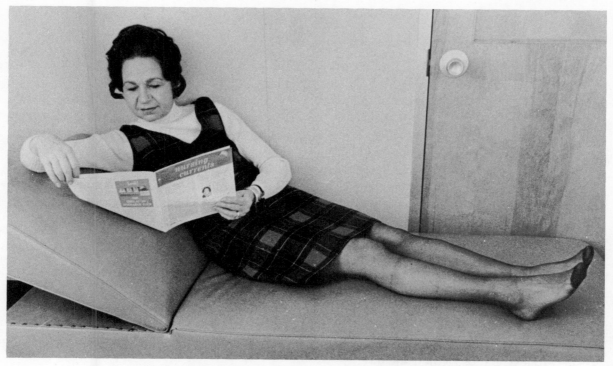

Those troubled by varicose veins or other circulatory problems should avoid standing still for long periods of time and should elevate their feet whenever possible.

contraceptives is lessened if the woman does not have high blood pressure. Any persistent pain in the leg, especially in the calf or behind the knee, deserves the attention of a physician. Anyone with varicose veins or anyone taking oral contraceptives should be especially attentive to these symptoms.

Pneumothorax

Another less common lung condition is spontaneous *pneumothorax* or collapse of a lung. This most commonly occurs in the second and third decade of life and presents itself with the sudden development of pain in the chest and breathlessness. The collapse occurs because of a sudden leak of air from the lung into the chest cavity.

The lung is ordinarily maintained in an expanded state by the rigid bony thorax, but if air leaks out into the space between the thorax and the lung, the lung collapses.

This condition is rarely very serious but the patient needs to be observed to be sure that the air leak does not become greater with further lung collapse.

Treatment

Often a tube has to be placed in the chest, attached to a suction pump, and the air pumped out from the space where it has collected. When the air is removed the lung expands to fill the thoracic cage again. Some individuals tend to have several recurrences. Since the reason for the collapse is poorly understood, there is no satisfactory method of preventing these recurrences except by surgery. This is rarely required. In a person with a proven propensity for recurrence it is usually advisable to open the chest and produce scarring of the lung surface so that it becomes fixed to the thoracic cage. Although it is usually successful, even this procedure does not always solve this bothersome problem.   PBB

DISEASES OF
THE ENDOCRINE GLANDS

Glands are organs that produce and secrete substances essential for normal body functioning. There are two main types of glands: the *endocrine* and the *exocrine*. The endocrines or *ductless* glands send their secretions directly into the bloodstream. These secretions, which are biochemically related to each other, are called *hormones*. The exocrines, such as the sebaceous or sweat glands, the mammary or milk glands, and the lachrymal or tear glands, have ducts that carry their secretions to specific locations for specific purposes.

The exocrine glands are individually discussed elsewhere in connection with the various parts of the body where they are found. This section is devoted to diseases of the ductless glands, which include:

• The *pituitary*, which controls growth and the activity of the adrenal, thyroid and sex glands

• The *thyroid*, which controls the rate of the body's chemical activity or metabolism

• The *adrenals*, which affect metabolism and sex characteristics

• The *male gonads* or testicles; the *female gonads* or ovaries

• The *parathyroids*, which regulate bone metabolism.

Unlike the exocrine glands, which can function independently of each other, the endocrines form an interrelated system. Thus a disorder in one of them is likely to affect the way the others behave. Glandular disorder can sometimes be anatomical, but it is usually functional. Functional disease can result in the production and release of too little or too much of a particular secretion.

When too much of a hormone is being secreted, the prefix *hyper-* is used for the condition, as in *hyperthyroidism*. When too little is being secreted, the prefix *hypo-* is used, as in the word *hypofunction*, to indicate that a gland operates below normal.

Abnormalities of the endocrine glands that cause changes in their functioning are responsible for a wide variety of illnesses. These illnesses are almost always accompanied by symptoms that can be recognized as distinctly abnormal. Prompt and accurate diagnosis can usually prevent the occurrence of irreversible damage. For many people with glandular disorders, treatment may have to be lifelong. They can feel well and function almost normally, but they must follow a program of regulated medication taken under a doctor's supervision.

Anterior Pituitary Gland

The anterior pituitary gland, also called the *hypophysis,* is located in the center of the brain. It produces two types of secretions: a growth hormone and hormones that stimulate certain other glands.

The anterior pituitary gland is subject to neurochemical stimulation by the *hypothalamus,* a nearby part of the brain. This stimulation results in the production of the hormones that promote testicular and ovarian functioning, and does not occur normally until around 12 years of age in girls and 14 in boys. The beginning of this glandular activity is known as the onset of *puberty.*

Puberty is sometimes delayed for no apparent reason until age 16 or 17. Since the hypothalamus is affected by emotional factors, all of the endocrine glands governed by the anterior pituitary can also be affected by feelings. Psychological factors can therefore upset the relationships in the glandular system and produce the physical symptoms of endocrine disorders.

It is extremely rare for the anterior pituitary to produce too much or too little of

THE ENDOCRINE GLANDS

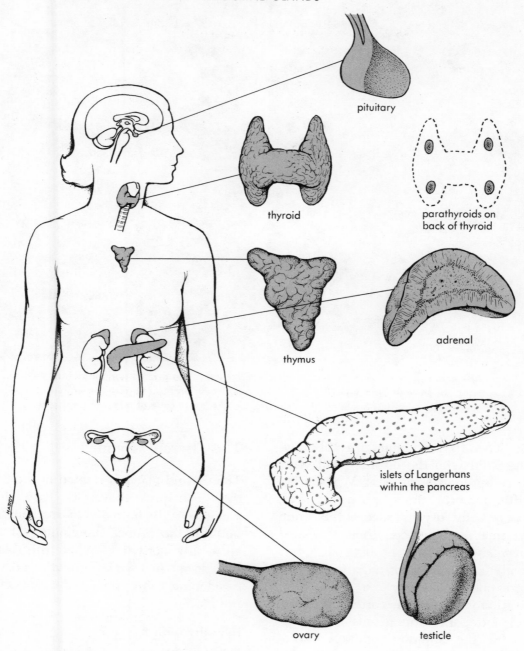

pituitary

thyroid

parathyroids on
back of thyroid

thymus

adrenal

islets of Langerhans
within the pancreas

ovary

testicle

its hormones, but sometimes hypofunction may follow pregnancy because of thrombosis or changes in the blood vessels.

A truly hypofunctioning anterior pituitary gland can cause many serious disturbances: extreme thinness, growth failure, sexual aberration, and intolerance for normal variations in temperature. When ap-

propriate diagnostic tests determine the deficiency, the patient is given the missing hormones in pill form.

Absence of the growth hormone alone is unknown. Most cases of *dwarfism* result from other causes. However, excess production of the growth hormone alone does occur, but only rarely. If it begins before

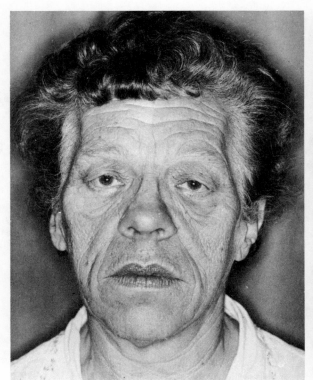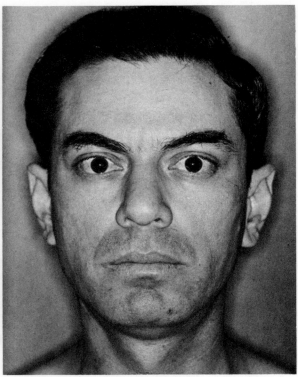

(*Left*) Acromegaly, a result of the excessive production of the growth hormone after puberty, causes enlarged head, hands, feet, and body organs. (*Right*) Hyperthyroidism produces a staring quality in the eyes and weight loss in spite of increased appetite.

puberty when the long bones are still growing, the child with the disorder will grow into a well-proportioned giant. When it begins after puberty, the head, hands, feet, and most body organs except the brain slowly enlarge. This condition is called *acromegaly*. The cause of both disorders is usually a tumor, and radiation is the usual treatment.

The thyroid, adrenal cortex, testicles, ovaries, and pancreatic glands are target glands for the anterior pituitary's stimulating hormones, which are specific for the functioning of each of these glands. Therefore, a disorder of any of the target organs could be caused either by an excess or a deficiency of a stimulating hormone, creating a so-called *secondary disease*. There are various tests that can be given to differentiate primary from secondary disorders.

The Thyroid Gland

The thyroid gland is located in the front of the neck just above its base. Normal amounts of the hormone *thyroxin* are necessary for the proper functioning of almost all bodily activities. When this hormone is deficient in infancy, growth and mental development are impaired and *cretinism* results.

Hypothyroidism

In adulthood, a deficiency of thyroxin hormone results either from too little iodine in the diet, from the thyroid's having been surgically removed, or from other reasons. In *hypothyroidism,* the metabolic rate is slower than normal, the patient has no energy, his expression is dull, his skin is thick, and he has an intolerance to cold weather.

Treatment consists of increasing the amount of iodine in the diet if it is deficient, or giving thyroid hormone medication. Normal metabolic functioning usually follows, especially if treatment is begun soon after the symptoms appear.

Hyperthyroidism

An excess amount of thyroid hormone secretion is called *hyperthyroidism* and may relate to emotional stress. It causes physical fatigue but mental alertness, a staring quality in the eyes, tremor of the hands, weight loss with increased appetite, rapid pulse, sweating, and intolerance to hot weather.

Long-term treatment is aimed at decreasing hormone production with the use of a special medicine that inhibits it. In some cases, part of the gland may be removed by surgery; in others, radiation treatment with radioactive iodine is effective.

Hyperthyroidism may recur long after successful treatment. Both hypothyroidism and hyperthyroidism are common disorders, especially in women.

Other Thyroid Disorders

Enlargement of part or all of the thyroid gland occurs fairly often. It may be a simple enlargement of the gland itself due to lack of iodine, as in *goiter,* or it may be caused by a tumor or a nonspecific inflammation. Goiter is often treated with thyroxin, but it is easily prevented altogether by the regular use of iodized table and cooking salt. Treatment of other problems varies, but surgery is usually recommended for a tumor, especially if the surrounding organs are being obstructed.

The Adrenal Glands

The adrenals are paired glands located just above each kidney. Their outer part is called the *cortex.* The inner part is called the *medulla* and is not governed by the anterior pituitary. The cortex produces sev-

eral hormones that affect the metabolism of salt, water, carbohydrate, fat, and protein, as well as secondary sex characteristics, skin pigmentation, and resistance to infection.

An insufficiency of these hormones can be caused by bacterial infection of the cortex, especially by *meningococcus;* by a hemorrhage into it; by an obstruction of blood flow into it; by its destruction because of tuberculosis; or by one of several unusual diseases.

In one type of sudden or acute underfunctioning of the cortex, the patient has a high fever, mental confusion, and circulatory collapse. Unless treated promptly, the disorder is likely to be fatal. When it persists after treatment, or when it develops gradually, it is called *Addison's disease* and is usually chronic. The patient suffers from weakness, loss of body hair, and increased skin pigmentation. Hormone-replacement treatment is essential, along with added salt for as long as hypofunction persists.

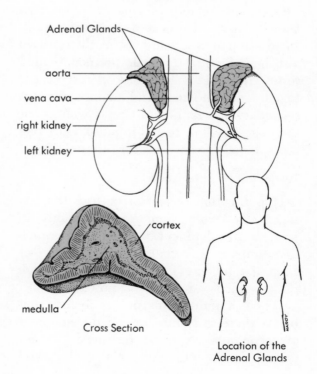

THE ADRENAL GLANDS

Adrenal Glands

aorta

vena cava

right kidney

left kidney

cortex

medulla

Cross Section

Location of the Adrenal Glands

The formation of an excess of certain cortical hormones—a disorder known as *Cushing's syndrome*—may be caused by a tumor of the anterior pituitary gland, which produces too much specific stimulating hormone; or by a tumor of one or both of the adrenal glands. It is a rare disease, more common in women, especially following pregnancy. Symptoms include weakness, loss of muscle tissue, the appearance of purple streaks in the skin, and an oval or "moon" face.

Treatment involves eliminating the overproducing tissue either by surgery or irradiation and then replacing any hormonal deficiencies with proper medication.

An excess of certain other cortical hormones because of an increase in cortical tissue or a tumor can result in the early onset of puberty in boys, or in an increase in the sexuality of females of any age. Surgical removal of the overproducing tissue is the only treatment.

Male Sex Glands

The male sex glands or *gonads* are the two testicles normally located in the *scrotum*. In addition to producing sperm, the testicles also manufacture the male hormone called *testosterone*. This hormone is responsible for the development and maintenance of secondary sex characteristics as well as for the male *libido* or sexual impulse. Only one normal testicle is needed for full function.

Testicular Hypofunction

Hypofunction of one or both of the testicles can result from an abnormality in prenatal development, from infections such as mumps or tuberculosis, from injury, or from the increased temperature to which undescended testicles are exposed.

When hypofunction occurs before puberty, there is failure in the development of secondary sex characteristics. The sex organs do not enlarge; facial, pubic, and

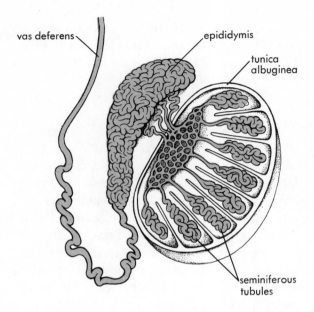

THE TESTICLE

vas deferens
epididymis
tunica albuginea
seminiferous tubules

armpit hair fails to appear; and the normal voice change does not occur. Fertility and libido also fail to develop. A person with this combination of abnormalities is called a *eunuch*.

If the disorder is secondary to anterior pituitary disease, it is called *Froehlich's syndrome*. When it occurs after puberty, the body changes are less striking, but there may be a loss of fertility and libido. The primary disease is usually treated by surgery, and testosterone may be given. If the disorder is secondary to anterior pituitary disease, the gonad-stimulating hormone should be administered.

Testicular hypofunction is rare because it results only when both testicles are damaged in some way. Although mumps may involve the testicles, it is rarely the cause of sterility, even though this is greatly feared. Even so, everyone should be immunized against mumps in infancy.

It is advisable to wear an appropriate athletic supporter to protect the testicles when engaged in strenuous athletics or when there is a possibility that they might be injured. However, nothing that restricts scrotal movement should be worn regularly,

1		Jacob Hudgins
2		Josh Hudgins
3		Brittany Ballard
4		Samantha Burton
5		Thomas, Burton
6		Justin Freeman
7		Sammy Hill
8		James Rivas
9		Kelli Shaver
10		Ellie McCoy
11		Daniel Hadden
12		Trevor Sligh
13		Jacob Williams

since movement is essential for the maintenance of constant testicular temperature.

A sudden decrease in sexual drive or performance may be caused by disease, trauma, or emotional factors. In certain cases administering male hormones may relieve the condition. However, a decrease in sexual drive is one of the natural consequences of aging. It is not a disease and should not be treated with testosterone.

Testicular Hyperfunction

Testicular hyperfunction is extremely rare and is usually caused by a tumor. Before puberty, the condition results in the precocious development of secondary sex characteristics; after puberty, in the accentuation of these characteristics. Such a tumor must be removed surgically or destroyed by irradiation.

Cancer can develop in a testicle without causing any functional change. It is relatively uncommon. When it appears, it shows up first as a painless enlargement. The cancer cells then usually spread quickly to other organs and have a fatal result. Prompt treatment by surgery and irradiation can sometimes arrest the condition.

Since an undescended testicle may become cancerous, it should be repositioned into the scrotum by surgery or removed.

Female Sex Glands

The female gonads are the *ovaries,* situated on each side of and close to the uterus or womb. In addition to producing an *ovum* or egg each month, they manufacture the female hormones *estrogen* and *progesterone,* each making its special contribution to the menstrual cycle and to the many changes that go on during pregnancy. Estrogen regulates the secondary sex characteristics such as breast development and the appearance of pubic and axillary hair.

The periodicity of the menstrual cycle depends on a very complicated relationship

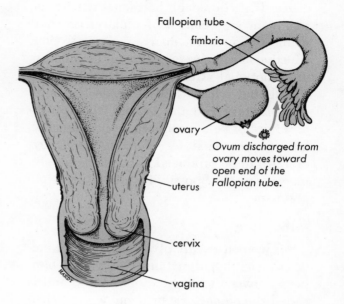

FUNCTION OF THE OVARIES

Fallopian tube

fimbria

ovary

Ovum discharged from ovary moves toward open end of the Fallopian tube.

uterus

cervix

vagina

between the ovaries and the anterior pituitary. Birth control pills, most of which contain estrogen and progesterone, interrupt this relationship in such a way that no ovum is produced and pregnancy therefore should not occur.

Changes in normal ovarian hormone function create problems similar to changes in normal testicular hormone function, except of course for the female-male differences. In general, the diseases responsible for these changes are the same in males and females. However, changes in female hormone function are very often caused by emotional stress or by other unspecific circumstances.

Ovarian Hypofunction

Hypofunction of the ovaries may cause failure to menstruate at all or with reasonable regularity. A disruption of the menstrual cycle is an obvious indication to the woman past puberty that something is wrong. Less obvious is the reduction or complete loss of fertility that may accompany the disorder.

Both menstrual and infertility problems should be evaluated by a trained specialist, preferably a gynecologist, to find out their cause. If it should be hormonal deficiency, treatment may consist of replacement hormone therapy. In many cases, however, effective treatment consists of eliminating the emotional stress that has affected the stimulation relationship between the anterior pituitary and the ovaries, thereby inhibiting hormone production. Occasionally, hormone treatment for infertility causes several ova to be produced in the same month, increasing the possibility of a multiple pregnancy.

Menopause

All women eventually develop spontaneous ovarian hypofunction. This usually happens between the ages of 45 and 50 and is called the *climacteric* or *menopause*. When it happens before the age of 35, it is called premature menopause.

Normal menopause results from the gradual burning out of the ovaries so that estrogen is deficient or absent altogether. Most women experience very few changes or symptoms at this time other than the cessation of menstruation, usually preceded by progressive irregularity and reduction of flow.

A few women become excessively irritable, have hot flashes, perspire a great deal, gain weight, and develop facial hair. Such women, as well as those who have premature menopause, are likely to benefit greatly from estrogen replacement therapy for a few years. The question of whether all menopausal women should be treated with estrogen for the rest of their lives is not yet completely answered. At the present time, most physicians feel that the treatment should be given only when menopause symptoms are causing special discomfort.

Ovarian Hyperfunction

Hyperfunction of the ovaries after puberty is one cause of increased menstrual flow during or at the end of each cycle. This is called functional bleeding and is due to excess estrogen. The disorder is treated with progesterone, which slows down estrogen production. In cases where this treatment fails, it is sometimes necessary to remove the uterus by an operation called a *hysterectomy*.

Some diseases of the ovaries, such as infections, cysts, and tumors, do not necessarily cause functional changes, but they may call attention to themselves by being painful, or a doctor may discover them during a pelvic examination. Treatment may be medical, surgical, or by irradiation, depending on the nature of the disorder.

A rather common cause of short-lived ovarian pain is connected with *ovulation*, which occurs about 14 days before the next expected menstrual period. This discomfort is called *mittelschmerz*, which is German for "middle pain," and can be treated with aspirin or any other simple analgesic.

The Pancreas

The pancreas, a combined duct and endocrine gland, is to some extent regulated by the anterior pituitary. See *Diabetes Mellitus*, p. 573, for a discussion of the pancreas and diabetes.

Posterior Pituitary Gland

The posterior lobe of the pituitary gland, the parathyroid glands, and the adrenal medulla are not governed by the anterior pituitary gland. The posterior pituitary produces a secretion called *antidiuretic hormone* which acts on the kidneys to control the amount of urine produced. A deficiency of this hormone causes *diabetes insipidus*, which results in the production of an excessive amount of urine, sometimes as much as 25 quarts a day. (A normal amount is about 1 quart.) The natural consequence of this disorder is an unquenchable thirst. It is an extremely rare disease, the cause of which is unknown, although it may result from a brain injury or tumor. Treatment involves curing the cause if possible. If not, the patient is given an antidiuretic hormone.

The Parathyroid Glands

The parathyroid glands are located in or near the thyroid, usually two on each side. They are important in the regulation of blood calcium and phosphorus levels and therefore of bone metabolism. Hypofunction of this gland almost never occurs except when it has been removed surgically, usually inadvertently during a thyroid operation. In underfunctioning of the parathyroid, blood calcium levels fall and muscle spasm results. The patient is usually given calcium and replacement therapy with parathyroid hormone to correct the disorder.

Hyperfunction is rare and is slightly more common in women. A benign tumor or *adenoma* is the usual cause. The amount of calcium in the blood rises as calcium is removed from the bones, which then weaken and may break easily. The excess calcium is excreted in the urine and may coalesce into kidney stones, causing severe pain. Treatment for hyperfunction of the parathyroid consists of surgical removal of the affected gland.

The Adrenal Medulla

The medulla of the adrenal glands secretes two hormones: *epinephrine* (or *adrenaline*) and *nor-epinephrine*. Although they contribute to the proper functioning of the heart and blood vessels, neither one is absolutely indispensable. Disease due to hypofunction of the medulla is unknown. Hyperfunction is a rare cause of sustained high blood pressure. Even more rarely, it causes episodic or paroxysmal high blood pressure accompanied by such symptoms as throbbing headache, profuse perspiration, and severe anxiety. The disorder is caused by a tumor effectively treated by surgical removal. Cancer of the adrenal medulla is extremely rare and virtually incurable.

Changes in hormone production can be caused by many intangible factors and are often temporary disorders. However, persistent or recurrent symptoms should be brought to a doctor's attention. The accurate diagnosis of an endocrine disease depends on careful professional evaluation of specific laboratory tests, individual medical history, and thorough examination. No one should take hormones or medicines that affect hormone production without this type of evaluation, since their misuse can cause major problems.   DST

DIABETES MELLITUS

A lot of people have diabetes and they live a long time with it. In the United States there are around four million *diabetics,* or people who have diabetes. About a third of them at any one time are undiagnosed. This figure constitutes about 2 percent of the population, and ranges from .01 percent of people under 24 years of age to 7 percent of those over 64.

Diabetes can develop at any age. Susceptibility gradually increases up to age 40, and then rapidly increases. After age 30 it more commonly affects women than men.

History of Diabetes

Diabetes has been known for several thousand years. Because people with this disease, when untreated, may urinate frequently and copiously, the Greeks named it diabetes, meaning "siphon." In the late seventeenth century the name *mellitus,* meaning sweet was added. In early days, diagnosis was made by tasting the urine. The sweetness is caused by the presence of sugar (*glucose*) in the urine; its presence distinguishes diabetes mellitus from the much rarer *diabetes insipidus*, an entirely different problem. See under *Diseases of the Endocrine Glands,* p. 566, for a discussion of diabetes insipidus.

Discovery of insulin: Late in the nineteenth century, when diabetes was well recognized as an abnormality in carbohydrate metabolism, several scientists discovered that the experimental removal of certain cells, the *islets of Langerhans,* from the pancreas, produced diabetes in dogs. This observation led to the 1921 discovery and isolation of *insulin* by two Canadian doctors, Frederick Banting and Charles Best. Insulin is a hormone produced by these islets. Injection of insulin proved to be the first and remains the most effective means of treating diabetes. And so began a real revolution in improving the outcome of this disease. Previously death occurred in a few years for almost every diabetic. Often death was much quicker, especially for people who were under 30 years of age when they developed diabetes—since this age group tends to have a more severe form of the disease. Since 1921 new knowledge and techniques have made it possible to do more and more for diabetics.

An early pioneer in the treatment of diabetes with insulin was Dr. Elliott Joslin of Boston. Dr. Joslin realized that the diabetic patient needed to have a full understanding of his disease so that he could take care of himself. He knew that the diabetic, with the chronic abnormality of a delicate and dynamic metabolic process, could not be cared for successfully solely by knowledgeable physicians. The patient and his family had to be informed about the disease and had to make day-to-day decisions about managing it.

In many ways this marked the beginning of what have become ever increasing efforts to educate patients about all their diseases, especially chronic ones. The results have been rather remarkable.

Characteristics of Diabetes

The fundamental problem in diabetes is the body's inability to metabolize glucose, a common form of sugar, fully and continually. This is a vital process in creating body cell energy. Glucose is a chemical derivative of the carbohydrate in foods after they have been ingested. Carbohydrates are mostly of plant origin and may be called starch, saccharide, sucrose, or simply sugar. Glucose is stored under normal conditions in the form of *glycogen,* or animal starch, in the liver and muscles for later use, at which time it is reconverted to glucose.

Need for insulin: Insulin is necessary for both the storage and reconversion of glucose. The metabolic failure may come about because of an insufficiency of insulin, an inability of the body to respond normally to it for a number of complex chemical reasons, or combinations of both. In any event, the failure to metabolize glucose results in an abnormal accumulation of sugar in the bloodstream.

This failure is somewhat similar to starvation. A starved person eats no food, whereas the diabetic eats food but cannot use the carbohydrate in it and cannot get sufficient energy from the protein and fat content of food. After the starving person has used his previously stored glycogen, which the diabetic without insulin cannot do, the body has to metabolize its stored fat for energy. This results in a loss of weight and is often an early indication of diabetes.

A by-product of fat metabolism is the formation of *ketone bodies* (chemical com-

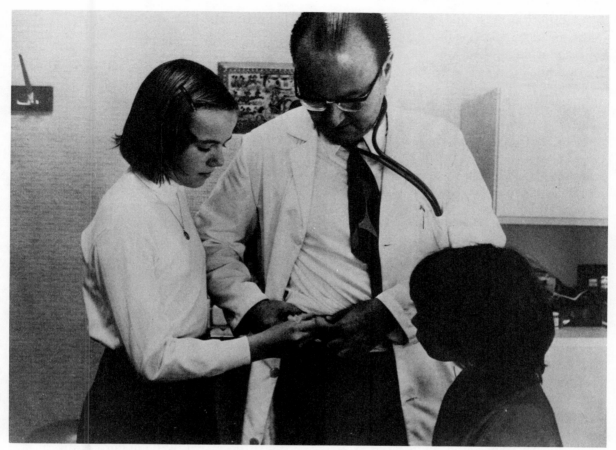

This doctor, a diabetic himself, shows diabetic children how to make an insulin injection.

pounds) which, when excessive, cause a condition known as diabetic *acidosis*. This can cause coma and death if not treated with insulin and the right kind of intravenous fluids. Before insulin was discovered, this was the way most diabetics died.

Excess urine production: As glucose accumulates above normal levels in the diabetic's bloodstream it is filtered by his kidneys and remains in the urine. Additional amounts of urine are produced to contain the excess glucose. This situation results in copious and frequent urination which in turn causes dehydration and an often insatiable thirst. These are classically the first signs of the presence of diabetes.

This is diabetes described largely in terms of changes in carbohydrate metabolism. But protein and fat metabolism are also involved, as are almost invariably some changes in the nerves, muscles, eyes, kidneys, and blood vessels.

No one knows why diabetes develops. In some ways diabetes resembles premature aging, and the causes of diabetes, if known, might shed some light on the causes of aging.

The body's need to obtain energy from glucose and to convert glucose to glycogen and vice versa is continuous but always changing quantitatively. Meeting these needs requires constantly fluctuating amounts of effective insulin. Nondiabetics produce these amounts no matter what they eat or do, thus maintaining a steady state of metabolism. Diabetics, however, cannot achieve this steady state simply by taking insulin. They must control their diets and their activities; most diabetics—80 percent —also need to take insulin or an oral diabetic agent daily. And they have to change the amounts of these medications from time to time.

Diabetes is not an all-or-nothing phenomenon. It can be mild, moderate, or severe, and can fluctuate in degree in any one individual over a long period of time, or even from day to day. Very little is really known about the reasons for these differences and changes. It is known, however, that diabetes generally gets worse in the presence of illness, particularly infections (even colds). It is also affected adversely by hyperfunctioning diseases of the anterior pituitary, thyroid, and adrenal glands, by emotional and physical stress, and during pregnancy.

Diabetes Diagnosis

The diagnosis of diabetes is not ordinarily a difficult one. Especially in children, the symptoms of rapid weight loss, extreme hunger, generalized weakness, frequent and copious urination, and insatiable thirst make it easy to recognize. Finding glucose in the urine along with increased levels of glucose in the blood generally confirms the diagnosis. However, glucose in the urine does not always indicate the presence of diabetes. A few people with unusual kidney function have glucose in their urine with normal blood levels, a condition known as *renal glycosuria.*

Moreover, an adult with diabetes may not have such a definite set of symptoms for months or years after he has actually developed the disease. Instead he may have vague fatigue or persistent skin infections. A woman may have a persistent genital itch that a physician might suspect is due to diabetes. Proof is provided by urine and blood tests. Glucose in the urine at the time of a routine physical examination might provide the first clue. Once diagnosed, treatment should be begun.

Treatment of Diabetes

Diet

The diet of a diabetic, although a major part of his treatment, is similar to what a normal person of the same age should eat. However, some radical dietary changes may be ordered if the previous diet has not been a proper one. This is particularly true in regard to reducing the calories in food eaten by overweight diabetics.

Diet is the only treatment needed by many adult diabetics, particularly those who are obese when they develop the disease, provided they can lose and not regain their excess weight. Since obese people are more likely to develop diabetes, they should have urine or blood sugar tests yearly after the age of 40. But it is more important for them to make every effort to lose weight before they become diabetics.

Individualized diets: Each diabetic's diet has to be individualized to a certain extent. This is done originally by the physician when the diagnosis is made and periodically thereafter. The physician must learn the eating habits, customs, and preferences of his diabetic patient. Since eating is so much a part of the patient's personality and has such great psychological importance, its pattern should be changed radically only when necessary.

Certain principles that may not involve major changes should be kept in mind. For example, the diet should conform to the patient's customary cultural and ethnic pattern. It should not make him feel weak and without energy. If it does, he needs more food and more insulin.

Some nonobese diabetics, especially elderly ones, need only to eliminate sugar, soft drinks, and pastry from their diets. A mild diabetic often needs only to reduce the amount of carbohydrate in his diet and replace it with fats and proteins. Alcohol can be a part of a diabetic's diet under certain circumstances, which he should dis-

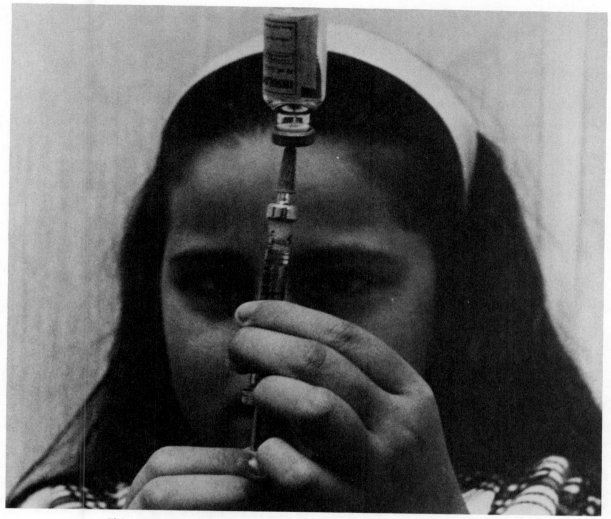

This nine-year-old girl has learned to control her diabetes by regulating her diet carefully and giving herself daily insulin injections.

cuss with his physician. Sugar-free foods and beverages enable a diabetic to enjoy some of life's minor luxuries.

Children should, if possible, have diets that are similar to those of their friends, although they must be helped to understand that they should avoid eating foods containing concentrated sugars, like soda pop, candy, jams, and jellies.

Diet guides: Most physicians have available printed diet guides to help their patients adjust their diets as needed. These indicate the number of calories and amount of protein, carbohydrate, and fat per household measure in all foods. See also under *Nutrition and Weight Control,* p. 295, for additional reading on this subject.

When to eat is another matter, and this often necessitates some changes in eating habit patterns, especially for people taking insulin. Most important is regularity in relation to the patient's rest-activity time patterns. In general, almost half of the day's carbohydrates should be eaten at lunch, since this is usually when activity and energy expenditure are greatest. The remainder should be divided between breakfast and dinner.

Insulin

Insulin is prepared commercially in the United States from beef or pork pancreas. It has to be given by injection, usually *subcutaneous injection,* just beneath the skin, since it is destroyed by gastric secretions when taken by mouth. Its dosage is measured by units, and it is prepared as 40, 80, or 100 units per cubic centimeter (cc), labeled respectively U40, U80, or U100.

The method of preparation also determines the timing of its action, and it is classified into three basic types:

TYPE OF INSULIN	TIME (HOURS) OF ACTION AFTER INJECTION		
	Onset	Peak	Duration
Rapid	½–1	2–8	4–14
Intermediate	2–4	6–12	10–26
Prolonged	4–8	12–24	24–36

There are two or three different insulin preparations of each type—rapid, intermediate, and prolonged.

Ideally insulin injected once a day should more or less mimic the normal insulin action of a nondiabetic. That is the purpose of the intermediate and long-acting insulins, with which a rapid insulin is sometimes combined. Many diabetics are able to take insulin only once a day, particularly when their diet and activity pattern is sufficiently constant. Others, however, require two or more injections. The usual time to take insulin is before breakfast. This should be the same time every day. Second injections are often taken at suppertime.

A diabetic's basic insulin dose has to be established initially according to the severity of his disease. The dose is determined largely by his blood and urine glucose levels, the physician's judgment, and trial and error. Once established, the dosage has to be assessed daily and adjusted as necessary on the basis of the amount of sugar in the urine, diet, activity, and other factors that affect insulin utilization.

Many diabetics take the same dose daily for years; others need to readjust theirs constantly. The number of units taken per day

INJECTION OF INSULIN DOSE

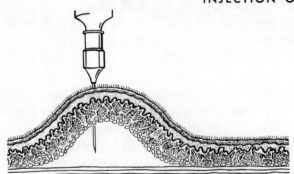

1. Wipe site of injection with cotton swab dipped in alcohol.
2. With one hand, pinch up skin at injection site. Place syringe perpendicularly to the skin and quickly insert needle for its entire length in order to insure injection of sufficient depth (see illustration). The more rapidly the needle is inserted, the less the pain will be. Stainless-steel needles are preferred.
3. Inject insulin dose.

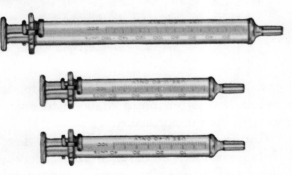

Insulin is measured in units, not in cubic centimeters (cc.), and doses are administered with specially marked insulin syringes. The syringes shown here, on which only one scale is used, are approved by the American Diabetes Association. Markings are always in red for U40 and in green for U80 concentrations. In 1973, the U100 concentration was introduced in the hope of eventually replacing the U40 and U80 syringes and thus establishing a uniform, stronger concentration for all diabetics who require insulin.

varies greatly from person to person, but probably most diabetics take between 10 and 40 units a day. The cost generally is less than one cent a unit. Insulin comes in ten-cc vials that must be refrigerated until first used. Thereafter they can be kept at room temperature.

Self-medication: Most diabetics self-inject their insulin. One can learn the technique of self-injection by practicing injecting an orange before trying it on oneself. The needle should always be sharp. It is important to change the exact site of the injection from day to day. Too frequent use of the same site may impair insulin absorption. The especially calibrated syringe and the needle can be either presterilized and discarded after one use, or they can be reused after resterilization by boiling for five minutes.

Insulin Shock

When injected insulin is active in the body system it must be matched by a sufficient amount of blood sugar. If not matched because of too much insulin, too much exercise, or too little ingested carbohydrate, the blood sugar level falls, a condition known as *hypoglycemia,* and the brain is deprived of an essential source of energy. This is most apt to occur at the time of the insulin's peak activity.

The first sign of an insulin reaction or *insulin shock* is usually mild hunger. Then come, and rather quickly, sweating, dizziness, palpitation, shallow breathing, trembling, mental confusion, strange behavior, and finally loss of consciousness. Prompt treatment is important. A lump of sugar or a piece of candy taken when symptoms first begin to appear will usually provide enough glucose to abort the reaction.

It is sometimes necessary to give intravenous glucose to counter insulin shock. This terminates the reaction almost immediately. Diabetics who use insulin should always have a lump or two of sugar or some

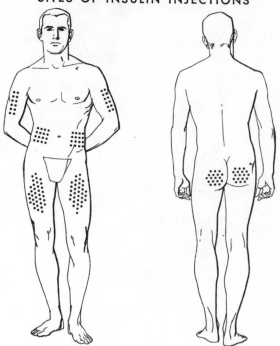

SITES OF INSULIN INJECTIONS

Change the site daily for best absorption of insulin.

candy with them and learn to recognize an oncoming insulin reaction. In general they should eat a small snack of glucose of some sort about the time their insulin activity reaches its peak.

Insulin reaction or shock can happen to any diabetic taking insulin. It is one of the liabilities of insulin therapy. Repeated and prolonged episodes of insulin reaction can be damaging to the brain. All diabetics, and especially those taking insulin, should have an identification bracelet or necklace indicating they have diabetes so that anyone examining them in an unconscious state can quickly realize the probable cause of their unconsciousness. This can be supplemented by a card in the wallet or purse with additional details. These are available from the Medic Alert Foundation, Turlock California, at a very modest cost. It is also vital that at least a few persons with whom the diabetic regularly associates know about his disease so that they can take prompt action if they see problems developing.

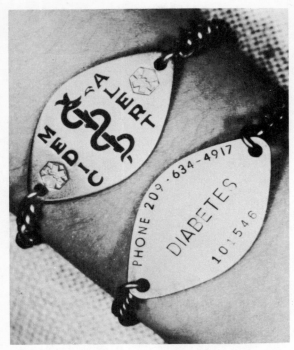

All diabetics who take insulin should wear an identifying necklace or bracelet so that the cause of unconsciousness can be recognized at once and properly treated. This emblem may be purchased for a slight charge from the Medic Alert Foundation, Turlock, California 95380, a nonprofit organization.

Oral Drugs

Oral *hypoglycemic drugs* have been available since the late 1950s. They are mainly helpful in controlling mild diabetes that develops in people 45 and over. However, younger people can occasionally be maintained on these drugs rather than on insulin. They stimulate the release of *endogenous* (self-produced) *insulin* from the pancreas or foster insulin activity in other ways. Chemically composed of *sulfonylurea,* they are remotely related to sulfa drugs but are not true sulfas. An entirely different oral hypoglycemic agent is *DBI* (*phenformin*). Some doctors urge that such drugs be prescribed only in cases that cannot be controlled effectively by other techniques.

For these drugs to work, some of the islet cells must be producing insulin or be capable of producing it. They either work well or not at all. The dose varies from one to eight tablets taken before meals and throughout the day. They cost a few cents a tablet. Insulin reactions do not occur although some diabetics take insulin also and are thereby vulnerable to insulin reactions. The decision about treating a given diabetic with these pills, insulin, or both, has to be left to the patient's physician.

Diabetic Coma

Prolonged *hyperglycemia,* or excess sugar in the blood, from insufficient insulin activity can cause *diabetic coma.* This condition involves the increasing buildup of ketone bodies, the by-product of fat metabolism, which creates an *acidotic* condition (chemical imbalance in the blood, marked by an excess of acid). When this has been present for several days, perhaps a week or longer, symptoms begin to develop that are similar to those associated with the onset of diabetes. They include excessive urination and thirst, dry and hot skin, drowsiness, and finally, coma. The earliest stage of the problem is called *diabetic ketosis;* a slightly later stage is known as *diabetic acidosis.* From the beginning there are increasing amounts of glucose as well as ketone bodies in the urine. The unconscious patient will have deep, labored breathing, and a fruity odor to his breath.

Diabetic acidosis resembles an insulin reaction, although they can be distinguished from one another. If you find a diabetic in coma and you do not know the cause, assume the cause is an insulin reaction and treat him initially with sugar. This will give immediate relief to an insulin reaction but will not affect diabetic acidosis.

Diabetic acidosis occurs for many reasons. The patient does not take his insulin or oral hypoglycemic drugs for several days. He may take too little insulin because he is confused about the dosage. He may overeat or underexercise for a number of days, perhaps because he feels ill or has a cold.

EXOPHITHALMIC GOITER

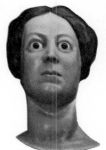

(Left) The thyroid gland secretes a hormone called thyroxin which has a profound influence upon metabolism and growth. If too much thyroxin is produced, a condition known as hyperthyroidism results. The patient suffers from nervousness and restlessness; he perspires excessively, feels too warm, and loses weight. His heart beats rapidly and forcefully. He becomes very weak and sleeps poorly. The eyes may protrude and the thyroid may become enlarged, as in this illustration, a condition known as exophthalmic goiter.

THE THYROID GLAND AND DISEASES THAT AFFECT IT

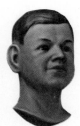
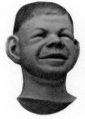

CRETINISM

If the deficiency in thyroid secretion occurs before birth, it may lead to cretinism, a condition marked by arrested physical and mental development. The cretin, pictured on the left, typically has a pudgy face and thick, coarse skin. The model on the right shows the change in appearance of the cretin after taking thyroid extract regularly for two years.

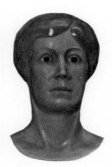

SIMPLE GOITER

Goiter refers to the enlargement of the thyroid gland. Although it may result from overproduction of thyroxin (exophthalmic goiter), it more commonly results from too little production of thyroxin caused by a lack of iodine in the diet. In this case the enlargement may be enormous. Although disfiguring, many goiters are present for years without producing symptoms. They are often removed to insure against the possibility of cancer or of a toxic substance developing from the goiter. The models illustrate the appearance of a patient before and after an operation for removal of a simple goiter.

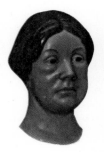
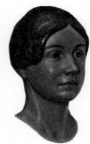

MYXEDEMA

When the thyroid gland becomes abnormally underactive, a condition known as hypothyroidism results. One form of this condition is called myxedema, in which the patient feels cold, sleepy, and slowed in his movements. He complains of weakness and fatigue. He perspires too little, his voice often becomes harsh, and the hands or face becomes puffy. Pictured on the left is a woman with myxedema. The model on the right shows the same woman after taking thyroid extract for one month.

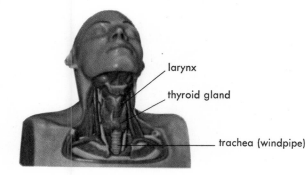

larynx

thyroid gland

trachea (windpipe)

THE EYE

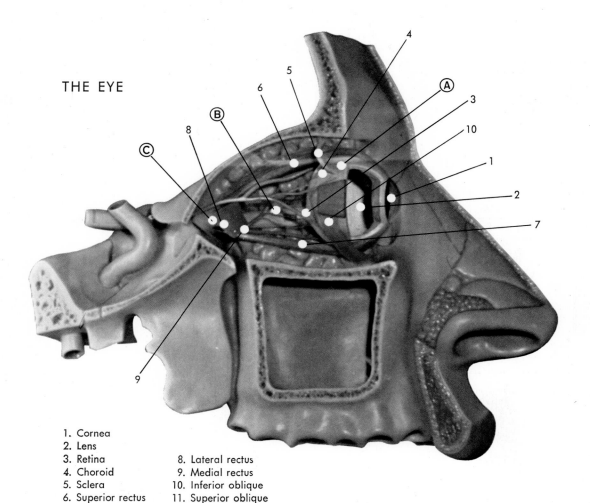

1. Cornea
2. Lens
3. Retina
4. Choroid
5. Sclera
6. Superior rectus
7. Inferior rectus
8. Lateral rectus
9. Medial rectus
10. Inferior oblique
11. Superior oblique
   (not seen from this angle)

A cut-away view of the right eye and that part of the skull, including the eye socket, in which it is located. The three main parts of the eye are: A) The eyeball, which includes, 1) the cornea—the transparent outer covering in front of the eyeball; the iris—which determines the color of the eye; and the pupil—the circular opening in the center of the iris which appears as a dark spot. 2) the lens, which changes shape and adjusts itself for correct focusing of objects closer or farther away from the eye. 3) The retina, the innermost and light-sensitive layer of the eyeball. 4) The choroid, which contains blood vessels. 5) The sclera, or so-called white of the eye. B) The optic nerve, which connects the retina with the brain. C) The set of six eye muscles, which includes, 6) superior rectus, 7) inferior rectus, 8) lateral rectus, 9) medial rectus, 10) inferior oblique, 11) superior oblique.

HOW THE EYE WORKS

The eye works somewhat like a camera, since it, like the camera, is made up of a light-tight box having an opening in front fitted with a lens and a light-sensitive film on the back.

In the camera the correct focusing for objects of various distances is accomplished by moving the back of the camera closer to or farther away from the lens.

In the human eye, however, the focusing for objects at various distances is accomplished by the change of the shape of the lens which takes place automatically.

SENSE OF VISION

Lachrymal Gland and its Function

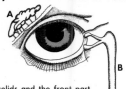

The eyelids and the front part of the eyeball are continuously lubricated by the secretion (tears) of the lachrymal gland (A). The superfluous moisture is drained into the nasal cavity by way of the nasolachrymal duct (B).

Accommodation of the Eye

Flattened lens   Thickened lens

Our eyes focus by changing the lens thickness —accommodation. The ciliary muscle (red) contracts the elastic lens.

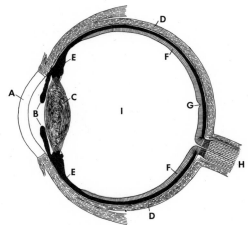

Cross Section of Eyeball Showing:

A. Cornea
B. Iris
C. Lens
D. Sclera

E. Chorioid
F. Retina
G. Macula lutea
H. Optic nerve

I. Vitreous body

Eye Muscles

Lewis "Grey's Anatomy"
Courtesy Lea & Febiger, Publisher

The movement of the eyeball is performed by six muscles for each eye. The innervation of all these muscles is perfectly synchronized so that they always cause coordinated movements.

Iris

A   B

Shown above are two views of the iris, front (A) and cross section (B). The iris can, by means of muscles, increase and decrease the diameter of its central opening (pupil).

Dark Adaptation

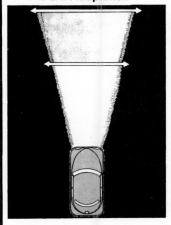

In darkness our sight improves gradually, but if a strong light strikes our eyes, as the headlights of an oncoming car at night, our vision instantly becomes greatly reduced.

Blind Spot Demonstration

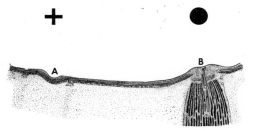

If you close your left eye, look at the cross with your right eye, and move the book slowly toward your face, the black dot will disappear. The image of the cross is then centered on the macula lutea (A) and the dot on the outlet of the optic nerve (B).

Binocular Vision

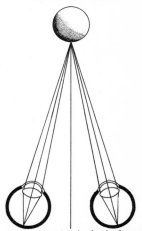

In order to perceive depth, simultaneous vision with both eyes is necessary. If we look at a ball with both eyes, we will see it as a sphere; one eye only will show it as a disk.

The Normal Eye

The normal eye gives a sharp image of a far object with a resting lens.

When such an eye looks at a close object, sharp image is secured by thickening the lens.

The Nearsighted Eye

In the nearsighted eye, longer than normal, far objects appear blurred.

The condition is rectified by a concave lens placed in front of the eye.

When looking at a close object, sharp vision is possible without thickening the lens.

The Farsighted Eye

In the farsighted eye, shorter than normal, near objects appear blurred.

If the lens thickens, a sharp image can usually be formed without glasses.

A convex lens relieves the eye lens from this strain.

The Older Eye

The older lens loses its ability to thicken. Only far objects are seen clearly.

It will be impossible to see nearby objects sharply without glasses.

A convex lens will correct this defect.

SENSES

HEARING

Eardrum and Auditory Bones

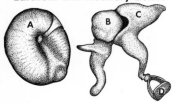

A. Eardrum   C. Anvil

B. Hammer   D. Stirrup

Cochlea and Semicircular Canals

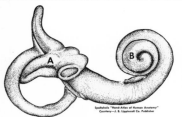

A. The Cochlea
B. The Semicircular canals

Spalteholz "Hand-Atlas of Human Anatomy"
Courtesy—J. B. Lippincott Co. Publisher

Cross Section of the Organ of Hearing

1. External ear proper	7. Eustachian tube
2. External auditory canal	8. Cochlea
3. Eardrum	9. Semicircular canals
4. Hammer	10. Auditory and
5. Anvil	vestibular nerve
6. Stirrup	11. Spinal cord

Orientation in Space

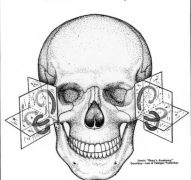

Lewis "Gray's Anatomy"
Courtesy—Lea & Febiger Publisher

This picture shows a human skull and the relative position of the semicircular canals greatly enlarged and diagrammatic. If the head is moved in any direction, the corresponding semicircular canals (which are filled with a liquid) will be stimulated and this stimulus will be transmitted to the brain through the vestibular nerve. In this way, even with closed eyes, we are able to distinguish the position in which our head is situated (vertical, horizontal. etc.).

Increase in Pressure

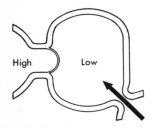

High   Low

If pressure in the external air increases (as in descending airplanes), the eardrum is pushed in and causes a feeling of pressure or pain. Air must be pumped into the middle ear, as by repeated swallowing, to secure equal pressure on both sides of the eardrum.

Physiology of Hearing

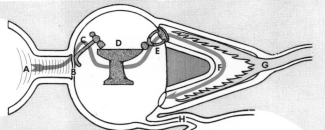

Sound waves (A) vibrate the eardrum (B), causing the hammer (C), anvil (D), and stirrup (E) to agitate the liquid in the cochlea (F) and thus stimulate an impulse through the auditory nerve (G). Pressure in the chamber which houses the hammer, anvil, and stirrup is maintained equal to atmospheric pressure by passage of air through the Eustachian tube (H). Pressure on both sides of the eardrum (B) must be equalized to permit free vibration. The red arrow indicates the route followed by the vibrations.

Decrease in Pressure

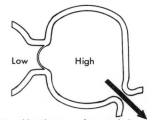

Low   High

In sudden decrease of external air pressure (as in ascending airplanes and elevators) the eardrum bulges out because of the increased air pressure in the middle ear. In such conditions air moves out of the middle ear by way of the Eustachian tube. This is usually not a painful process.

TOUCH

The intricate nerve endings (A) which give rise to the sense of touch are located right under the epidermis of the skin and are in direct contact with higher nervous centers.

TASTE

The sense organ of taste is mostly localized in the so-called circumvallated papillae of the tongue (A). (B) shows a microscopic picture of a so-called taste bud.

SMELL

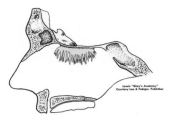

Lewis "Gray's Anatomy"
Courtesy—Lea & Febiger Publisher

The end organ of the sense of smell is located in a dense nervous texture in the upper part of the nasal cavity.

Treatment: In its early stages ketosis generally can be treated by the patient himself with directions from his physician, usually by telephone. The fundamentals of this treatment involve taking rapid-acting insulin—every diabetic should keep a bottle of this on hand—every three or four hours until the urine has less glucose and no longer contains ketone bodies. Ketone bodies can be tested in the urine along with glucose. If there is a treatable underlying cause for the acidosis, such as an infection, it should be treated as well. In the later stages, hospital treatment with larger amounts of insulin, often given intravenously, and specific intravenous fluid therapy is essential.

Diabetes Control

An occasional insulin reaction is almost unavoidable, but diabetic acidosis occurs mainly because the diabetes was not well controlled. Good control means feeling well with only small amounts or no sugar in the urine. This is possible for most but not all diabetics. A few diabetics can never achieve good control for a variety of reasons relating largely to the vagaries of this disease.

Personal Glucose Tests

The amount of glucose in the urine provides a kind of barometer of diabetic control. The amount in the blood at a given point in time provides a better barometer but is more difficult to check for obvious reasons. Therefore all diabetics should test their urine daily and sometimes more often, particularly in the beginning or when they are having control problems.

The ordinary urine specimen contains urine collected in the bladder over a period of several hours or overnight. The glucose in it is an average indication of what the blood sugar has been during a previous period. To get an idea of the blood sugar level at the time of the urine test, the urine

that has accumulated in the bladder must first be discarded. Then a second specimen of urine should be passed about a half hour later and that specimen tested for glucose.

Several types of tests are available for this purpose. Some utilize chemically treated paper which, when dipped in urine, turns different colors to indicate varying amounts of glucose in the urine. Others use tablets that change to different colors when dropped into small amounts of urine. Adjustments in diet, activity, and insulin or oral hypoglycemic agents can be made on the basis of these test results. It costs a few cents to do each test.

Making Lifelong Adjustments

Once a diabetic has learned the fundamentals of his diet, his insulin or oral hypoglycemic agent medication, and has stabilized sufficiently his daily physical activities, he is well on his way to leading a normal life. There are a certain number of psychological roadblocks with which the diabetic has to cope.

First is the hard business of adjusting to the disease and coming to accept the fact that it can be lived with even though there is no cure. Initial depression is understandable and common. It does not persist. Then comes the often difficult task of regularizing one's life in terms of eating schedules, taking insulin, testing the urine, and exercising regularly.

Not many diabetics can maintain good control if they go to a Saturday night party, postpone their dinner time by four or five hours, and sleep until noon on Sunday. Maintaining one's usual schedule while traveling is another obstacle. The diabetic may feel that people treat him differently from the way they used to treat him or from the way they treat others. He will have to get used to seeing his physician frequently and regularly and having blood drawn to determine his blood sugar. He will have to spend a certain amount of money for insulin or oral hypoglycemic drugs, syringes and needles, urine-testing materials, special sugar-free foods, and medical care.

Self-pity and then rebellion against these factors are not unusual, especially in children. And with rebellion comes an increased likelihood of insulin reactions or diabetic ketosis. Some diabetics use their disease as a way to manipulate others and thus create trying interpersonal relationships. The good physician is aware of all of this and will give his patient the opportunity to verbalize his feelings.

Those with whom the diabetic lives—parents, siblings, spouse, and children—are also affected in various ways. The family's food style may be changed to some extent. Parents may have a sense of guilt about what they erroneously presume to be their part in the child's development of diabetes. They may have difficulty differentiating normal adolescent moods from those associated with the diabetic's fluctuating carbohydrate metabolism. They may become controlling and coddling or rejecting and resentful. Either reaction pattern will affect the child adversely. Parents should be helped to understand the disease as well as its effect on their child.

Pregnancy and Diabetes

Pregnancy is a very special time in any woman's life, but it is particularly special for a diabetic and her unborn child. Diabetes is not a factor of any magnitude as far as conception is concerned, but pregnancy affects the diabetic's carbohydrate metabolism dramatically. In general there is an increase in blood glucose levels and an ever-increasing need for insulin. However, there can be periodic and unpredictable reductions in insulin need. Therefore, urine glucose and blood glucose need to be tested more frequently than under ordinary circumstances.

The urine should be tested three or four times a day and the blood glucose at every visit to the obstetrician. With good management during a diabetic's pregnancy, her baby has an excellent chance of being as normal and healthy as that of the nondiabetic mother.

Diabetes in Later Life

The association between aging and diabetes relates largely to a gradual loss of elasticity in the cells of the blood vessels, kidneys, eyegrounds (the inner sides of the backs of the eyeballs), and nerve tissues. These cellular changes may not become apparent for many years after the development of diabetes. However, occasionally they are present before or appear several years after the diabetes is recognized. This is particularly apt to be true in older people who develop diabetes.

The nerve-tissue changes can cause a diminished sensation to touch and pain and sometimes a loss of motor function of the extremities as well as sexual impotence. The eyeground changes damage the retina in various ways and can cause varying degrees of loss of vision. In about eight percent of cases this progresses to blindness.

The changes in the kidneys affect their filtration functions, causing *albuminuria,* a loss of protein from the blood serum into the urine and the development of high blood pressure in roughly 23 percent of diabetics. The vascular changes, which are rather diffuse, contribute to the specific organ changes noted above, and frequently cause a reduction in blood supply to the legs and heart muscle. This ultimately causes heart damage in perhaps 20 percent of diabetics. Medicine can do much to reduce the effects of these many changes but cannot cure them.

Some degree of prevention is possible, and good diabetic control generally is thought to contribute to a reduction and delay in the development of these complications. Since the nerve and vascular changes make the feet particularly vulnerable to infections that can be serious and even lead to amputation—gangrene occurs in about three percent of diabetics—proper and daily care of the feet is essential to prevent the development of infections. The older diabetic should be careful to keep his feet clean and dry and cut his toenails frequently and evenly.

Early Detection

Anyone who does not have diabetes might very well wonder whether he or she is at all likely to get it, and, if so, what can be done to prevent it. One answer is clear. If you are obese, whatever your age, try to lose weight. This is especially important if you have grandparents, parents, brothers, sisters, or children who developed diabetes in middle age or earlier. It is important also if you are a mother who has had babies weighing nine or more pounds at birth.

A fairly simple laboratory test, called a *glucose tolerance test* (GTT), has been developed to identify a person who is prediabetic. The subject either swallows a drink containing 100 grams of glucose or is given the same amount intravenously. Thereafter his blood sugar is determined at set intervals over a three-to-six-hour period. If his blood sugar level remains abnormally high for too long, he is said to be a prediabetic or to have *chemical diabetes.*

All adults should have their urine tested at least once a year for the presence of sugar. Some adults and younger persons should have more frequent urine tests and perhaps periodic glucose tolerance tests. Both of these possibilities have to be determined individually by the physician who provides that individual's care.

Genetically, diabetes has many characteristics of a Mendelian recessive inherited disease. Theoretically the chances are one

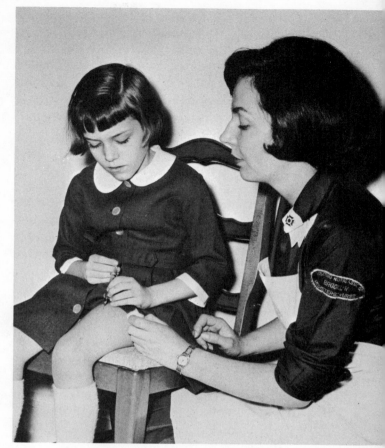

This diabetic child is being given a lesson in the proper way to self-administer daily insulin injections.

in four of a child developing diabetes if one parent has the disease; it is almost inevitable if both have it. These are obviously important factors for diabetics to consider before they have children, particularly when both prospective parents have diabetes.

The person who develops diabetes today has a far better chance for a normal life than a patient of only a generation or two ago. The development of insulin therapy in the 1920s and oral hypoglycemic drugs in the late 1950s has made it possible for victims of a still very serious disease to add many active, productive years to their lives. Current research in the field of carbohydrate metabolism offers the promise of still more effective control of this insidious ailment in future years.   DST

DISEASES OF THE EYE AND EAR

Most people never experience any impairment of the senses of smell, taste, and touch. But it is lucky and unusual to reach old age without having some problems connected with sight or hearing or both.

The Eyes

All sensations must be processed in the brain by a normally functioning central nervous system for their proper perception. In addition, each sensation is perceived through a specific sense organ. Thus sight is dependent on at least one functioning eye.

The eye is an optical system that can be compared to a camera, because the human lens perceives and the retina receives an image in the same way that a camera and its film does. Defects in this optical system are called errors in refraction and are the most common type of sight problem.

Myopia

Nearsightedness or *myopia* is a refractive error that causes faraway objects to be seen as blurred and indistinct. The degree of nearsightedness can be measured by testing each eye with a Snellen Test Chart. Normal vision is called 20/20. This means that at 20 feet the eye sees an image clearly and accurately.

Eyesight of less-than-normal acuity is designated as 20/50 or 20/100 and so on. This means that what the deficient eye can see accurately at a distance of 20 feet or less, the normal eye can see accurately at 50 or 100 feet.

Myopia is the most common of all the refractive errors and results from an elongation of the eyeball. The cause of this abnormality is unknown, but it prevents the image from being focused on the retina. Those who are affected by myopia usually develop it between the ages of 6 and 15. They are likely to become aware of the condition when they can no longer see as well as they used to in school or at the movies or as well as their friends can.

Myopia is rarely severe and generally does not get progressively worse, although in a few extreme cases, it can lead to blindness. Individually prescribed eyeglasses or contact lenses can correct the refractive error and produce normal vision.

HOW EYEGLASSES CORRECT MYOPIA

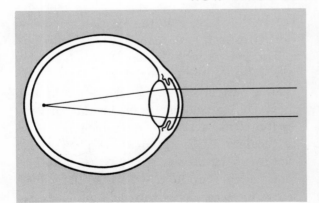 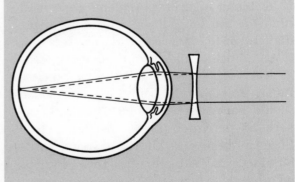

In a myopic or nearsighted eye (*left*), the images focus in front of the retina, either because the eyeball is too long or because the lens is shaped defectively. (*Right*) The concave eyeglass lens separates the images before they reach the eye so that they focus on the retina.

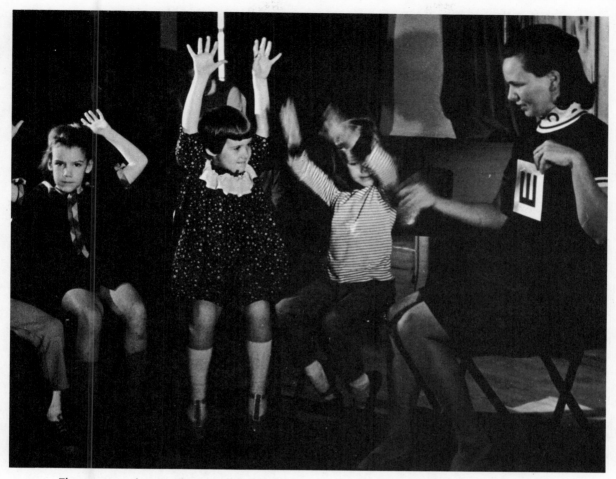

These pre-readers are being asked which way the bars point—up, down, or to which side. Once the "game" is understood, each child can be tested individually at a prescribed distance with an eye chart consisting of such shapes in place of the letters of the alphabet.

Farsightedness and Astigmatism

The opposite of myopia is *hypermetropia* or farsightedness, which results from a shortening of the eyeball. The two conditions may be combined with *astigmatism,* in which vertical and horizontal images do not focus on the same point, mainly because of some abnormality of the front surface of the cornea. Properly fitted glasses can correct all of these deficiencies.

Presbyopia

A fourth refractive error combines with the other three to make up about 80 percent of all visual defects. It is known as *presby-opia* or old-sight and results from an inability of the lens to focus on near objects. Almost everyone is affected by presbyopia some time after the age of 40, because of the aging of the lens itself or of the muscles which expand and contract it. The condition is usually noticed when it becomes necessary to hold a book or newspaper farther and farther away from the eyes in order to be able to read it. Although presbyopia is a nuisance, it can be easily corrected with glasses.

All these conditions represent variations in the sight of one or both eyes from what is considered the norm. Since seating distance from a school blackboard, the size of print, and the distance at which signs must be read are all based on what is considered to be normal vision, eye defects are handicaps, some mild and some severe.

Many people can function normally without glasses if the defects are minor. But since uncorrected refractive errors can cause headaches and general fatigue as well as eye aches and eye fatigue, they should receive prompt medical attention.

Color Blindness

Color blindness is a visual defect that occurs in about eight percent of men but is extremely rare in women. It is hereditary and usually involves an inability to differentiate clearly between red, green, and blue. It is a handicap for which there is no known cure at the present time.

Glaucoma

Glaucoma is a serious problem that affects about two percent of those people who are over forty. It is caused not only by the aging process, but also and more impor-

tantly by anatomical changes inside the eye that prevent the normal drainage of fluid. The pressure inside the eye is therefore increased, and this pressure causes further anatomical change that can lead to blindness.

Glaucoma may begin with occasional eye pain or blurred vision, or it may be very insidious, cause no symptoms for years, and be discovered only at an eye examination. Glaucoma is the number one cause of blindness, and an annual check for its onset by a specialist is particularly recommended for everyone over forty. The test is quick, easy, and painless, and should symptoms appear, early treatment, either medical or surgical or both, can reduce the likelihood of partial or complete loss of sight.

Cataracts

Another serious eye problem is the development of *cataracts*. These are areas in the lens which are no longer transparent. The so-called *senile cataract* is common among elderly people because of degenerative changes in the lens. The condition causes varying degrees of loss of vision which are readily noticed by the patient. If the vision is reduced a great deal, the entire lens can be removed surgically and appropriate glasses can be provided.

Detached Retina

Among the most serious eye disorders is the condition known as *separated* or *detached retina*. It occurs when fluid from inside the eye gets under the retina (the inner membrane at the back of the eye, on which the image is focused) and separates it from its bed, thus breaking the connections that are essential for normal vision. The most common cause of the detachment is the formation of a hole or tear in the retina. However, the condition may also develop following a blow to the head or to the eye, or because of a tumor, nephritis, or high blood pressure.

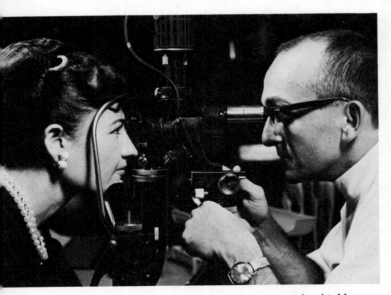

The biomicroscope or slit lamp provides highly concentrated illumination and magnification for the detection of foreign bodies, the studies of eye diseases and abnormalities, and the fitting of contact lenses.

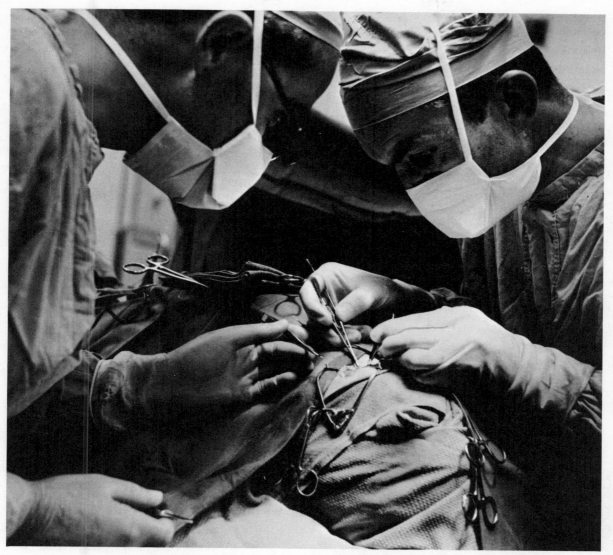

Thanks to the advanced state of knowledge of the anatomy of the eye, modern surgery is often successful in correcting defects and in preventing blindness, such as that caused by cataracts.

The symptoms of the onset of retinal separation are showers of drifting black spots and frequent flashes of light shaped like pinwheels that interfere with vision. These disturbances are usually followed by a dark shadow in the area of sight closest to the nose.

A retinal detachment is treated by surgical techniques in which the accumulated fluid is drained off and the hole in the tissue is sealed. About 60 percent of all cases are cured or considerably improved after surgery. The earlier the diagnosis, the more favorable is the outcome. Proper post-operative care usually involves several weeks of immobilization of the head so that the retinal tissue can heal without disturbance.

Trauma

Like any other part of the body, the eye can be injured by a major accident or *trauma*, although it is somewhat protected by the bones surrounding it. Trauma can cause most of the problems previously de-

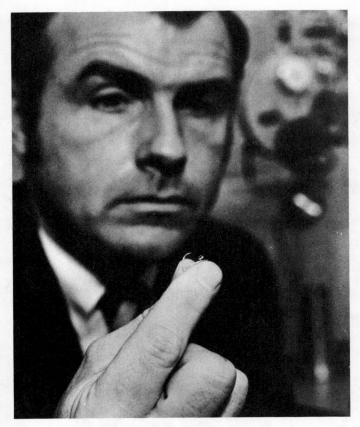

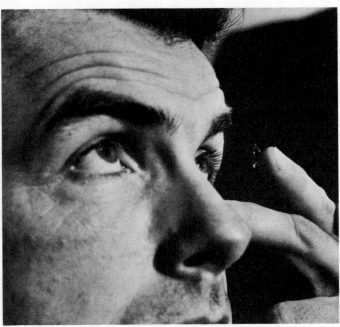

Soft plastic contact lenses (*top and bottom*) are extremely flexible and readily adapt their shape to fit the contours of the eye. Unlike hard lenses, hydrophilic lenses adhere directly to the moist cornea.

scribed. In addition, small objects can get into the eye easily, and particles of soot and other wind-borne dirt can cause great discomfort. The tearing that results from the irritation usually floats foreign substances away, but occasionally they have to be removed by an instrument.

When a particle in the eye or under the eyelid is not easily dislodged and begins to cause redness, it should be removed by someone qualified to do so. The eye should never be poked at or into by untrained hands.

Leaving contact lenses in the eye for too long can cause discomfort which lasts for quite a while even after they have been taken out. Bacterial or viral infections of the outer surface of the eye such as *conjunctivitis* or *pinkeye,* or of the eyelids, are quite common and should be treated by a doctor if they are extensive or chronic.

Contact Lenses

Contact lenses, which are fitted directly over the iris and pupil of the eye in contact with the cornea (the tissue covering the outer, visible surface of the eye) are preferred by some people for the correction of vision defects. In some cases of severe astigmatism, nearsightedness, or following cataract surgery, contact lenses can be more effective than eyeglasses, but the chief reason for their popularity has been cosmetic. They are practically invisible. Hard plastic contact lenses adhere to the eye by suction: a partial vacuum is created between the inner surface of the lens and outer surface of the eyeball. Unfortunately, particles of dust can get under the lens and cause extreme discomfort. For this reason, many contact lens users habitually wear sunglasses when out of doors in sooty urban streets.

Recently, soft plastic contact lenses have been introduced commercially. These lenses are *hydrophilic* (literally, water-loving) and adapt their shape to the shape of the moist

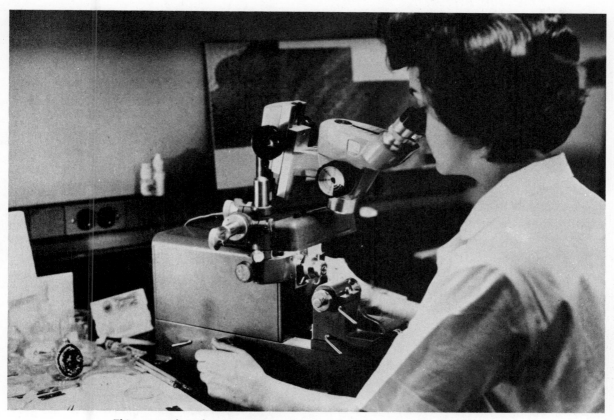

This research technician is preparing eye tissue sections in measurements smaller than $\frac{1}{1000}$th of a millimeter as part of a study of corneal disease.

cornea, to which they adhere. Thus, they are more easily fitted, and patients seldom experience discomfort in adjusting to them. It is virtually impossible for dust particles to get underneath them. However, the soft lens must be sterilized daily; it scratches or tears easily; and it is limited at present to the correction of only certain kinds of nearsightedness. It is also relatively expensive. Further technological improvements are likely to make it more widely applicable, however, and reduce the cost. The soft lens has already proved to be valuable therapeutically in the treatment of certain eye disorders, and some eye specialists believe that its potentialities have only begun to be explored. At present, neither soft nor hard lenses are recommended for 24-hour-a-day use; they should be removed before going to bed.

Diseases Which Affect Vision

In addition to the various disorders involving only the eye, there are a number of generalized diseases that affect vision. Among these are arteriosclerosis, diabetes mellitus, and hypertension or high blood pressure, which often cause abnormalities in the blood vessels of various parts of the eye. These abnormalities can lead to tissue changes which cause the patient to see spots or to notice that his vision is defective.

Diseases of the brain, such as multiple sclerosis, tumors, and abscesses, although rare, can result in double vision or loss of lateral or central vision. Any sudden or gradual changes in vision should be brought to a doctor's attention promptly, since early diagnosis and treatment is usually effective and can prevent serious deterioration.

The Ears

The ear, like the eye, is a complicated structure. Its major parts consist of the auditory canal, middle ear, and inner ear. Hearing results from the perception of sound waves whose loudness can be measured in decibels and whose highness or lowness of pitch can be measured by their frequency in cycles per second.

Sound waves usually travel through the auditory canal to the eardrum or *tympanic membrane,* vibrating it in such a way as to carry the vibrations to and along the three interlocking small bones in the middle ear to the inner ear. Here the vibrations are carried to the auditory nerve through a fluid-filled labyrinth called the communicating channel.

An abnormality at any of these points can produce a hearing deficiency. Normal hearing means the ability to hear the spoken voice in a relatively quiet room at a distance of about 18 feet. How well a person hears can be tested by an audiometer, which measures decibels and frequency of sound.

Wax Accumulation

A very common cause of hearing deficiency is the excessive accumulation of wax in the auditory canal, where it is continually being secreted. When the excess that blocks the passage of sound waves is

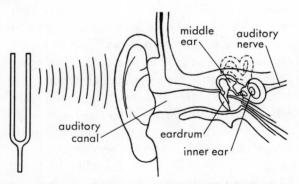

Sound waves stimulate the eardrum, whose vibrations are communicated to the three bones of the middle ear, then to the spiral inner ear and auditory nerve.

removed—sometimes by professional instrumentation—hearing returns to normal. Anyone whose hearing is temporarily impaired in this way should avoid the use of rigid or pointed objects for cleaning out the accumulated wax.

Infection

Infections or other diseases of the skin that lines the auditory canal can sometimes cause a kind of local swelling that blocks the canal and interferes with hearing. Although such a condition can be painful, proper treatment, usually with antibiotics, generally results in a complete cure.

A major cause of hearing deficiency acquired after birth is recurrent bacterial infection of the middle ear. The infecting organisms commonly get to the middle ear through the *Eustachian tube,* which connects the middle ear to the upper throat, or through the eardrum if it has been perforated by injury or by previous infection.

The infection can cause hearing loss, either because it becomes chronic or because the tissues become scarred. Such infections are usually painful, but ever since treatment with antibiotics has become possible, they rarely spread to the mastoid bone as they used to in the past.

Disorders Caused by Pressure

The Eustachian tube usually permits the air pressure on either side of the eardrum to equalize. When the pressure inside the drum is less than that outside—as occurs during descent in an airplane or elevator, or when riding through an underwater tunnel, or during skin diving—the eardrum is pushed inward. This causes a noticeable hearing loss or a stuffy feeling in the ear which subsides as soon as the pressure equalizes again. Yawning or swallowing usually speeds up the return to normal.

When the unequal pressure continues for several days because the Eustachian tube is blocked, fluid begins to collect in the middle

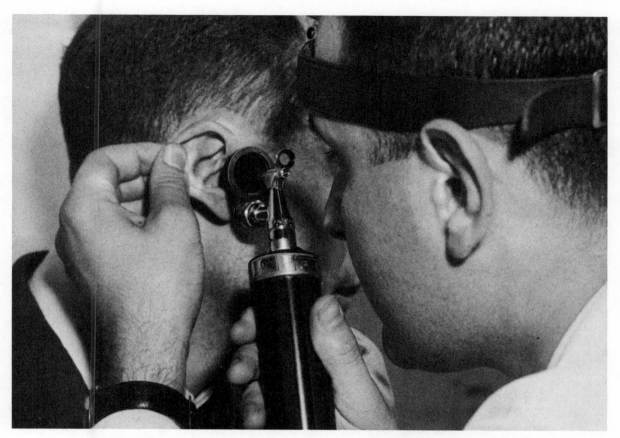

A physician examining a patient's eardrum with an otoscope for signs of infection.

ear. This is called *nonsuppurative otitis media* and can cause permanent hearing damage.

Eustachian tube blockage is more commonly the result of swelling around its *nasopharyngeal* end because of a throat infection, a cold, or an allergy. Nose drops help to open up the tube, but sometimes it may be necessary to drain the ear through the eardrum or to treat the disorder with other surgical procedures.

Otosclerosis

A very common cause of hearing loss that affects about 1 in 200 adults—usually women—is *otosclerosis*. This disorder is the result of a sort of freezing of the bones in the middle ear caused by an overgrowth of tissue. The onset of the disorder usually occurs before age 30 among about 70 per-

cent of the people who will be affected. Only one ear may be involved, but the condition does get progressively worse. Although heredity is an important factor, the specific cause of otosclerosis is unknown. In some cases, surgery can be helpful.

Injury

A blow to the head, or a loud noise close to the ear such as the sound of a gun shot or a jet engine, especially when repeated often, can cause temporary and sometimes permanent hearing defects. Anyone who expects to be exposed to damaging noise should wear protective earmuffs. Injury to the auditory nerve by chemicals or by medicines such as streptomycin can also cause loss of hearing. For further information about the potential and actual dangers of noise, see *Noise Pollution,* p. 369.

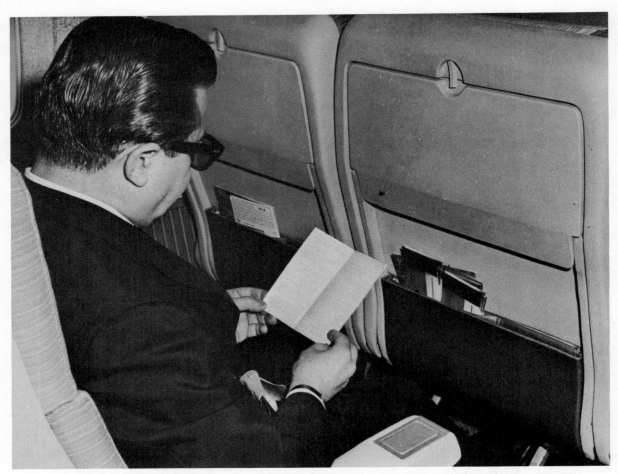

Motion sickness is usually caused by a combination of up-and-down and lateral movements, such as those on a bumpy airplane ride, on the sensitive organ of equilibrium of the inner ear.

Ringing in the Ears

Sometimes people complain of hearing noises unrelated to the reception of sound waves from an outside source. This phenomenon is called *tinnitus* and occurs in the form of a buzzing, ringing, or hissing sound.

It may be caused by some of the conditions described above and may be relieved by proper treatment. In many cases, however, the cause is unknown and the patient simply has to learn to live with the sounds and ignore them.

Impairment of Balance

The *labyrinths* of the inner ear are involved not only in hearing but also in controlling postural balance. When the labyrinths are diseased, the result can be a feeling of *vertigo* or true dizziness. This sensation of being unable to maintain balance is quite different from feeling lightheaded or giddy.

Vertigo can be an incapacitating disorder. Sometimes it is caused by diseases of the central nervous system such as epilepsy or brain hemorrhage, but more often by inflammation sometimes caused by infection of the labyrinth. It can be sudden and recurrent as in *Ménière's disease*, or somewhat gradual and nonrecurrent. It may or may not be accompanied by vomiting or hearing loss. Treatment for the condition varies depending on the cause.

Deafness

Deafness at birth or in a very young baby is an especially difficult problem because hearing is necessary for the development of speech. Although the deafness itself may be impossible to correct, its early recognition and management can usually prevent muteness from developing.

Many communities now have special schools for deaf children, and new techniques and machines are constantly being devised for helping them to learn how to speak, even if imperfectly. Any doubt about an infant's ability to hear should therefore be brought to a doctor's attention immediately.

Deafness at birth can be caused by a maternal infection such as rubella (German measles) during pregnancy. Since children

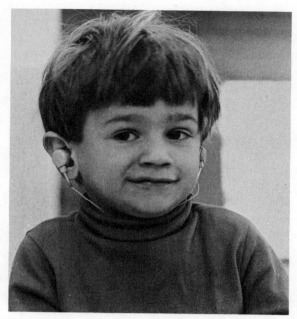

This youngster was born with a hearing defect because his mother had rubella during early pregnancy.

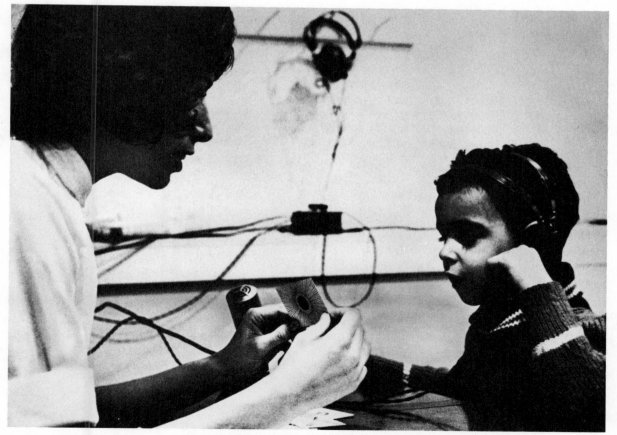

A speech therapist using a microphone and ear phones to help a child with a hearing disability.

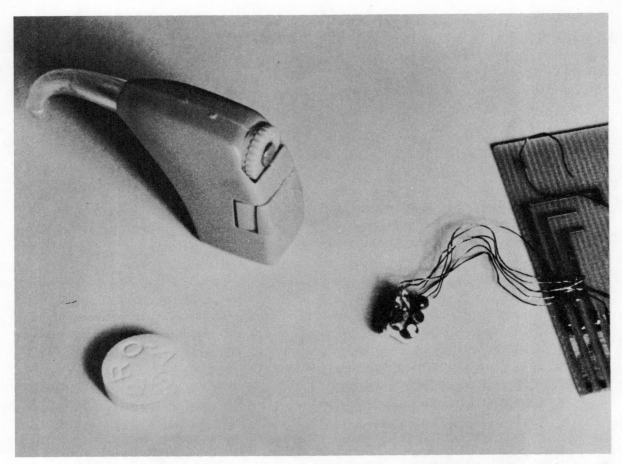

Some serious hearing defects can be corrected by a hearing aid such as the one illustrated above (pictured with an aspirin tablet to indicate relative size). With the aid of transistors, the hearing aid (*see below*), picks up sound waves, amplifies them, and transmits sound to the cochlea of the inner ear through the bones of the skull itself. This is why a hearing aid can work even when the drum or the ossicles of the middle ear are seriously damaged.

are often the ones who spread this disease, youngsters should be immunized against it.

Hearing aids: Hearing loss that cannot be treated medically or surgically can often be compensated for by an accurately fitted hearing aid. This device, which now comes in many sizes, shapes, and types, converts sound waves into electrical impulses, amplifies them, and reconverts them into sound waves. A hearing aid can be placed in the auditory canal for air conduction of sound waves, or it can be worn behind the ear for bone conduction. See under *Aging and What To Do About It,* p. 188, for further information about hearing aids.   DST

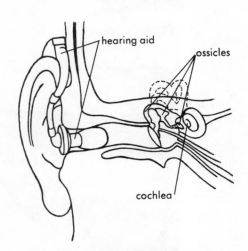

How a Hearing Aid Works
by Bone Conduction

DISEASES OF THE URINOGENITAL SYSTEM

The parts of the urinogenital tract that produce and get rid of urine are the same for men and women: the kidneys, ureters, bladder, and urethra. To understand some of the problems that can arise from diseases of the urinary tract, it is necessary to know a few facts about the anatomy and function of these parts.

The two kidneys are located on either side of the spinal column in the back portion of the abdomen between the last rib and the third vertebrae of the spine. They are shaped like the large beans named after them but are considerably larger.

Their function is to filter and cleanse the blood of waste substances produced in the course of normal living and, together with some other organs, to maintain a proper balance of body fluids. The kidneys do this job by filtering the fluid portion of the blood as it passes through them, returning the necessary solids and water to the bloodstream, and removing waste products and excess water, called *urine*. These products then flow into the *ureters*, the ducts that connect the kidneys and the bladder.

The *bladder* holds the urine until voiding occurs. The duct from the bladder to the urinary opening is called the *urethra*. In the male, it passes through the penis; in the female, through the anterior wall of the vagina.

Symptoms of Kidney Disorders

Normal kidney function can be disrupted by bacterial or viral infection, by tumors, by external injury, or by congenital defects. Some of the common symptoms that may result under these circumstances are:

• *Anuria*—inability to produce or void urine

• *Dysuria*—pain, often of a burning quality, during urination

• Frequency—abnormally frequent urination, often of unusually small amounts

• Hesitancy—difficulty in starting urination

• Urgency—a very strong urge to urinate, often strong enough to cause loss of urine

• *Oliguria*—reduced production of urine

• *Polyuria*—voiding larger than normal amounts of urine

• *Nocturia*—frequent voiding at night

• *Hematuria*—voiding blood in the urine.

Since any of these symptoms may indicate a disease of the urinary tract, their appearance should be brought to the attention of a doctor without delay.

THE ANATOMY OF THE KIDNEY

The cortex is the darker, outer part of the kidney. The medulla, the inner part, includes the renal pyramids and the straight tubules associated with them.

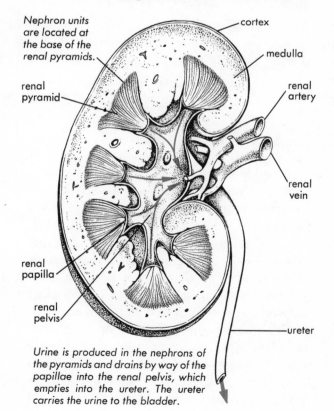

Nephron units are located at the base of the renal pyramids.

cortex

medulla

renal pyramid

renal artery

renal vein

renal papilla

renal pelvis

ureter

Urine is produced in the nephrons of the pyramids and drains by way of the papillae into the renal pelvis, which empties into the ureter. The ureter carries the urine to the bladder.

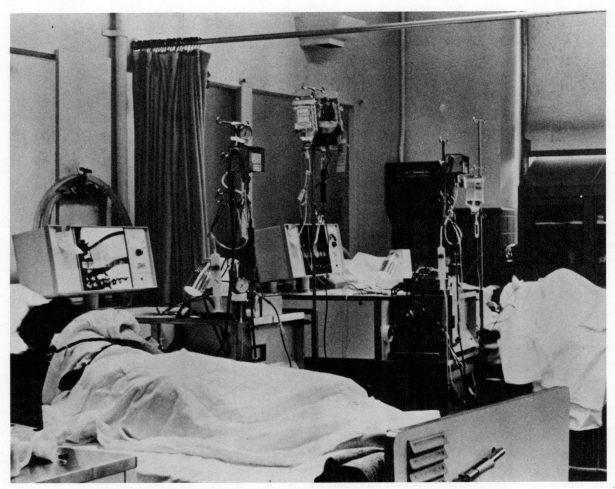

A hospital hemodialysis room. The machines cleanse the patients' blood of waste products which their kidneys can no longer remove.

Acute Kidney Failure

The sudden loss of kidney function over a period of minutes to several days is known as acute kidney failure. It may be caused by impairment of blood supply to the kidneys, by severe infection, by nephritis (discussed below), by poisons, and by various other conditions that injure both kidneys.

The body can function adequately throughout a normal lifespan with only one healthy kidney, but if both are impaired sufficiently over a short period of time, there will be symptoms of acute kidney failure: production of a decreased amount of urine (*oliguria*) sometimes with blood in it; fluid retention in body tissues, a condition known as *edema;* increasing fatigue and weakness; nausea and loss of appetite.

If damage to the kidneys hasn't been too severe, the patient begins to have a *diuresis,* or greater than normal urine output. When this happens—usually after one or two weeks of reduced urine output—he is kept on a restricted diet and reduced fluid intake after recovery until normal kidney function returns.

Dialysis: A new, promising research tool and method of treatment is based on an artificial kidney that cleanses the patient's blood during the period when his own kidneys are not functioning properly. The procedure, known as *dialysis*, still quite expensive and not in widespread use, removes dangerous waste products and excess fluids from the patient's bloodstream. It is the accumulation of waste products and fluids that probably cause the symptoms of acute kidney failure and that can be fatal if not removed in one way or another.

Causes

Heredity is rarely a factor in acute kidney failure, although people born with one kidney or with congenital defects of the urinary tract may lack the normal reserve capacity to prevent it. It is also unusual for external injury to result in a loss of function in both kidneys. However, severe internal shock accompanied by a reduction of blood flow to the kidneys can cause acute kidney failure.

Prevention and Treatment

Acute kidney failure can occur at any age. Prevention hinges on the proper control of its many causes. About 50 percent of patients with this disease may succumb to it; in cases of severe kidney failure involving widespread destruction of tissue, mortality may be almost 100 percent.

When acute kidney failure occurs as a complication of another serious illness, its prevention and treatment are usually managed by doctors in a hospital. If the patient is not already under a doctor's supervision when he has the characteristic symptoms, he should immediately be brought to a medical facility for diagnosis and treatment.

Chronic Kidney Failure and Uremia

Many progressive kidney diseases can eventually lead to a group of symptoms called *uremia*. Other diseases, such as severe high blood pressure, diabetes, and those leading to widespread damage of kidney tissue, can also cause uremia.

In this condition, as in acute kidney failure, waste products and excess fluid accumulate in the body and cause the symptoms of chronic kidney failure. Certain congenital defects in the urinogenital system such as *polycystic kidney disease,* in which cysts in the kidneys enlarge slowly and destroy normal kidney tissue, may lead to uremia. Hereditary diseases such as hereditary nephritis may cause chronic kidney failure, but this is uncommon. Injury is also rarely the cause of uremia.

Although kidney failure is more likely to occur in older people because of the decreased capacity of the body to respond to stress, uremia can occur in any age group if kidney damage is severe enough. The onset of uremia may be so gradual that it goes unnoticed until the patient is weak and seems chronically ill. Voiding unusually large amounts of urine and voiding during the night are early symptoms.

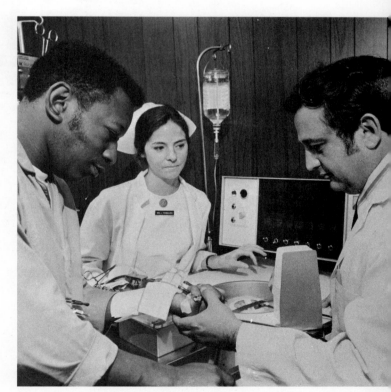

A patient receives instruction that will enable him to undergo dialysis at home with a kidney machine.

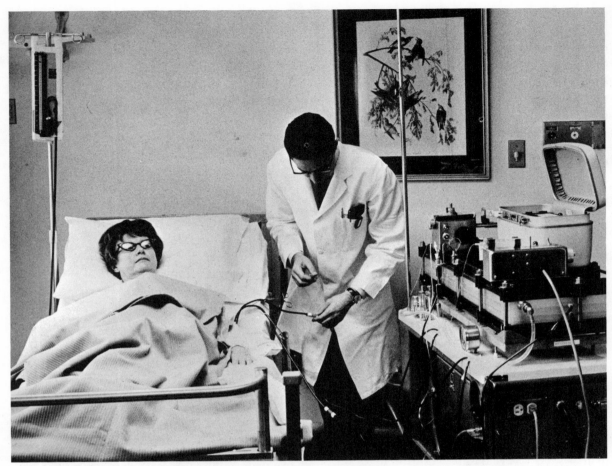

A home dialysis machine in operation. Some hospitals have set up programs for instructing patients in home dialysis, which is considerably less expensive than in-hospital treatment.

Sleepiness and increasing fatigue set in as the kidney failure progresses, and there is a loss of appetite accompanied sometimes by nausea and hiccups. As the disease gets more serious, increasing weakness, anemia, muscle twitching, and sometimes internal bleeding may occur. High blood pressure is another characteristic symptom. Because of fluid retention, there will often be marked signs of facial puffiness and swelling of the legs.

Kidney damage that leads to chronic kidney failure is irreversible and the outlook for the victim of uremia is poor. When the technique of dialysis becomes more practical, it may save many lives. At the present time, there are only limited facilities for its application and the costs are too high for the average family to sustain. The patient must be dialyzed with the artificial kidney unit two or three times a week, usually for six to eight hours at a time. Although the technique does not cure uremia, it can keep the patient comfortable provided that his diet is carefully restricted and supervised. One approach that promises to be helpful in reducing the excessive cost is the development of home dialysis programs prepared with the cooperation of hospitals having departments specializing in kidney disease. Home dialysis is not suitable for everyone, but the overall costs are approximately one-third those of hospital dialysis.

Surgical Kidney Transplant

Some people suffering from kidney disease may benefit greatly from the surgical transplant of a donor's kidney. The donor kidney may be taken from a live relative or from someone recently deceased. The organ is removed from the donor's abdomen, usually flushed with a salt solution, and then re-attached to a large artery and vein in the recipient's abdomen and to his ureter.

The successfully transplanted kidney functions just as the patient's own did when he was healthy, removing wastes and excess fluids from his bloodstream and excreting the resulting urine through the bladder. The recipient of a kidney transplant must take special medication to prevent the rejection of the newly installed organ by his own body tissues. With proper medical care, recipients have lived for many years with their transplanted organs.

Nephritis

Nephritis is a disorder characterized by inflammation of the *glomeruli* of the kidneys. The glomeruli are tiny coiled blood

A kidney transplant can enable the recipient to live a relatively normal life for many years.

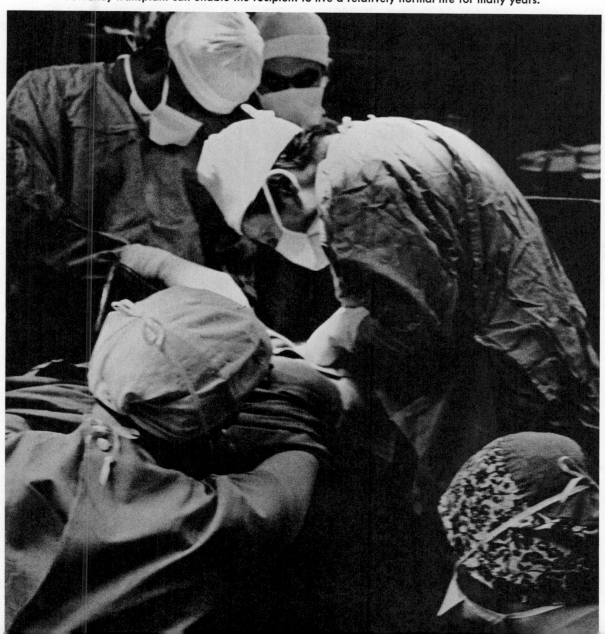

vessels through which the liquid portion of the blood is filtered as it enters the outer structure of the kidneys. There are about one million of these tiny blood vessels in each kidney. The fluid from the blood passes from them into many little ducts called *tubules*. Water and various substances are secreted into and absorbed from the liquid in the tubules. The final product of this passage of filtered fluid from the glomeruli through the tubules to the ureters and then to the bladder is urine. It contains the excess fluid and waste products produced by the body during normal functioning.

When the glomeruli become inflamed, the resulting disease is called *glomerulonephritis*. There are several forms of this disease. One type is thought to be caused by the body's allergic reaction to infection by certain streptococcal bacteria. Another type sometimes accompanies infection of the valves of the heart. The relationship between glomerulonephritis and strep infections is not fully understood at present, and the same may be said for nephritis that is connected with allergic reaction to certain drugs or heart valve infections.

Glomerulonephritis may occur ten days to two weeks after a severe strep throat infection. For this reason, any severe sore throat accompanied by a high fever should be seen and diagnosed by a doctor. Prompt treatment with antibiotics may decrease the possibility of kidney involvement.

Nephritis Symptoms

The inflammation and swelling of the glomeruli causes a decrease in the amount of blood that the kidney is able to filter. As a result of the slowing down of this kidney function, the waste products of metabolism as well as excess fluid accumulate in the body instead of being eliminated at the normal rate.

In a typical case, a person will develop a severe sore throat with fever and a general feeling of sickness. These symptoms will disappear, but after one or two weeks, there will be a return of weakness and loss of appetite. The eyes and the face may become puffy, the legs may swell, and there may be shortness of breath—all because of the retention of excess fluid in the body. The amount of urine is small and the color is dark brown, somewhat like coffee. Abdominal pain, nausea, and vomiting may occur, always accompanied by fatigue. In most cases, the blood pressure increases, leading to headaches.

Although there is a hereditary type of nephritis, the more common types of the disease have other causes. When the disease is suspected, the doctor examines a specimen of urine under a microscope and

NEPHRON

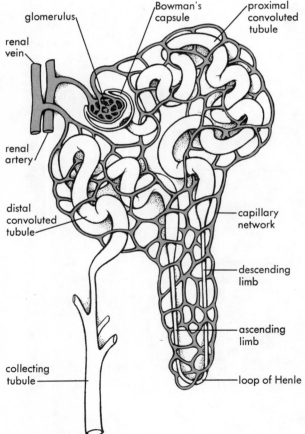

glomerulus

Bowman's capsule

proximal convoluted tubule

renal vein

renal artery

distal convoluted tubule

capillary network

descending limb

ascending limb

collecting tubule

loop of Henle

looks for red blood cells. These cells, which usually do not pass through the walls of the normal glomerulus in large numbers, do pass through the damaged walls of the inflamed blood vessels characteristic of nephritis. Evidence of decreased kidney function is also found by special blood tests.

Nephritis occurs in all age groups. Children under ten have an excellent chance of recovery, about 98 percent. In adults, from 20 to 50 percent of the cases may be fatal or may progress to chronic nephritis, which often leads to uremia and death.

Treatment

It is absolutely essential for anyone with a streptococcal infection, which may lead to acute glomerulonephritis, to receive prompt and proper treatment. Penicillin is considered the most effective antibiotic at present.

Once acute nephritis is present, the treatment consists of bed rest, some fluid restriction, and protein restriction if kidney failure occurs. If there is a total loss of kidney function, a specially restricted diet is prescribed. Complete lack of urine output —*anuria*—may last as long as ten days, but the patient can still make a full recovery if the treatment is right. Usually a gradual return of kidney function occurs over a period of several months.

Nephrosis

The *nephrotic syndrome,* commonly referred to as *nephrosis,* is a disease in which abnormal amounts of protein in the form of *albumin* are lost in the urine. Albumin consists of microscopic particles of protein present in the blood. These particles are important in maintaining the proper volume of fluids in the body, and they have other complicated functions as well. The loss of albumin in the urine affects the amount that remains in the blood, and it is this imbalance, together with other body changes,

that results in the retention of excess fluid in the tissues, thus causing facial puffiness and swelling of the legs.

The disease is caused by damage to the glomeruli, but at the present time the exact nature of the damage is uncertain. It may be caused by an allergic reaction, by inflammation, or it may be a complication of diabetes. The nephrotic syndrome may also appear because of blood clots in the veins that drain the kidneys.

Although the disease is more common among children than among adults, it may affect a person of any age. The main symptom is painless swelling of the face, legs, and sometimes of the entire body. There is also loss of appetite, a tired, rundown feeling, and sometimes abdominal pain, vomiting, and diarrhea.

Recovery from nephrosis varies with age. Over 50 percent of child patients are completely free of kidney ailments after the first attack. Adults are more likely to develop some impairment of kidney function, or the disease may become chronic, with accompanying high blood pressure. In some people, protein loss may continue over the years, although the kidneys function in an apparently normal manner without any visible symptoms.

Treatment

Treatment of the nephrotic syndrome has been greatly helped by the use of the adrenal hormones known as *steroids.* The treatment is effective for about two-thirds of child patients and for about one-fourth to one-third of adults. Some patients may relapse after therapy is completed, sometimes years after such therapy has been discontinued. For this reason, steroids are sometimes continued after initial treatment but in reduced dosage, to avoid some of the unpleasant side effects such as acne and facial swelling.

Unlike the dietary treatment for uremia, a high protein diet is used with nephrotic patients so that the protein loss can be replaced. Salt intake is usually restricted because salt contributes to fluid retention and may cause high blood pressure or heart failure. If fluid retention doesn't respond to steroid treatment, other medicines called *diuretics,* which increase urinary output, are used.

Anyone with unusual swelling of the face, limbs, or abdomen should see a physician promptly. Even though the swelling is painless, it may be the first sign of the onset of a serious kidney problem.

Infection in the Urinary Tract

Infection in the urinary tract is a common disorder that can be serious if the kidneys themselves are involved.

THE FEMALE URINARY SYSTEM

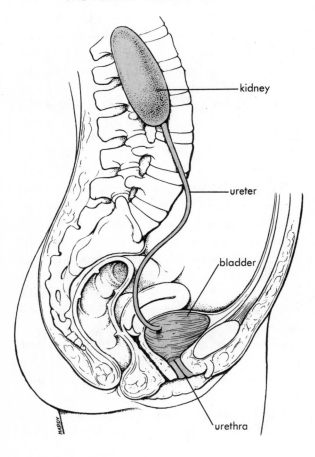

kidney

ureter

bladder

urethra

Cystitis

Infection of the bladder is called *cystitis.* The symptoms include a burning sensation when urine is passed, the frequent need to urinate, occasionally blood in the urine, and sometimes difficulty in starting to urinate. Cystitis is rarely accompanied by high fever.

The problem may be recurrent and is more usual with women than men, probably because the female urethra is shorter and closer to the rectum, permitting bacteria to enter the bladder more easily. These bacteria multiply in the urine contained in the bladder, causing irritation to the bladder walls and producing the symptoms described above.

Cystitis should be treated promptly because the infection in the bladder can easily spread to the kidneys, with serious consequences. Treatment usually consists of antibiotics after urine analysis and culture have determined the type of bacteria causing the infection. Cystitis and other kidney infections are especially common during pregnancy because of the body changes that occur at this time. At no time is cystitis itself a serious disease, but it must be diagnosed and treated promptly to avoid complications.

Other Causes of Infection

Infection of the bladder and kidneys may occur because of poor hygiene in the area of the urethra, especially in women. It is also caused by some congenital defects in the urinary tract or by the insertion of instruments used to diagnose a urinary problem.

Sometimes bacteria in the bloodstream can settle in and infect the kidneys. Patients with diabetes seem to be more prone to urinary infections—indeed to infections generally—than other people. Any obstruction to the flow of urine in the urinary tract, such as a kidney stone, increases the possibility of infection in the area behind the obstruction. Damage to the nerves controlling the bladder is another condition that increases the chances of infection in that area.

Pyelonephritis

Infection in the kidneys is called *pyelonephritis*. Although it sometimes occurs without any symptoms, a first attack usually causes an aching pain in the lower back, probably due to the swelling of the kidneys, as well as nausea, vomiting, diarrhea, and sometimes severe pain in the front of the abdomen, on one or both sides, depending on whether one or both kidneys are involved. Fever may be quite high, ranging from 103 to 105 degrees, often accompanied by chills.

Although the symptoms of pyelonephritis may disappear in a few days without treatment, bacterial destruction of the kidney tissue may be going on. This silent type of infection can eventually disrupt normal kidney function and result in a chronic form of the disease, which in turn can lead to uremia. If the disease is not halted before this, it can be fatal.

Anyone with symptoms of acute pyelonephritis must have prompt medical attention. In order to diagnose the disease properly, the urine is analyzed and the number and type of bacteria in the urine are determined. The disease is brought under control by the right antibiotics and by administering large amounts of fluids to flush out the kidneys and urinary tract, thus decreasing the number of bacteria in the urine. In its chronic form the disease is much more difficult to cure, since bacteria that are lodged deep in the kidney tissue do not seem to be susceptible to antibiotics and are therefore almost impossible to get rid of.

Kidney Stones

Another cause of infection in the bladder and kidneys is obstruction in the urinary tract by *kidney stones*. These stones, crystallizations of salts that form in the kidney tissue, may be quite small, but they can grow large enough to occupy a considerable part of one or both of the kidneys. The smaller ones often pass from the kidney through the ureters to the bladder, from which they are voided through the urethra. However, obstruction of the flow of urine behind a kidney stone anywhere in the urinary tract usually leads to infection in the urine. This type of infection may lead to attacks of acute pyelonephritis.

Removal of stones: For this reason, unless the stone causes no symptoms of infection, it must be removed. Removal may be accomplished by flushing out the urinary tract with large fluid intake or by surgical methods. Any accompanying infection is treated with antibiotics.

Why kidney stones form in some people and not in others is not clearly understood. Because of metabolic disorders, certain substances may build up in the body. The increased excretion of these substances in the urine as well as excessive amounts of calcium in the blood may encourage kidney-stone formation. People who have gout are also likely to develop them.

Renal colic: Sometimes the formation and passage of stones cause no symptoms. However, when symptoms do occur with the passage of a kidney stone, they can be uncomfortably severe. The pain that results from the passage of a stone through the ureter, referred to as *renal colic,* is usually like an intense cramp. It begins in the side or back and moves toward the lower abdomen, the genital region, and the inner thigh on the affected side. The attack may last for a few minutes or for several hours. Sometimes bloody urine may be passed accompanied by a burning sensation.

Kidney stones are more likely to form in middle-aged and older people than in young ones. A history of stones is sometimes found in several generations of a family, since the metabolic disorders encouraging their formation have a hereditary basis.

Treatment for an acute attack of renal colic usually relieves the pain several hours after the patient has taken medication and fluids. If they are not promptly treated, kidney stones may lead to serious infection and eventual impairment of function.

Tumors of the Urinary Tract

Benign and malignant tumors of the kidney are not common problems. However, anyone with pain in the midback, blood in the urine, or a mass in the abdomen should have the symptoms diagnosed. If a malignant tumor is discovered early enough, it can be removed with the affected kidney, and normal function can be maintained by the healthy kidney that remains.

Malignant kidney tumors are most often found in children or adults over 40, and more often in men than in women. A tumor of any type can usually be diagnosed by X-ray studies. Where this technique is inadequate, an operation is necessary to search for the suspected growth. About one-fourth of all patients with a malignant kidney tumor live for more than ten years after surgery.

A malignant tumor of the bladder is a serious problem since it obstructs kidney drainage and may cause death from uremia. The main symptom is the painless appearance of blood in the urine, although sometimes a burning sensation and a frequent need to urinate are also present. Treatment usually includes surgical removal of the bladder and radiation treatment of the affected area to destroy any malignant cells that remain after the operation.

Some malignant bladder tumors grow very slowly and do not invade the bladder wall extensively. Surgical treatment for this type, called *papillary tumors*, is likely to be more successful than for tumors of the more invasive kind.

The Prostate Gland

The *prostate gland,* which contributes to the production of semen, encircles the base of the male urethra where it joins the bladder. When it begins to enlarge, it compresses the urethra and causes difficulty in voiding. Urination may be difficult to start, and when the urine stream appears it may be thinner than normal.

Since urine may remain in the bladder, there is the possibility of local infection that may spread to the kidneys. If the kidneys become enlarged because of this type of obstruction, a condition of *hydronephrosis* is said to exist. This disease can cause impaired kidney function and lead to uremia.

Benign Prostatic Enlargement

Enlargement of the prostate gland occurs in about half the male population over 50, and the incidence increases with increasing age. The condition is called *benign prostatic enlargement* and must be treated surgically if sufficient obstruction is present. For temporary relief, a catheter can be inserted into the bladder through the urethra, allowing the urine to drain through the catheter and out of the body. If surgery is necessary, the entire prostate may be removed or only that part of it that surrounds the urethra.

Symptoms of benign prostatic enlargement are quite distinctive: increased difficulty in voiding; an urge to continue to urinate after voiding has been completed; burning and frequent urination, caused in part by infection from urine retained in the bladder.

The cause of benign prostatic enlargement is thought to be a change during the aging process in the hormones that affect prostate tissue, but the exact nature of the change and its effect is not clear. It is likely that hormone-containing medicines will eventually be developed that will prevent or reverse prostate tissue growth.

THE MALE URINARY SYSTEM

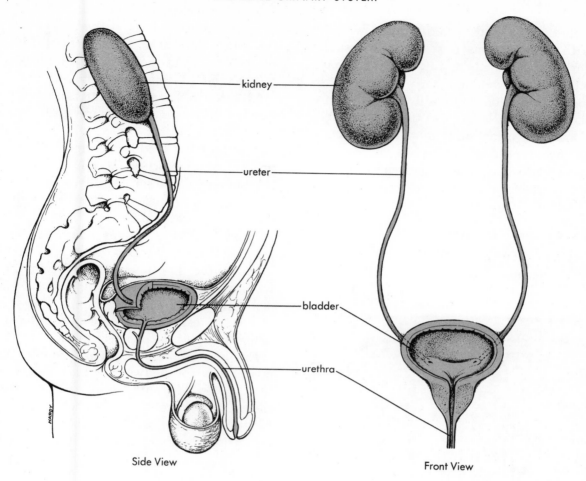

kidney

ureter

bladder

urethra

Side View   Front View

Cancer of the Prostate

Cancer of the prostate is a common type of malignancy in older men. It accounts for about 10 percent of male deaths from cancer in the United States. The disease may be present without any symptoms or interference with normal function and is therefore difficult to diagnose. A very high proportion of men over 80—probably more than 50 percent—has been found to have had cancer of the prostate at autopsy.

When symptoms are present, they are likely to be the same as those of benign prostatic enlargement. The disease can be diagnosed only by a biopsy examination of a tissue sample taken from the prostate dur-

ing surgery. If malignancy is found, the gland is surgically removed when feasible to do so; the testes are removed too so that the level of male hormones in the body is lowered.

Male hormones increase the growth of malignant prostate tissue, but since female hormones slow it down, they may be administered after a diagnosis of prostate malignancy. If the tumor has spread to bone tissue, radiation treatment of the affected areas may slow down cancerous growth and relieve pain.

Men over 40 should have a rectal examination once a year, since tumors of the prostate and benign prostatic enlargement can often be diagnosed early in this way.

Bedwetting

Enuresis, the medical term for bedwetting, is the unintentional loss of urine, usually during sleep at night. Infants do not have sufficiently developed nervous systems to control urination voluntarily until they are about two-and-a-half or three years old. Controlling urination through the night may not occur until after the age of three. A child who wets his bed recurrently after he has learned to control urination has the problem of enuresis.

Causes and Treatment

There are many causes of enuresis. It may occur because of a delay in normal develop-

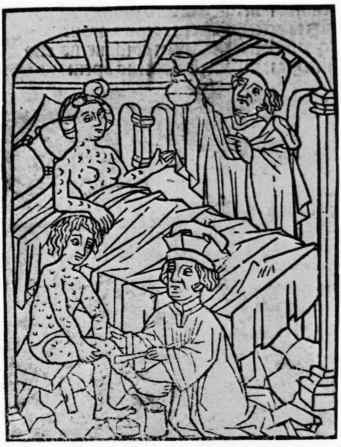

A 15th-century woodcut illustrating the treatment of venereal disease patients who display the body rashes that are characteristic of secondary-stage syphilis.

ment or as a result of emotional stress. About 15 percent of boys and 10 percent of girls are bedwetters at the age of 5. By 9, about 5 percent of all children still have the problem, but most children outgrow it by the time they reach puberty.

Children who are bedwetters should be examined to rule out any physical abnormality in the urinary tract. Obstruction at the neck of the bladder where it joins the urethra or obstruction at the end of the urethra may cause uncontrollable dribbling of urine, but this usually occurs during the day as well as at night.

Disease of the nerves controlling the bladder, sometimes hereditary, can cause loss of urine. It can also occur in children who are mentally retarded or mentally ill, or because of an acute or chronic illness. In the latter cases, the problem disappears when the child regains his health.

Emotional problems: If all physical abnormalities for bedwetting have been explored and eliminated as possible causes, the emotional problems of the child and his family should be examined. An understanding attitude rather than a hostile or punitive one on the part of the parents is extremely important in helping a child who is a bedwetter. He may be anxious about school or angry at a favored younger child, or he may feel insecure about parental acceptance. In such cases, an effort to bring the child's hidden feelings into the open and to deal with them sympathetically usually cause the problem to disappear.

Venereal Disease

Venereal diseases are those which are transmitted by sexual contact. The most common are syphilis and gonorrhea, although several others are transmitted in the same way. Since they are highly contagious and can cause serious complications, the symptoms should be treated by a doctor without any delay.

Syphilis

Syphilis is caused by the type of microscopic organism known as a *spirochete*. The spirochete cannot survive outside the body for more than a brief period unless it is frozen. It is transmitted through the membranes of the reproductive system by direct sexual contact or through a break in the skin.

Primary stage: Such transmission leads to an initial sore, usually an ulcerated area called a *chancre,* on the penis, vagina, or any other area in contact with the spirochetes, including the fingers, lips, or breasts. The primary lesion, as the chancre is called, is usually a single one and not painful, although there are occasional exceptions. Any sore in the genital region should be examined by a physician. If the sore is actually a chancre, a specimen examined under a microscope will contain the spirochetes that cause syphilis. Certain blood tests also reveal the presence of the disease, but they require a waiting period before they turn positive.

Secondary stage: There are no symptoms when the spirochetes enter the body, but the chancre usually appears about three to six weeks later. It heals without treatment, sometimes leaving a scar. About six weeks after its appearance, there is usually a skin eruption that takes various forms. The rash signals the onset of the secondary stage of syphilis. The rash may consist of many small pigmented spots or wider areas of darkened pigmentation, often involving the entire body, including the palms, soles, and face. The rash may be accompanied by itching.

All the affected areas contain spirochetes and are therefore infectious. In addition to the rash, there are general symptoms of illness at this stage, such as sore throat, fatigue, headaches, fever, muscle pain, and sometimes temporary loss of scalp hair.

In some cases, the infected person does not experience either the primary or sec-

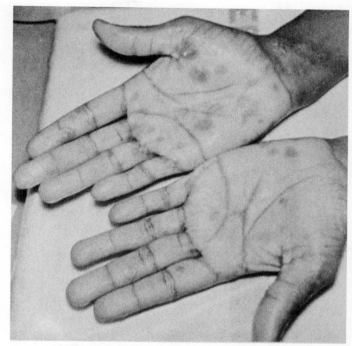

The onset of the secondary stage of syphilis is often signaled by a rash covering the entire body, including the palms of the hands and the soles of the feet.

ondary phase of the illness, and there may be no history of symptoms until the onset of the third stage of syphilis, many years after the first contact with the spirochete. However, a blood test will be positive in almost all cases of secondary syphilis.

Tertiary stage: The characteristic rash and other symptoms of secondary syphilis will also disappear without treatment in the same way as the chancre of the primary stage. Then a stage of latent syphilis may occur in which the spirochete is present for many years—sometimes for an entire lifetime—without doing further harm or causing further symptoms.

In many cases, however, the syphilis spirochetes seriously damage various organs, particularly the heart and brain. These late effects that appear years after the first untreated infection are called tertiary syphilis.

Neurosyphilis affects the brain and spinal cord, causing progressive loss of the mental faculties, eventual insanity, and death. Damage to the aorta, the main artery leading from the heart, can cause heart failure and the formation of an *aneurysm*, in which the wall of the aorta becomes weak and swollen. The rupture of such an aneurysm is likely to be fatal.

Although the devastating effects of tertiary syphilis are rarely seen today, they can result from lack of treatment or inadequate treatment of the early stages of the disease. Therefore, symptoms of primary or secondary syphilis, or knowledge of contact with a possible source of infection, makes medical attention absolutely essential.

Ninety percent of the deaths from syphilis are the result of the involvement of the heart and nervous system. Almost any part of the body may be involved in the tertiary stage, but even when the disease is this advanced, proper treatment can greatly improve the function of the damaged organ.

Children born of mothers having syphilis during pregnancy may have congenital syphilis at birth. These children require a great deal of special care if they are to survive the effects of this disease.

Treatment: Penicillin is extremely effective in killing the syphilis spirochete and should be called a wonder drug if only for this special role. However, proper and early treatment for the many forms of syphilis is a problem for many doctors, since the entire responsibility for seeking medical attention rests with the person exposed to the disease.

The possibility of catching or transmitting syphilis can be lessened by the use of a prophylactic condom. It is because of the widespread use of the contraceptive pill and the decreased use of the condom that the incidence of syphilis is presently on the rise. Even under these circumstances, without the protection afforded by the condom, washing the genital region thoroughly with soap and water after sexual relations will reduce the possibility of infection. Penicillin in the proper dosage immediately after suspected contact with syphilis will prevent infection altogether in most cases.

Gonorrhea

Gonorrhea is among the most common bacterial infectious diseases in the United States today. It is caused by a bacterium called the *gonococcus*. Infection with this organism causes the formation of pus composed of dead white blood cells and tissues on the lining of the genital tract. The urethra, the Fallopian tubes in women, the prostate in men, and other parts of the reproductive system of either sex may be subject to the infection, which causes a heavy white discharge from the penis and sometimes from the vagina.

In women, the infection may cause fever and low abdominal pain with or without the discharge. Since gonorrhea may occur without any symptoms at all, unsuspected damage to the female reproductive system can eventually lead to sterility. Infections of the joints and other parts of the body may occur if the gonococcus spreads through the bloodstream, but these complications are rare so long as penicillin is administered promptly.

The discharge from the urethra in the male usually occurs three to seven days after contact with an infected partner. Symptoms include a severe burning sensation during urination, a heavy white discharge, and occasional lower abdominal pain. A testicle may become swollen when infected.

The disease is diagnosed by a microscopic examination of the discharge. If the gonococcus is present, penicillin is administered. In cases where the gonococcus strain is resistant to this treatment, various other antibiotics are tested in the laboratory on a culture of the resistant bacteria. Immediate and adequate treatment is essential to prevent the complications of sterility and the spread of infection.   SEW

CANCER

Cancer has always figured uniquely in the diseases of mankind. For centuries people spoke of it only in whispers, or not at all, as if the disease were not only dreadful but somehow shameful as well. Today, the picture is changing, and rapidly. This decade may see the time—undreamt of only scant years ago—when half of those stricken by cancer will survive its ravages. And much of the mystery that cloaked the disease in an awful shroud has been dissipated, although the last veils remain to be stripped away.

Of course, cancer remains a formidable enemy. Close to a million Americans are suffering from it; an estimated 335,000 will die of it annually. Of all those Americans now alive, some 52 million—one in four—will be stricken; and some 34 million will die. Cancer is the greatest cause of lost working years among women, and ranks third after accidents and heart disease in denying men working years.

But in context, the picture is not as bleak as it might seem. At the beginning of the century, survival from cancer was relatively rare. At the end of the 1930s, the five-year survival rate (alive after five years) was one in five or less. Ten years later it had shot up to one in four, and in the mid-fifties to one in three. This figure has remained relatively stable because the survival rate for some of the more widespread cancers has leveled off despite the best efforts of physicians to devise better forms of treatment. For such cancers, which include those of the breast, colon, and rectum, improvements will come through earlier detection and even prevention. Dr. Richard S. Doll, Professor of Medicine at Oxford University, has said that we could prevent 40 percent of men's cancer deaths, and 10 percent of women's, simply by applying what we already know. For example, according to the president of the American Cancer Society,

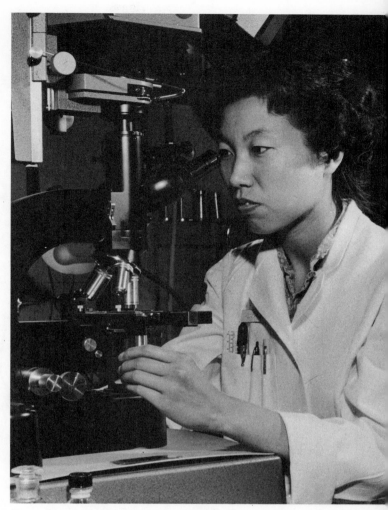

Continuing medical research has led to encouraging progress in the war against cancer. Here a scientist screens a slide in a study relating to cellular division.

roughly one-sixth of the total cancer deaths in 1969 would not have occurred if it had not been for cigarette smoking.

Still, considerable progress is being made on many fronts in the war against cancer. These range from advances in early detection to breakthroughs in treatment. The last 20 years have seen a 50 percent dip in the death rate from cervical cancer, mostly because of widening acceptance of the Pap test, which can detect the disease at a very early stage. At the same time, children with acute lymphocytic leukemia, which used to be invariably fatal in weeks or months, have benefited from new therapies, with at least half now surviving three years, some more than five years, and a few on the verge of being pronounced "cured." Similar advances have been made in a cancer of the lymph system called *Hodgkin's disease.*

The mortality rates for some forms of cancer are dropping for no known reason. Stomach cancer, for example, produces only indigestion as an early symptom, so most patients do not get the benefit of early diagnosis. The result is a rather poor five-year survival rate. There are an estimated 17,000 new cases each year, and an estimated 15,000 deaths. Nevertheless, the mortality rate for stomach cancer has dropped about 40 percent in the last 20 years; nobody knows why.

What Is Cancer?

Cancer would surely be easier to detect and treat if it were a single entity with a single simple cause. But it is not. Experts

NORMAL CELLS

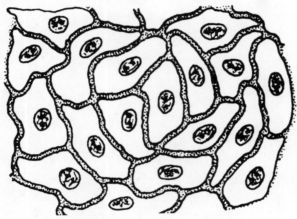

1. Cell surface bonding is strong.
2. Cells remain in place.
3. Electrical voltage level is high.
4. Cells divide at a low rate.

MALIGNANT CELLS

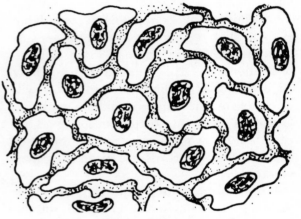

1. Cell surface bonding is very weak.
2. Cells spread and invade normal tissue.
3. Electrical voltage level is low.
4. Cells divide at a rapid pace.

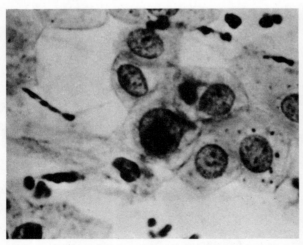
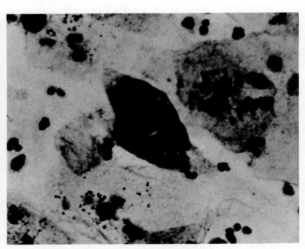

Cancer begins when normal body cells lose their normal growth and development controls and begin to proliferate, often very rapidly and without any apparent limit to growth.

agree that there are actually some 200 different diseases that can be called cancers. They have different causes, originate in different tissues, develop for different reasons and in different ways, and demand vastly different kinds of treatment. All have one fatal element in common, however: in every case, normal cells have gone wild and lost their normal growth and development controls.

The cancer may start with just one or a few cells somewhere in the body which undergo a change and become malignant, or cancerous. The cells divide and reproduce themselves, and the cancer grows.

Most cancers arise on the surface of a tissue, such as the skin, the lining of the uterus, mouth, stomach, bowel, bladder, or bronchial tube in the lung, or inside a duct in the breast, prostate gland, or other site. Eventually, they grow from a microscopic clump to a visible mass, then begin to invade underlying tissues. As long as the cells remain in one mass, however, the cancer is localized. But at some later phase, in a process called *metastasis,* some of the cancer cells split off and are swept into the lymph channels or bloodstream to other parts of the body. They may be captured for a while in a nearby lymph node (a stage called regional involvement), but unless the disease is arrested, it will rapidly invade the rest of the body, with death the almost certain result. Some cancers grow with an almost malevolent rapidity, some are dormant by comparison. Some respond to various therapies, such as radiation therapy; others do not. About half of the known types of cancer are incurable at almost any stage. Of the remaining half, it is obviously imperative to diagnose and treat them as early as possible.

The cancers described above, arising in *epithelial* (covering or lining) tissue are called *carcinomas* as a group. Another class of malignant tumors, similar in most basic respects, is the *sarcomas,* which originate in connective tissue such as bones and muscles. A third group of cancers—*leukemia* and the *lymphomas*—are diseases of the blood-forming organs and the lymphatic system, respectively, and are not tumors. They arise and spread in a basically different way.

What Causes Cancer?

What makes the first cell turn malignant? We know a great deal about the factors that can produce cancer in human beings. They include a large number of chemical agents including those in tobacco smoke; ionizing radiation such as that from X rays, nuclear bombs, and sunlight; injury or repeated irritation; metal or plastic implants; flaws in the body's immune reaction; genetic mistakes; parasites; and—we think—viruses. It is this last factor that is generating perhaps the most interest among scientists today. We know that viruses cause a variety of cancers in animals; yet they have never been proved responsible in human cancer, although they have been linked to at least six different ones. Recently, researchers discovered an enzyme in a virus believed to cause cancer and also in the tissues of leukemia patients. This enzyme may be the key to the mechanism by which a virus induces a malignant change in normal cells.

Six Major Cancer Sites

Obviously, it is impossible to discuss all the forms of cancer in a work of this scope. The following material deals with what the American Cancer Society describes as the six major sites of cancer: lung, breast, colon-rectum, uterus, skin, and oral. They are the cancers that offer the greatest opportunity for saving lives, either through prevention (as in lung cancer) or through early diagnosis and therapy. Together, they add up to 60 percent of all cancer cases in this country and 50 percent of all deaths.

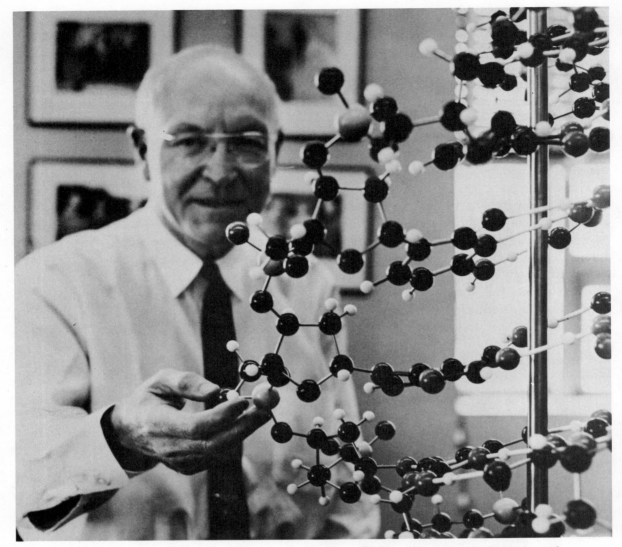

Many viruses are known to cause cancer in animals, and although this has not been proved in human cancer, it is one of the most widely-held theories of the cause of leukemia today. One of the foremost scientists in this field is Dr. Wendell Stanley, of the University of California, Berkeley, shown here with a three-dimensional model of the DNA molecule. DNA occurs in the nucleus of all cells and is found in most viruses, including those known to cause cancer.

Lung Cancer

Lung cancer kills more Americans than any other cancer. The average annual death toll for recent years is over 50,000 men and over 10,000 women. It represents 17 percent of all cancers in men, 4 percent of all cancers in women. And there has been a steady increase in the incidence of lung cancer in both men and women over the last 35 years—especially so in men, among whom the mortality rate has gone up 15 times. In 1965, women accounted for 1 in 8 lung cancer mortalities; the figure now is 1 in 6. The current chances of being cured of this disease are no more than 5 or 6 percent.

Causes of lung cancer: Lung cancer is one of the most preventable of all malignancies. Most cases, the majority of medical experts agree, are caused by smoking cigarettes. The U.S. Public Health Service has indicted smoking as "the main cause of lung cancer in men." Even when other agents are known to produce lung cancers—uranium ore dust or asbestos fibers, for example—cigarette smoking enormously boosts the risk among uranium miners and asbestos workers. In fact, the incidence of lung cancer in such

men is higher than the rate expected by merely adding the two probabilities together.

Various theories have been proposed to explain the mechanism by which smoking causes cancer in human beings; none has been proved. But it is known that the lungs of some cigarette smokers show tissue changes before cancer appears, changes

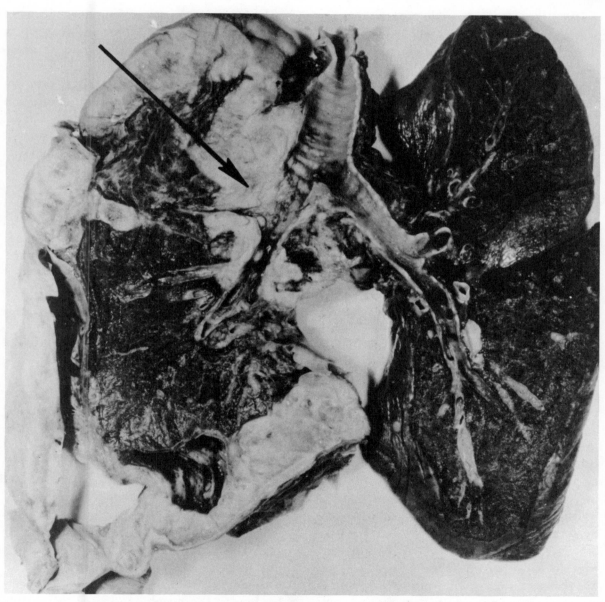

Although scientists do not yet understand the exact way in which cigarette smoking causes cancer, the cause-and-effect relationship has been established. Shown here are the lungs of a heavy smoker, with the arrow indicating the site of cancer.

apparently caused by irritation of the lining of the *bronchi*—the large air tubes in the lung. Physicians believe these changes can be reversed before the onset of cancer if the source of irritation—smoking—is removed. This is why a heavy smoker who has been puffing away for many years but then stops smoking has a better chance of avoiding lung cancer than one who continues smoking.

Until recently, the evidence linking cigarette smoking and lung cancer was purely statistical, although overwhelming. No one had succeeded in producing lung cancer in laboratory animals by having them smoke. In 1970, however, the American Cancer Society announced that lung cancer had been induced in beagle dogs specially trained to inhale cigarette smoke.

Cigarette smoking has also been implicated in other kinds of lung disease, including the often-fatal emphysema, and in cardiovascular diseases. To any sensible person, then, the options would seem clear; if you don't smoke, don't start. If you do smoke, stop. If you can't stop, cut down, and switch to a brand low in tars and nicotine—suspected but not proved to be the principal harmful agents in cigarette smoke.

Detection: If many lives could be saved by preventing lung cancer in the first place, others could be saved by early detection. By the time most lung cancers are diagnosed, it is too late even for the most radical approach to cure—removal of the afflicted lung. Experts estimate that up to ten times the present cure rate of five percent could be achieved if very early lung cancers could be spotted. They therefore recommend a routine chest X ray every six months for everyone over 45.

Symptoms: Although some early lung cancers do not show up on an X-ray film, they are the ones that usually produce cough as an early symptom. For this reason, any cough that lasts more than two or three weeks—even if it seems to accompany a

cold or bronchitis—should be regarded as suspicious and investigated in that light. Blood in the sputum is another early warning sign that must be investigated immediately; so should wheezing when breathing. Later symptoms include shortness of breath and pain in the chest, fever, and night sweats.

Breast Cancer

Breast cancer is the commonest form of cancer and the leading source of death from cancer among American women. Indeed, it is the leading cause of death from all causes among women aged 40–44. It produces an estimated 70,000 new cases, and an estimated 31,000 deaths annually. Of all American women living, based on current projections, 6 out of every 100 will one day contract the disease.

Cancer of the breast may occur as early as the teens, but this is rare; it is found most often in women of middle age and beyond, dropping to second place in cause of cancer death only in women who are aged 75 or over.

Symptoms: Its first symptom is often a lump in the breast, usually quite painless. (Pain in the breast is rarely caused by cancer.) The lump may appear anywhere in the breast, but the most frequent site is the upper, outer quarter. Such lumps are not necessarily malignant—chances are that any given one, especially in a woman below 45, is not. From 65 to 80 percent of all women whose breast tissue is sampled (biopsied) for tumor are found to have a benign condition.

If the tumor is allowed to grow unchecked, it may cause pulling of the skin from within, visible as a flattening of the breast or a dimpling of the skin, or a sinking, tilting, or flattening of the nipple. Less frequently, the tumor starts in the ducts leading to the nipple, and causes irritation of the skin of the nipple and a moist discharge, which eventually forms a scab.

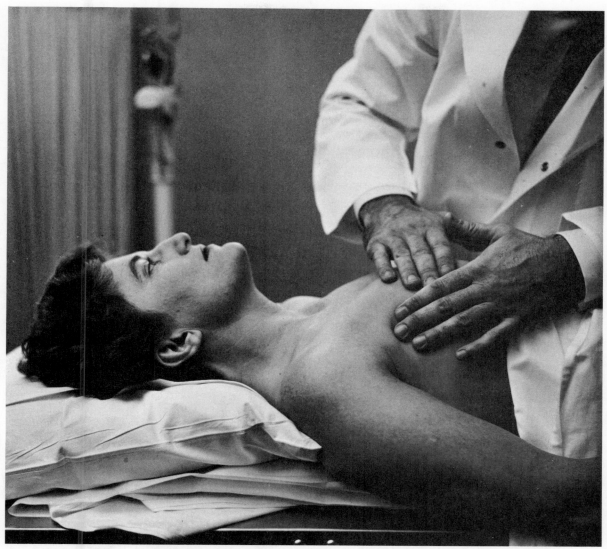

A doctor giving a breast examination for cancer. Early detection saves the lives of thousands of women, but breast cancer is still the leading source of cancer death among American women.

It is vital—literally a matter of life and death—for a woman to report any such symptom to her doctor immediately. For breast cancer is, fortunately, one of those varieties of cancer that can be cured in the large majority of cases, provided it is detected early enough. If breast cancer is treated while it is still restricted to the breast, the five-year survival rate (in other words, the proportion of women who are alive five years later, essentially cured) is 85 percent. But if treatment begins after the malignancy has spread to the lymph node in the armpit, the five-year survival rate is only about 35 percent.

Detection: Some 95 percent of all breast cancers are discovered by the woman herself, when she notices a lump. But in far too many instances, she reports it when the lump has become quite large—about two inches across—whereas careful self-examination can disclose lumps only one-half inch across or even smaller. This difference in size represents, in typical patients, a time lapse of 6 to 12 months—that's about how long it takes the tumor mass to grow that amount. Those months have meant for many, many women the difference between life and death.

The American Cancer Society and the National Cancer Institute recommend that every woman follow a prescribed method of self-examination just after the menstrual period, continuing every month after the change of life. The procedure consists of carefully looking at and feeling the breasts, and takes only a few minutes. A detailed description of the proper procedure is available in pamphlet form from the Superintendent of Documents, U.S. Government Printing Office, Washington, D.C. 20402 for ten cents. Ask for Public Health Service Publication No. 1730. A film entitled "Breast

Self-Examination," produced by the American Cancer Society and the National Cancer Institute, is also available.

To detect breast cancer at an even earlier stage, that is, when the tumor is considerably less than a half-inch in diameter, more sophisticated methods are used. Two that are now in standard medical practice are mammography and thermography.

Mammography is a specialized form of X raying, and can detect very small abnormal tumor masses. The Health Insurance Plan of Greater New York conducted a test program, after which it reported the following: in a group of 31,000 women who were mammographed regularly, the mortality rate of those who contracted breast cancer was cut to 18.1 percent, compared to 33.7 percent mortality in a control group of women

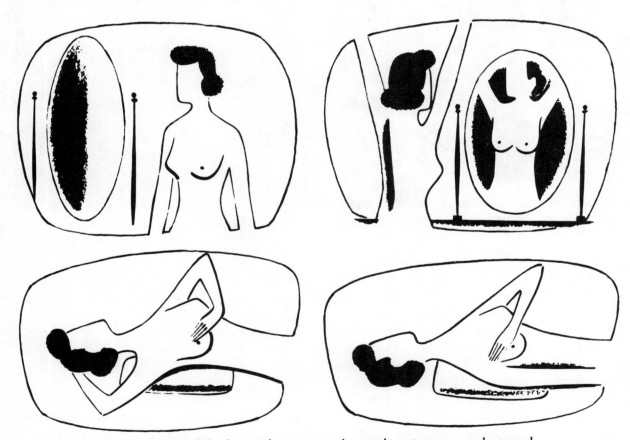

Self-examination of the breasts has uncovered many breast cancers early enough for cure. It consists of careful scrutiny of the breasts with arms lowered and then raised, and palpation, or feeling, with the flat of the fingers while lying on the back.

who used self-examination only. The same Health Insurance Plan is embarked on testing thermography and evaluating its usefulness compared with mammography.

Thermography measures the surface temperature of the skin of the breast with heat-sensitive devices and an infra-red camera. Most breast cancers cause a rise in temperature at the surface. Some authorities have suggested that a combination of the two methods, perhaps once a year, together with monthly self-examination, could detect virtually all breast cancers at a very early stage.

Several other detection techniques are under investigation, but are in the experimental stage as yet. They include a device that relies on *xerography*—a method used in copying machines, and ultrasonic probing with very-high-frequency sound waves.

Therapy: Once it is discovered, breast cancer is treated primarily by surgery, with the possibility of other therapies such as radiation, drugs, hormones, or a combination of these.

The usual approach, after cancer has been diagnosed, is a surgical procedure called a *radical mastectomy,* in which the affected breast, the underlying chest muscles, and the lymph glands in the armpit (into which the breast drains) are all removed. The aim is to block the possible spread of malignant cells throughout the body via the lymph system.

Male and female sex hormones and other hormones such as cortisone also help control breast cancer in some cases, and so may radiation therapy and certain powerful chemical agents. Because of the relation of sex hormones to breast cancer, a physician may recommend that the patient's ovaries be surgically removed. Some of these therapies may be used in conjunction with the mastectomy, or they may be called on to arrest the spread of advanced cancer in inoperable cases or where surgery has come too late.

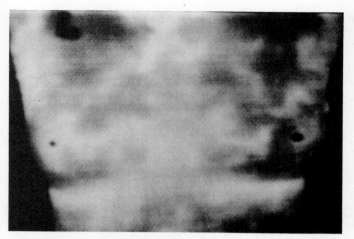

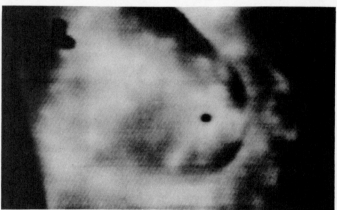

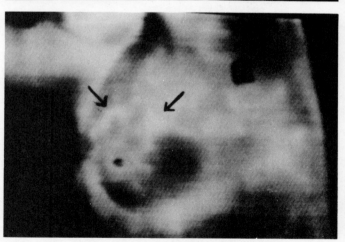

Thermograms, pictures of heat radiation of body tissues, can sometimes reveal the presence of a breast tumor that could not be discovered by touch. The tissue of tumors has a distinctively higher temperature than normal tissue. (*Top*) A typical thermogram, with lightest shades reflecting warmest areas. The other thermograms show an abnormal pattern of temperature elevation in both breasts. Arrows point to a hot quadrant and a dilated vein produced by the lesion.

You might want to know cancer's seven warning signals. So if you spot one you'll get the message.

And the message is—see your doctor. Pronto.
Sure a signal can be a false alarm. But then again, it just might be the real thing. And if it is, the sooner you act, the better the chance to beat cancer.
These are the signals to be on the lookout for:

1. Unusual bleeding or discharge.
2. A lump or thickening in the breast or elsewhere.
3. A sore that does not heal.
4. Change in bowel or bladder habits.
5. Hoarseness or cough.
6. Indigestion or difficulty in swallowing.
7. Change in size or color of a wart or mole.

Be alert to these signals. If one lasts more than two weeks, see your doctor.

End of message.

**american
cancer
society**

The American Cancer Society's poster points out suspicious symptoms that should not be ignored.

Over the years, some doctors have felt that the radical mastectomy is *too* radical. Although most women adjust to its consequences eventually, the operation is a drastic one. (There are local and national clubs of mastectomy patients to help women having a difficult physical or psychological transition.) The doubting doctors believe that a simple mastectomy, perhaps assisted by irradiation of the lymph nodes, would show just as good a cure rate with much less pain and disfigurement. In a simple mastectomy, only the breast itself is removed, and the muscles of the chest wall and lymph glands in the armpit are left intact.

To resolve the issue, a scientifically controlled experiment involving hundreds of women will be carried out under the auspices of the National Cancer Institute. Surgeons will perform both types of operation, using carefully screened groups. Within three years, perhaps less, we should have some clear indication of whether the radical operation really offers any greater chances of success.

Causes of breast cancer: Why do some women get breast cancer whereas most do not? There are many tantalizing clues but no answers yet. For example, the occurrence of the disease is very high in the United States, Canada, and several northern European countries, but very low in Japan. It is also rare in Japanese women living in the United States. Some researchers believe the reason may lie in a higher thyroid activity in Japanese women, which in turn affects their hormone balance. A study is now underway to learn whether women with greater than normal risk of developing breast cancer can be identified by the hormones they excrete.

Other investigators have reported that viruses may be a causative agent of breast cancer in some cases. Two kinds of virus-like particles have been found in human breast tumors and in the milk of breast cancer patients. Work along these lines might make possible the use of drugs or other biological agents to interfere with the reproduction of the virus.

Colon-Rectum Cancer

Cancer of the colon (large intestine) and rectum is the second leading cause of cancer death in the United States. Each year it claims an estimated 46,000 lives, and produces about 75,000 new cases—more than any other kind of cancer except skin cancer. It afflicts men and women about equally. The five-year survival rate from this form of cancer, usually after surgery, is 69 percent where the cancer was localized and 39 percent where there was regional involvement. However, authorities now believe that this rate could be upped to some 75 percent through early enough diagnosis and prompt treatment.

Symptoms: It is important, then, to be alert to the early symptoms of these cancers. Cancers of the colon often produce changes in bowel habits that persist longer than normal. The change may be constipation or diarrhea, or even both alternating. Cancers of the colon also often produce large quantities of gas, which cause abdominal discomfort ranging from a feeling of overfullness to pain, intermittent at first and then coming as regular cramps.

Both colon cancer and rectal cancer may also cause bleeding. Sometimes such bleeding is evidenced in the stool or on the tissue (the most frequent first sign of rectal cancer); but if the bleeding is slight and occurs high enough up the colon, it may not be visible at all. After a period of weeks, however, the persistent bleeding causes anemia in the patient.

All such symptoms should be investigated promptly. Unfortunately, many persons tend—or prefer—to ignore them. Chronic constipation, for example, or gas, is easy to dismiss for the nuisance that it usually is. Even rectal bleeding, which de-

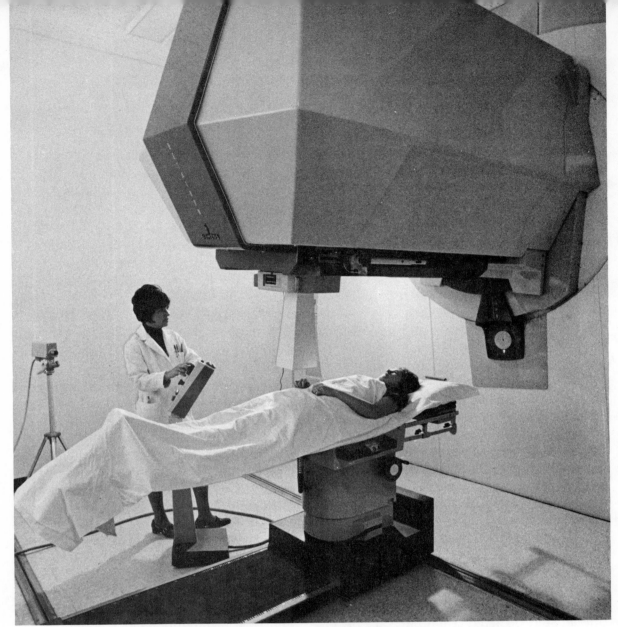

This powerful betatron at the Boston University Medical Center, used to treat cancer by irradiation, has a capacity of 42 million electron volts.

mands immediate medical consultation, is ignored by hemorrhoid sufferers, who fail to realize that hemorrhoids and cancer, though unrelated, can and sometimes do exist in the same persons at the same time.

Detection: For these reasons, the key to successful and early diagnosis of colon and rectum cancer lies in making a *proctoscopy* part of the regular annual health checkup. In this procedure, performed in a doctor's office, a lighted tube called a *proctoscope* is passed into the rectum. Through it, the

doctor can examine the walls visually for signs of tumor. If the physician thinks it advisable to check the sigmoid colon also, the procedure is called a *proctosigmoidoscopy,* and a similar instrument called a *sigmoidoscope* is used. The American Cancer Society now recommends that everyone over age 40 have a proctoscopy or proctosigmoidoscopy in routine annual checkups.

Therapy: The indicated treatment for colon-rectum cancer is surgical removal of the affected part of the bowel. Adjacent portions and related lymph nodes may also be removed, and if the surgeon sees that the cancer is widespread, he may have to perform extensive surgery. This may require that he create a *colostomy*—a temporary or permanent opening in the abdominal wall through which solid wastes may pass. Although this method of voiding the bowels is somewhat inconvenient at first, most colostomy patients adjust to it very easily and lead perfectly normal, active, and healthy lives. The wall of prudish silence that used to surround the disease and the colostomy is fortunately crumbling, and there is even an organization of 8,000 members called the United Ostomy Association that keeps up with current information on diet, colostomy equipment, and other problems the members have in common.

Radiotherapy is sometimes used before the operation (occasionally to make surgery possible) and sometimes afterward to treat recurrence of the cancer. Various chemical agents have been found useful in treating colon-rectum cancer that has spread to the lymph nodes or more widely.

Uterine Cancer

Uterine cancer is the third most deadly form of the disease in women. It kills an estimated 13,000 annually, and is diagnosed in an estimated 42,000. More than two-thirds of these cancers occur in the cervix, or neck, of the uterus; the rest occur in the corpus, or body, of the uterus.

Symptoms: Symptoms of cervical cancer are abnormal bleeding or other vaginal discharge and, of course, appearance of a visible tumor itself. But by the time these

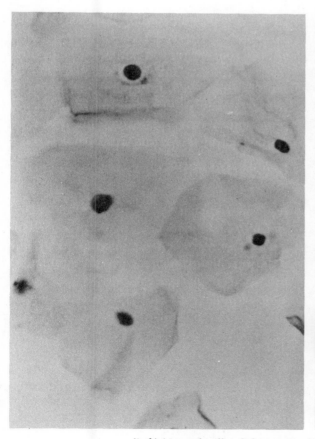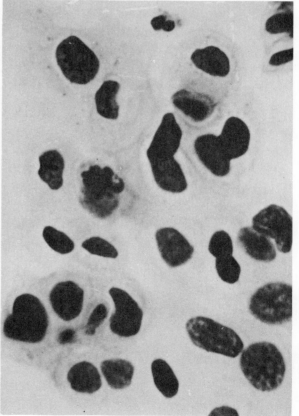

(*Left*) Normal cells of the cervix. (*Right*) Cancer cells of the cervix.

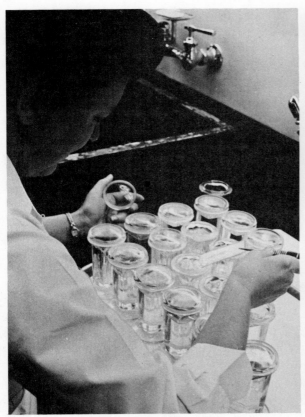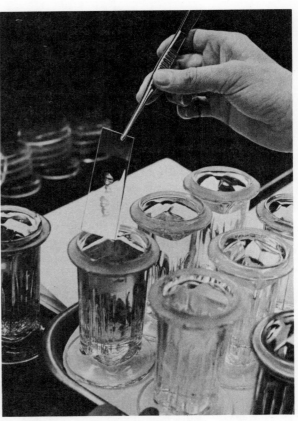

Cells cast off from the cervix are fixed on glass slides, which are then put through a series of stains, as shown above, to facilitate screening under a microscope. The pathologist's diagnosis of cancer is based upon an analysis of tissue and body fluids.

symptoms have manifested themselves, the cancer is usually well advanced, and the cure rate has dropped significantly.

Detection: This is yet another cancer that results in many, many needless deaths. There now exists a simple and effective test that can detect the predominant form of early cervical cancer. This is the famous *Pap test* (or *Pap smear*), named after Dr. George N. Papanicolaou, who developed it. It consists of a microscopic examination of cells that are normally cast off by the cervix and collected from the vagina. Collection of the cells in a doctor's office is fast and painless. The Pap test can detect abnormal changes in tissue five to ten years earlier than symptoms of cancer begin to appear. The significance of this fact is seen by looking at the five-year survival rates.

If the cervical cancer is localized, the patient has an 81 percent chance of recovery; if the cancer has spread to regional lymph nodes, the chances drop to 45 percent. The Pap test is now required of adult women on admission to most U.S. hospitals. Most uterine cancers occur in women over 40, but all adult women should make sure they get a Pap test at least once a year—preferably twice a year.

Recently, a vaginal irrigation smear technique, which can be self-administered by a woman (with the sample then sent along to a physician or laboratory) has been developed. Although this technique is not as reliable as a physician's own examination and cell collection, it may prove very useful where doctors are few and far between. Commercial laboratories in this country are now developing do-it-yourself kits for this technique, including pipettes, solutions, and instructions.

Therapy: Cervical cancer is usually treated by surgery, or by external irradiation—most often by X rays—and may be followed by internal radiotherapy using a variety of radioactive materials.

Cancers of the body of the uterus occur in the membrane lining, the *endometrium.* This cancer is also treated by irradiation, followed by surgical removal of the uterus and ovaries. But either radiotherapy alone or surgery alone may be used, depending on the individual case. Some synthetic hormones related to the female hormone progesterone may also be used to accompany irradiation and surgery in endometrial cancer.

Causes of uterine cancer: Studies made among various populations of women indicate that environmental factors may well play some role in cervical cancer. It appears that sexual intercourse is important in the development of the disease. It is not the frequency that counts, but rather the number of different partners. Further, there is a very low occurrence of cervical cancer among Jewish women, whose partners are usually circumcised. From these and other observations, authorities theorize that the disease is actually transmitted via a virus that thrives in male *smegma,* a secretion that accumulates under an intact foreskin. Indeed, viruses have been found in smegma that are related to the herpes viruses that cause fever sores and shingles. This theory of viral origin has by no means been proved. In general, those women who have the highest risk from cervical cancer have the lowest risk from breast cancer, and vice versa.

Skin Cancer

With 115,000 new cases predicted for each coming year, skin cancer is the largest single source of malignancy in the United States. The five-year survival rate, however, is 92 percent; there are an estimated 5,200 deaths from this disease per year.

Symptoms: Experts believe that many of these deaths could be avoided if only patients promptly reported to their doctors any sores that refuse to heal, or changes in warts or moles.

Therapy: Fortunately, almost all skin cancers remain localized, and can either be removed surgically or with an electric needle, or treated by irradiation with X rays or radioactive sources.

Causes of skin cancer: Skin cancer is one of the easiest cancers to avoid entirely, for

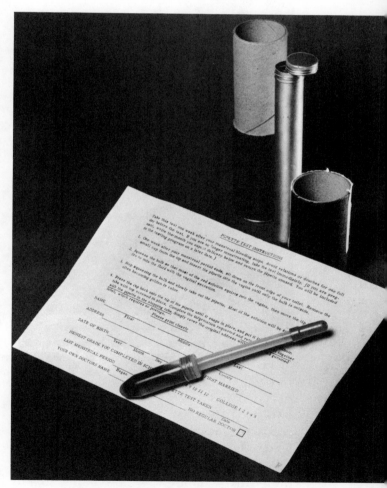

A self-administered method of taking vaginal smears for detection of uterine cancer has been developed for those women who cannot get to a doctor regularly for examination. The kit comes with simple directions.

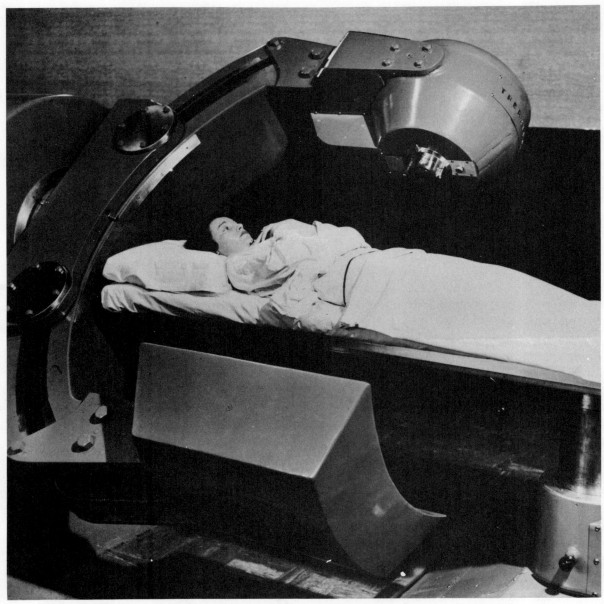

This cobalt therapy unit may be rotated a full 360 degrees. The cancer is centered in the path of bombardment of radiation, while the surrounding tissues receive only a fraction of the radiation, thus preserving them from harm while producing maximum effect on the cancer site.

most are caused by prolonged and repeated exposure to ultraviolet radiation in sunlight; they usually appear after age 40. Fair-skinned individuals who burn readily, rather than tanning, are more vulnerable to this source of skin cancer than the rest of the population. Geographic location is also important. Skin cancer occurs more frequently in the southern belt of states, particularly in the brilliantly sunny Southwest.

Chemicals, too, can cause skin cancer. Before the relationship was discovered, the disease was an occupational hazard for many thousands of unprotected workers who dealt with arsenic and various derivatives of coal and petroleum.

Oral Cancer

Cancers of the mouth and lips strike an estimated 14,000 persons in the United States each year and kill a shocking 7,000. Shocking because anyone with the aid of a mirror and a good light can see into his mouth and therefore spot even very small cancers early in their development. Five thousand of these deaths are among men; the disproportion may stem from the same source as the disproportion in lung cancer deaths between men and women—smoking.

Symptoms: Any sore, lump, or lesion of the mouth or lips should be regarded as suspicious if it persists more than two weeks without healing, and a doctor or dentist should then be consulted without delay. The five-year survival rate for localized mouth cancers—when they are usually no larger than the little fingernail—is 75 percent. But if regional involvement occurs, the rate falls to 25 percent.

Detection: Just as the Pap test screens for cervical cancer by scraping up sloughed off cells which are then examined under a microscope, so one day your dentist may routinely scrape mouth cells to detect oral cancer. When more than 40,000 patients were screened over a five-and-one-half year period at the Western Tennessee Cancer Clinic, about 230 cases of oral cancer were diagnosed, of which 35 percent would have been missed otherwise.

Right now, a weekly or monthly personal inspection of your mouth is the best detective method available. The American Cancer Society has materials explaining the best way to conduct such an examination.

Therapy: Oral cancers are treated by surgical removal or by irradiation.

Causes of oral cancer: No one can pinpoint the causes of oral cancer definitely, but there are a number of leading suspects. They are smoking, in all its forms; exposure to wind and sun (for lip cancer); poor mouth hygiene; sharp or rough-edged teeth or improperly fitted, irritating dentures; dietary inadequacies; and constant use of very hot foods and liquids.   **AF**

CHAPTER 10

Alcohol

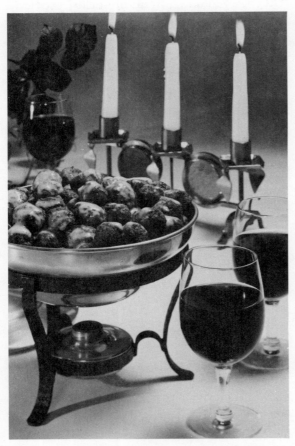

Alcoholic drinks have been used as food and medicine and in religious ceremonies for thousands of years.

Alcoholic beverages have an ancient history. Long before man began to keep records of any kind, they were valued as food, medicine, and ceremonial drinks. When people nowadays have a beer with dinner, or toast newlyweds with champagne, or share wine at a religious festival, they are observing traditions that have deep roots in the past.

The consumption of alcoholic beverages has always been a fact of American life. Most Americans drink, either occasionally or often. Most drinkers are usually in control of what they are doing and are none the worse for their habit. However, of the estimated 90 million drinkers in this country, about 9 million have some kind of problem with alcohol.

Some people have the idea that anyone with an alcohol problem is sinful, or has a weak character, or wants to thumb his nose at the law. Scientists have come to believe that *alcoholism* is a disease and should be treated as such. In 1956, the American Medical Association officially termed alcoholism an illness and a medical responsibility.

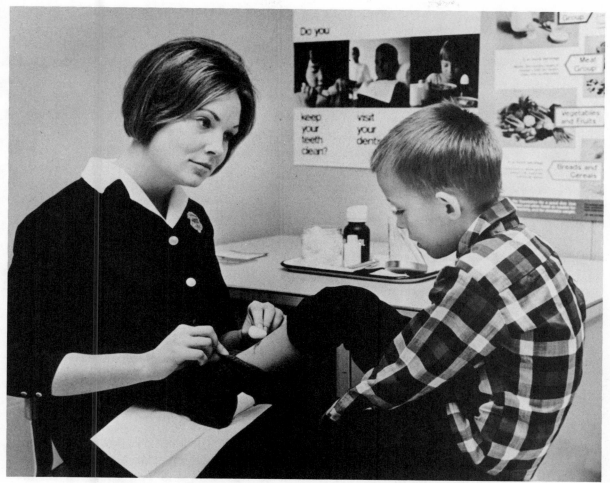

Denatured alcohol is ethyl alcohol made unfit to drink but useful as a coolant (as in anti-freeze), a solvent, or a disinfectant. Here a school nurse uses some to daub a scraped shin.

In the following pages, alcohol is examined as the neutral spirit that it truly is. Some people have a sickness involving food; others can't be trusted with a car. Alcohol too can be properly used or hopelessly abused.

What Is Alcohol?

The alcohol in beverages is chemically known as *ethyl alcohol*. It is often called *grain alcohol*. It is produced by the natural process of *fermentation:* that is, when certain foods such as honey, fruits, grains, or their juices remain in a warm place, airborne yeast organisms begin to change the

sugars and starches in these foods into alcohol. Although ethyl alcohol is in itself a food in the sense that its caloric content produces energy in the body, it contains practically no essential nutriments.

Methyl alcohol, also called *wood alcohol* because it is obtained by the dry distillation of maple, birch, and beech, is useful as a fuel and solvent. It is poisonous if taken internally and can cause blindness and death. Other members of the same family of chemicals, such as *isopropyl alcohol,* are also used as rubbing alcohols—that is, they are used as cooling agents and skin disinfectants, and they too are poisonous if taken internally.

How Alcoholic Beverages Evolved

Fermentation: In all times and places, man has made use of those local products that lend themselves to fermentation. One of the earliest alcoholic beverages was probably mead, made from honey. Wines originated from fruits and berries, beers from grains. Palm leaves, bananas, cactus, corn, sugar cane, and rice are among the natural products that provide fermented drinks for social and religious occasions.

Distillation of Alcohol: Distilled alcoholic beverages appear to be the result of a process discovered in the Arab world some time around the year 800. *Distillation* consists in separating the compound parts of a substance by boiling them until they become vapors. The vapors are then condensed into separate liquids. Since alcohol has a lower boiling point than water, it can be separated from water in this way. Soon after the process of distillation was discovered, it was applied to wine to make brandy and to the various beers based on rye, corn, and barley to make whiskies.

The earliest distilled beverages were produced during the Middle Ages by monks. The different monasteries guarded their secret formulas involving medicinal herbs and spices—as the makers of Benedictine and Chartreuse continue to do—and sold their products to physicians.

Still later, the nobility worked out complicated routines for the use of alcoholic beverages to enhance the taste of foods, such as directions concerning which wine complemented which food and what time of day suited a particular beverage. The poor at this time usually drank the fermented beverages that came easily to hand.

Changes in Drinking Habits

The Europeans who came to the New World brought their drinking customs with them. Even the most rigid Puritans took the view that since drinking was sanctioned by the Scriptures, moderate drinking was no sin. But as the early settlers began to move westward, established drinking habits changed.

For the frontiersmen, barrels of wine and beer were too heavy to transport. Corn "likker" and rum—more potent and easily carried in small jugs—became the favored drinks of the pioneers. Saloons began to spring up and public drunkenness became more and more of a problem.

The temperance movement was born out of a need to reestablish moderation in drinking—not total abstention. Eventually, however, it was instrumental in imposing Prohibition on the whole country. The era of Prohibition lasted for about 12 years. By the time it came to an end in 1933, it was obvious that when the majority of the population wants to drink alcoholic beverages, the law is not likely to stop them.

Present-Day Drinking Trends

On a per capita basis, Americans drink twice as much wine and beer as they did a century ago, and half as much distilled spirits. Where the drinking takes place has changed, too. There's less hard drinking in saloons and more social drinking at home and in clubs. The acceptance of drinking in mixed company has made it more a part of social situations than it used to be.

Here are some facts about the current consumption of alcoholic beverages in the United States:

• Drinking is more common among men than among women, but the gap keeps closing.

• It is more common among people who are under 40.

• It is more common among the rich than among the poor. A recent study indicated that in the income group of $3,000 or less, 45 percent are drinkers; in the group earning $10,000 or more, 85 percent drink.

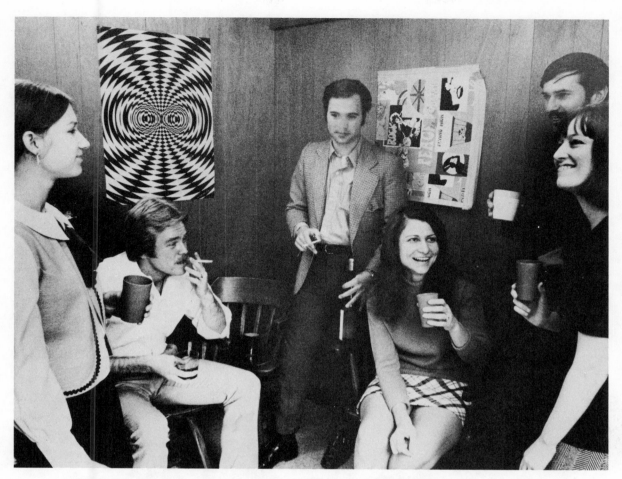

Drinking habits of Americans change markedly from one generation to the next. Today, more people drink at home and in clubs, especially in social situations. More women are drinking, though drinking is still more common among men than among women.

• There are more drinkers among the educated than among the uneducated. About 45 percent of those who didn't complete eighth grade drink, whereas 90 percent of all college graduates drink.

• Drinking is more common in metropolitan areas than in rural areas.

• Beyond the age of 45, the number of drinkers steadily declines.

Teen-Agers and Alcohol

One fact emerges clearly and consistently from all the surveys of teen-age drinking in all parts of the country: the drinking behavior of parents is more closely related to what children do about drinking than any other factor. It is more influential than their friends, their neighborhood, their religion, their social and economic status, or their local laws.

Depending on the part of the country investigated, from 71 percent to 92 percent of the nation's teen-agers have tasted an alcoholic beverage at one time or another. The older the teen-ager who drinks, the more often he does so. After 17, the percentage of young people who drink is the same as that of the adult percentage.

Most high school students drink only on holidays or special family occasions. College students drink at their own parties.

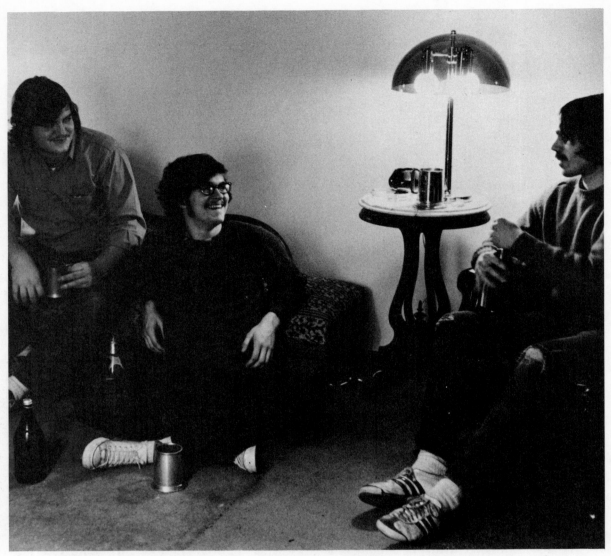

Depending on the region of the country, between 71 and 92 percent of American teen-agers have taken an alcoholic drink. Many teen-agers have beer in their own homes or in their friends' homes.

Solitary drinking is rare, and so is drinking in parked cars. Most youngsters have beer, and less often, wine in their own homes or in the homes of friends. Only about one in ten drinks away from home against parental wishes. However, the rebels drink more and get drunk more often than those who drink with their parents' consent.

It is not true that high school students who drink occasionally are more likely to be delinquent or maladjusted. They play as important a role in all student activities as do the abstainers. In the group with grades over 90 percent, half drink and half don't. The statistics connected with automobile accidents involving teen-agers show that alcohol is negligible as a cause compared to faulty judgment and faulty cars.

In general, drinking is an activity connected with growing up. For boys, it represents manhood, for girls, sophistication. Since adult drinking is a widespread custom, teen-agers adopt the established patterns as they progress towards maturity.

Young Problem Drinkers

Teen-age drinking behavior studied in many different states shows that 2 to 5 out of every 100 young people who drink are misusing alcohol. This is the group that drinks in defiance of parental or school authority. It includes young people from families with mixed feelings about drinking and from families where adults drink heavily but forbid their children to do so until they are 21.

Constituents of Alcoholic Beverages

The way any alcoholic drink affects the body depends chiefly upon how much alcohol it contains. The portion of alcohol can range from less than 1/20th of the total volume—in the case of beer—to more than one half—in the case of rum. It is a general rule that distilled drinks have a higher alcohol content than fermented ones.

The five basic types of beverages are beers, table wines, dessert or cocktail wines, cordials and liqueurs, and distilled spirits. The labels of beers and wines usually indicate the percentage of alcohol by volume. The labels of distilled spirits indicate *proof.*

Proof: The proof number is twice the percentage of alcohol by volume. Thus a rye whisky which is 90-proof contains 45 percent alcohol; 80-proof bourbon is 40 percent alcohol and so on. The word *proof* used in this way comes from an old English test to determine the strength of distilled spirits. If gunpowder soaked with whisky

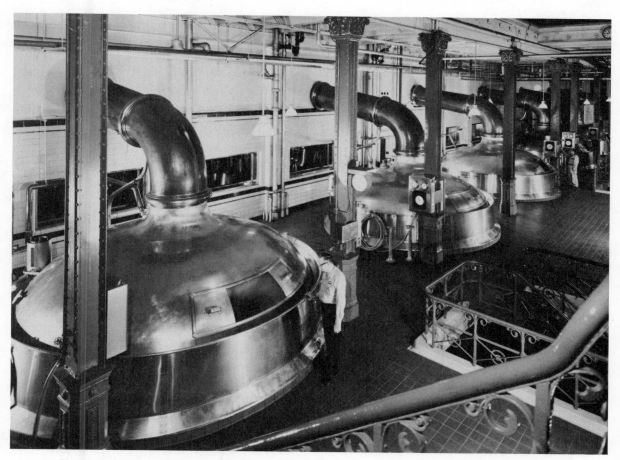

Huge copper brew kettles in a Milwaukee brewery. Each kettle has a capacity of 1,550 gallons.

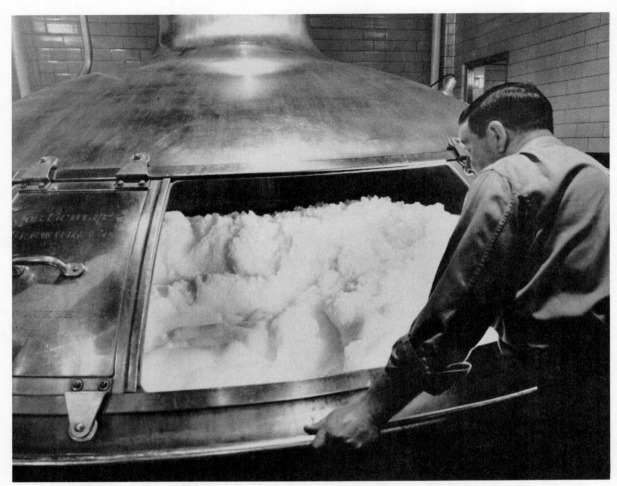

A mixture of grains and water is boiled in the brewing process, creating huge billows of foam.

would still ignite when lighted, this was "proof" that the whisky contained the right amount of alcohol. The amount, approximately 57 percent, is still the standard in Canada and Great Britain. Any distilled beverage containing less is labeled "underproof."

Many alcoholic beverages contain additional substances such as minerals, sugars, and vitamins. The list below describes the contents of the best-known beverages.

Beers: Light beer, known as lager or pilsner, dark beer, ale, stout, and porter vary in alcohol content from 3 percent to 8 percent. Beers are also rich in carbohydrates.

Table wines: Red and white table wines have an alcohol content of about 12 per-

cent. Although the age and origin of a particular type of wine affects its aroma, taste, and especially its price, the physiological effect on the wine drinker is essentially the same. Red table wines are higher in acids, potassium, and vitamins such as riboflavin; white table wines, including champagne, have a higher content of sugar, sodium, and thiamine. The sugar content can range from as little as 0.2 percent in a dry red wine to 10 percent in a vintage sauterne. Some kosher wines contain enough added sugar to bring the content up to 20 percent.

Cocktail and dessert wines: In aperitif drinks such as sherry and vermouth, and in such dessert wines as port and marsala, the alcohol content ranges from about 15 percent to 20 percent. The amount of sugar can be as low as 0.1 percent in dry sherry or as much as 20 percent in marsala. These wines are lower in iron, potassium, and sodium than are table wines, but higher in various vitamin B compounds.

Other fermented drinks: Apple cider contains from 4 percent to 14 percent alcohol; mead or honey wine from 10 percent to 20 percent, and sake, the Japanese rice wine, about 15 percent.

Liqueurs and cordials: These are usually very sweet, containing as much as 50 percent sugar, and are flavored with fruit, herbs, and spices. Alcohol content can reach as much as 30 percent.

Brandy: The oldest of the distilled spirits, brandy is still made from grape wine and usually has an alcohol content of 50 percent. Apple brandy, known as applejack in the United States and as calvados in France, may be 55 percent alcohol.

Whisky: Whisky-making probably began in Ireland as early as the 12th century, spread to Scotland, and eventually reached Canada and the United States. The technique for preparing all types of whisky is

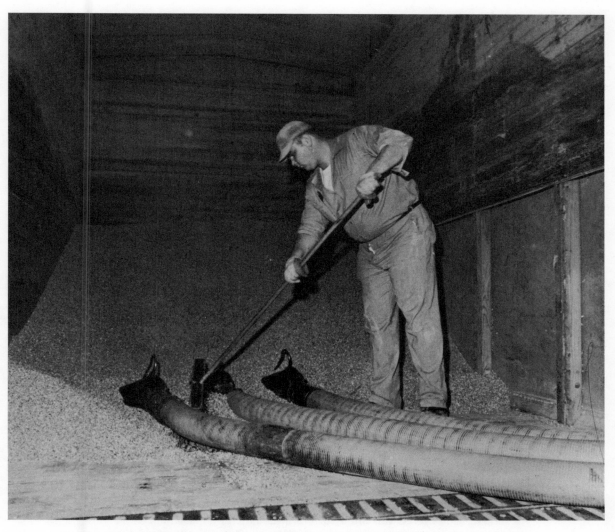

The process of making whisky begins with the receipt of grain. Here the grain inside a railway car is being unloaded by an "airveyor" system that operates by suction.

essentially the same. Production begins with a strong beer derived from a fermented grain such as rye, corn, or barley. The beer is distilled, and the distillate is stored in charred oak barrels. Scotch, Irish, Canadian, rye, and bourbon whiskies range from 80- to over 100-proof.

Rum: The basic ingredient in rum is fermented molasses or sugar-cane juice, and the distillate may be flavored with a dessert wine, spices, or fruit extract. Caramel or burnt sugar is often added for color. Rums range from 80-proof to as much as 150-proof.

Gin and vodka: These are made from any fermentable carbohydrate and are essentially redistilled alcohol with some flavor added. Since the product is bottled without aging, it is the least expensive of the distilled spirits. It ranges from 80- to 100-proof.

How Alcohol Affects the Body

The overall effects of alcoholic beverages on the body and on behavior vary a great deal depending on many factors. Although the concentration of alcohol in the drink is

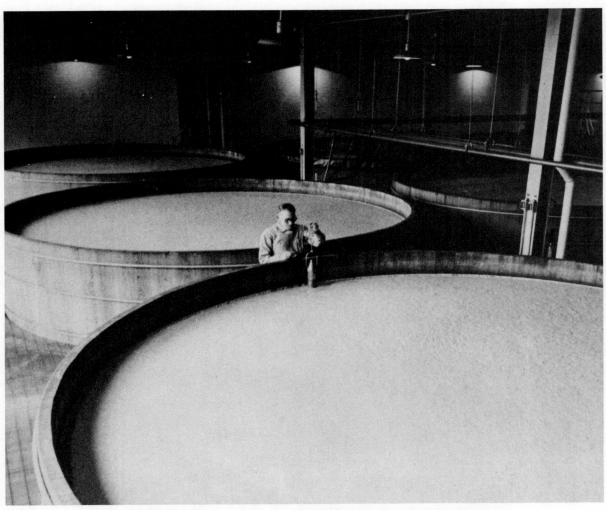

These huge cypress vats are used to provide natural fermentation of the grain. The strong beer that results will be distilled to make the spirits that, after being aged in charred oak barrels, will become whisky.

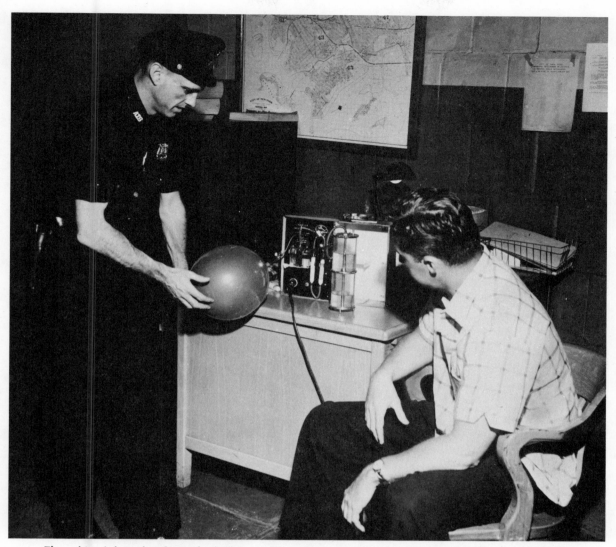

The subject's breath inflates the balloon, whose contents are analyzed, revealing how much alcohol is in the bloodstream of the subject. A similar device, called a breathalyser, is widely used in Great Britain, where it has been effective in reducing the incidence of driving while intoxicated.

the chief factor, other significant factors are: how quickly the drink is consumed; the other components of the drink; how much the person has eaten before or while drinking; his weight, physical condition, and emotional stability.

One factor remains constant: if the bloodstream that reaches the brain contains a certain percentage of alcohol, there are marked changes in reaction. As the percentage increases, the functioning of the brain and central nervous system is increas-

ingly affected. As the alcohol is gradually metabolized and eliminated, the process reverses itself.

Alcohol Concentration in the Blood

If at any given time the blood contains a concentration of about 3/100 of one percent (.003 percent), no effects are observable. This amount will make its way into the bloodstream after drinking a highball or cocktail made with one and one-half ounces of whisky, or two small glasses of table wine, or two bottles of beer. It takes about two hours for this amount of alcohol to leave the body completely.

Twice that number of drinks produces twice the concentration of alcohol in the bloodstream—0.06 percent—with an accompanying feeling of warmth and relaxation. By the time the drinker has had three cocktails or highballs in quick succession without any food, a marked change sets in. Depending on individual and group behavior patterns, the drinker becomes either much noisier or much quieter; his speech gets sloppier or more precise, and his general attitude is likely to be either unusually affectionate or unusually hostile.

If the concentration of alcohol in the bloodstream reaches 0.12 percent, there is a noticeable lack of coordination in standing or walking, and if it goes up to 0.15 percent, the physical signs of intoxication are obvious, and they are accompanied by an impairment of mental faculties as well.

A concentration of as much as 0.4 percent can cause a coma, and of 0.7 percent, paralysis of the brain centers that control the activities of the lungs and heart, a condition which can be fatal.

Alcohol affects the brain and nervous system in this way because it is a depressant and an anesthetic. In small amounts, it acts as a sedative. In larger amounts, it depresses the brain centers that control behavior. In still larger amounts, it causes paralysis, unconsciousness, and death.

How Alcohol Moves Through the Body

Although it is negligible in nourishment, alcohol is an energy-producing food like sugar. Unlike most foods, however, it is quickly absorbed into the bloodstream through the stomach and small intestines without first having to undergo complicated digestive processes. It is then carried to the liver, where most of it is converted into heat and energy. From the liver, the remainder is carried by the bloodstream to the heart and pumped to the lungs. Some is expelled in the breath and some is eventually eliminated in sweat and urine. From the lungs, the alcohol is circulated to the brain, where it affects the central nervous system in the manner already described.

People who use good judgment when drinking rarely, if ever, get drunk. The safe and pleasurable use of alcoholic beverages depends on the following factors:

The concentration of alcohol in the beverage: The higher the alcohol content in terms of total volume, the faster it is absorbed. Three ounces of straight whisky—two shot glasses—contain the same amount of alcohol as 48 ounces (or 4 cans) of beer.

Sipping vs. gulping: Two shots of straight whisky can be downed in two minutes, but the same amount diluted in two highballs can be sipped through an entire evening. The former makes trouble, and the latter makes sense, because during the elapsed time, the body has a chance to keep getting rid of the alcohol.

Additional components of the drink: The carbohydrates in beer and wine slow down the absorption of alcohol into the blood. Vodka mixed with orange juice travels much more slowly than a vodka martini.

Food in the stomach: The alcohol concentration in two cocktails consumed at the peak of hunger before dinner can have a nasty effect. Several glasses of wine with a meal or a brandy sipped after dinner get to the bloodstream much more slowly and at a lower concentration. The sensible drinker doesn't drink on an empty stomach. The wise hostess doesn't prolong the cocktail hour before dinner.

The Hangover

The feeling of discomfort that sometimes sets in the morning after excessive drinking is known as a hangover. It is caused by the disruptive effect of too much alcohol on the central nervous system. The symptoms of nausea, dizziness, heartburn, and a feeling of apprehension are usually most acute several hours after drinking and not while there is still any appreciable amount of alcohol in the system.

Although many people believe that "mixing" drinks—such as switching from whisky drinks to wine—is the main cause of hangovers, a hangover can just as easily be induced by too much of one type of drink or by pure alcohol. Nor is it always the result of drinking too much, since emotional stress or allergy may well be contributing factors.

Some aspects of a hangover may be caused by substances called *congeners*. These are the natural products of fermentation found in small amounts in all alcoholic beverages. Some congeners have toxic properties that produce nausea by irritating certain nerve centers.

In spite of accumulated lore about hangover remedies, there is no certain cure for the symptoms. Neither raw eggs, oysters, alkalizers, sugar, black coffee, nor another drink has any therapeutic value. A throbbing head and aching joints can be relieved by aspirin and bed rest. Stomach irritation can be eased by bland foods such as skim milk, cooked cereal, or a poached egg.

Alcohol and General Health

As a result of new studies of the effect of alcohol on the body, many myths have been laid to rest. In general, it is known that in moderate quantities, alcohol causes the following reactions: the heartbeat quickens slightly, appetite increases, and gastric juices are stimulated. In other words, a drink makes people "feel good."

Tissue Impairment

Habitual drinking of straight whisky can irritate the membranes that line the mouth and throat. The hoarse voice of some heavy drinkers is the result of a thickening of vocal cord tissue. As for the effect on the stomach, alcohol doesn't cause ulcers, but it does aggravate them.

It used to be thought that drinking was the direct cause of cirrhosis of the liver. It now appears that this disease, as well as many deficiency diseases formerly attributed to alcohol, are caused by some form of malnutrition. Laboratory experiments have shown that a daily intake of twenty bottles of a sweet carbonated soft drink is as likely to cause liver impairment as the consumption of a pint of whisky a day.

There is no evidence to support the belief that port wine or any other alcoholic beverage taken in moderation will cause gout. Studies in California show that 60 percent of all patients with this disease had never drunk any wine at all.

The moderate use of alcoholic beverages has no proven permanent effect on brain or nerve tissue. Laboratory scientists, however, continue to investigate the possibility of a direct link between alcohol consumption and brain and nerve tissue damage. While it is true that brain damage has been observed in chronic alcoholics, the impairment is generally attributed to the absence from the diet of essential proteins and vitamins.

Alcohol and Immunity to Infection

Moderate drinkers who maintain proper health habits are no more likely to catch viral or bacterial diseases than nondrinkers. Heavy drinkers suffering from malnutrition have conspicuously lower resistance to infection. However, it has been shown by recent research that even well-nourished heavy drinkers have a generally lower immunity to infection than normal. When the blood-alcohol level is 0.15 percent or above, the alcohol appears to paralyze the activities of disease-fighting white blood cells.

Alcohol and Life Expectancy

It is difficult to isolate drinking in itself as a factor in longevity. A study made some time ago reports the shortest life span for heavy drinkers, a somewhat longer one for those who don't drink at all, and the longest for moderate drinkers. In this connection, it has been pointed out that those who drink sensibly are likely to have equally good judgment in other health matters.

Alcohol and Sex Activity

Alcohol in sufficient quantity depresses the part of the brain that controls inhibitions; this liberating effect has led some people to think that alcohol is an aphrodisiac. This is far from the truth, since at the same time that alcohol increases the sexual appetite, it decreases the ability to perform. In excessive amounts, it unfortunately causes enough impairment of judgment, particularly among the young, to be the indirect cause of many unwanted pregnancies. There is no proof, however, that drinking even in large quantities can cause sterility or defective children.

Alcohol as an Irritant

There are many otherwise healthy people who can't drink alcoholic beverages of any kind, or of a particular kind, without getting sick. In some cases, the negative reaction may be psychological in origin. It may be connected with a disastrous experience with drunkenness in the teen years, or with an early hatred for a drinker in the family. Some people can drink one type of beverage but not another because of a particular congener, or because of an allergy to a particular grain or fruit.

People suffering from certain diseases should never drink any alcoholic beverages unless specifically told to do so by the doctor. Among these diseases are peptic ulcers, kidney and liver infections, and epilepsy.

Alcoholic Beverages as Medicine

At practically all times and in many parts of the world today, alcoholic beverages of various kinds have been and are still used for medicinal purposes. This should not be taken to mean that Aunt Sally is right about the curative powers of her elderberry wine, or that grandpa knows best when he says brandy is the best cure for hiccups.

European doctors prescribe wine, beer, and occasionally distilled spirits—each in specific doses—for their value in treating specific disorders. American doctors did the same until the Prohibition era. During that time, such prescriptions were seriously abused in the same way that prescriptions for amphetamines and barbiturates are currently abused. Today an American physician may recommend a particular alcoholic beverage as a tranquilizer, a sleep-inducer, or an appetite stimulant.

Alcohol with Other Drugs and Chemicals

Many people use carbon tetrachloride as a spot remover and cleaning agent in the home. This chemical can be extremely dangerous if the fumes are inhaled over a long period. If they are inhaled after alcohol consumption, the body absorbs the poison more quickly and the consequent damage to the liver, kidneys, and nervous system is much greater.

Alcoholic beverages should be avoided by anyone taking barbiturates or other sedatives. See under *Drug Use and Abuse*, p. 651, for a discussion of barbiturates.

Alcohol and Driving

Recent studies of traffic accidents indicate that considerably more than half of those that are fatal are the result of drunken driving.

Although small amounts of alcohol affect reflex responses, there appears to be no deterioration in response and judgment when the blood-alcohol content is below 0.05 percent. According to the law in most states, a blood-alcohol content beyond 0.15 percent is legal ground for prosecution. In most European countries, this limit is set at 0.10 percent.

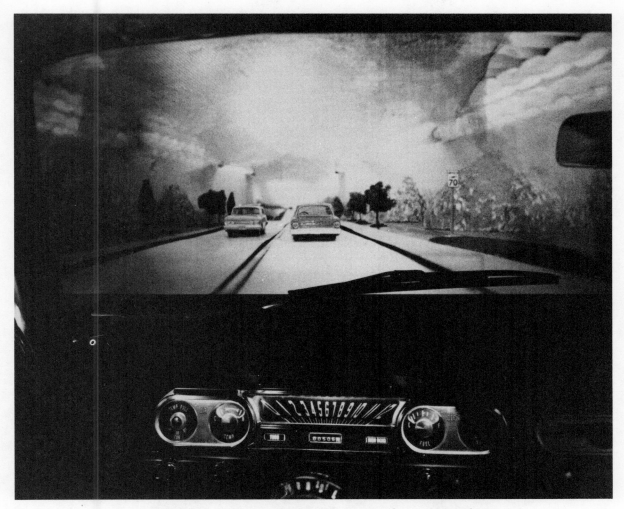

Driver's view from inside a specialized driving simulator, designed to test driver reaction and behavior while under the influence of alcohol or drugs.

For many people, coordination, alertness, and general driving skills are impaired at blood-alcohol levels below the legal limit. There are some people who become dangerous drivers after only one drink. Attempts are constantly being made, but so far with less than perfect success, to educate the public about the very real dangers of drunken driving.

Alcohol Problems

The obvious proof that a deep confusion exists about the place of alcoholic beverages in American life is the fact that only one amendment to the Constitution has ever been repealed: the Prohibition Amendment. The conflict continues to express itself in the bewildering range of laws in different states.

Local laws: In Texas, it is illegal to buy a drink in a public place. In Vermont, only state-operated stores can sell distilled beverages by the bottle. In some states, bars can't have a liquor license unless they also serve food, but in North Dakota, they may not serve hamburgers, sandwiches, milk, or coffee.

Often the local laws governing such matters are enacted through the support of interests that would seem to be opposed to each other. In many areas with dry statutes, church and temperance groups have voted with bootleggers to defeat the legal sale of alcoholic beverages.

Alcohol education is required in all states. Yet teachers are rarely given guidelines to make the education effective. Are they supposed to encourage complete abstinence? Should the problem be thrown at the physical education department with a chart that shows liver damage? Should there be open discussions on the social and psychological causes of problem drinking?

Until comparatively recently, people with drinking problems had few places to turn for help. When they got obstreperous in public, they were put in jail. When they

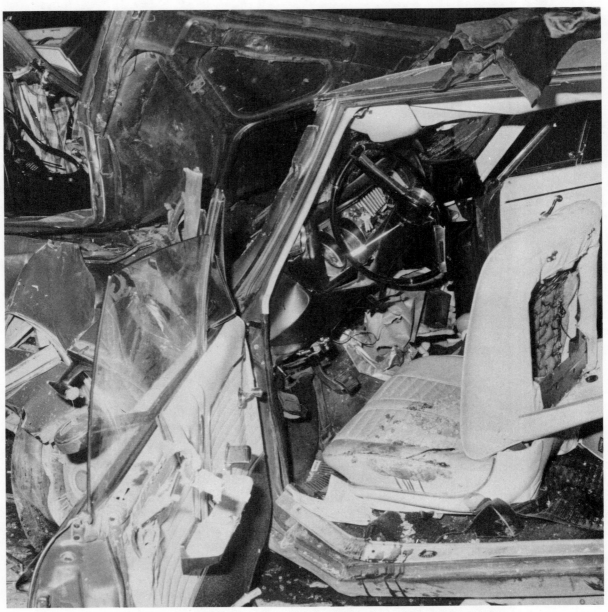

Some people become dangerous drivers after only one drink. More than half of the traffic fatalities in the United States result from drunken driving.

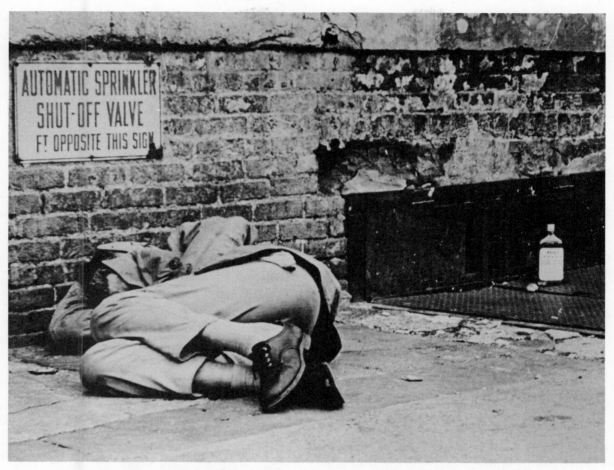

Though an all-too-familiar sight in some parts of our cities, the homeless, skid row alcoholic is not typical of alcoholics in general. Only about five percent of alcoholics are derelicts.

deteriorated physically, they were put in a hospital. And when their brains were sufficiently affected, they were sent off to a state or private asylum.

Changing attitudes: The situation has changed somewhat over the past 30 years. The concern of government agencies, of the medical profession, and of industry has led to efforts to create a broad and effective program for dealing with problem drinking, for educating the public, and for shaping a national policy about the use of alcoholic beverages.

What Is Problem Drinking?

In 1961, the National Institute of Mental Health under the jurisdiction of the U.S. Department of Health, Education and Welfare, established a commission to study the problems related to alcohol. In its report, published in 1966, the commission, which was composed of specialists in medicine, psychiatry, and sociology, defined problem drinking as "the repetitive use of beverage alcohol causing physical, psychological, or social harm to the drinker or to others."

The commission further defined alcoholism as "the condition in which an individual has lost control over his alcoholic intake in the sense that he is consistently unable to refrain from drinking or to stop drinking before getting intoxicated."

Specialists have pointed out that excessive use of beverage alcohol is the most important drug abuse problem in the United States today. Of the approximately 90 million Americans who drink, 1 out of 10 has problems related to drinking. Of the nine million who need some help with problem drinking, about half are addictive alcoholics, and of this number, only about 5 percent are homeless, jobless or skid row alcoholics. Most people with drinking problems are otherwise respectable members of society.

Alcoholism as a Disease

The American Medical Association, the World Health Organization, and more recently the courts, now recognize the type of alcoholism involving loss of control over drinking behavior as a disease. More specifically, it has come to be considered a complex illness best described as a drug dependency.

The leadership of the medical profession points out that although the liquor industry is expanding and the per capital consumption of alcoholic beverages is increasing, there is no reason to assume an increase in alcoholism. It is also true that some ethnic groups have a conspicuously higher rate of addictive alcoholism than others. The rate among Irish-Americans is high and so is the rate among white Anglo-Saxon Protestants; the rate is low among Italian-Americans, and lower still among the Chinese and Jews in this country.

Possible Causes of Alcoholism

Before examining some of the complicated factors that lead to the development of alcoholism, a few popular misconceptions should be disposed of. Alcohol doesn't cause alcoholism any more than sugar causes diabetes. Alcoholism isn't caused by a particular beverage. Nor is it an inherited illness.

Physiological causes: Although several physiological factors seem to be involved in the progression of alcoholism, no single one can be pointed to as the cause of the disease. Among the theories now being investigated are the following: abnormal sugar metabolism; disorder of the endocrine glands; dietary deficiencies.

Psychological causes: Up to this point, there is no conclusive evidence that there is such a thing as an alcoholic or a prealcoholic personality. Common traits of emotional immaturity and strong dependency needs have been observed in patients. However, it is still not certain whether these conditions forerun or follow excessive alcohol use. The neurotic patterns that alcoholics share with each other they also share with nonalcoholics suffering from personality disturbances.

Many psychiatrists believe that emotional traumas and deprivation suffered in childhood can eventually cause certain poorly adjusted adults to seek relief through alcohol from such feelings as anxiety, hostility, extreme guilt, and a deep sense of inferiority.

Sociological factors: Practically all studies of alcoholism in this country indicate that ethnic groups vary dramatically in their rate of problem drinkers. A great deal of attention has therefore been focused recently on *learned attitudes* towards alcoholic beverages and how they affect drinking patterns.

It has been found that in low-incidence groups, the attitude toward drinking is clearly defined, understood by all the members of the group, and drunkenness is consistently disapproved of and viewed as unacceptable. In these groups, alcoholic beverages are introduced to children in the home with no emotional overtones and are used in family situations, at meals, or for religious celebrations.

In the high-incidence groups, there is usually a great deal of conflict about alcohol. The basic rules aren't clearly defined, and there are no clear-cut standards for acceptable and unacceptable drinking behavior. In such groups, drinking is more often looked on as a way of drowning one's sorrows; solitary drinking is therefore more common.

Recognizing the Danger Signals of Problem Drinking

Because different groups have different standards about drinking and drunkenness, it is extremely important for families to have a clear idea of some of the recognizable symptoms of problem drinking. A man or woman—or a teen-ager—with several of the following symptoms needs professional help before the situation becomes unmanageable:

• Using alcohol as a way of handling problems or escaping from them

• An increasing use of alcohol with repeated occasions of unintended intoxication

• Sneaking drinks or gulping them rapidly in quick succession

• Irritation, hostility, and lying when the subject of excessive drinking is mentioned

• Marital, financial, and job problems that can be traced to alcohol

• A noticeable deterioration in appearance, health, and social behavior

• Arrests for drunkenness or drunken driving

• Persistent drinking in spite of such symptoms as headaches, loss of appetite, sleeplessness, and stomach trouble.

Symptoms of Chronic Alcoholism

Excessive drinking over a long period is often accompanied by nutritional deficiencies that show up in liver disorders, anemia, and lowered resistance to infection. Chronic alcoholism is often accompanied by disorders of the central nervous system. There may be tremors of the hands; eye function may deteriorate; bladder control may suffer. Changes in behavior result from a decrease in inhibition control: excessive cheerfulness quickly turns into weeping; moods of self-hatred alternate with moods of hos-

tility to others. The attention span grows shorter, and there are increasing lapses of memory.

Delirium tremens: Chronic alcoholics occasionally suffer from episodes of hallucination during which they may "see things" and hear accusing voices. Such episodes are different from the acute disorder known as *delirium tremens,* or the *DTs.* This mental and physical disturbance is accompanied by nausea, confusion, the sensation that something is crawling on the skin, and hallucinations involving fantastic, brightly-colored animals. The condition is caused by rapid lowering of blood alcohol levels in very heavy drinkers, usually at a time of withdrawal from alcohol.

Delirium tremens is a medical emergency requiring prompt treatment and sometimes hospitalization.

Where to Go for Help With an Alcohol Problem

Resources for the diagnosis and treatment of problem drinkers are more readily available than they used to be. Detailed information about agencies that treat alcoholism in a particular community will be supplied by the North American Association of Alcoholism Programs, 323 Dupont Circle Building, Washington, D.C. 20036.

Alcohol Information Center: Although more help is available in metropolitan than in rural areas, many places now have their own Alcoholism Information Center, listed in phone directories under that name.

Business: Many large business and industrial firms as well as unions have medical programs that can help in identifying an alcohol problem. Some group health insurance plans provide coverage for long-term treatment as well as for hospitalization.

Alcoholics Anonymous: One of the oldest agencies offering help is Alcoholics Anonymous. Founded in the 1930s, it now has

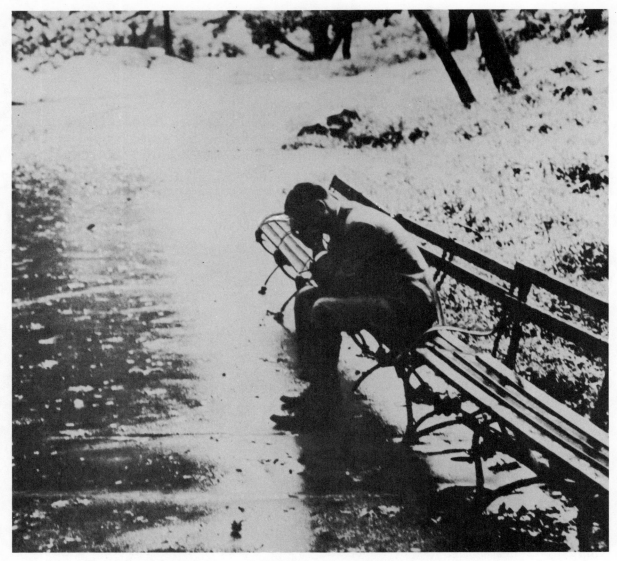

The realization that one is an alcoholic is hard to accept, but it is the first step toward eventual rehabilitation. The change of habit and often of life style can be less lonely by seeking help from one of the organizations dedicated to helping alcoholics.

chapters throughout the United States. Its program has been successful with those problem drinkers willing to seek help on their own.

Family doctor: Family doctors have been alerted to the need for dealing with alcohol problems as part of their regular medical practice. They should be called on for individual care as well as for information about special alcoholism programs in the community.

Some Methods of Treatment

The kind of treatment to which a problem drinker will respond depends on many factors: the extent of his dependence on alcohol, his general health, his attitudes toward treatment, and the cooperation of his family, friends, and community.

It is only in recent years that general hospitals have begun to admit people suffering from alcoholism in the same routine way that they admit other sick people. A study at Massachusetts General Hospital indicates that when an alcoholic patient is received with courtesy and sympathy, he is much more likely to cooperate in the prescribed treatment.

Currently, various medicines are being used to help the patient break his drinking pattern. Tranquilizers are used to reduce tensions and to get the patient calm enough to begin some form of psychotherapy.

The purpose of exploring the patient's past is to dig up buried conflicts and try to resolve them so that he can accept himself without self-hatred and face his real problems as a sober adult. It is customary to include the patient's family in the therapeutic sessions from time to time.

A model treatment program: An outstanding example of team treatment of alcoholics is being practiced at a state clinic in Georgia. Because the director of the project felt that an alcoholic was a person sick in body, mind, and soul, he consolidated the services of medical doctors, psychiatrists, and clergymen of various faiths. The program has been described as follows:

> After physical evaluation, the patient undergoes psychiatric, social, and vocational screening in an attempt to determine his recovery potential. Medical management and treatment prescription is begun immediately and continued throughout the contact. A series of orientation procedures follows: the patient sees appropriate films, attends personal interviews and counseling sessions, and participates in group meetings. Each week, there are 69 group meetings together with 16 staff group meetings. A network of occupational, recreational, and vocational activities designed to aid self-expression is woven into the program. The patients themselves form a therapeutic community, earlier members sponsoring the newer and more frightened. This "acceptance attitude therapy" is an important factor in orienting and strengthening the new patient. After leaving the clinic, all patients are urged to attend group meetings regularly for at least two years in the outpatient clinic, or at a local chapter of Alcoholics Anonymous or at a community-based clinic, and to continue indefinitely if possible.

Chances for Recovery

The word "cure" is rarely used in connection with alcoholics, since a cure implies complete control over alcohol intake. Even the arbitrary goal of permanent abstention is achieved by only a small number of treated patients.

Leading therapists consider that treatment has been successful when the patient can reestablish and maintain a good family life, a good work record, and a respectable place in his community by controlling his drinking most of the time. There is no doubt that the sooner a problem drinker is treated, the greater his chances for recovery.

Help with Family Problems

Alcoholics usually disrupt family life in one way or another. In some cases, they remain alcoholics because of an unhealthy family situation. It is therefore recommended that family members seek help and support from outside agencies that can take a detached view of the problem.

Mental health clinics, family service agencies, and church-sponsored groups are among the community organizations that can be called on for assistance. Relatives and friends of alcoholics can join one of the Al-Anon Family Groups that work with Alcoholics Anonymous. The Al-Teen Groups are specifically set up for the children of problem drinkers.

Laws to Cure Alcohol Problems

Neither here nor in any European country has it been possible to eliminate the use of alcoholic beverages by the enactment of national laws. As for the various state laws, they bear practically no relation to the extent and nature of the use and abuse of alcohol. Regulations aimed at controlling the legal minimum drinking age are extremely difficult to enforce and may even be irrelevant. Neither France nor Italy has a minimum drinking age. France has one of the highest rates of alcohol problems of any European country and Italy has one of the lowest.

Since 1882, when Vermont voted to make alcohol education compulsory in the public schools, every state has enacted a similar law. Yet even though this education has consisted chiefly of stressing the dangers of alcohol, a majority of the students grew up to be drinking adults. The reason for the failure of a negative approach to drinking has been summarized by Dr. Robert Straus, Professor of Behavioral Science at the University of Kentucky, a leading figure in the field of alcohol studies. This is what he says:

> It is as if driver-education classes in schools would be concerned only with the gorier aspects of speeding and reckless driving. This might frighten a few students, but it would not produce many who know how to handle an automobile safely. With the emphasis placed solely on alcoholism, alcohol might similarly frighten a few students, but it would not produce many who knew about drinking, or how to handle alcohol safely.

Alcohol Education

As research in all areas connected with problem drinking goes forward, new ways are being examined to enlighten the American people about the differences between a safe and sensible approach to alcohol and a damaging one.

At Home

Since most basic attitudes are instilled in the home, each family has the responsibility for clear thinking and clear-cut behavior about alcoholic beverages. Those people who abstain completely out of re-

ligious or moral principle obviously hope that their children will do the same. To present drinking, however, simply as an evil or a sinful activity may only succeed in making it more attractive, especially to teen-agers. If total abstention is recommended, it should be for reasons that make sense to youngsters, particularly if they are exposed to other attitudes in the homes of friends whom they respect.

On the other hand, no one should be made to feel inferior because he doesn't drink. Alcoholic beverages aren't essential to good health or the good life. They in no way add to anyone's masculinity, sophistication, or social status.

In families where drinking is part of the pattern, it appears that the most wholesome attitudes result from a clear agreement about the acceptable and unacceptable use of alcoholic beverages. If children are taught that drinking is first and foremost a social activity, they are less likely to see alcohol as a solution to personal misery.

Groups with especially low rates of alcohol problems have clear standards not only about drinking but also about drunkenness. Children in these groups get the idea that drunkenness is never sanctioned and never excused. Someone who is drunk isn't laughed at or argued with. The consensus, clearly stated and frequently implied, is that anyone who gets drunk simply doesn't know how to behave and therefore there must be something wrong with him.

New Approaches

"It is a historical medical fact that almost no condition has been eradicated by treating casualties."—Dr. M. E. Chafetz, Director of Clinical Services, Massachusetts General Hospital.

Many educators are trying to present a more realistic and sensible picture of drinking than the negative one that was presented in the past. Some schools are considering alcohol education as part of courses where it is relevant: not only in health, hygiene, and safety, but also in history, geography, science, and literature.

A current government pamphlet prepared especially for teen-agers is an excellent starting point for classroom discussions. It is called "Thinking About Drinking" and is a lively presentation of the latest findings in alcohol research. It can be ordered by mail by writing to the Superintendent of Documents, U. S. Government Printing Office, Washington, D. C. 20401. The price for individual copies and for orders of a hundred is available on request. The pamphlet is officially referred to as Children's Bureau Publication No. 456.

Whether in politics, sex education, or alcohol education, it is the duty of teachers to put aside personal bias so that young people can trust them as a source of information and reliable guidance. A presentation of alcohol that clarifies its use as food, that discusses standards of behavior, and that encourages young people to think about what's really good for them, achieves better results in the long run than scare tactics.

In the Community

Wherever possible, guidelines should be agreed on for drinking at parties and in public. Hosts should never press additional drinks on guests who have had enough already. They should never permit a guest who is "high" to drive his own car home.

Alcohol education programs for community presentation are available on request from the National Institute on Alcohol Abuse and Alcoholism, Rockville, Maryland 20852. Such programs can be presented in schools, churches, and community centers by committees including doctors, ministers, educators, social workers, and young people. Meetings should encourage questions from the audience and discussion so that prejudices and misconceptions about alcohol and its abuse can be handled by authorities who know the facts.

Hopefully, general enlightenment will eventually lead to a code of behavior about alcohol that has wide acceptance. Such a code will go a long way toward eliminating a great deal of personal misery and a major national health problem.   HMacL

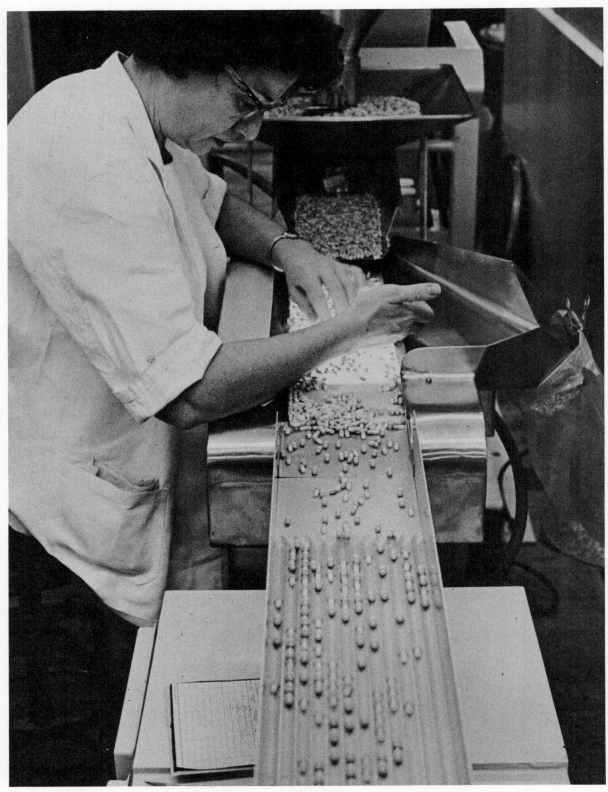

Americans consume 34 million pounds of aspirin annually, nearly ten million pounds of vitamins, and nearly three million pounds of tranquilizers and barbiturates.

CHAPTER 11

Drugs

The drug problem is obviously concerning more and more people these days. Most of the adults who are upset about drugs have young people and the so-called dangerous drugs in mind. But many authorities think we should really examine our whole American society for the "pill-happy" context in which the drug explosion is taking place.

For example, Dr. W. Walter Menninger of the Menninger Foundation has said:

> . . . in recent years, the American people have annually consumed nearly 2.5 billion gallons of alcoholic beverages, 34 million pounds of aspirin, nearly 10 million pounds of vitamins, nearly three million pounds of tranquilizers and barbiturates—and the medicine cabinets in American homes have never been so full.

We are constantly bombarded by television commercials promising us instant relief from even minor pain, as if brief discomfort were somehow immoral. Dr. Joel Fort, former Consultant on Drug Abuse to the World Health Organization, called us—

> a drug-prone nation . . . the average "straight" adult consumes three to five mind-altering drugs a day, beginning with the stimulant caffeine in coffee, tea, or Coca Cola, going on to include alcohol and nicotine, often a tranquilizer, not uncommonly a sleeping pill at night and sometimes an amphetamine the next morning. . . .

What Is a Drug?

Some people are surprised to hear aspirin, coffee, tobacco, and whisky described in the same context as marihuana. The definition of a drug varies with the user; however, here is the one accepted by pharmacologists: a drug is any substance that changes body form or function. In the much narrower medical sense, a drug is a substance used to diagnose, treat, or prevent illness. The drugs we take for medical purposes fall into two broad categories: over-the-counter and prescription (or *ethical*) drugs.

Over-the-Counter Drugs

Over-the-counter drugs are sold and consumed by us in enormous quantities—from headache remedies to cold nostrums, laxatives to tonics, acne ointments to vitamins. Many physicians think that Americans indulge in far too much self-diagnosis and self-dosing, with the risk that serious conditions may go undetected and untreated, and even be aggravated by the medicine being used.

In general, good practice is to use over-the-counter drugs as seldom as possible, for short-term, minor illness, being careful to choose medicines of proven effectiveness: taking a couple of aspirins for a headache is a good example. The U.S. Public Health Service offers these guidelines:

> Self-prescribed drugs should never be used continuously for long periods of time . . . a physician is required for: abdominal pain that is severe or recurs periodically; pains anywhere, if severe, disabling, persistent, or recurring; headache, if unusually severe or prolonged more than one day; a prolonged cold with fever or cough; earache; unexplained loss of weight; unexplained and unusual symptoms; *malaise* lasting more than a week or two.

The Food and Drug Administration (FDA), a branch of the Public Health Service, is responsible for establishing the safety and usefulness of all drugs marketed in this country, both over-the-counter and prescription. You can be assured that over-the-counter drugs are safe for you to use, provided you take them in strict accordance with the label instruction, which will tell you the appropriate dose, among other things, and carry warnings against prolonged or improper use, such as "discontinue if pain persists" or "do not take if abdominal pain is present." This labeling information is regulated by the FDA.

From time to time the FDA decides that a particular over-the-counter product is useless for its advertised function and seeks to have it removed from the market or its advertising changed. A recent example is the ruling that mouthwashes are ineffective in eliminating that most dread of all maladies—bad breath. However, the fact that a patent remedy may be useful in some cases

doesn't mean that it is necessary, or even good, for you personally. Your own doctor should tell you whether you really need vitamins and tonics; buffered aspirin or a combination of aspirin with other ingredients; cough drops and syrups; reducing tablets; hemorrhoid ointments; and other over-the-counter favorites.

Prescription Drugs

Prescription drugs are in theory at the opposite pole from over-the-counter drugs. They require medical supervision for safe use and so may only be sold, by law, to persons holding a doctor's prescription. A prescription drug is a uniquely personal product; it must be used only by the one for whom it was prescribed. It is meant to be taken in consultation with your doctor.

The label may or may not carry directions, size of dose, name of drug, warnings—at the option of the physician. Therefore, you must make sure you understand exactly how your doctor wants you to take the medication. If the labeling is skimpy, write down what you need to know. Some drugs cannot be refilled without a new prescription. Even it it can be refilled, do not do so without checking first with your doctor. You may no longer need it, and it may do you harm.

Similarly, it is a good idea to keep only those medicines you are currently taking. Destroy old prescriptions; they may decompose in time. Resist the powerful temptation to play doctor by passing on the unused part of one of your medications to a friend whom you feel certain has the same thing you did. Also resist treating one child with another child's prescription without the doctor's approval.

Some drugs have undesirable side effects in some individuals, even though they have been judged safe for general use. The reason they are marketed is that their special therapeutic properties far outweigh the potential for adverse reactions. Your doctor

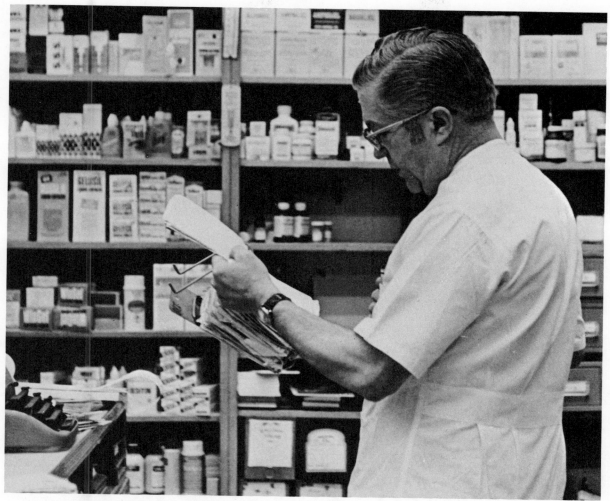

A prescription drug is selected by a physician according to the individual needs of a particular patient, and should not be used by anyone other than the person for whom it is prescribed.

may warn you in advance of the possibility of such reactions. If you think you are having a reaction that is not normal—gastric distress following a drug taken for muscle pain, for example—call your doctor immediately. If you can't reach him, discontinue the drug until you get his advice.

A few individuals are aware that they are allergic or have severe reactions to certain drugs, such as penicillin, or vaccines made from poultry eggs. These persons should of course alert their doctor and pharmacist to their allergies.

The problem of selecting the right drug for your case is not an easy one; 90 percent of prescriptions written today are for drugs that didn't exist ten years ago. You can help your doctor by taking them exactly as ordered.

Drug Use and Abuse

Among the drugs that may be prescribed for you are some that possess a tremendous capability for abuse. They include: *stimulants,* such as amphetamines; *depressants,* such as sleeping pills and tranquilizers; and *narcotic* painkillers, such as morphine and codeine. When abused—that is, when taken in any way other than according to a doctor's strict instructions for medical use —they constitute the worst part of our burgeoning national drug problem.

The second part of this chapter will discuss the abuse of these drugs, as well as others for which there is no present regular medical use, such as marihuana and the hallucinogens.

Stimulant Drugs

The Amphetamines

The *amphetamines,* first synthesized in the 1920's, are powerful stimulators of the central nervous system.

The major forms of the drug are: amphetamine (Benzedrine), the more powerful dextroamphetamine (Dexedrine), and methamphetamine (Methedrine, Desoxyn).

Despite a great deal of publicity to the contrary, there seems to be no scientific evidence that Methedrine is more powerful than Dexedrine.

Legitimate use of amphetamines: The legitimate use of amphetamines in medicine and their great capacity for abuse both stem from the same property—the ability to speed up the body's systems, and especially the central nervous system. The general street name given to these drugs is "speed," which some abusers restrict to Methedrine.

Doctors prescribe amphetamines mostly to curb the appetite of patients who are dieting, and to counteract mild depression. More rarely, they use it to treat *narcolepsy* —a disease in which the patient is overwhelmed by bouts of sleep—and to counteract the drowsiness caused by sedatives.

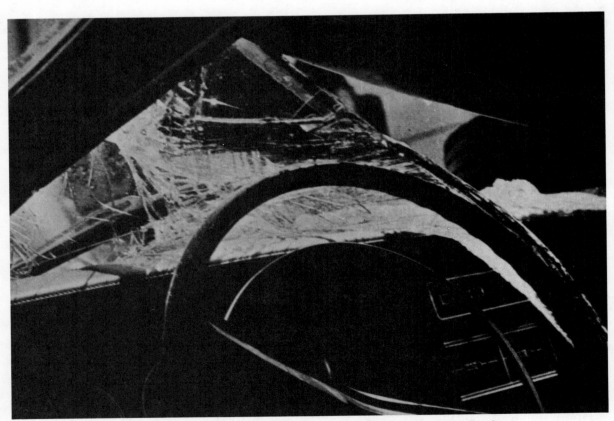

The let-down from amphetamines can be dangerous, especially for long-haul truck drivers, some of whom use the drug to fight off fatigue.

One paradoxical use that has been getting much publicity recently is the use of amphetamines and an amphetaminelike drug (Ritalin) to treat certain kinds of children who—probably because of mild brain damage—are extremely overactive and excitable. For reasons imperfectly understood, the drug calms them instead of stimulating them. For all these uses, amphetamines are called for in approximately eight percent of all prescriptions written in this country, according to one estimate.

Amphetamine abuse: The consumption of amphetamines, however, is far greater than the prescription books indicate. Some ten billion tablets are produced in this country annually, enough for 50 doses for every man, woman, and child. Of this amount, probably half is diverted into illicit channels. Underground laboratories manufacture even more, especially methamphetamine.

Who uses this enormous quantity of drugs, and why? At one end of the range of users is the student cramming for an exam, the housewife trying to get through the day without collapsing from exhaustion, the businessman who has tossed and turned all night in a strange hotel bedroom and needs to be alert for a vital conference the next morning.

Effects: For many of these people, the drugs are obtained legally, by prescription. There is no question whatever that used judiciously, amphetamines can bring the desired results without any problems to the user or to society. They can improve performance, both mental and physical, over a moderate period of time, by delaying the deterioration in performance that fatigue normally produces. This has been especially useful when an individual has been temporarily required to carry out routine duties under difficult circumstances and for extended times. Thus some astronauts have used amphetamines, under long-range medical supervision, while in space. There

A student who is "high" on amphetamines may write his answer in an examination booklet all in one indecipherable line, or he may find, much to his surprise, that his examination booklet is entirely blank.

is also no question that for some people amphetamines can bring feelings of self-confidence, well-being, alertness, and an increased ability to concentrate and perform at the peak of their powers.

But some individuals may have completely different reactions to amphetamines, including an increase in tension ranging from the merely uncomfortable to an agonizing pitch of anxiety. Some experience unpleasant physical symptoms that are generally linked only to fairly high doses. These include dry mouth, sweating, palpitations, and a rise in blood pressure.

Moreover, since the drugs merely defer the effects of fatigue, the benefits are fleeting, and the let-down from amphetamines can be both severe and dangerously inconvenient, especially for someone like a long-haul truck driver. Some authorities believe that many truck accidents derive from the effects of amphetamine abuse.

Also, the feelings of self-confidence about improved performance are often highly deceptive. Because of certain freak effects of amphetamines, performance may actually have deteriorated sharply or vanished entirely. Stories abound of students who have crammed all night for a final and then written what they thought to be a masterly paper, only to learn that their examination book is blank, or written all on one dense line.

Most serious, the repeated use of amphetamines may lead to an utterly different kind of drug experience and an exceedingly dangerous one. Amphetamine users quickly develop tolerance to the drug. Even those who use amphetamines as appetite suppressants or minor mood elevators usually find that after a few days or weeks the dose must be increased to attain the same results. Psychological dependence, for some individuals, can build rapidly, with the results that the user becomes "hooked"—dependent on the drug.

Speed freak: The *speed freak* may be someone who started using amphetamines as diet or pep pills, or someone out for kicks from the beginning. Whatever the origin, greatly increased tolerance and iron-strong psychological dependence compel him to take large quantities of the drugs. Pill-popping and snorting (sniffing powdered amphetamine) have, for most speeders, been superseded by injecting large doses of a methamphetamine, usually Methedrine, directly into a vein.

The speed freak uses a hypodermic because the Methedrine thus given has an immediate, electric effect on his body. He experiences an almost instant *rush*—a surge of powerful physical feelings that make his skin tingle, make him feel suddenly a hundred times more alive.

The price for this gorgeous rush is a stiff one by any standard. The heavy user cannot sleep, sometimes going for ten days or two weeks with only a kind of half-sleep. During this time he tends to be suspicious without cause, aggressive, and frantically active. If the "run" (the time on an amphetamine high) is a long one, if the dose is large, or if the speed freak is a chronic user, then his belligerence may phase into confusion and fear, or paranoia with illusions and hallucinations. High-dose users are apparently regularly skirting incidents of murder or mayhem. In this context, "speed kills" may have some truth; but death from overdose is actually rare.

During his high, the user is obviously not capable of much meaningful activity; his life is riveted to the sensations of the drug. In fact, one of the hallmarks of a methamphetamine binge is the "hangup" in which the "meth-head" repeats some action over and over again—like a phonograph needle stuck in a groove. He may shower all day long, or mindlessly dismantle and reassemble the same piece of equipment, or sing the same song or note endlessly.

At the end of his run is the crash: depression, extreme fatigue, debilitated physical condition (he has probably been unable to eat or sleep), irritability. There is a great temptation to ease the descent of the crash by using barbiturates to come down from the high, or simply to take more stimulants and get back into the next run as soon as possible.

Some experts believe that this reaction is actually a set of withdrawal symptoms; most disagree, and hold that amphetamines do not create true physical dependence, as the barbiturates and narcotics do.

Prolonged amphetamine abuse: But prolonged amphetamine abuse is in itself harmful to the body, unlike heroin abuse (short of fatal overdoses). It has caused permanent brain damage in experimental animals, and may do so in human users. One researcher has said: "Speed is a hundred times more dangerous than heroin." Recovery usually follows, however, if the speeder can stop.

The Commissioner of the U.S. Food and Drug Administration, Dr. Charles C. Edwards, reacted to the situation in August, 1970, by announcing legal moves to cut the use of amphetamines and criticized the drug industry for allegedly shirking its responsibilities. He said that drug makers produced enormous quantities of amphetamines, which had "significant potential for abuse," even though the drugs had very limited medical usefulness; the excess, he charged, entered illicit channels. An agency statement noted that a reputable study had shown the drugs had only a short-term effect in suppressing appetite and that there was no real evidence that they could cope with overweight in the long run.

Amphetaminelike Stimulants

Several drugs, although chemically unrelated to the amphetamines, have very similar effects on the body: they are strong stimulants of the central nervous system. The two most important ones in this country are methylphenidate (Ritalin) and phenmetrazine (Preludin). Preludin has been widely touted as a diet pill. Both drugs seem to be as prone to abuse and as dangerous as the amphetamines. In Sweden, the "shooting" (injection) of Preludin is a major national problem.

Cocaine

Cocaine is the principal active ingredient of the coca plant, whose leaves are chewed by millions of Andean Indians as a mild stimulant. Cocaine itself is a powerful stimulant to the central nervous system.

In its crystalline form, cocaine is a white powder that looks like moth flakes. It is called *snow, girl, coke,* and by a dozen or more other names. A cocaine user is a *snowbird.* Generally, he sniffs it or injects it into a vein, with results similar to those from amphetamines. Snowbirds, however,

don't seem to develop tolerance, and thus don't need to increase the dosage. An overdose of cocaine can kill the user by depressing heart and lung functions.

A classic recipe for many years has been the speedball, a combination of heroin and cocaine that is injected. The shot yields a sudden rush in the genitals or lower abdomen (from the cocaine) followed by a long daze (from the heroin). Because cocaine is costly and often hard to get, many addicts have been switching to heroin-methamphetamine combinations.

Depressant Drugs

Depressant drugs (the downs), are those that depress the central nervous system. They have a sedative, or calming, effect. Apart from alcohol—probably the most widely used and abused depressant—they consist mainly of barbiturates, which are both *sedative* and *hypnotic* (sleep-producing), and those, called *tranquilizers,* that can calm without producing sleep. Some 14 to 18 percent of all prescriptions written by physicians in this country are for sedatives and tranquilizers. By far the largest number of these prescriptions call for barbiturates.

Barbiturates

The *barbiturates,* hypnotic and sedative derivatives of barbituric acid, have been used by physicians for almost 70 years.

Legitimate use of barbiturates: In legitimate medical practice, barbiturates are prescribed for any of the following: to overcome insomnia, to reduce high blood pressure, to treat mental disorders, to alleviate anxiety, to sedate patients both before and after surgery, and to control the convulsions accompanying epilepsy, tetanus, and the administration of certain other drugs. The Food and Drug Administration has conducted a survey showing that during one representative year a million pounds of

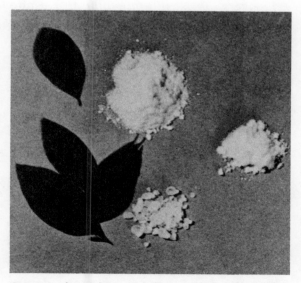

Cocaine, shown here with leaves of the coca plant, resembles moth flakes when in its crystalline form.

barbiturates were made available—enough to furnish 24 doses to every living soul in the country.

The barbiturates have widely varying effects, but they can usually be sorted according to how long-lived their action is: long-acting, short-acting, and ultra-short-acting. (The last category includes the shot the dentist gives you intravenously for instant oblivion: thiopental or Pentothal.) When barbiturates are abused, it is generally the short-acting variety, because these drugs also start their action quickly.

Barbiturate abuse: Who abuses barbiturates, and why? Basically, barbiturate abusers fall into four categories, with some overlap.

The "silent abuser" takes sleeping pills first simply to get some sleep, probably with a doctor's prescription, then to deal with tension and anxiety. These users are usually middle-aged or older, do not take any other drugs, and confine their problem to the privacy of their own homes. For them, barbiturates produce a state of intoxication very close to that from an alcoholic binge, with slurred speech, confusion, poor judgment and coordination, and sometimes wild emotional swings, from combative irritability to elation. These users eventually wind up getting their drugs primarily through illicit channels. They may become so trapped in the cycle of sedation and hangover that they literally spend their lives in bed in a kind of permanent half-sleep, interrupted only to rise for more drugs, and, occasionally, food.

The second group of abusers takes barbiturates, strangely enough, for stimulation. This effect appears in some long-time users of the drug who have developed a high tolerance to it. In others, the drug gives an apparent boost because it releases inhibitions. This may be the kind of sensation sought by such groups as high school students and U.S. soldiers in Vietnam. The latter used Binoctal, a French barbiturate sold among the Vietnamese as a headache remedy.

A third group, probably consisting mostly of young people who are into the drug scene and taking a variety of drugs, uses barbiturates to counter the effects of an amphetamine spree, to come down from a high. This establishes a vicious cycle of dependence that has been called a seesaw of stimulation and sedation. This kind of abuse shows up among some motorcycle gangs that are notorious for aggressive behavior. Some drug abusers take the barbiturate-amphetamine combination in the same swallow to obtain their effects simultaneously. The combination is known as a set-up. In New York, some users inject themselves with a mixture of heroin, Methedrine, and Tuinal (amobarbital and secobarbital). This cocktail is called, with some justification, a "bombita."

Finally, heroin (and other narcotics) users may use barbiturates for two reasons: as a substitute when heroin is temporarily unavailable, or combined with heroin to prolong its effect. In one hospital surveyed in 1964, 23 percent of the narcotics users said they were also dependent on barbiturates.

Dangers of barbiturate abuse: Despite popular belief, barbiturate abuse is far more dangerous than the abuse of narcotics. Indeed, many physicians hold barbiturates to be the most perilous of all drugs. Chronic abuse brings psychological dependence and increased tolerance. The continued use of large doses in turn leads to physical dependence of a particularly anguishing kind.

Abrupt withdrawal from barbiturates is far more dangerous than cold-turkey withdrawal from heroin. It begins with anxiety, headache, muscle twitches, weakness, nausea, and sharp drops in blood pressure. If the user stands up suddenly he may faint. These symptoms develop after one day of withdrawal. Later, delirium and convulsions resembling epileptic seizures can develop. If the withdrawal is not performed under medical supervision, an absolute must with barbiturates, these convulsions may be fatal. By contrast, withdrawal from narcotics may be unpleasant, but does not involve convulsions. A supervised withdrawal from barbiturates may take as long as two months.

Even discounting the hazards of withdrawal, abuse of barbiturates is extremely dangerous. Unintentional overdose, which is often fatal, may occur very easily. If someone takes a regular dose to achieve sleep and then remains awake, or awakens shortly thereafter, he may be so confused that he will continue to take repeated normal doses until he is severely poisoned or dead. Fatal reactions are also possible if he mixes barbiturates and alcohol. Each drug reinforces the depressant or toxic effect of the other, often with deadly effects on respiration. Moreover, tolerance does not increase the lethal dose of barbiturates, as it does with narcotics. Every year there are some three thousand deaths from barbiturate overdose, accidental or intentional. More deaths result from barbiturates than from any other drug.

Other Drugs of the Barbiturate Type

Other depressants that are chemically unrelated to the barbiturates but have similar effects are glutethimide (Doriden), ethchlorvynol (Placidyl), ethinamate (Valmid), and methyprylon (Noludar). These, too, when abused, bring tolerance and psychological and physical dependence, as well as withdrawal symptoms.

Tranquilizers

Current since the early 1950s, these drugs, unlike the barbiturates, can allay anxiety without inducing sleep. The tranquilizers fall into two groups, major and minor, depending on their influence on *psychoses*, severe mental disorders.

The minor tranquilizers are generally ineffective in dealing with such mental disease, but are used in treating emotional tension and sometimes as muscle relaxants. It is this group that is subject to abuse, for unlike the major tranquilizers—reserpine and phenothiazine, for example—their use induces tolerance and physical dependence as well as psychological dependence. Sudden withdrawal can be dangerous if large doses of these drugs have been taken. They include meprobamate (Miltown, Equanil), chlordiazepoxide (Librium), and diazepam (Valium). So far, abuse of these drugs does not seem to be widespread.

Narcotic Drugs

Narcotics are drugs that relieve pain and induce sleep and stupor by depressing the central nervous system. Legally, they include *opium* and its derivatives (*morphine, codeine, heroin*) and the so-called synthetic opiates, such as *meperidine*, and *methadone*. (Federal law classifies cocaine as a narcotic, but it bears no resemblance to these drugs; it is actually a stimulant.)

Opium

The seedpods of the opium poppy, *Papaver somniferum*, produce a brownish

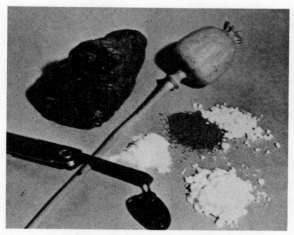

An opium poppy displayed with derivatives: crude and smoking opium, codeine, heroin, and morphine.

gummy resin that yields narcotic effects when it is eaten or smoked. Opium has been used extensively in many lands and many cultures; not until relatively recently did its addictive characteristics become known. Of the more than two dozen active compounds, called *alkaloids,* that can be isolated from opium, the two most important are morphine and codeine.

Morphine

Morphine, the first alkaloid to be extracted from a plant, was isolated from opium in 1805 and later synthesized in pure form. In the illicit drug market it appears as a white powder called *M, dreamer,* or *Miss Emma.* Its more formal name stems from Morpheus, god of dreams, son of the god of sleep. It is a remarkably effective painkiller. It is also addicting.

During the Civil War, Army physicians believed that by injecting morphine with the recently developed hypodermic syringe, they could avoid addiction in their patients. They were wrong, and 45,000 soldiers left the Army with the soldiers' disease, *morphinism.* The civilian population was also being exposed to opiates, mostly in the form of uncontrolled patent medicines. In the years following the war, perhaps one and one-quarter million Americans, four percent of the population, were snared in some variety of opiate abuse. Then, at the end of the century, a substance was synthesized from morphine (by adding acetic acid to it) that seemed at first to cure addiction both to opium and to morphine. The name of the wonder drug—heroin.

Heroin

Today the problem of narcotics abuse focuses on heroin. (There are still some morphine abusers, mostly doctors and nurses.) Called *H, horse, junk, smack,* and *scag,* heroin (or diacetylmorphine) is several times more powerful than morphine.

Effects: All of the opiates produce a dulling of the senses to external events, a feeling of well-being, a reduction of fear, hunger, tension, anxiety, and pain. Heroin offers one an immediate escape from any and all problems. Because the drug depresses the central nervous system, the user also becomes sleepy and lethargic; "nodding" is one of the symptoms of heroin abuse. Some possible side effects are nausea, flushing, constipation, slowing of respiration, retention of urine, and eventually, malnutrition through loss of appetite.

The degree to which heroin's agreeable effects are felt depends in part on how the user takes it. Sniffing is the mildest form of abuse, followed by skin-popping (subcutaneous injection), and then by mainlining (injecting directly into a vein),

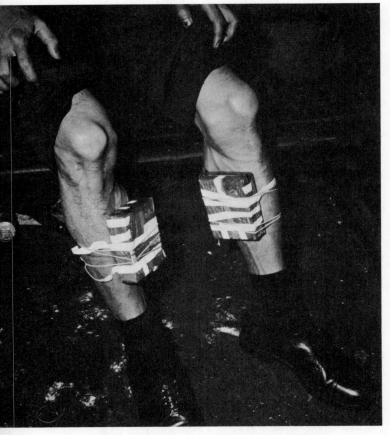

Narcotics smugglers use ingenious hiding places. This seaman was discovered carrying two packets of heroin out of Hong Kong, a drug traffic center.

which is the mode used by almost all those dependent on heroin.

Dependence on heroin: A high and rapid tolerance to heroin is one of its hallmarks, with the regular user requiring ever-larger doses to produce the same degree of euphoria. In the chronic user, it produces both psychological and physical dependence. The former is far more important, and its shackles are the harder to break. With the need to take larger doses, the cost of the habit increases, and the addict's life becomes increasingly centered on the desperate cycle of obtaining enough money for the drug (often by criminal means), injecting it, relaxing for a few hours, and then starting again.

The addict may be driven as much by the need to avoid withdrawal symptoms, or even the thought of them, as by the search for escape. Yet, strangely, the addict may fear a greatly exaggerated monster. It is true that withdrawal for a heavy, chronic heroin user can be difficult and painful, with anxiety, sweating, yawning, muscle aches, vomiting, and diarrhea. But the experience is more likely to be no worse than recovering from a bad cold.

The explanation is that heroin as sold today on the street is "cut" or diluted with milk sugar, quinine, or baking soda. A *bag* or *deck* of powdery white junk may contain a mere 1 to 5 percent heroin. On this kind of habit, most addicts will have very mild withdrawal symptoms.

Unfortunately, pushers sometimes begin selling decks of more than 30 percent pure heroin. For the unwary addict, the tremendously more potent doses can spell grave illness or death. In New York City, where perhaps half of the nation's heroin addicts are concentrated, more than 900 persons have died from heroin abuse in a single year, 224 of them nineteen or younger. One was twelve. Heroin is now the leading cause of death in New York within the 15 to 35 age group.

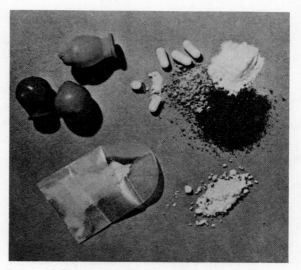

Forms of heroin. The heroin sold on the streets is greatly diluted, but varies so much in potency that addicts risk grave illness and death from overdoses.

The notion that one shot of heroin inevitably leads to addiction is a myth; many have certainly experimented with the drug without becoming addicted, and there are even some individuals who "joy-pop" (shoot on weekends or occasionally for kicks), or take a certain amount every day, without developing tolerance or physical dependence. Nevertheless, the majority of people who use heroin regularly do apparently become addicted, and although some of these may be able to break the habit themselves, most need some kind of help. For reasons not yet determined, many addicts who reach maturity, about age 35, spontaneously get off the heroin treadmill without treatment.

Treatment for heroin addicts: There is little agreement among experts on what kinds of therapy for heroin addiction stand most chance for success. One of the most promising yet controversial methods is the substitution of controlled doses of methadone, a synthetic opiate, for heroin. The substitution apparently allows the addict to lead a stabilized life, but he is still addicted —to methadone. A methadone program is now under way in New York.

Other forms of treatment concentrate on group psychotherapy, often in live-in communities modeled after the West Coast's *Synanon.* Some experts believe that only a multi-pronged attack, combining chemical treatment, psychiatry, user communities, and rehabilitation by social services, will prove effective. As of now, the five-year cure rate for heroin addicts is only about one-third that for alcoholics.

Codeine

Codeine is a modest pain-reliever that can be produced from gum opium or can be converted from morphine. Called *schoolboy* in the streets, it has much milder effects than either morphine or heroin, and is an ingredient in some popular nonprescription cough syrups.

Methadone

Methadone, called *Dolly* after its trade name Dolophine, is a synthetic opiate that does not produce the euphoria of heroin, but is addicting nevertheless. It is being used in several drug therapy pilot programs.

Other Synthetic Opiates

Prescription pain-relievers such as Demerol, Dilaudid, Pantopon, and other synthetic opiates can become addicting if used indiscriminately. They occasionally appear on the drug scene.

The Hallucinogens: LSD and Others

LSD (lysergic acid diethylamide) is one of a group of drugs legally classed as *hallucinogens*—agents that cause the user to experience hallucinations, illusions, and distorted perceptions.

LSD

LSD is a colorless, tasteless, odorless compound, as plain-looking as water. What makes it truly remarkable is its potency. A single effective dose requires, on the average, only 100 millionths of a gram. A quantity of LSD equivalent to two aspirin tablets would furnish 6,500 such doses.

LSD may not be made legally except for use in certain well-supervised experiments. Doctors are using it to treat alcoholism and some mental disease, without convincing results. But on the illicit market it is provided in vials of liquid, or as capsules or tablets. It is consumed in sugar cubes, candy, cookies, on the surface of beads, even in the mucilage of stamps and envelopes. One dose is enough to provoke a 4 to 18 hour *trip,* a hallucinogenic experience.

It is this trip that made LSD, at least for a while in the 1960s, a focus of almost idolatrous interest. Many, including well-known public figures, claimed that LSD and other *psychedelic* (mind manifesting) drugs were consciousness-expanding. That is, they were supposed to enhance the tripper's appreciation of everything in the world around him, increase his creativity, open the doors to mind-bending mystical or religious experiences, and perhaps bring about profound changes, hopefully for the better, in his personality.

Indeed, some trippers reported just such results—although several studies suggest the improvements are illusory. In many groups, it became a distinction to be an *acid-head,* a user of lysergic acid. The people who flocked to the LSD banner were mostly from the educated white middle class, including large numbers of high school and college students. One authority estimates that something under one percent of the total population have experimented with LSD.

Today, the peak popularity of this drug is past, although it is still an important part of the drug scene. The reason: as more and more people experienced the drug, and as more intensive research was carried out, disquieting things came to the surface—dangers, previously unsuspected, of LSD use.

Effects: When an individual takes LSD, he is prepared for a certain amount of minor physical discomfort: a rise in temperature, pulse, and blood pressure; the sensation of hair standing on end; some nausea, dizziness, and headache. About an hour after the drug is first taken, the psychedelic part of the trip begins, with striking impact on the senses. Vision is affected the most profoundly. Walls may seem to sway and buckle. Colors become more intense, more beautiful; those in a painting may seem to merge and stream. Flat objects become three-dimensional. The other senses also seem to become more acute.

On a bad trip, all these sensations can add up to a terrifying experience. The hallucinations can be horrible as well as bizarre. Deep depression, anxiety, and fright can alternate with insight and ecstasy. A tripper may panic because he fears he is losing his mind.

Some bad trips have ended in the psychiatric ward, with the tripper suffering from a severe mental disorder, a *psychosis*. This sometimes results from an effect peculiar to LSD: a severe distortion of a person's body image (his mental picture of his own body). If a tripper sees himself without a head, for example, his panic may be extreme. Sometimes these psychotic episodes, or breaks, clear up within a day or two. Sometimes they last for months or years.

Certain trips have ended even more badly. Convinced that they could literally float through the air, trippers have waltzed through high windows and fallen to their deaths. Others have walked in front of trains or cars, apparently in the belief that they were invulnerable.

It is impossible to say how frequent or rare these adverse reactions are in LSD users, because the overwhelming majority of trips are made illegally and thus without professional supervision. It seems likely that those whose emotional balance is already precarious are those most prone to develop psychotic reactions. But many experts contend that the drug's effect on any given person is completely unpredictable. One reason is that no one really knows exactly how LSD works inside the body to affect the mind and how it can be so potent in such microscopic amounts. The upshot is that abusing LSD, according to a former FDA Commissioner, is like playing "chemical Russian roulette."

LSD does not cause physical dependence, although tolerance does develop; psychological dependence doesn't seem to be severe. Apparently, no one has died as a result of a lethal dose of LSD.

Research on hazards: Some recent research suggests that the drug may have toxic effects on some cells of the human body. One set of studies indicates that there may be a link between LSD use and breaks in chromosomes that could conceivably lead to leukemia or to birth defects in trippers' children. As of now, however, there is no conclusive scientific evidence on which to base a final judgment.

One long-term study, recently concluded, is more definite. Dr. Cheston M. Berlin, of George Washington University, followed 127 pregnancies in women who had taken LSD before or during the pregnancy. The study turned up this statistic: children of LSD users are 18 times more likely to have birth defects than the average. Dr. Berlin said that although his study does not prove conclusively that LSD causes birth defects, "we are more suspicious than ever before."

Other Hallucinogens

Many other substances, both natural and synthetic, are being used as hallucinogens. Most of them produce effects similar to those of LSD, but are less potent. Here is a list of some in common use.

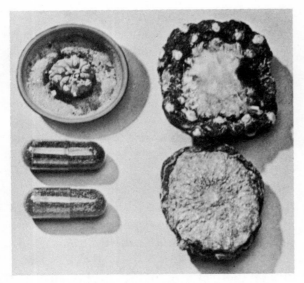

Mescaline is the active ingredient in the peyote cactus. Buttons are consumed either whole or ground.

Mescaline: Mescaline is the active ingredient of *peyote,* a Mexican cactus that has been used by American Indians for centuries to attain mystical states in religious ceremonies. Users consume cactus "buttons" either ground or whole; mescaline itself may be had as a powder or a liquid. Mescaline can also be synthesized in the laboratory.

Psilocybin and psilocin: Psilocybin and psilocin come from the Aztec hallucinatory mushroom, *Psilocybe mexicana,* which grows in southern Mexico and has been eaten raw by the natives from about 1500 B.C. Both derivatives can be made in the laboratory.

DMT: DMT, or dimethyltryptamine, has been called the businessman's high, because its effects may last only 40 to 50 minutes. It can be smoked (tobacco or parsley is soaked in the liquid) or injected, which results in a powerful wave of exhilaration. It is an ingredient of various plants native to South America, and has long been used by Indian tribes in the form of intoxicating drinks or snuff, often very dangerous. In the United States, however, DMT is synthesized from tryptamine in the laboratory.

DOM or STP: DOM or STP is a synthetic compound originally developed by the Dow Chemical Company as a possible agent for the treatment of mental disorders, but never released. When manufactured illicitly, it was given the name STP, so the story goes, for Serenity, Tranquility, Peace. It is powerful, produces vivid hallucinations, and seems to last as long as LSD. But it is also extremely poisonous. It can bring on fever, blurred vision, difficulty in swallowing, and occasionally death from convulsions. It can also cause manic psychoses lasting for days.

Marihuana

Marihuana may be, after alcohol, the most widely used drug in our country. One estimate is that 40 million Americans have tried it. It is certainly the most controversial. We are in the midst of a great debate over whether marihuana (commonly called *pot* or *grass*) is really a dangerous drug at all, or only a mild intoxicant.

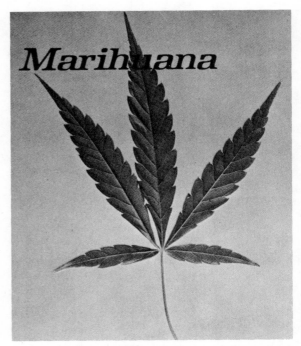

The Indian hemp (*Cannabis sativa*), from whose flowering tops marihuana is obtained, is a tall, weedy plant that grows freely in many parts of the world.

In the summer of 1970, for example, the U.S. Department of Agriculture issued a booklet on marihuana that called abuse of the drug a "major menace . . . [that] frequently leads to dangerous forms of addiction and dependencies." Just a few days later, Dr. Roger O. Egeberg, then Assistant Secretary of Health, Education and Welfare and thus the senior federal health official, said that on the available evidence, "marihuana is not a narcotic, its use does not lead to physiological dependence under ordinary circumstances, and . . . there is no proof that it predisposes an individual to go on to more potent and dangerous drugs."

The Marihuana Plant

Marihuana is a Mexican-Spanish word originally applied to a poor grade of tobacco, and only later meaning a smoking preparation made from the hemp plant. The Indian hemp (*Cannabis sativa*) is a tall, weedy plant related to the fig tree and the hop. It grows freely in many parts of the world and provides drug preparations of one kind or another (the general term is cannabis) to some 300 million people. But the quality and strength of these drugs depend on where the plant is grown, whether it is wild or cultivated, and especially on how the preparation is made.

Drugs are obtained almost solely from the female plants. (The males produce the fiber for hemp.) When the female plants are ripe, in the heat of summer, their top leaves and especially the clusters of flowers at their tops produce a minty, sticky, golden-yellow resin, which eventually blackens. It is this resin that contains the active principles of the drug. And obviously, the pure resin of carefully cultivated plants is the most potent form of cannabis. It is available in cakes, called *charas* in India, and as a brown powder, called *hashish* in the Middle East.

A small but increasing quantity of hashish is smuggled here. But it is the weakest form of cannabis, made from the tops,

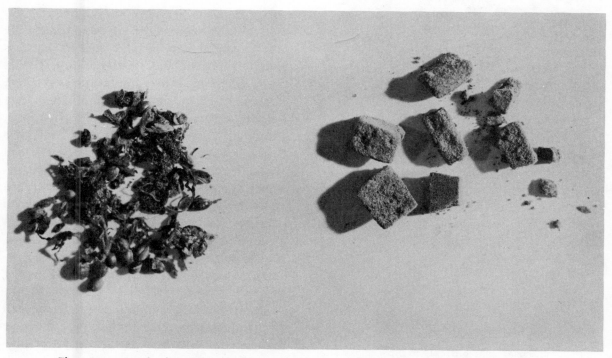

The pure resin of cultivated cannabis plants is the most potent form. As a brown powder in the Middle East, it is called hashish; in India, available in cakes, it is called charas.

leaves, and often stems of low-resin plants, that is smoked in this country as marihuana. Some experts have ranked hashish from four to ten times as powerful as marihuana.

Scientists have not yet succeeded in establishing exactly what substances in the cannabis plant produce its drug effects in man, nor how. Three of the resin's ingredients are chemical compounds called cannabinol, cannabidiol, and tetrahydrocannabinol (*THC*), the last actually a group of related substances. THC is probably the most important active principle in the hemp plant, but most chemists believe it is not the only one.

Effects: What happens when a marihuana cigarette is smoked? If the smoker is a novice, if he doesn't know what to expect, or how to inhale properly, nothing at all

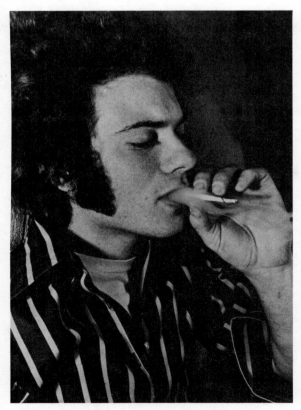

Marihuana smokers inhale deeply to draw smoke into the lungs. Whether the reaction is pleasant or not depends to some extent on the mood of the smoker.

may be noticeable, apart from the lingering sweetish smell of burning rope that the reefer exudes. If he is feeling insecure about smoking, he may experience a feeling of panic, usually controllable with some reassurance. More serious reactions have been reported among marihuana smokers, including toxic psychosis with confusion and disorientation, but these are rare. Also, experimenters using large doses of marihuana, hashish, and THC have induced what they termed hallucinations and psychotic reactions in their subjects.

For the experienced smoker, however, the usual reaction is to feel about half way between elation and sleepiness, with some heightened or altered perceptions (of sound and color, for example), and a greatly slowed-down sense of time. The smoker can usually control the extent of his high and does not feel tempted to smoke beyond the point he wishes to reach. He often experiences mild headache or nausea.

Special properties of marihuana: Marihuana seems to be in a class by itself as a drug. It resembles both stimulants and depressants in some of its actions. It certainly has psychedelic effects, but it is far less potent than the hallucinogens and differs from them in other important ways. (A standard text on pharmacology lists it as a "miscellaneous" drug.) It is not a narcotic, although it is classified as such under laws in some states. It does not produce physical dependence, nor does its use entail tolerance; some users, in fact, find that with regular use they need less marihuana to produce the desired high. There seems, in general, to be slight to moderate psychological dependence among regular users— less, in some experts' opinion, than among regular users of alcohol or tobacco.

None of these general observations can be presented as gospel; there simply have not been enough scientific studies performed to say we know very much positively about marihuana.

Extent of use: Facts about the incidence of marihuana use in this country are as hard to come by as solid data on its effects. In June, 1970, Dr. Stanley F. Yolles, then director of the National Institute of Mental Health, estimated that some 20 million Americans had used the drug at least once. Dr. Yolles also estimated that its use had peaked at 50 percent in some high schools, that 65 percent of the students who experiment with it stop after one to ten trials, that 25 percent become social users, and that 10 percent become habitual users. Almost all authorities, even those who want to legalize marihuana, are in agreement on one point: it should be kept out of the hands of minors.

One very special area where the spread of marihuana is of concern is among the U.S. armed forces. One Army neuropsychiatric team, headed by Dr. Joel H. Kaplan, estimated that 50 to 80 percent of the Army's enlisted men in Vietnam tried marihuana at least once, with some 10 to 20 percent being regular users of marihuana or other drugs. The plant grown in Vietnam was far more potent in cannabis than the American variety, which led to obvious problems with men whose lives depended on their alertness. Acute psychotic episodes were reported to have occurred among numbers of servicemen after smoking this potent marihuana in Vietnam.

Continuing research: The most serious indictment of marihuana as a dangerous drug stems from recent research at St. John's University in New York. When pregnant mice and rats "smoked" marihuana, some 20 percent of their offspring had birth defects such as cleft palate. Moreover, the defects were transmitted to the next two generations, indicating genetic damage. Drug experiments on rodents cannot be regarded as conclusive as far as human drug use is concerned, but they do suggest the need for further study of the effects of marihuana on human beings.   AF

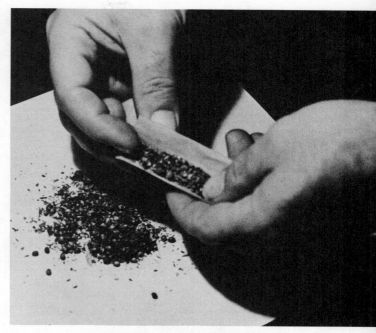

Marihuana being rolled into a cigarette, called a joint. Authorities have estimated that some 20 million Americans have used the drug at least once.

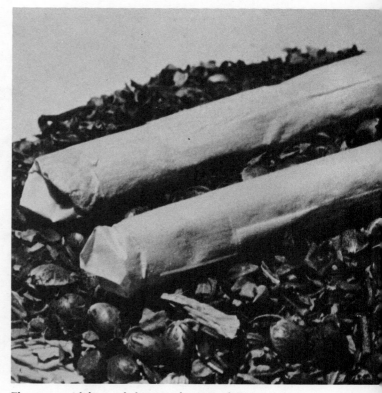

The most widely used drug in the United States outside of alcohol is marihuana, shown here in its form of hemp leaves and in hand-rolled cigarettes.

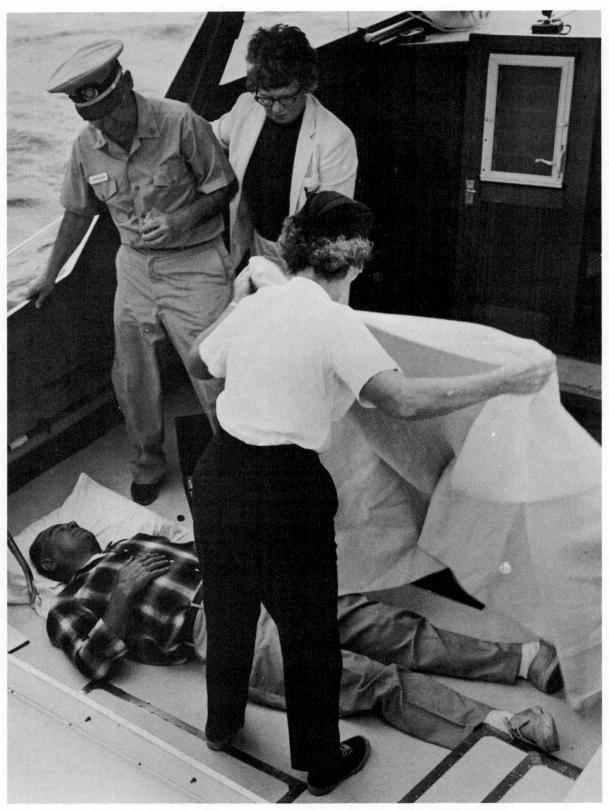

The victim of a serious accident should be kept flat on his back while help is being summoned.

Medical Emergencies

The following pages deal with various medical emergencies that require immediate action of the right kind. In cases involving severe bleeding, poisoning, asphyxiation, suffocation, or shock, administering first aid until hospitalization is possible can make the difference between life and death.

In others, such as an epileptic seizure or an attack of croup, danger and discomfort can be kept at a minimum by doing the right thing until professional help is available.

Anyone attempting any kind of rescue procedures will do so with considerably more confidence if he has a clear notion of the order of importance of various problems. Over and above all technical knowledge about such things as tourniquets or cardiac massage is the ability of the rescuer to keep a cool head so that he can make the right decisions and delegate tasks to others who wish to be helpful.

Cessation of Breathing

The medical emergency which requires prompt attention before any others is *cessation of breathing*. No matter what other injuries need treatment, mouth-to-mouth resuscitation as described on page 673 should be administered immediately. With a certain amount of practice, this technique can be mastered by every member of the family. It is now possible to obtain a plastic device called an *airway* especially designed with

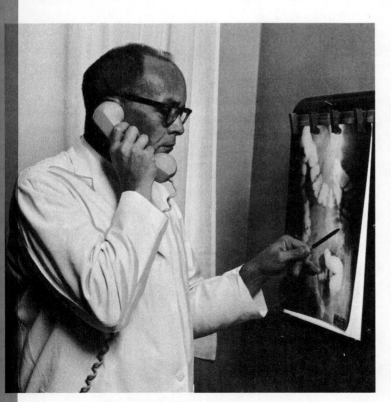

Although emergencies are best handled in a hospital, a doctor's advice on the phone can be indispensable when the nearest hospital is not easily accessible.

a breathing tube for the victim and a mouthpiece for the rescuer, so that direct mouth-to-mouth contact can be eliminated. The airway is compact enough to fit into the glove compartment of a car or a portable first-aid kit.

Severe Bleeding

If the victim is not suffering from respiration failure or if breathing has been restored, *severe bleeding* is the second most serious emergency to attend to. Instead of wasting time trying to figure out how to apply a tourniquet and where the right pressure points are, the rescuer will be most effective if he simply applies direct and constant pressure on or around the wound, with a sterile bandage if possible, or with the flat of the hand until the proper supplies are available. See *Emergency procedures,* p. 670, for a more detailed discussion.

Shock

In any acute medical emergency, the possibility of the onset of *shock* must always be taken into account, especially following the fracture of a large bone, extensive burns, or serious wounds. If untreated, or if treated too late, shock can be fatal. See p. 685 for the proper procedures.

A crucial decision confronting anyone dealing with the victim of a serious accident is whether or not to move him. The best rule to follow is: unless he is in the path of immediate danger, keep him lying down. If he is conscious, reassure him that help is on the way, and that he must remain quiet rather than try to sit up or stand.

Calling for Help

Every household should have a card close by the telephone—preferably attached to an adjacent wall—that contains the numbers of various emergency services. In most communities, it is possible to call the police or the fire department simply by dialing the operator and asking for the police or reporting a fire. When this is done, the caller should immediately follow the request by clearly giving his name and address. In many large cities, there is a special three-digit number that can be dialed for reaching the police directly.

An ambulance can be summoned either by asking for a police ambulance, by calling the nearest hospital, or by having on hand the telephone numbers of whatever private ambulance services are locally available. Such services are listed in the classified pages of the telephone directory.

Practically all hospitals have emergency rooms for the prompt treatment of accident cases. If the victim is in good enough physical condition, he can be placed in a prone position in a family station wagon for removal to a hospital. However, under no circumstances should a person who has sustained major injuries or who has collapsed be made to sit upright in a car. First aid must be administered to him on the spot until a suitable conveyance arrives.

Every family should find out the telephone number of the nearest Poison Control Center and note it on the emergency number card. These centers are usually staffed to handle calls throughout the day and night and can provide information for emergency treatment. See p. 686 for an alphabetical listing of poisons and their antidotes.

Reaching a Doctor

Emergencies of a crucial nature are usually better handled in a hospital than by a visiting physician, since they are likely to require oxygen or blood transfusions. However, there are many situations in which a doctor's guidance on the phone can be extremely helpful and reassuring.

Since there are times when the family physician may not be available by phone,

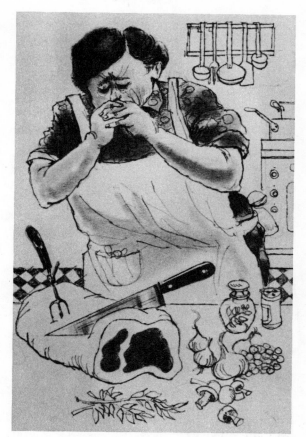

The use of sharp knives and cooking fires make the kitchen a good place to store first-aid equipment.

it's a good idea to ask him for the names and phone numbers of doctors who can be called when he can't be reached. In many communities, it is also possible to get the services of a doctor by calling the County Medical Society.

A family on vacation in a remote area or on a cross-country trip by car can be directed to the nearest medical services by calling the telephone operator. If she can't provide adequate information promptly, ask to be connected with the nearest headquarters of the State Police.

Bleeding

Bleeding from minor cuts, scrapes, and bruises usually stops by itself, but even small injuries of this kind should receive at-

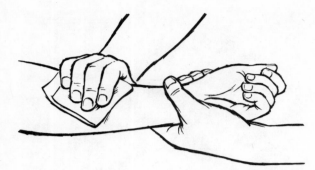

External bleeding can usually be controlled by the application of direct pressure on the wound with a clean cloth. When the bleeding has been controlled, an additional layer is added and bandaged in place.

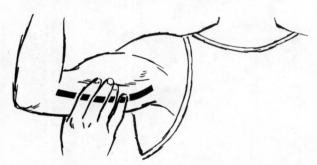

The two main pressure points in the top half of the body are located on the inner half of each arm, midway below elbow and armpit. Pressure applied compresses the brachial artery and diminishes blood flow to the rest of the arm beyond the pressure point.

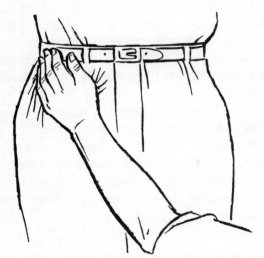

The two main pressure points below the waist are on the front, inner half of each thigh just below the groin. Pressure applied compresses the femoral artery against the pelvic bone and diminishes blood flow to the rest of the leg below the pressure point.

tention to prevent infection. The injured area should be washed thoroughly with soap and water, or if possible, held under running water. The surface should then be covered with a sterile bandage.

The type of wound known as a *puncture wound* may bleed very little, but is potentially extremely dangerous because of the possibility of tetanus infection. Anyone who steps on a rusty nail or thumbtack or has a similar accident involving a pointed object that penetrates deep under the skin surface should consult a physician about the need for anti-tetanus inoculation or a booster shot.

Severe external bleeding: Massive bleeding occurs when either an artery or a vein has been severed. Arterial blood is bright red and spurts rather than flows from the body, sometimes in very large amounts. It is also more difficult to control than blood from a vein, which can be recognized by its dark red color and steady flow.

Emergency procedures: The quickest and most effective way to stop bleeding is by direct pressure on the wound. If heavy layers of sterile gauze are not available, use a clean handkerchief, or a clean piece of material torn from a shirt, slip, or sheet to cover the wound. Then place the fingers or the palm on the hand directly on the bleeding area. The pressure must be *firm and constant* and should be interrupted only when the blood has soaked through the dressing. *Do not remove the soaked dressing.* Cover it as quickly as possible with additional new layers. When the blood stops seeping through to the surface of the dressing, secure it with strips of cloth until the patient can receive medical attention. This procedure is almost always successful in stopping blood flow from a vein.

If direct pressure doesn't stop arterial bleeding, two alternatives are possible: pressure by finger or hand on the pressure point nearest the wound, or the application of a tourniquet. No matter what the source of the bleeding, if the wound is on an arm or leg, elevation of the limb as high as is comfortable will reduce the blood flow.

Tourniquets: A tourniquet improperly applied can be an extremely dangerous device, and should only be considered for a hemorrhage that can't be controlled in any other way.

It must be remembered that arterial blood flows away from the heart, and that venous blood flows toward the heart. Therefore, while a tourniquet placed on a limb between the site of a wound and the heart may slow or stop arterial bleeding, it may actually increase venous bleeding. By obstructing blood flow in the veins beyond the wound site, the venous blood flowing toward the heart will have to exit from the wound. Thus, the proper application of a

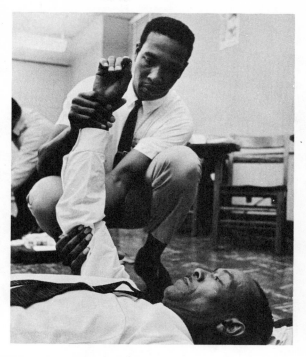

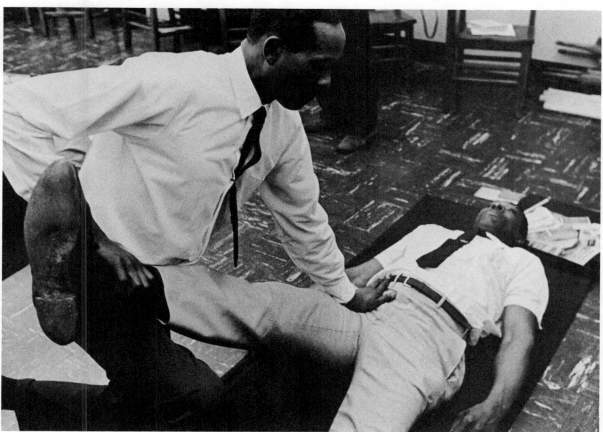

Pressure on the brachial artery (*top*) and femoral artery (*bottom*) is demonstrated. In both cases, the extremity is elevated to reduce blood flow to the site of the wound.

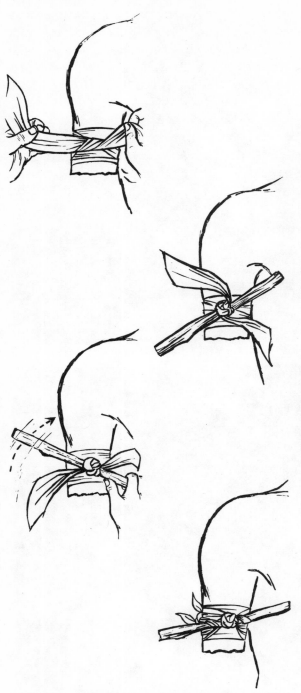

Severe arterial bleeding can be controlled by the correct application of a tourniquet. A long strip of gauze or other material is wrapped twice around the arm or leg above the wound and tied in a half-knot (*top, left*). A stick, called a windlass, is placed over the knot, and the knot is completed (*top, right*). The windlass is turned to tighten the knot (*bottom, left*), and finally, the windlass is secured with the tails of the tourniquet (*bottom, right*).

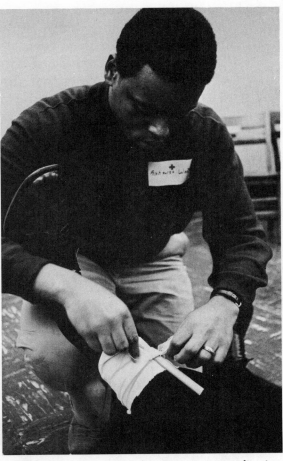

A Red Cross trainee practices tourniquet application. An improperly applied tourniquet can do a great deal of harm. A tourniquet should never be applied by someone unfamiliar with the correct techniques.

tourniquet depends upon an understanding and differentiation of arterial from venous bleeding. Arterial bleeding can be recognized by the pumping action of the blood and by the bright red color of the blood.

Once a tourniquet is applied, it should not be left in place for an excessive period of time, since the tissues in the limb beyond the site of the wound need to be supplied with blood.

Electric Shock

An electric shock from the usual 110-volt current in most homes can be a serious emergency, especially if the person's skin or clothing is wet. Under these circumstances, the shock may paralyze the part of the brain that controls breathing and stop the heart completely or disorder its pumping action.

Emergency treatment: It is of the utmost importance to break the electrical contact *immediately* by unplugging the wire of the appliance involved or by shutting off the house current switch. *Do not touch the victim of the shock while he is still acting as an electrical conductor.*

If the shock has come from a faulty wire out of doors and the source of the electrical current can't be reached easily, make a lasso of dry rope on a long sturdy dry stick. Catch the victim's hand or foot in the loop and drag him away from the wire. Another way to break the contact is to cut the wire with a dry axe.

If the victim of the shock is unconscious, or if his pulse is very weak, administer mouth-to-mouth respiration and cardiac massage until he can get to a hospital. See below and p. 674.

Precautions against electric shock: All home appliances should carry the label of the Underwriters' Laboratory (UL) which guarantees that they have been tested for shock hazard. The cords and plugs of all appliances should be examined regularly for fraying, wire exposure, or loose parts, and repaired promptly if necessary. If there are young children in the family, all unused but active electrical wall outlets should be completely covered with layers of masking tape.

Mouth-to-Mouth Respiration

This method of artificial respiration reestablishes breathing by forcing the rescuer's breath directly into the victim's lungs. It is more efficient than other methods because it supplies more air directly, the rise and fall of the chest can be watched, and the procedure can be carried on while the patient is being transported to the hospital in an ambulance or station wagon.

Speed is of the essence in preparing someone for mouth-to-mouth respiration. He should be placed on his back, face up, with head to one side. His mouth may have to be opened forcibly, and foreign matter such as chewing gum, food, or false teeth should be removed. The inside of the mouth down to the throat should be wiped clean by a cloth or handkerchief wrapped around the rescuer's fingers. Then proceed as follows:

1. Tilt the head as far back as it will go, with the jaw pushed upward so that the lower teeth are in front of rather than under the upper ones.

2. Open the mouth, or if the teeth are clenched shut, move the lower lip down.

3. The rescuer then takes a deep breath, opens his mouth wide while the breath is still in his lungs, and puts his mouth firmly over the victim's mouth. At the same time, he presses his cheek against the victim's nostrils, or pinches them shut to prevent air leakage.

OBSTRUCTED

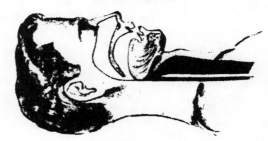

OPENED

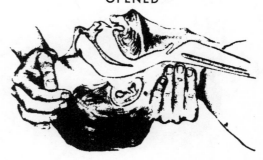

The first step in artificial respiration is the creation of an open air passage. With the victim lying on his back, the head is tilted back as far as possible. One hand lifts up at the neck, while the heel of the other hand pushes down on the forehead.

4. The rescuer blows his breath forcefully into the victim's mouth, and when he sees the chest rise, the rescuer removes his mouth so that the victim can exhale. If the chest doesn't rise, tilt the head farther back and force another breath into the mouth.

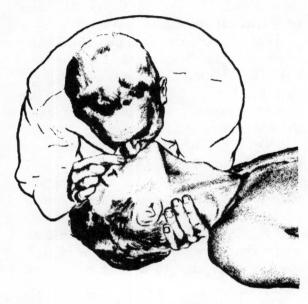

If breathing does not start, pinch the victim's nose shut, take a deep breath, seal your mouth around the victim's mouth, and blow until the chest rises.

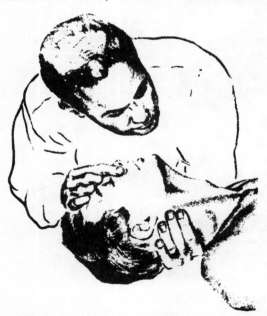

As soon as the victim's chest rises you must raise your mouth to let him exhale and to take another deep breath yourself. Repeat every five seconds.

5. When the victim has completed an exhaled breath, the rescuer repeats the process about every three seconds.

FURTHER SUGGESTIONS

1. The rescuer can avoid dizziness by making sure that he exhales the *full force* of each breath into the victim's mouth.

2. Tension and fatigue can be minimized if the rescuer's hands and back are in a relaxed position.

3. To make sure that the victim's chest and abdominal movements indicate true breathing, listen closely for the sound of exhaled breath or feel for the exhaled air with the fingers.

External Cardiac Massage

If as a result of severe electric shock the victim is not only unconscious but also shows signs of heart stoppage, he should be given cardiac massage at the same time that another rescuer is administering mouth-to-mouth resuscitation. Both procedures can be carried on in the moving vehicle taking him to the hospital.

It is assumed that he is lying down with his mouth clear and his air passage unob-

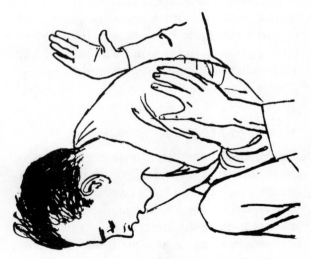

If the victim's lungs do not inflate, roll the victim on his side and strike him between the shoulder blades to dislodge whatever is blocking the airway.

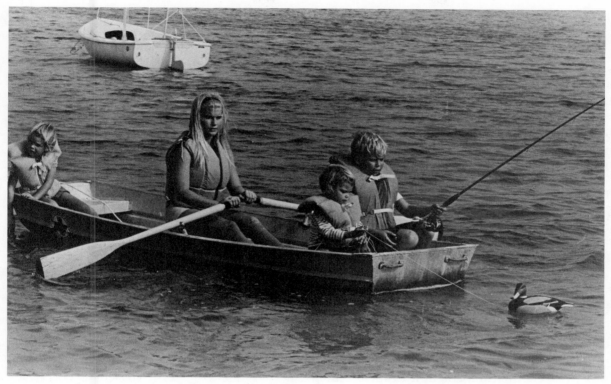

Children should always wear life jackets while boating, whether they know how to swim or not. Many tragedies can be prevented by taking this precaution.

structed. The massage is given in the following way:

1. The heel of one hand with the heel of the other crossed over it should be placed on the bottom third of the breastbone and pressed firmly down with a force of about 80 pounds so that the breastbone moves about two inches toward the spine. Pressure should not be applied directly on the ribs by the fingers.

2. The hands are then relaxed to allow the chest to expand.

3. If one person is doing both the cardiac massage and the mouth-to-mouth respiration, he should stop the massage every half minute and administer four deep breaths to the victim.

4. The rate of cardiac massage should try to simulate restoration of the pulse rate. This is not always easily accomplished, but compression should reach at least 35 to 40 times per minute.

Drowning

Anyone attempting to rescue a distressed swimmer who is far away from shore should have the proper training and credentials for doing so. Too many double deaths have occurred because of good intentions and inadequate skill.

Rescue: A child or adult who appears to be drowning near shore, or near a boat from which he has fallen, can be rescued even by someone who can't swim. The rescuer can lie prone and extend his hand or foot, or he can extend the longest available pole or branch or an oar to pull the bather to safety.

If the swimmer is too far from shore to be reached in this way, a ring buoy attached to a long rope can be tossed in his direction. If a rowboat is available, row to the victim as quickly as possible and extend an oar that will bring him around to the stern so that he can hang on while being brought to shore.

Emergency treatment: If normal breathing has been impaired, administer mouth-to-mouth respiration, described on p. 673, at once.

Prevention: Drowning is one of the major causes of accidental death. As in many major accidents, the chief contributing factor is poor judgment.

Obstruction in the Windpipe

Many people die each year from choking on food; children incur an additional hazard in swallowing foreign objects. Most of these victims could be saved through quick action by nearly any other person.

Food choking usually occurs because a bit of food becomes lodged at the back of the throat or at the opening of the trachea, or windpipe. The victim cannot breathe or speak. He may turn pale or blue before collapsing. Death can occur in four or five minutes.

The Heimlich Maneuver

This lifesaving technique works simply by squeezing the volume of air already trapped in the victim's lungs so that the piece of food pops out of the throat.

The rescuer stands behind the victim and grasps his hands firmly over the victim's abdomen, just below the rib cage. He makes a fist with one hand and places his other hand over the clenched fist, then forces the fist sharply inward and upward against the victim's diaphragm, compressing the lungs. If necessary, the maneuver should be repeated until the air passage is unblocked.

The Heimlich maneuver has been used successfully by persons who were alone when they choked on food; some pressed their own fist into their abdomen, others forced the edge of a chair or sink against their abdomen.

The obstruction may also be released by a combination of gravity pull and coughing. If the patient is a child, he should be held upside down by his legs and given a series of quick, hard blows with the fist on his back between the shoulder blades. If the person is an adult and holding him by the heels isn't practical, he should lie face down on a bed or table, with the upper half of his body suspended in the direction of the floor so that he can receive the same type of blows.

Obstruction caused by allergic reaction: There are a few people who are critically allergic to the sting of wasps, bees, or yellow jackets. This sensitivity causes the vocal

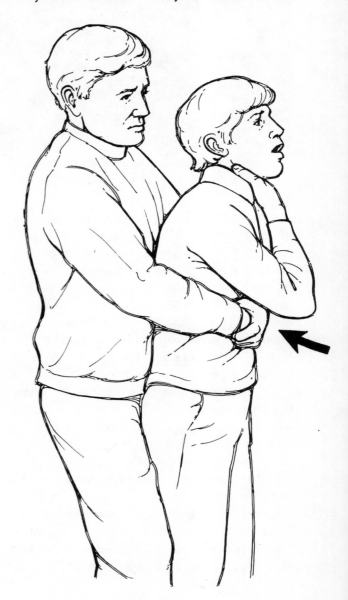

FIRST AID

ARTIFICIAL RESPIRATION
(Mouth-to-Mouth Method)

The most effective method of artificial respiration is the mouth-to-mouth method. If it is not practicable to use this method for restoring breathing, however, the back pressure-arm lift method illustrated on the following page should be employed. If the victim is not breathing begin artificial respiration at once. Wipe out quickly any foreign matter visible in the mouth, using your fingers or a cloth wrapped around your fingers.

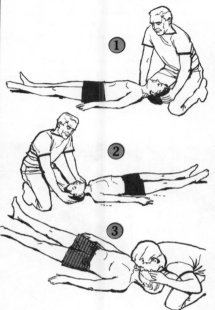

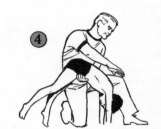

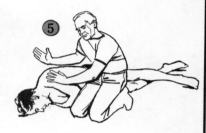

Tilt victim's head back. (Fig. 1)

Pull or push the jaw into a jutting-out position. (Fig. 2)

If victim is a small child place your mouth tightly over his mouth and nose and blow gently into his lungs about 20 times a minute. If victim is an adult (see Fig. 3), cover the mouth with your mouth, pinch his nostrils shut, and blow vigorously about 12 times a minute.

If unable to get air into lungs of victim, and if head and jaw positions are correct, suspect foreign matter in throat. To remove it, suspend a small child momentarily by the ankles or place child in position shown in Fig. 4, and slap sharply between shoulder blades.

If the victim is adult place in position shown in Fig. 5, and use same procedure.

WOUNDS

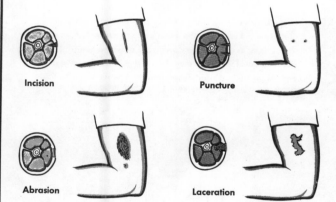

Incision

Puncture

Abrasion

Laceration

BURNS

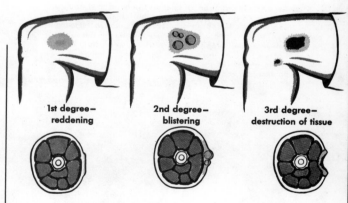

1st degree— reddening

2nd degree— blistering

3rd degree— destruction of tissue

A wound is a break in the skin. Wounds may be divided into four types: Incisions are made by sharp cutting instruments and tend to bleed freely. Punctures are caused by penetrating instruments and usually do not bleed freely. Abrasions are made by rubbing or scraping off the skin. They are sometimes called floor or mat burns. Lacerations result when the skin is torn by a blunt instrument. Wounds require good first aid and possibly medical care since they may result in infection and/or loss of blood.

Burns may be caused by contact with hot liquids or solids, certain chemicals or exposure to radiation such as sunshine. Burns are classified according to the degree, that is the depth, to which the body tissues are injured. Because of pain and other factors, shock usually results if the burn is at all extensive. Burns also frequently become infected. The first aider's duties are therefore, to relieve pain, prevent infection, and treat shock. If the burn is extensive or deep, a physician's services are always needed.

Courtesy— American National Red Cross "American Red Cross First Aid Text Book"

Edited by Ervin, Gordon and Hayman

Published by A. J. Nystrom & Co., Chicago

FIRST AID

Artificial Respiration by the Back Pressure-Arm Lift Method

Reproduced by permission of The American National Red Cross, Washington, D. C.

If breathing stops because of electro-cution, drowning, sedative poisoning, gas poisoning, suffocation, or poliomy-elitis, start artificial respiration immedi-ately. Don't delay—seconds count. As soon as possible send someone for a physician.

There should be a slight inclination of the body in such a way that fluid drains better from the respiratory passage. The head of the subject should be extended, not flexed forward, and the chin should not sag lest obstruction of the respiratory passages occur. A check should be made to ascertain that the tongue or foreign objects are not obstructing the passages.

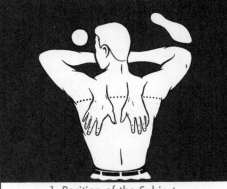

1. Position of the Subject

Place the subject in the face-down, prone position. Bend his elbows and place the hands one upon the other. Turn his face to one side, place-ing the cheek upon his hands.

These aspects can be cared for when placing the subject into position or shortly thereafter, between cycles. A smooth rhythm in performing artificial respiration is desirable, but split second timing is not essential. The cycle should be repeated 12 times per minute at a steady uniform rate. The compression and expansion phases should occupy about equal time, the release periods being of minimum duration. Shock should receive adequate attention, and the subject should remain recumbent after resusci-tation until seen by a physician or until recovery seems assured.

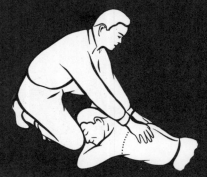

2. Position of the Operator

Kneel on either the right or left knee at the head of the subject, facing him. Place the knee at the side of the subject's head, close to the forearm. Place the opposite foot near the elbow. If it is more comfortable, kneel on both knees, one on either side of the subject's head. Place your hands upon the flat of the subject's back in such a way that the heels lie just below a line running between the armpits. With the tips of the thumbs just touching, spread the fingers downward and outward.

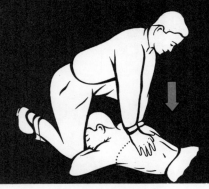

3. Compression Phase

Rock forward until the arms are approximately vertical and allow the weight of the upper part of your body to exert slow, steady, even pressure downward upon the hands. This forces air out of the lungs. Your elbows should be kept straight and the pressure exerted almost directly downward on the back.

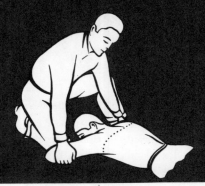

4 Position for Expansion Phase

Release the pressure, avoiding a final thrust, and commence to rock slowly backward. Place your hands upon the subject's arms just above his elbows.

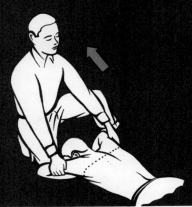

5. Expansion Phase

Draw his arms upward and toward you. Apply just enough lift to feel resistance and tension at the subject's shoulders. Do not bend your elbows, and as you rock backward the subject's arms will be drawn toward you. Then drop the arms to the ground. This completes the full cycle. The arm lift expands the chest by pulling on the chest muscles, arching the back, and relieving the weight on the chest.

cord tissue to swell to the point where breathing may become impossible. Anyone with this type of allergy who is stung should be rushed to a hospital immediately.

A person who becomes aware of having this type of allergy should consult with a physician about the kind of medicine to carry for use in a crisis.

Burns

If someone has been severely burned, get medical help immediately or call an ambulance so that the victim can get hospital treatment. *Don't* treat the burned area with any salves or ointments. Cut the charred clothing away from the injured part of the body, but *don't* pull at any fabric or anything else that has stuck to the burn. Cover the injured areas of skin with several layers of dry sterile gauze. If this isn't available, rip up pieces of newly laundered sheet and use them as temporary dressing. If the victim of the fire has gone into shock, use the emergency treatment described on p. 685.

Degrees of Burns

The degree of a burn depends on how deep into the skin the damage has reached. *First-degree burns* affect the epidermis only, causing the surface of the skin to redden and blister. Even though this type of burn is superficial, it can be serious if it covers a large area of the body, particularly in the case of children. Either petroleum jelly or a paste of baking soda and water may be applied to the burn and loosely covered with a sterile gauze. Exposure of the burn to very cold water or cold compresses has been found to reduce the pain of minor burns.

A *second-degree burn* is deeper than a first-degree burn, damaging both the epidermis and the dermis. The skin is red and charred. A *third-degree burn* is deeper still, damaging the epidermis, dermis, and the

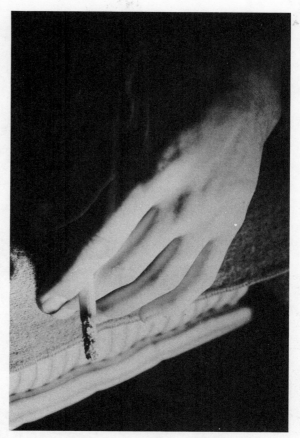

Many severe burns and tragic fires have been caused by smokers who fell asleep with a lighted cigarette.

subcutaneous tissue below. Frequently, only a physician can be sure of how deep the burn is, and then only after very careful inspection. Anything beyond a first-degree burn requires prompt emergency treatment. In administering aid to the victim of major burns, the following steps are recommended:

1. Have the patient lie down and call a physician. Apply dry dressings of sterile gauze over the burned areas.

2. If the patient is conscious and can swallow, give him fluids.

3. If the burn is extensive, wrap him in a clean sheet and call a hospital ambulance. Do not try to remove clothing from a severely burned area; cut around it instead. Do not apply oily substances, antiseptics, or absorbent cotton.

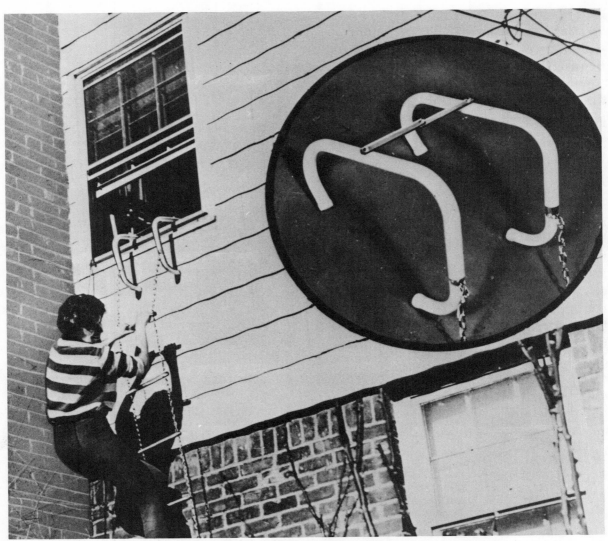

A lightweight aluminum escape ladder that fastens securely to a windowsill is important to have in the house in case of fire.

In cases of chemical burns, the affected area should be bathed immediately with soap and water until the chemical has been removed. If the burn is extensive, call for professional medical help and check the patient for shock. For treatment of shock, see p. 685.

Fire

Fire is one of the greatest hazards in the home, especially because so many people lose their heads when they see something or someone burning. In practically all cases, cool judgment and prompt action can prevent major disaster.

The most important thing to remember if someone's hair or body is on fire is to grab the thickest piece of material nearest to hand and cover the flame with it. Smothering fire with a coat, rug, or blanket is usually quicker and more effective than wasting time getting enough liquid to do the job.

Only if absolutely no other method is available for extinguishing flames should an attempt be made to beat out a flame with bare hands. Severe injury can result both to the victim and the rescuer in such cases.

Fire extinguishers: A fire extinguisher that is simple to operate is an essential part of household equipment. Two of the safest and most effective means of putting out small fires are water and sand. A hose connected to a special faucet for this purpose can be stored under the sink ready for emergency use. Several fire buckets filled with sand can be stored in a utility closet, pantry, or on the back porch.

Don't use water to put out flames caused by burning fat, oil, or solvents. One of the quickest ways to extinguish a fire in a pan of burning oil is to drop a lid on it immediately. Another method is to sprinkle the fire with the contents of a box of bicarbonate of soda that should be kept on the kitchen shelf for such emergencies.

Chemical fire extinguishers in aerosol cans should be kept in the kitchen, basement, and garage, since they are easy to use and effective against flaming oil, grease, gasoline, and chemical solvents. Avoid the use of extinguishers that contain carbon tetrachloride, and make sure that children understand that no extinguisher is meant to be played with.

Fire safety: Every household should be carefully checked for fire hazards.

Even when a fire begins, the proper and prompt use of an extinguisher can usually put it out. However, if the flames aren't brought under control immediately, the most important thing to do is get everyone out of the house and then notify the fire department.

The National Safety Council makes these additional recommendations:

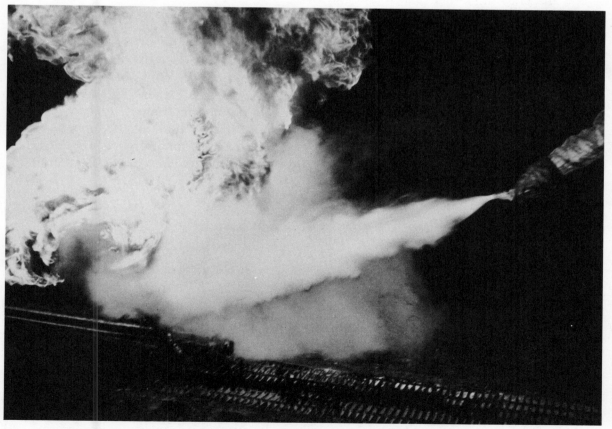

In this laboratory test, two gallons of gasoline have been ignited in an iron tub to test the performance of a foam extinguisher. A chemical extinguisher should be kept in the kitchen.

1. A sleeper who is awakened by the smell of smoke during the night should not open the bedroom door until he has felt it to find out whether it is warm. If the door temperature feels normal, it should be opened slowly and carefully. If the door feels warm from the inside, *do not* open it. If there is no fire escape attached to the bedroom window, a rope can be created by twisting and tying the bed linens to a bedpost or some other secure support. If jumping is absolutely necessary, the mattress should be thrown out the window first. Sliding out backwards, hanging on the sill, and then letting go is a much safer way to escape than leaping out face forward.

2. If the situation is such that when the door is opened slowly, there are no flames in the hall but there is dense smoke, a wet cloth should be tied over the nose and mouth, and crawling rather than walking or running should be used as a method of escape. During a fire, the air is clearer and cooler close to the floor.

3. Anyone whose clothing is on fire *should not run.* The most effective way to smother the flames is to use a rug, blanket, or heavy coat as a wrap and roll slowly on the floor.

4. Everyone in the family, as well as household help and baby-sitters, should know exactly how to report a fire by telephone. The fastest procedure should be checked with local authorities.

5. City dwellers should locate the fire alarm box closest to their dwelling and know how to use it in an emergency. Instructions are printed conspicuously on the box.

6. In the event of a serious fire, no time should be wasted fighting it or even reporting it until everyone is safely outside the building.

7. Every family should schedule fire drills on a regular basis so that each person knows the best escape routes, particularly from a bedroom. There should also be a prear-ranged meeting place outside the house in the event of fire so that no one is tempted to return to a burning building for someone who is already safely outside.

Sunstroke (Heatstroke)

Sunstroke, a more serious emergency than *heat exhaustion* (discussed below), is characterized by an acutely high body temperature caused by the cessation of perspiration. The patient's skin becomes hot, dry, and flushed, and he may suffer collapse. Should the skin turn ashen gray, a physician must be called immediately. Prompt hospital treatment is recommended for anyone showing signs of sunstroke who has previously had any kind of heart damage.

The following emergency treatment should reduce the patient's body temperature as quickly as possible and prevent damage to the internal organs:

1. Place him in a tub of very cold water.

2. Take his temperature by mouth, and when it has dropped to 100°F., remove him to a bed and wrap him in cold, wet sheets.

3. If possible, expose him to an electric fan or an air conditioner.

Sunstroke is best avoided by reducing physical activity and forgoing very vigorous sports during periods of high heat and high humidity.

Heat Exhaustion (Heat Prostration)

Heat exhaustion occurs when the body is exposed to high temperatures and large amounts of blood accumulate in the skin as a way of cooling it. As a result, there is a marked decrease in the amount of blood that circulates through the heart and to the brain. The patient becomes markedly pale and is covered with cold perspiration. Breathing is increasingly shallow and the pulse weakens. In acute cases, fainting occurs.

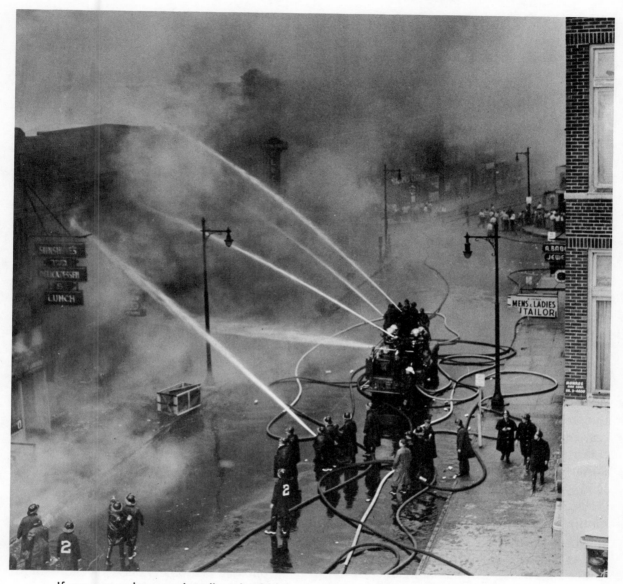

If you ever wake up and smell smoke, feel the door before opening it. If it does not feel warm, open it slowly and carefully. If it does feel warm, do not open it; get out another way.

The following emergency treatment is usually effective:

1. Place the patient in a reclining position, loosen or remove his clothing, and apply cold, wet cloths to his wrists and forehead.

2. If he has fainted and doesn't recover promptly, smelling salts or spirits of ammonia should be placed under his nose.

3. When the patient is conscious, give him salt tablets and cool, sweetened tea or coffee as a stimulant. Don't try to force any liquids into the patient's mouth while he is not fully conscious. Don't offer him any alcoholic beverages.

Falls

Any accident involving a fall—whether tripping on the stairs, slipping on ice, or stumbling on a street curb—may result in broken bones. Many serious falls occur in

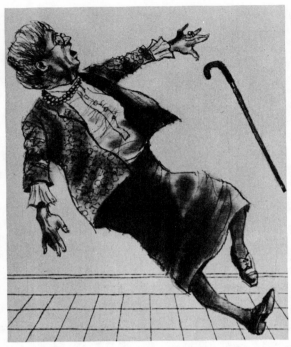

Older people are particularly subject to falls. Good lighting and nonslippery floors should be the rule.

and around the home, particularly to the very young and the old.

Fractures: Any break in a bone is called a *fracture*. The break is called an *open* or *compound fracture* if one or both ends of the broken bone pierce the skin. A *closed* or *simple fracture* is one in which the broken bone doesn't come through the skin.

It is sometimes difficult to distinguish a strained muscle or a sprained ligament from a broken bone, since sprains and strains can be extremely painful even though they are less serious than breaks. However, when there is any doubt about the type of injury resulting from a fall, it should be treated as though it were a simple fracture and the following precautions should be taken:

1. Don't try to help the person who has fallen to move around or to get up unless he has slowly tested out the injured part of his body and is sure that nothing has been broken.

2. If he is in extreme pain, or if the injured part has begun to swell, or if by running the finger lightly along the affected bone a break can be felt, *don't* move him. Under no circumstances should he be crowded into a car if his legs, hip, ribs, or back are involved in the accident. Call for an ambulance immediately, and until it arrives, treat the person for shock as described on p. 685.

Splinting: In a situation where it is imperative to move someone who may have a fracture, the first thing to do is to apply a splint so that the broken bone ends are immobilized.

Splints can be improvised from anything rigid enough and of the right length to support the fractured part of the body: a metal rod, board, long cardboard tube, tightly rolled newspaper or blanket. If the object being used has to be padded for softness, use a small blanket or any other soft material, such as a jacket.

The splint should be long enough so that it can be tied with a bandage, torn sheet, or neckties beyond the joint above and below the fracture as well as at the site of the break. If a leg is involved, it should be elevated with pillows or any other firm support after the splint has been applied. If the patient has to wait a considerable length of time for professional help to arrive, the splint bandaging should be checked from time to time to make sure it isn't too tight.

Concussion: Some falls, especially those involving children, can result in a severe blow to the head or the base of the spine, which may cause *concussion*. Concussion, which causes the functioning of the brain to be temporarily impaired, resulting in unconsciousness if only of momentary duration, may or may not be associated with a skull fracture. In either case, the emergency treatment is the same. The victim may lose consciousness for a more prolonged period, and his breathing is likely to be conspicuously rapid or slow. If he is conscious, he is likely to complain of stabbing head pains, dizziness, faulty vision, and nausea.

PLACING AN INJURED PERSON ON A STRETCHER

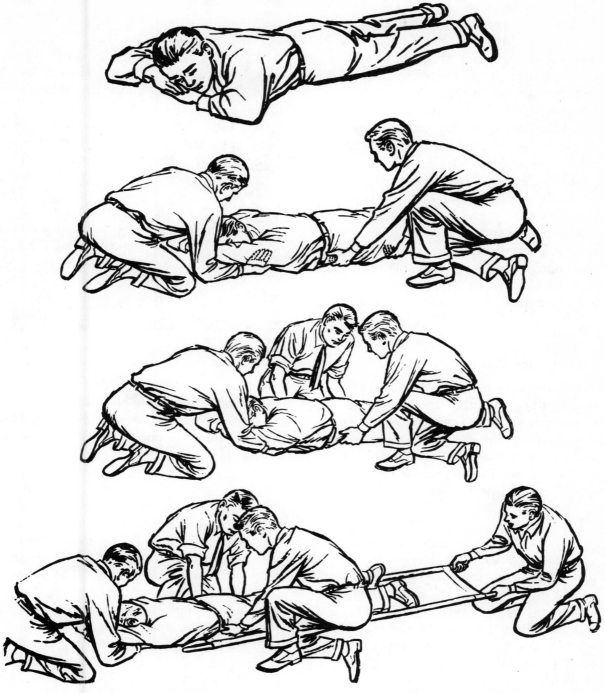

If an injured person must be moved, he should be placed in a prone position with hands under chin (*top*). Carrier 1 kneels at the victim's head, carefully places upturned palms under the mid-forearms of the injured person; carrier 2 grasps the victim's hipbone with one hand and kneecap with the other (*second from top*). Carrier 1 slides his hands to the victim's armpits, and carrier 3 crouches opposite carrier 2 and also grasps victim's hipbone and kneecap (*third from top*). At a given signal, the three carriers lift the victim's body as a unit about five or six inches from the ground, providing enough clearance for a stretcher to be slid underneath (*bottom*).

Treatment: If these symptoms occur, a doctor must be called immediately, and the patient kept absolutely still and covered. If there are visible head wounds, they should wait for professional attention. Under no circumstances should any effort be made to shake or slap the patient into consciousness, nor should he be given any kind of stimulant. If breathing is conspicuously impaired, mouth-to-mouth respiration should be administered as described on p. 673.

Most cases of concussion are neither permanently damaging nor fatal, but the victim does take from a few days to a few weeks to recover completely. However, professional attention is necessary even if the condition is only suspected, because there may be delayed reactions to a head injury even though there are no immediate symptoms.

Strains and Sprains

Two types of injuries less serious than fractures but considerably more common are strains and sprains. They occur to the muscles, joints, tendons, and ligaments, and since in some cases they can be sufficiently uncomfortable to be incapacitating, they should receive prompt treatment.

Strain

When a muscle is stretched because of misuse or overuse, the interior bundles of tissue may tear, or the tendon which connects it to the bone may be stretched. This condition is known as *strain.* It occurs most commonly to the muscles of the lower back when heavy weights are improperly lifted, or in the area of the ankle as the result of a sudden twist or undue pressure.

Treatment: Resting the affected area and taking aspirin usually relieves any acute pain. The application of heat and gentle massage are also effective measures. In severe cases of strained back muscles, a physician may have to be consulted for

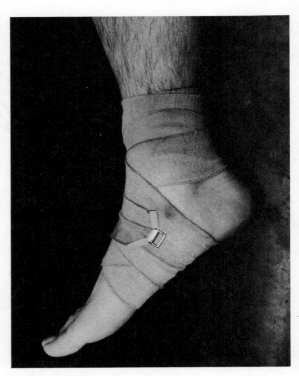

An elastic bandage provides temporary support for healing ankle muscles following a strain or sprain.

strapping. For a strained ankle, a flexible elastic bandage can be helpful in providing the necessary support until the injured muscle heals.

Sprain

A *sprain* occurs when a joint is wrenched or twisted in such a way that the ligaments holding it in position are ruptured, possibly damaging the surrounding blood vessels, tendons, nerves, and muscles. This type of injury is more serious than a strain and is usually accompanied by pain, sometimes severe, soreness, swelling, and discoloration of the affected area. Most sprains occur as a result of falls, athletic accidents, or improper handling of heavy weights.

Treatment: Emergency treatment for a sprain consists of prompt rest, the application of cold compresses to relieve swelling and any internal bleeding in the joint, and elevation of the affected area. Aspirin is recommended to reduce discomfort. If the swelling and soreness increase after such treatment, a physician should be consulted to make sure that the injury is not a fracture or a bone dislocation.

Shock

Shock is an emergency condition in which the circulation of the blood is so disrupted that all bodily functions are affected. It occurs when blood pressure is so low that insufficient blood supply reaches the vital tissues. This type of shock is not to be confused with electric shock (see p. 672) or with insulin or diabetic shock (see p. 579).

Types of Circulatory Shock and Their Causes

• *Low-volume shock* is a condition brought about by so great a loss of blood or blood plasma that the remaining blood is insufficient to fill the whole circulatory system. The blood loss may occur outside the body, as in a hemorrhage caused by injury to an artery or vein, or the loss may be internal because of the blood loss at the site of a major fracture, burn, or bleeding ulcer. Professional treatment involves replacement of blood loss by transfusion.

• *Neurogenic shock,* manifested by *fainting,* occurs when the regulating capacity of the nervous system is impaired by severe pain, profound fright, or other overwhelming stimulus. This type of shock is usually relieved by having the patient lie down with his head lower than the rest of his body.

• *Allergic shock,* also called *anaphylactic shock,* occurs when the functioning of the blood vessels is disturbed by a person's sensitivity to the injection of a particular foreign substance, as in the case of an insect sting or certain medicines.

• *Septic shock* is brought on by infection from certain bacteria that release a poison which affects the proper functioning of the blood vessels.

• *Cardiac shock* can be caused by any circumstance that affects the pumping action of the heart.

Symptoms: Shock caused by blood loss makes the patient feel restless, thirsty, and cold. He may perspire a great deal, and although his pulse is fast, it is also very weak. His breathing becomes labored and his lips turn blue.

Emergency treatment: A doctor should be called immediately if the onset of shock is suspected. Until medical help arrives, the following procedures can alleviate some of the symptoms:

1. With a minimum amount of disturbance, arrange the patient so that he is lying on his back with his head somewhat lower than his feet. Loosen any clothing that may cause constriction, such as a belt, tie, waistband, shoes. Cover him warmly against possible chill, but see that he isn't too hot.

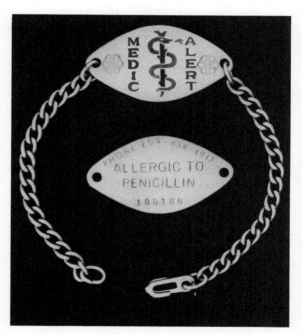

Some people are so severely allergic to certain medications that exposure to them can produce unconsciousness and, if not treated promptly, even death. To alert others, emblems identifying the allergy are available for a slight charge from the nonprofit Medic Alert Foundation, Turlock, California 95380.

2. If his breathing is weak and shallow, begin mouth-to-mouth respiration as described on p. 673.

3. If he is hemorrhaging, try to control bleeding as described on pp. 668 and 670.

4. When appropriate help and transportation facilities are available, quickly move the patient to the nearest hospital or health facility in order to begin resuscitative measures.

5. *Do not* try to force any food or stimulant into the patient's mouth.

Asphyxiation by Gas

Before attempting to revive someone overcome by toxic gas poisoning, the most important thing to do is to remove him to the fresh air. If this isn't feasible, all windows and doors should be opened to let in as much fresh air as possible.

Any interior with a dangerous concentration of carbon monoxide or other toxic gases is apt to be highly explosive. Therefore, gas and electricity should be shut off as quickly as possible. *Under no circumstances should any matches be lighted in an interior where there are noxious fumes.*

The rescuer needn't waste time covering his face with a handkerchief or other cloth. He should hold his breath instead, or take only a few quick, shallow breaths while bringing the victim to the out-of-doors or to an open window.

If possible, someone should call the police or the fire department for an oxygen inhaler while another person administers mouth-to-mouth respiration to the victim as described on p. 673.

Poisoning

Most cases of poisoning occur as a result of swallowing a substance that can be fatal if it isn't neutralized, diluted, or removed from the stomach *at once*. If the nature of the poison is known, the list below gives the specific treatment for it. If the poison taken is not known, the following preparation, which is called the universal antidote, should be given:

The universal antidote: 2 parts activated charcoal, 1 part tannic acid, 1 part magnesium oxide to make up 1 tablespoon to be mixed into half a glass of warm water. This combination can be bought at any pharmacy and should be kept in the household medicine cabinet at all times.

Other suggestions: If the container from which the poison has been swallowed is at hand, check the label for the specific antidote.

In all cases of poisoning, call the doctor at once. If he isn't immediately available, call the nearest Poison Control Center. These centers are open 24 hours a day. Look the number up in your telephone directory and jot it down with other emergency numbers. The Directory of Poison Control Centers is available for 20¢ from the National Clearinghouse for Poison Control Centers, Public Health Service, U.S. Department of Health, Education, and Welfare, Washington, D.C. 20201.

Do not attempt to induce vomiting unless the nature of the poisoning calls for it as a treatment. If vomiting is indicated, it can be induced by 2 to 4 glasses of any of the following *emetics:*

1 teaspoon of dry mustard *or*
1 teaspoon of salt *or*
1 teaspoon of baking soda

stirred into a glass of warm water. If none of these products is quickly available, give 2 to 4 glasses of warm, soapy water. If vomiting doesn't occur promptly, induce it by placing the forefinger on the base of the patient's tongue and pressing down gently. When the patient begins to vomit, see that his head is lower than his body to prevent strangulation.

If breathing is irregular, administer mouth-to-mouth respiration as described on p. 673.

In cases where poisons have been inhaled, such as carbon monoxide or gas fumes, place the patient in the fresh air and wrap him in blankets to prevent chill. Loosen all clothing and apply mouth-to-mouth respiration if necessary.

The treatment for snakebite poisoning is described on p. 690.

Emergency Treatment for Some Common Household Poisons, Listed Alphabetically

Acetone products such as nail polish remover, varnish solvents, rubber cement: Induce vomiting, follow with large amounts of warm water or milk, and repeat the emetic used to induce vomiting. When the vomitus

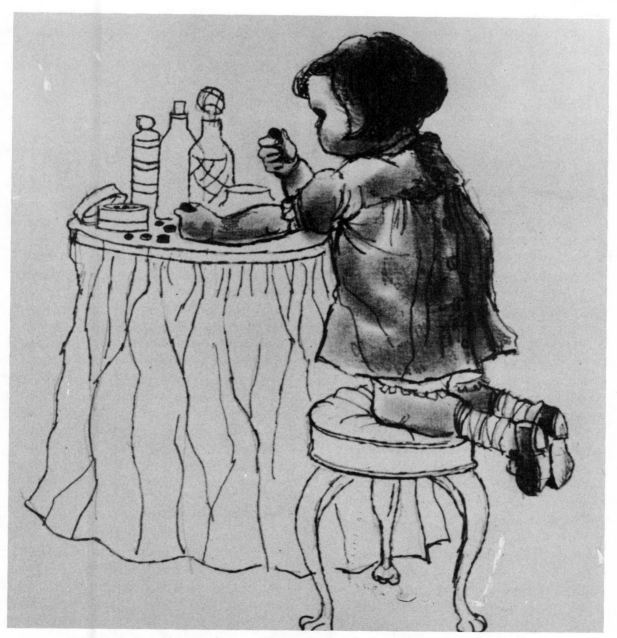

If a poisonous substance has been swallowed and the container is available, check the label for a specific antidote, administer it at once, and call a doctor immediately.

(vomited matter) is clear, give strong tea or black coffee and keep the patient warm and quiet.

Ammonia and quicklime: Do not induce vomiting. Have the patient swallow half a cup of lemon or orange juice or vinegar diluted in a glass of water. Follow with 3 egg whites stirred into a glass of water *or* ½ cup of cooking oil *or* 1 to 2 glasses of milk.

Arsenic products such as rat poison, paris green, weed killer: Induce vomiting and follow with the universal antidote *or* 2 tablespoons of Epsom salts in 2 glasses of warm water. Repeat the emetic and follow with 3 egg whites in a glass of water *or* 1 to 2 glasses of milk.

Aspirin: Follow the same procedure as for acetone. Parents should avoid the use of candy-coated aspirin for children. To tell them that any medicine is just like candy is courting disaster.

Benzine, furniture polish, gasoline, lighter fluid, naphtha: Do not induce vomiting. Give 3 egg whites in a glass of water *or* ½ cup of cooking oil *or* 2 glasses of milk. Follow with strong tea or coffee and keep patient warm.

Boric acid or borax: Induce vomiting and follow with the universal antidote *or* large amounts of warm milk or water. Repeat several times.

Camphor or camphorated oils: Induce vomiting and follow with 2 tablespoons of Epsom salts in 2 glasses of water. Repeat emetic and follow with large glass of milk.

Carbolic acid, creosol, Lysol, disinfectants: Give 2 tablespoons of Epsom salts in 2 glasses of water. Induce vomiting and follow with 3 egg whites in water *or* flour or cornstarch diluted to a drinkable mixture in water.

Codeine, paregoric, morphine, and cough medicines containing opium derivatives: Induce vomiting and follow with large amounts of milk or water. Repeat emetic. Keep the patient awake and moving about,

and see that he drinks large quantities of strong hot tea or coffee.

Iodine: Give large quantities of bread or cornstarch diluted to a paste in water. Follow with an emetic to induce vomiting. Repeat both procedures until the vomit is colorless.

Kerosene: Same treatment as benzine.

Lead paints, dyes, insecticides: Same treatment as arsenic.

Lye or styptic pencil: Same treatment as ammonia.

Methyl alcohol, wood alcohol, methanol: Induce vomiting, follow with 1 to 2 tablespoons of baking soda diluted in 2 to 3 glasses of water. Repeat emetic and follow with a tablespoon of baking soda in a glass of warm milk or water. Keep the patient lying down and covered.

Rust removers containing hydrofluoric acid: Do not induce vomiting. Give ½ cup milk of magnesia stirred into ½ cup of water *or* 2 tablespoons of baking soda in a glass of water. Follow with 3 egg whites in a glass of water *or* ½ cup of cooking oil *or* a large glass of milk.

Sleeping pills or sedatives containing barbiturates such as phenobarbitol or chloral hydrate: Induce vomiting and follow with large amounts of milk or water. Repeat both procedures several times and then give strong hot tea or coffee. Make every effort to keep the patient awake and moving about.

Turpentine: Same treatment as rust removers.

Firearm Accidents

Bullet wounds, whether accidental or purposely inflicted, can range from those that are superficial and external to those that involve internal bleeding and extensive tissue damage.

Emergency procedure: A surface bullet wound accompanied by bleeding should be covered promptly with sterile gauze to pre-

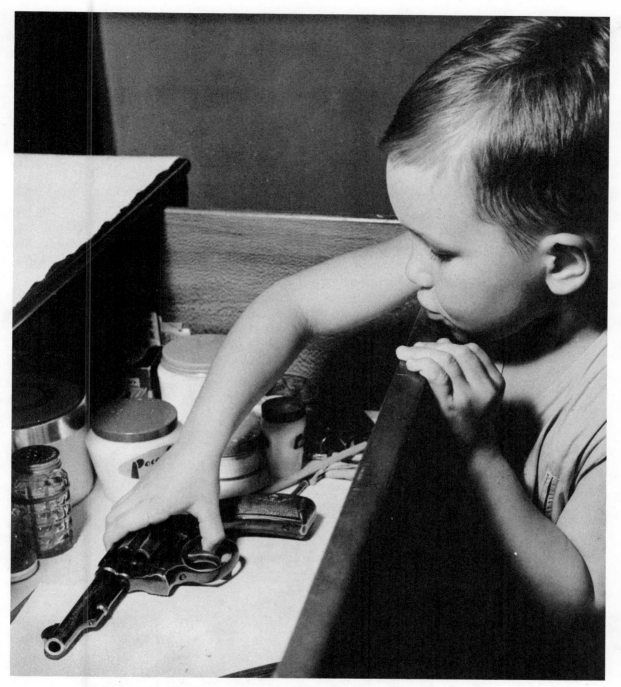

If firearms must be kept in the house, they should be kept well out of the reach of children and under lock and key, and they should never be stored when loaded.

vent further infection. The flow of blood should be controlled as described on p. 670. *Don't* try to clean the wound with soap or water. Wait for the doctor's instructions before applying any medicines.

If the wound is internal, keep the patient lying down and wrap him with coats or blankets placed over and under his body. If respiration has ceased or is impaired, give mouth-to-mouth respiration as described on p. 673, and treat him for shock as described on p. 685. Get an ambulance.

Any gunshot injury *must* be reported to the police.

Preventing firearm accidents: Most gunshot accidents occur at home as a result of carelessness. Families who own firearms *of no matter what type* should therefore observe the following rules, especially if there are children in the house:

1. A loaded gun should never be kept indoors.

2. Even before a hunting trip, a gun should never be loaded in the house or in a car.

3. Guns should be stored in a locked cabinet and ammunition stored elsewhere so that both are inaccessible to children.

4. Adults should *never* show off or play with a gun in the presence of children, nor should irresponsible remarks be made in their presence about shooting.

5. A child who is afraid of a gun should not be encouraged to handle one.

Snakebites

Of the many varieties of snakes found in the United States, only four kinds are poisonous: copperheads, rattlesnakes, moccasins, and coral snakes. The first three belong to the category of pit vipers and are known as *hemotoxic* because their poison enters the bloodstream. The coral snake, which is comparatively rare, is related to the cobra and is the most dangerous of all because

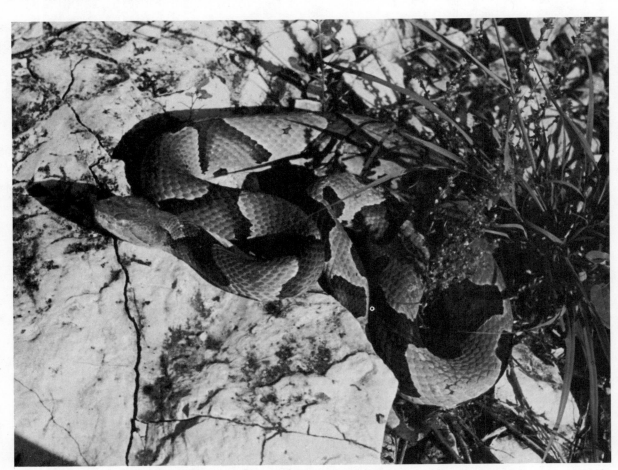

The poisonous copperhead, widely distributed in upland areas of the east and midwest, is colored with chestnut-brown hourglass shapes against a tan background.

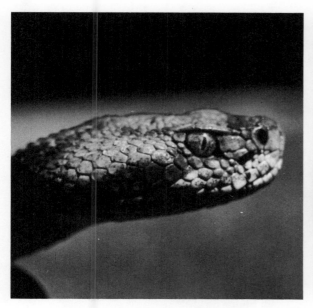 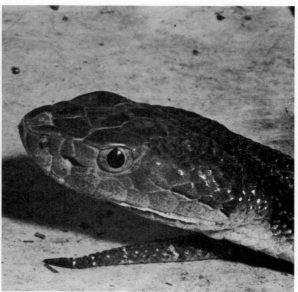

Two pit vipers: (*left*) a timber rattlesnake and (*right*) a copperhead. Note the pit between eye and nostril. A pit viper's eyes are like a cat's eyes; the pupils narrow to vertical slits in sunlight, become large and round at night. Nonpoisonous snakes have round pupils at all times.

its venom is *neurotoxic*. This means that the poison transmitted by its bite goes directly to the nervous system and the brain.

How to differentiate between snakebites: Snakes of the pit viper family have a fang on each side of the head. These fangs leave characteristic puncture wounds on the skin in addition to two rows of tiny bites or scratches left by the teeth. A bite from a nonpoisonous snake leaves six rows—four upper and two lower—of very small bite marks or scratches and no puncture wounds.

The marks left by the bite of a coral snake do not leave any puncture wounds either, but this snake bites with a chewing motion, hanging on to the victim rather than attacking quickly. The coral snake is very easy to recognize because of its distinctive markings: wide horizontal bands of red and black separated by narrow bands of yellow.

Symptoms: A bite from any of the pit vipers produces immediate and severe pain and darkening of the skin, followed by weakness, blurred vision, quickened pulse, nausea, and vomiting. The bite of a coral snake produces somewhat the same symptoms, although there is less local pain and considerable drowsiness leading to unconsciousness.

Treatment for a poisonous bite: If a doctor or a hospital is a short distance away, the patient should receive professional help *immediately*. He should be transported lying down, either on an improvised stretcher or carried by his companions—with the wounded part of his body lower than the rest. He should be advised to move as little as possible.

If several hours must elapse before a doctor or a hospital can be reached, the following procedures should be applied promptly:

1. Keep the victim lying down and as still as possible.

2. Tie a constricting band *above* the wound between it and the heart and tight enough to slow but not stop blood circulation. A handkerchief, necktie, sock, or piece of torn shirt will serve.

3. Sterilize a knife or razor blade in a flame and make shallow cuts through the wound and puncture marks in a crisscross

pattern. The cuts should be just deep enough to draw blood.

4. Suck out the venom as rapidly as possible. It will be mixed with blood and will not be toxic if swallowed.

5. This procedure should be continued until the swelling subsides and the other symptoms decrease.

Animal Bites

Wild animals, particularly bats, serve as a natural reservoir of rabies, a disease that is almost always fatal unless promptly and properly treated. But the virus may be present in the saliva of any warm-blooded animal. Domestic animals should be immunized against rabies by vaccines injected by a veterinarian.

Symptoms: Rabies is transmitted to humans by an animal bite or through a cut or scratch already in the skin. The infected saliva may enter through any opening, including the membranes lining the nose or mouth. After an incubation period of about ten days, a person infected by a rabid animal experiences pain at the site of infection, extreme sensitivity of the skin to temperature changes, and painful spasms of the larynx that make it almost impossible to drink. Saliva thickens and the patient becomes restless and easily excitable. By the time symptoms develop, death may be imminent. Obviously, treatment should begin promptly after having been exposed to the possibility of infection.

Treatment: The area around the wound should be washed thoroughly and repeatedly with soap and water, using a sterile gauze dressing to wipe fluid away from—not toward—the wound. Another sterile dressing is used to dry the wound and a third to cover it while the patient is taken to a hospital or doctor's office. A tetanus injection is also indicated, and police and health authorities should be promptly notified of the biting incident.

If at all possible the biting animal should be identified—if a wild animal, captured alive—and held for observation for a period of 10 to 15 days. If it can be determined during that period that the animal is not rabid, further treatment may not be required. If the animal is rabid, however, or if it cannot be located and impounded, the patient may have to undergo a series of daily rabies vaccine injections lasting from 14 days for a case of mild exposure to 21 days for severe exposure (a bite near the head, for example), plus several booster shots. Because of the sensitivity of some individuals to the rabies vaccines used, the treatment itself can be quite dangerous.

Insect Stings

Honeybees, wasps, hornets, and yellowjackets are the most common stinging insects and are most likely to attack on a hot summer day. Strongly scented perfumes or cosmetics and brightly colored, rough-finished clothing attract bees and should be avoided by persons working or playing in garden areas. It should also be noted that many commercial repellents do not protect against stinging insects. If one is stung, the insect's stinger should be scraped gently but quickly from the skin; don't squeeze it. Apply Epsom salt solution to the sting area. Antihistamines are often helpful in reducing the patient's discomfort. If a severe reaction develops, call a doctor. Bee venom is a dangerous poison, and in some allergic individuals a sting can have very serious and even fatal consequences if not treated promptly.

Heart Attack

A heart attack is caused by interference with the blood supply to the heart muscle. When the attack is brought on because of a blood clot in the coronary artery, it is known as *coronary occlusion* or *coronary thrombosis*.

Symptoms: The most dramatic symptom of a serious heart attack is a crushing chest pain that usually travels down the left arm into the hand or into the neck and back. The pain may bring on dizziness, cold sweat, complete collapse, and loss of consciousness. The face has an ashen pallor, and there may be vomiting.

Treatment: The patient *must not be moved* unless he has fallen in a dangerous place. If no doctor is immediately available, an ambulance should be called at once. No attempt should be made to get the victim of a heart attack into an automobile.

Until help arrives, give the patient every reassurance that he will get prompt treatment, and keep him as calm and quiet as possible. Don't give him any medicine or stimulants. If oxygen is available, start administering it to the patient immediately, either by mask or nasal catheter, depending on which is available.

Acute Angina Pectoris

Angina pectoris is a condition that causes acute chest pain because of interference with the supply of oxygen to the heart. Although the pain is sometimes confused with ulcer or acute indigestion symptoms, it has a distinct characteristic of its own, producing a feeling of heaviness, strangling, tightness, or suffocation. Angina is a symptom rather than a disease, and may be a chronic condition with those over 50. It is usually treated by placing a nitroglycerine tablet under the tongue.

An attack of acute angina can be brought on by emotional stress, overeating, strenuous exercise, or by any activity that makes excessive demands on heart function.

Emergency treatment: An attack usually subsides in about ten minutes, during which the patient appears to be gasping for breath. He should be kept in a semireclining position rather than made to lie flat, and should be moved carefully only in order to place pillows under his head and chest so that he can breathe more easily. A doctor should be called promptly after the onset of an attack.

Acute Asthma Attack

Asthma is an allergic condition in which the breathing mechanism is impaired in such a way that air remains trapped in the lungs, which prevents adequate fresh air from entering. The effort to expel the stale air results in the characteristic wheezing of an asthma attack, and the lack of oxygen causes the skin to take on a bluish pallor.

Symptoms: The onset of an attack, especially in children, is usually preceded by symptoms that can easily be mistaken for a cold: a stuffed nose, hard cough, and difficulty in breathing. A child prone to asthma attacks often has them at night, and as breathing becomes increasingly difficult, he may sit upright and cough in order to clear his chest.

Treatment: A doctor should be consulted about a first attack, chiefly for reassurance of the child and parents and for advice on how to make the patient more comfortable until the acute phase is over. Every effort should be made to find out the nature of the irritant that brings on the attacks so that their recurrence can be prevented. In many cases, the source of the allergy is something easily identified, such as pillow feathers or a pet cat. Some children outgrow the asthmatic condition with time, but when it becomes chronic, it can cause permanent lung damage. For further information, see *Allergic Asthma*, p. 552.

Croup

Croup is a breathing disorder usually caused by a virus infection and less often by bacteria or allergy. It is a common condition during childhood, and in some cases, may require brief hospitalization for proper treatment.

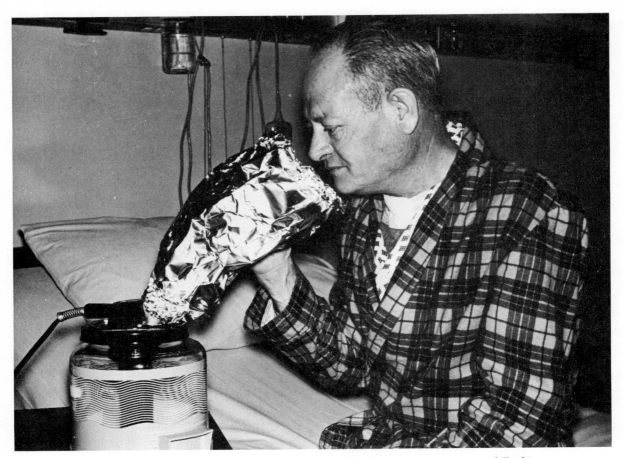

A bedside humidifier can help those with asthma, croup, or other respiratory difficulties.

Symptoms: The onset of a croup attack is likely to occur during the night with a sudden hoarse or barking cough accompanied by difficulty in breathing. The coughing is usually followed by choking spasms that sound as though the child is strangling. There may also be a mild fever. A doctor should be called immediately when these symptoms appear.

Emergency treatment: The most effective treatment for croup is cool moist air. Cool water vaporizers are now available as well as warm steam vaporizers. Another alternative is to take the child into the bathroom, close the door and windows, and let the hot water run from the shower and sink taps until the room is filled with steam.

It is also possible to improvise a croup tent by boiling water in a kettle on a portable hot plate and arranging a blanket over the back of a chair so that it encloses the child and an adult as well as the steaming kettle. A child should never be left alone even for an instant in such a makeshift arrangement.

If the symptoms do not subside in about 20 minutes with any of the above procedures, or if there is mounting fever, and if the doctor is not on his way, the child should be rushed to the closest hospital. Cold moist night air, rather than being a danger, may actually make the symptoms subside temporarily.

Unconsciousness

Unconsciousness is the condition which has the appearance of sleep, but is usually the result of injury, shock, or serious physical disturbance. A brief loss of consciousness followed by spontaneous recovery is called *fainting.* A prolonged episode of unconsciousness is a *coma.*

EMERGENCY PROCEDURES

1. Call a doctor at once. If none is available, get the person to the nearest hospital.

2. If the loss of consciousness is accompanied by loss of breathing, begin mouth-to-mouth respiration as described on p. 673.

3. Don't try to revive the patient with any kind of stimulant unless told to do so by a doctor.

Some causes of unconsciousness: Unconsciousness can be caused by a great many conditions. Among the more likely possibilities—with references to the pages where they are discussed—are the following:

alcoholic intoxication: p. 634
concussion: p. 682
diabetes or insulin shock: p. 579
electric shock: p. 672
epilepsy: p. 695
heart attack: p. 692
internal injury (falls: p. 681; firearm accidents: p. 688)
narcotic overdose: p. 657
poisoning: p. 686
shock: p. 685
suffocation: p. 676

Epilepsy

Epilepsy is a disorder of the nervous system that produces convulsive seizures. There are several types of epilepsy, most of which are now treated with medicines called *anticonvulsants.* Detailed information on the subject can be obtained by writing to the Epilepsy Foundation of America, 1419 H Street, N.W., Washington, D.C. 20005.

Types of seizures and their symptoms: In general, an epileptic seizure is characterized by a brief or prolonged period of unconsciousness accompanied by involuntary twitching and convulsive movements.

In the form of the disorder that produces minor seizures or *petit mal,* the loss of consciousness lasts for only a few seconds, during which there is twitching of the eye and mouth muscles.

In a major seizure or *grand mal,* the epileptic usually falls to the ground. Indeed, falling is in most cases one of the principal dangers of the disease. Then the epileptic's body begins to twitch or jerk spasmodically. His breathing may be labored, and saliva may appear on his lips. His face may become pale or bluish. Although the scene can be frightening, it is not truly a medical emergency; the afflicted person is in no danger of losing his life. For a more detailed discussion of this disease and its symptoms, see *Epilepsy,* p. 472.

Emergency procedures: Make the person suffering the seizure as comfortable as possible. If he is on a hard surface, put something soft under his head, and move any hard or dangerous objects away from him. *Make no attempt to restrain his movements, and do not force anything into his mouth.* Just leave him alone until the attack is over, as it should be in a few minutes. If his mouth is already open, you might put something soft, such as a folded hankerchief, between his side teeth. This will help to prevent him from biting his tongue or lips. If he seems to go into another seizure after coming out of the first, or if the seizure lasts more than ten minutes, call a doctor. If his lower jaw sags and begins to obstruct his breathing, support of the lower jaw may be helpful in improving his breathing.

When the seizure is over, the patient should be allowed to rest quietly. Some people sleep heavily after a seizure. Others awake at once but are disoriented or confused for a while. Treat the episode in a matter-of-fact way. If it is the first seizure the person is aware of having had, advise him to see his physician promptly. HMacL

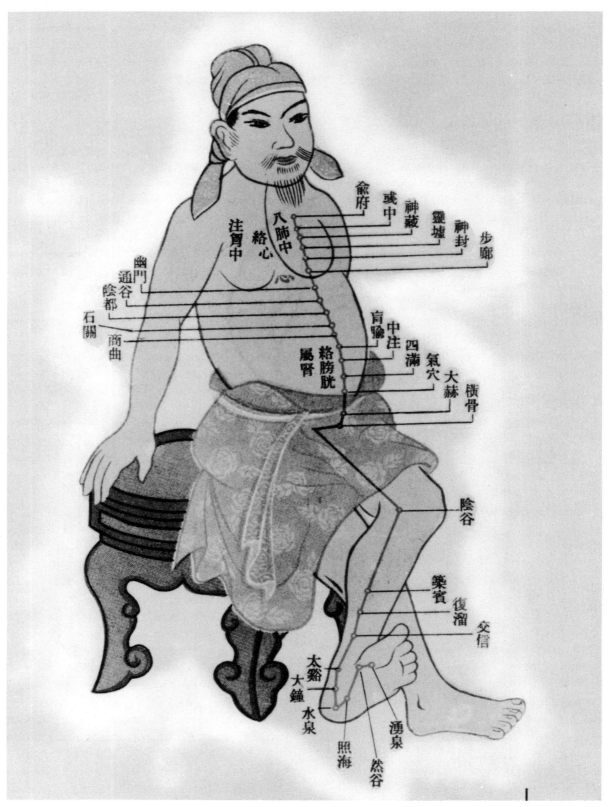

A Chinese drawing indicating a meridian along which acupuncture points are located.

The Ancient Art of Acupuncture

Acupuncture, the Oriental art of inserting needles through the skin for the treatment of physical and mental ailments, is so ancient that its true origin cannot be traced. Some Asian scholars believe that acupuncture may have started during the stone ages; most agree that acupuncture has been used as a form of medical practice for at least 5,000 years. Among the oldest known manuscripts from early Chinese cultures is The Yellow Emperor's Canon of Internal Medicine, written about 400 B.C., which contains a description of the relationships between acupuncture and the religious philosophy of Tao.

Taoism and the Balance of Forces

Taoism teaches that there is a balance of forces in nature. The function of acupuncture in this metaphysical concept of medicine is to restore the balance of forces within the body by either stimulating or calming the organ system that seems to be at the root of the disorder. The two primary forces are the Yin and the Yang, represented by female and male, negative and positive, passive and active, shadow and light, or the earth and the heavens. The two primary forces both oppose and complement each other in a relative manner so that the universe is in harmony when the Yin and the Yang are in) balance.

THE FIVE ELEMENTS

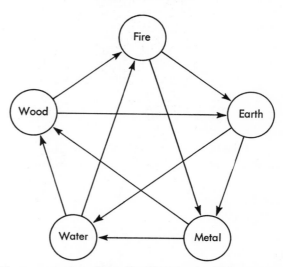

The arrows show how the Elements interrelate, e.g., fire governs metal but is in turn controlled by water.

697

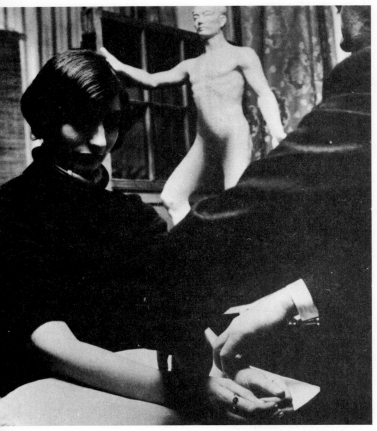

Before any needles are inserted, the practitioner takes a series of pulse readings from each wrist.

The Taoist concept also recognizes the Five Elements of nature. They are earth, fire, water, metal, and wood. Like Yin and Yang, the Five Elements are interdependent; each has its opposite, and each governs and is in turn governed by another element. Thus, water creates wood and wood creates fire, but metal overcomes wood and fire overcomes metal, and so on, in a five-sided cycle.

The Law of the Yin and the Yang and the Law of the Five Elements form the basis of traditional Oriental medical practices. Each organ of the body is either Yin or Yang; each organ is also associated with one of the Five Elements. The liver, regarded as the center of metabolic activity that makes life possible, is Yin and is also a wood element. The gallbladder, an ana-

tomical neighbor of the liver, is also a wood element but it is Yang. Wood is the only element of the five that is of an organic nature. In this context, the lungs and the upper digestive tract have functions of supplying oxygen and food for the liver's metabolic activity, the heart helps circulate the metabolic products, and the kidneys and lower digestive tract carry away by-products of metabolism.

When symptoms of a liver disease are revealed by a doctor's diagnosis, the role of acupuncture is to help restore the equilibrium of the organ. If the ailment is associated with a lack of energy, the energy may be restored by pricking the skin with an acupuncture needle at a specific point on the body—a point which may be far removed anatomically from the diseased organ. If the disease is diagnosed as evidence of an excess of energy, a somewhat different application of acupuncture therapy may be prescribed to calm the excess energy flow.

As the reader may have gathered by now, the practice of acupuncture is a complex art that requires a long period of study and training. Even before the first needle is inserted through the patient's skin, the practitioner makes a detailed examination that includes taking 12 pulse readings, six from each wrist at three different points. The examination may also require studying skin coloration and body odor, palpating the chest and abdomen, and listening to the voice of the patient.

Meridians

After the diagnosis is completed, one or more acupuncture needles are inserted at a point along a *meridian*—the term used to describe a pathway beneath the skin through which energy flows. Each organ system is associated with a meridian that extends to other areas of the body, which explains the rationale of treating a headache by inserting a needle in a toe. If both parts of the body are connected by a meridian, the energy flow in an organ can be stimulated or calmed by application of a needle to a point along the meridian even though the acupuncture point may be far removed from the site of the organic disorder.

According to traditional Chinese acupuncture texts, there are a dozen meridians and approximately 360 acupuncture points along those meridians. In recent years, practitioners have reported finding additional meridians and many more acupuncture points. A number of efforts have been made to explain the meridians and acupuncture points in terms compatible with scientific medical logic of the western world. It has been pointed out, for example, that meridians frequently follow the pathways of the body's major nerves and blood vessels.

Development of the Embryo

One theory proposed to explain acupuncture suggests that tissues in widely separated parts of the body may be related through the embryonic development of the various organs from three primary tissue layers. The human embryo is composed of an ectoderm (outer tissue layer) mesoderm (middle layer), and endoderm (innermost layer). The muscles and bones are derived from the mesoderm, as are the heart, the urinary organs, and the diaphragm, among other body parts. Also, during development of the embryo, the tiny arms and legs rotate so that skin and muscles originally on the side facing the body become tissues on the outer surface of the limb, and vice versa. The fact that body tissues migrate and shift positions during embryonic life is thus used to help explain why an acupuncture point on one part of the body might stimulate a seemingly unrelated body area. In other words, it is believed by some acupuncturists that body cells retain throughout adult life a relationship that dates back to the first days of the embryo.

Oval Cells

A North Korean report in the 1960s stated that acupuncture points had been examined microscopically and were found to consist of groups of oval cells, surrounded by blood capillaries, just below the skin. The report also said that blood-rich bands of tissues that followed the pathways or meridians also were found. However, the report was not verified by other investigators.

Needles and How They Are Manipulated

The needles used for acupuncture are usually made of stainless steel, although gold and silver needles also are used. The type of metal apparently is not as important as the manner in which the needle is applied. Modern acupuncture practices include such techniques as boiling or otherwise sterilizing the needles, and cleaning the acupuncture point with a small wad of cotton soaked in alcohol. But the medical personnel may or may not provide protection for the skin puncture after the needle is removed: leaving the puncture exposed is part of the method of treating certain disorders. Extreme care, however, is taken to avoid puncturing important blood vessels or nerve tracts which are near the acupuncture points. To insert the needle in skin that is close to the bone or where there is a minimum of muscle beneath the skin, the acupuncturist pinches a fold of skin between his fingers and aims the needle at an angle. The needle may in some cases be inserted at a 45-degree angle rather than directly downward into the flesh.

Although the acupuncture needle usually is inserted only a fraction of an inch, long needles sometimes are used to reach points that may be six inches beneath the skin. The depth of insertion is measured in *fens,* with a fen approximating one-tenth of an inch. In actual practice, the "inch" measure is based on the length of the middle bone of the middle finger. If the patient has a layer of fat beneath the skin, additional fens of insertion are applied to get the needle past the fatty tissue. As a precaution against the possibility that a needle will break during insertion, it usually is guided into place by the fingers of the hand that is not holding the needle.

Manner of Insertion

The needle is not simply inserted into an acupuncture point, although that was a common practice in traditional Chinese medicine. It is manipulated by moving the needle up and down rapidly while twirling the top between the thumb and fingers. Some acupuncturists manipulate the needle by scratching the needle surface in a rhythmic pattern while it is in place. The modern Chinese method, however, calls for an up-and-down twirling rhythm of about 120 cycles per minute.

A variation of the manual manipulation technique is to attach a source of low-voltage electricity to the needles and allow the electricity to provide a vibratory stimulation at a rate of 120 cycles per minute. The amount of electricity is small, from one-fourth to one-half ampere at six to nine volts. And the frequency of vibration of the needles can with some equipment be varied from 120 up to 180 cycles per minute if the medical personnel feel that a faster rate will produce certain desired effects. The electrical devices, called *pulsators*, operate on direct current.

Traditional acupuncture methods direct that the practitioner continue to check the various pulses while the needles are in

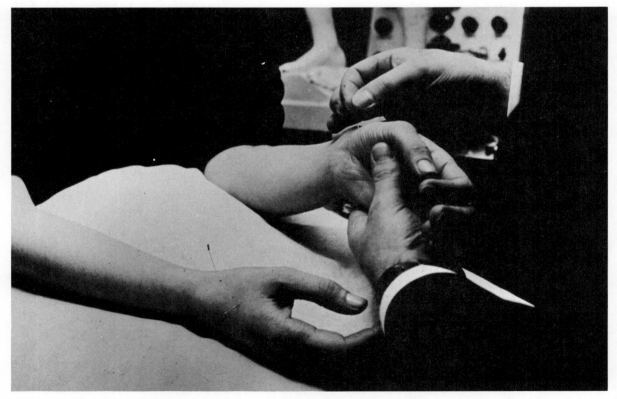

The patient illustrated on this page and the next is being treated for sinusitis. Needles are positioned in the hands and at the sides of the nose, (*continued next page*)

place. They are then removed when the pulses indicate that the meridians are in equilibrium. An acupuncturist's rule-of-thumb is that the pulses will return to normal within a few minutes if the illness is mild, but a serious illness will require a longer period of needling. Even in serious cases of disease the needle seldom is used for longer than a half-hour. Additional treatment may consist of *moxibustion,* or burning a pinch of an herb over an acupuncture point, with the heat providing the extra bit of therapy.

Effectiveness of
Acupuncture as Therapy

For reasons less well understood than acupuncture itself, the therapy seems to be more effective for some patients than others. Certain patients reportedly respond to the

needle treatment within a few seconds while others appear to receive no benefits from the therapy, even after repeated efforts to reduce the symptoms of an ailment. Some patients find the application of needles painful while others describe the feeling of the needle as similar to an injection of Novacaine ordinarily given by dentists: a numbness about the area of the needle prick.

A review of clinical reports in the *Chinese Journal of Medicine,* an English-language publication of the People's Republic of China, indicates that acupuncture in government hospitals produces varied results in the treatment of the same ailment. In the treatment of appendicitis in children, for example, acupuncture alone or acupunture supplemented by antibiotics controlled the symptoms in 87 of 93 of the cases; the patients were pronounced completely recov-

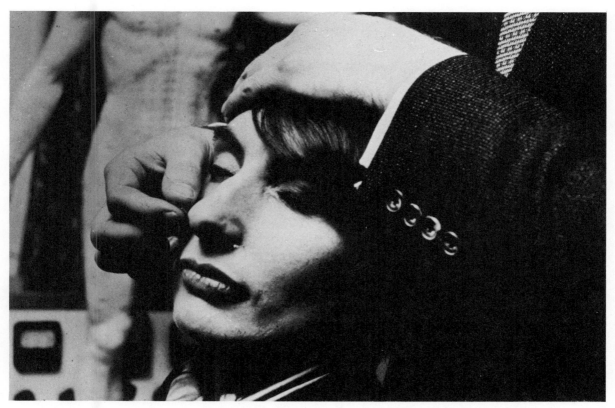

and are manipulated by the thumb and forefinger of the acupuncturist. A more modern technique utilizes an electric pulsator that sends a weak current through the needles.

ered and dismissed. In the remaining six cases, acupuncture apparently failed to control the symptoms and surgery was required to complete a cure. Each of the 93 children involved in the study was given acupuncture treatment at the beginning. But if the child continued to appear feverish and his white blood cell count increased, he was taken into the operating room for removal of the appendix by conventional western techniques.

In another report in the official organ of the Chinese Medical Association, a doctor reported on the successful use of acupuncture to treat headache and dizziness side-effects of ten patients who had been given spinal anesthesia during conventional surgical procedures. "This method proved to be much better than routine analgesics because of its simplicity and efficacy," the author reported.

The Use of Acupuncture as a Pain-Killer

Acupuncture has been most successful in the field of anesthesia, and it is probably because of the great strides reported in the use of needling to control pain during surgery that acupuncture has aroused the serious interest of many physicians in the western world. The loss of feeling of pain follows the insertion of the fine needles in the arms, legs, ears, nose, or face. It is applied with or without electrical stimulation. In some instances distilled water is injected into the acupuncture points to produce *analgesia,* or loss of pain. American observers of acupuncture anesthesia have reported that in many cases the patient is given a typical western sedative such as pentobarbital (just as he might before a conventional surgical procedure), before the acupuncture needles are applied. The rate of success in achieving analgesia has been reported at around 90 percent by the Chinese when the needles are used to produce anesthesia for operations. It is used in many different kinds of operations, ranging from the mending of broken bones to brain surgery, and including procedures in which the chest is opened to repair a heart defect or to remove a diseased portion of a lung.

According to a recent report in the Chinese *Peking Review,* some 400,000 operations have been performed with acupuncture anesthesia on patients ranging in age from children to adults in their 80s.

Advantages of Acupuncture Anesthesia

One advantage of acupuncture anesthesia reported by Chinese doctors is that in an operation on the eye muscles to correct a defect such as squinting, the patient can move the eyes at the request of the surgeon because he remains fully conscious. The surgeon is thus able to evaluate the results of his work while the patient is still on the operating table. When anesthetic drugs are used, success or failure of the operation cannot be determined until after the drugs wear off and the patient regains consciousness.

Similarly, when acupunctural anesthesia is applied in an operation on the thyroid gland in the throat, the surgeon and patient can talk freely during the operation. This permits the doctor to evaluate vocal functions that might be affected by the throat surgery. During open-chest surgery, the patient can be instructed to maintain abdominal breathing techniques to give the surgeon more freedom in surgical activity that involves the lungs. In orthopedic surgery involving the arms and legs, medical personnel can observe the functioning of muscles and tendons of the involved limb while the surgery is in progress.

Origin of Anesthetic Use

According to an official Chinese version of the development of acupuncture anesthesia, a patient in a Shanghai hospital was

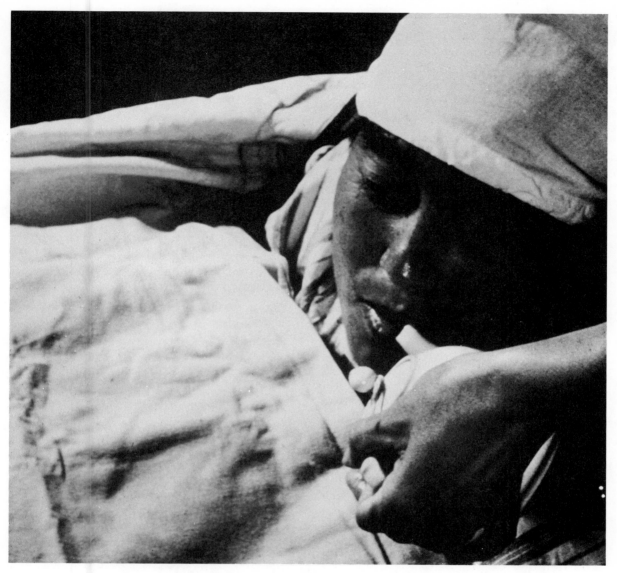

This patient, anesthetized by acupuncture needles, is drinking tea at the same time that an abdominal incision is being made prior to the removal of an ovarian cyst.

unable to swallow without pain after his tonsils had been removed by conventional surgical methods. The medical personnel inserted a needle in one of the traditional acupuncture points and the pain stopped immediately. The patient then ate a meal of meat dumplings without difficulty.

The medical workers reasoned that since needling could stop the throat pain of a patient who had just undergone conventional surgery, perhaps the use of acupuncture could be developed to replace western-type drugs as anesthetics during other tonsil operations. In their enthusiasm, the medical personnel began inserting needles at various acupuncture points in their own bodies to determine various degrees of pain relief. They also started application of acupuncture anesthesia in many kinds of surgery, applying as many as 100 needles at a time at various points in the bodies of patients undergoing lung operations. During that experimental period, according to the Chinese, it was not unusual to see four medical workers employed in an operating room for the sole purpose of manipulating the dozens of needles that had been inserted in the body of one patient.

Gradually, however, the medical personnel found that some acupuncture points were not necessary to produce anesthesia for a particular surgical procedure. The present practice is to use only a few needles, and in some cases only one needle, in key acupuncture points. Also, only one acupunctural anesthetist is required to manipulate the few needles by hand or to control the electric power source when that technique is used.

Although the Chinese themselves cannot offer adequate explanations of how acupuncture works, the procedure apparently has been successful in treating certain kinds of medical and psychiatric cases for many generations. It is perhaps useful to recall that physicians of the western world have prescribed drugs such as aspirin for many years without being able to explain how the chemical is able to relieve pain.

Acupuncture and Modern Medicine

Until the communist revolution in China, acupuncture was practiced as a kind of folk medicine, mainly by healers in rural areas who lacked the formal training provided by western-type medical colleges. Along with herbal medicine, acupuncture was in fact the only kind of therapy available to perhaps 90 percent of the hundreds of millions of Chinese who live in rural areas. Most of the available medical college

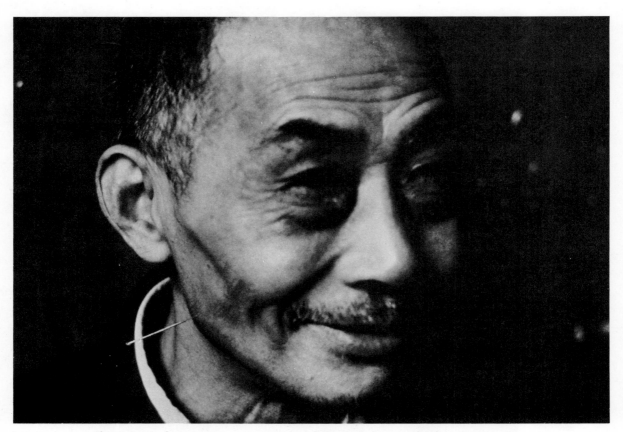

This man is being given acupuncture therapy for a toothache. Acupuncture has also reportedly been successful in treating headaches, including migraine.

graduates practiced in the cities, and the Chinese medical colleges produced only a handful of doctors each year to serve the largest nation on earth. For a period of nearly 40 years before the revolution the Peking Medical College averaged fewer than 30 graduates a year.

Both acupuncturists and herbal practitioners gained respectability in China after the communist revolution. Chairman Mao Tse-tung directed that both western scientific and traditional Chinese medical techniques be employed as a more effective means of meeting the health needs of the nation. The result has been an interesting blend of modern surgery and pharmaceuticals with acupuncture and herbs. Western observers have reported that each modern hospital in China maintains a large department in which the roots, leaves, and barks of various herb plants are stored and processed. Well-trained teams of pharmacologists, meanwhile, study the ancient herbs for identification of the active ingredients that apparently have therapeutic benefits for the patients. The government, in an effort to protect the patient against reckless experimentation, requires that before a doctor can prescribe acupuncture or herb treatments he must permit the herbs or needling to be applied to his own body.

Although it has been suggested that acupuncture may appear to be a success in the People's Republic of China because of some hypnotic effect related to the enthusiasm of the people for Chairman Mao, the Chinese have pointed out that acupuncture also has been used successfully on dogs, cats, rabbits, and other animals that are not likely to be influenced by the Cultural Revolution or the words of Chairman Mao. Acupuncture has also been employed for some years in Russia, Germany, France, and England, as well as in Taiwan, Japan, and other countries of the Orient, although the precise methods of application vary somewhat. The Russians involved in acupuncture

research not only agree with the Chinese that energy flows along the meridians, but claim that it can be detected by electronic instruments. Students of acupuncture outside of China also have reported evidence that when a meridian is severed the flow of energy does not extend beyond the point at which the tissue is cut.

Western-trained physicians who have watched acupuncture as practiced in China seem convinced that it can be effective, particularly as used to produce analgesia in surgery. As reported by American doctors who have visited mainland China, acupuncture anesthesia works better in surgery that involves those parts of the body above the waist, such as the lungs and heart. Other physicians, who were trained in the United States before returning to China to practice, claim that acupuncture has been effective in the treatment of migraine headaches and in controlling irregular heartbeats. Western doctors who have observed the use of acupuncture in the treatment of deafness, a common application of needling in China, reported that they were unable to judge the benefits of such therapy in terms of their own knowledge and experience.

One American doctor who has been trained in the techniques of acupuncture believes the method is compatible with standard western medicine in the treatment of a wide range of ailments. It is not recommended for the treatment of cancer, tuberculosis, or arthritis cases in which the disease has advanced to the point of permanent changes in the body tissues. As for the argument that there is a psychological effect in acupuncture that makes it appear to be more successful than it actually is, the supporters of needle therapy reply that psychology is a factor in the treatment of disease by almost any method. For this reason many western-trained physicians claim that placebos, or therapeutically ineffective sugar pills, provide relief from the symptoms of certain ailments.   KNA

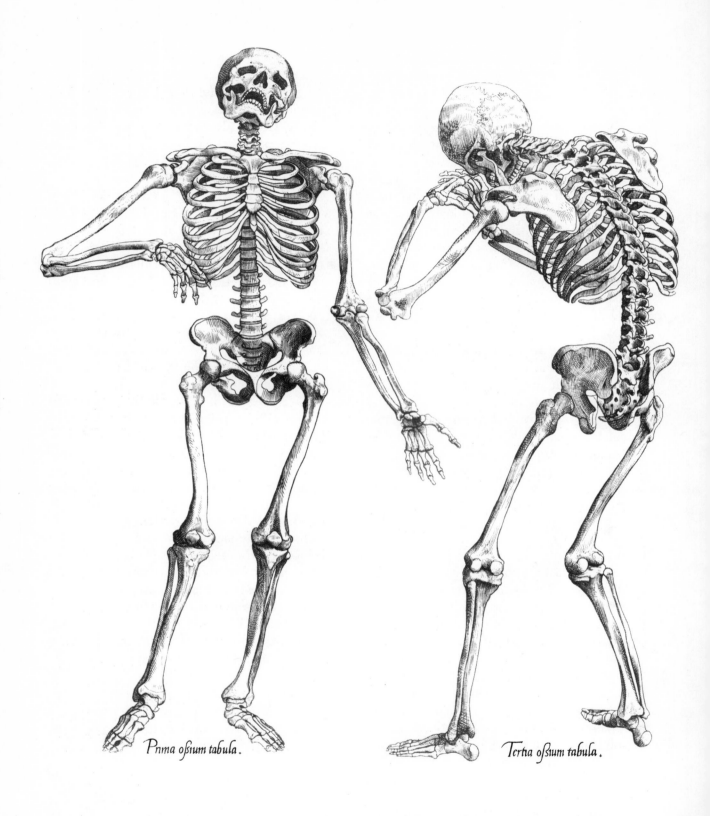

Prima ossium tabula.   *Tertia ossium tabula.*

These remarkable drawings are the work of the great 16th-century Belgian physician, Andreas Vesalius, who is widely regarded as the founder of modern anatomy.

Information Key: Glossary and Index

The *Thesaurus of Medical Terms* on pages 708–709 is designed to enable the reader to find the more technical terms that apply to a variety of health-related subjects. By locating the Key Word that applies to a particular subject and reading across the page, the pertinent adjective, study, specialist, and major disorders may be found. For example, if one wants to know the technical term for an eye doctor, one looks under the Key Word column for *eye,* and under *Specialist,* finds the words *ophthalmologist* and *oculist.* If one cannot recall the name of a common heart disease, one looks under *heart* in the Key Word column and finds, under Major Disorders, angina and other conditions listed. These disorders may in turn be looked up in the index and glossary following for definitions and page references to the text.

The index beginning on page 710 includes a glossary of over 2,000 terms. Regular figures following an index entry (e.g., 15, 28) refer to the text on the pages cited; italic figures (e.g., *15, 28*) refer to illustrations on the pages cited.

Entries are alphabetized letter by letter rather than by separate words. For example, *accidents* appears in the index before *accident victim.* The entry consists of the word or words that precede a comma, colon, parenthesis, or slant bar.

The colon (:) is used to introduce a definition or a cross-reference. The latter use is illustrated by the following item:

acoustic nerve: auditory nerve

The slant bar (/) is used to separate synonyms. Because of the relatively large number of synonyms used in medicine, it was felt that the repetition of synonyms at the page-reference entry would be valuable to the reader and serve to avoid possible confusion. In the entry below, the reader is informed that *acoustic nerve* is synonymous with *auditory nerve* and is directed to textual references on pages 76 and 77 and to illustrative references on pages 77 and 79.

> auditory nerve/acoustic nerve: nerve consisting of the cochlear nerve and the vestibular nerve and connecting the inner ear with the brain, conveying the sense of hearing and of equilibrium, 76, 77, *77, 79*

The *Information Key* includes 11 subindexes, headed by an entry in bold type and set off from the rest of the index by a gray tint. The subindexes are:

Age Groups
Circulatory System
Digestive System
Endocrine System
Musculature
Nervous System
Respiratory System
Sex
Skeletal System
Skin and Hair
Urinogenital System

The subindexes are designed to provide in a single place full information about a particular subject. Also, by scanning a subindex, the range of coverages provided may be estimated and items of interest may be found more easily than by searching through the entire index. Every entry in the subindexes appears also in the regular index, frequently with a definition as well. In order to keep the Information Key within manageable limits, definitions ordinarily appear only in the entry's regular alphabetic place, not in the subindexes.

THESAURUS OF MEDICAL TERMS

Key Word	Adjective	Study	Specialist	Major Disorders
allergy	allergic	allergology	allergist, allergologist	respiratory and skin disorders, e.g. asthma and contact dermatitis
anesthesia	anesthetic	anesthesiology	anesthesiologist	
blood	hemal	hematology	hematologist	anemia, leukemia, hemophilia
blood vessels	vascular	angiology	vascular surgeon	varicose veins, phlebitis
bone	osteal, osseous	orthopedics	orthopedist, orthopedic surgeon, orthopod	back disorders, fractures, trauma
brain See nervous system.				
cancer See tumor.				
causes of disease	etiologic, etiological	etiology	etiologist	
chest cavity	thoracic	thoracic surgery	thoracic surgeon	lung cancer, tuberculosis, emphysema
children	pediatric	pediatrics	pediatrician	all diseases children are subject to
colon and rectum	proctologic, proctological	proctology	proctologist	hemorrhoids, cancer of the rectum or colon
cosmetic surgery See plastic surgery.				
diet	nutritive	nutrition	nutritionist	malnutrition, obesity
digestive tract	gastroenteric	gastroenterology	gastroenterologist	digestive difficulties, ulcers, gallstones, inguinal hernia
disease	pathologic, pathological	pathology	pathologist	
ear	otologic, otological	otology	otologist	hearing or equilibrium disorders
ear, nose, and throat	otolaryngological	otolaryngology	otolaryngologist, ENT specialist	hearing or equilibrium disorders, laryngitis, upper respiratory infections
endocrine glands See glands.				
epidemics (geographical distribution of disease)	epidemic, epidemical	epidemiology	epidemiologist	forms of cancer, cholera, influenza
eye	ophthalmic	ophthalmology	ophthalmologist, oculist	glaucoma, cataract, detached retina
foot	pedal	podiatry, chiropody	podiatrist, chiropodist	arch troubles, bunions, ingrown toenails
gastrointestinal tract (GI tract) See digestive tract.				
general medicine			general practitioner (GP)	
genital tract (female) See reproductive system (female).				
genital tract (male) See urinogenital tract (male).				
glands (endocrine)	glandular	endocrinology	endocrinologist	diabetes, hyperthyroidism, hypothyroidism
hair See skin and hair.				
heart	cardiac, coronary, cardiologic, cardiological	cardiology	cardiologist, cardiovascular specialist	angina, coronary thrombosis (heart attack), atherosclerosis, hypertension

THESAURUS OF MEDICAL TERMS

Key Word	Adjective	Study	Specialist	Major Disorders
immunization	immunologic, immunological	immunology	immunologist	poliomyelitis, measles, smallpox
internal medicine			internist	
joints and muscles		rheumatology	rheumatologist	rheumatoid arthritis, osteoarthritis
kidney	renal, nephric	nephrology	nephrologist	nephritis, kidney failure
law and medicine		forensic medicine, forensic pathology		
liver	hepatic	hepaticology	hepaticologist	hepatitis
lung	pulmonary	internal medicine	internist	emphysema, lung cancer, tuberculosis
medicine *See* **general medicine, internal medicine, osteopathic medicine, rehabilitation.**				
mental illness	psychiatric	psychiatry	psychiatrist	neurosis, psychosis, psychosomatic disease
muscles *See* **joints and muscles.**				
nervous system	neural, neurologic, neurological, neuropathological	neurology, neuropathology	neurologist, neuropathologist, neurosurgeon	epilepsy, cerebral palsy, brain tumors, meningitis
nose *See* **ear, nose, and throat.**				
osteopathic medicine	osteopathic	osteopathy	osteopath	
plastic surgery		plastic surgery, cosmetic surgery	plastic surgeon, cosmetic surgeon	scars, burns, cosmetic improvements
radiology	radiologic, radiological, X-ray	radiology, roentgenology	radiologist, roentgenologist	
rectum *See* **colon and rectum.**				
rehabilitation		physical medicine	physical therapist	
reproductive system (female)	obstetric, obstetrical, gynecologic, gynecological	obstetrics, gynecology	obstetrician, gynecologist, ob-gyn specialist	pregnancy and its complications, infertility, fibroid tumors, dysmenorrhea, birth control, ovarian cysts
reproductive system (male) *See* **urinogenital tract (male).**				
skin and hair	dermal	dermatology	dermatologist	dermatitis, acne, psoriasis
surgery	surgical	surgery	surgeon	
throat (*See also* **ear, nose, and throat.**)	laryngologic, laryngological	laryngology	laryngologist	laryngitis, upper respiratory infections
tooth	dental, orthodontic, periodontal	dentistry, orthodontics, orthodontia, oral or dental surgery, periodontics, periodontia	dentist, oral or dental surgeon, orthodontist, periodontist, pediatric dentist	caries (tooth decay), periodontal disease, malocclusion, children's dental needs
tumor	oncologic	oncology	oncologist	cancer, benign tumors
urinary tract (female)	urologic, urological	urology	urologist	cystitis, nephritis
urinogenital tract (male)	urologic, urological	urology	urologist	kidney stones, nephritis, prostate problems
X ray *See* **radiology.**				

ankylosing spondylitis: spondylitis, rheumatoid

anorexia: loss of appetite, 319, 442

anovulatory: without ovulation

antacid: any alkaline substance that can neutralize stomach acidity caused by gastric juices, often prescribed in ulcer diets, 530

anterior: toward the front

anterior lobe hypophysis: the anterior part of the pituitary gland that produces growth hormones and hormones that stimulate other glands

anterior urethra: the meatus, or external opening, of the urethra in the penis

antibiotic(s): any of a large class of substances, such as penicillin and streptomycin, produced by various microorganisms and fungi that have the power to destroy or arrest the growth of other microorganisms, including many that cause infectious diseases, 347
and acne, 399
in agranulocytosis, 493
in bronchitis, 431
in colitis, 533
in ear infections, 434, 590
in influenza, 411
in meningitis, 476
in pyelonephritis, 603
in pyrogenic arthritis, 451
and rheumatic fever, 518
screening for, *440*
and tuberculosis, 545, 548

antibody: substance produced by the body to counteract infection and in response to specific antigens, 69, 515
in rheumatic fever, 516
and Rh factor, 152, 492

anti-clotting compounds: anticoagulant

anticoagulant: substance that retards clotting of the blood, *485*, 495
in stroke prevention, 499

anticonvulsant: medicine used to control epileptic seizures

antidiuretic hormone: *vasopressin*

antidote: in poisoning, *687*
universal, 686

anti-freeze, *627*

antigen: any of several substances, including toxins, enzymes, and proteins, that cause the development of antibodies when introduced into an organism, 515

antihelmintic: drug or remedy used to destroy intestinal worms, or helminths, 534

antihemophilic factor/AHF: substance that causes clotting and stops bleeding in hemophiliacs, 485, 486, *487*

antihistamine: any of a number of drugs that counteract the nasal engorgement and vasoconstrictor action of histamine in the body, often used in the treatment of hay fever, 411, 552
in asthma, 554

anti-honking ordinances, 374

antimetabolite: chemical that interferes with cell metabolism
in psoriasis, 400

antiperspirant: astringent preparation which acts to diminish or prevent perspiration, 381

antitoxin: antibody produced in response to the presence of a specific toxin, which it neutralizes

anuria: inability to urinate, 595
in glomerulonephritis, 601

anus: the opening at the lower extremity of the alimentary canal, *44, 49, 49,* 55

anvil/incus: the middle of the three ossicles of the middle ear, the bone between the hammer and the stirrup, 76, 78, *79*

anxiety, 219, 262
and sexual problems, 265

aorta: the large artery originating from the left ventricle of the heart that forms the main arterial trunk from which blood is distributed to all of the body except the lungs, *32, 33, 40,* 41, 57, *67, 569*

aortic valve: the membranous valve between the left ventricle of the heart and the aorta, 516
artificial, *502, 503*

Apgar system: system of rating the health of newborn babies, 163

aphasia: partial or total loss of the power of articulate speech due to a disorder in the cerebrum of the brain, 499

aphrodisiacs, 183

apoplexy: stroke

appendectomy: surgical removal of the vermiform appendix, 55, 533

appendicitis: inflammation of the vermiform appendix characterized by pain in the right lower abdomen, nausea, and vomiting, 55, 437, 533
acupuncture in, 701–702

appendicular skeleton: *skeleton*

appendix vermiformis: vermiform appendix, *44, 49,* 55, 533

appetite
of adolescent, 315
of infant, as guide to needs, 301
loss of: anorexia

appetite stimulators, 196

apple juice, nutrients in, 309

apples, nutrients in, 309

apple sauce, nutrients in, 309

apricots, nutrients in, 309

aqueous humor: the clear, limpid alkaline fluid that fills the anterior chamber of the eye from the cornea to the lens, *73, 75*

arachnoid: the middle of the three membranes that envelop the brain and spinal cord

arches, fallen, 421

arch supports, 422

areola: the dark circular area around the nipple of a breast or around a pustule

arms(s)
muscles of, *15*
relief of tension in, 171

arrhythmia: variation from the normal heartbeat, 508

arsenic, 365

arsenic products, 688

arterial: having to do with or carried by the arteries

arterial bleeding, control of, *672*

arterial blood, 671

arteriogram: X-ray picture of an artery

arteriography: technique of injecting an opaque substance into the coronary arteries and observing the material by X ray as it runs its course through the heart muscle, 506

arteriole: small artery, esp. one that leads to a capillary, 33, *33,* 512

arteriosclerosis: thickening and hardening of the walls of an artery, with impairment of blood circulation, 91, 502
cerebral, 478

arteritis: inflammation of an artery, 494

artery: any of a large number of muscular, tubular vessels conveying blood away from the heart to all parts of the body, *32, 33, 33*
adult teeth, *5*
axillary, *32*
brachial, *671*
carotid, *33*
coronary, 41
femoral, *32, 671*
hardening of, 91, 502
iliac, *32*
peroneal, *32*
pulmonary: artery that delivers oxygen-poor blood from the heart to the lungs, 40, *40,* 56, 57, *57*
radial, *32*
renal, *32,* 81, *81, 82,* 595, *600*
subclavian, *32*
tibial, *32*
ulnar, *32*

artery-capillary-vein sequence, *33*

arthritis: inflammation of a joint, characterized by pain, swelling, and tenderness, 11, 205–206, 449–451, *450, 451.* See also *osteoarthritis.*
hemophilic: painful swelling and bleeding in joint cavities, 486
in hip, 457
and nail deformity, 389–390
pyrogenic: form of arthritis characterized by fever, 451
rheumatoid, 205, 449, *449*
juvenile, 450
spinal, 461–462
traumatic, 453

artificial pneumothorax: *pneumothorax*

artificial respiration: artificial maintenance of respiration in someone who has ceased to breathe, esp. mouth-to-mouth resuscitation, 673, *673, 674*

asbestos workers, lung cancer in, 356

ascaris: roundworms

ascorbic acid/vitamin C: white, odorless, crystalline compound found in citrus and other fresh fruits and green leafy vegetables, and also made synthetically, that prevents scurvy, 297
and common cold, 343, 411–412
deficiency of, 524
for infant, 301

aseptic meningitis: meningitis, aseptic

asparagus, nutrients in, 305

asphyxiation: loss of consciousness caused by too little oxygen in the blood, generally as a result of suffocation by drowning or the breathing in of noxious gases, 686

aspirate: to withdraw by suction

aspirin: analgesic drug that has fever-reducing properties, widely used to treat symptoms of the common cold, rheumatoid arthritis, and many other conditions
in arthritis, 205, 450
in backaches, 415
for common cold, 411
consumption of, *648*
in earache, 434
in headache, 414
as poison, 688
in rheumatic fever, 517
in writer's cramp, 425
assimilation: the process by which digested food is made an integral part of the solid or fluids of an organism, 51
asthma: chronic respiratory disorder characterized by recurrent paroxysmal coughing caused by spasms of the bronchi or diaphragm, and due in many cases to an allergic reaction, 550, 552–554
acute attack, 693
allergic, *553*
two main types of, 550
astigmatism: distorted vision caused by an uneven curvature of the cornea, 121, 585
asymptomatic: condition in which antibodies for a disease are present in the blood but no symptoms of the disease can be observed. Compare *symptomatic.*
atherosclerosis: hardening of the inner walls of the arteries, resulting in a loss of elasticity, and accompanied by the deposit of fat and degenerative tissue changes, 343, 416, 496–497, *496*, 502–503
athetosis: derangement of the nervous system in which the hands and feet, esp. the fingers and toes, keep moving or twitching, 470
athletes
injuries to, 454
lungs of, *62*
athlete's foot: ringworm of the foot, caused by a parasitic fungus, 395–396, *395*, 439
prevention of, 208
athletic supporter, 570
atrioventricular block: disruption of normal transmission of signals between the upper and lower chambers of the heart, as from scar tissue, that may affect blood flow to the brain and cause blackouts or convulsions, 521
atrium (*pl., atria*)/auricle: one of the two upper chambers of the heart, which receive blood from the veins and transmit it to the ventricles, 40
left, *40*, 56
right, *40*, 56
atrophy: the wasting or withering away of the body or any of its parts, as from disease or lack of use
bone: decalcification
attention, child's craving for, 230–231
attenuated: weakened in strength, as a microorganism for use in a vaccine
attitudes, learned, in alcoholism, 642
audiologist: one who specializes in

the treatment of those with hearing problems, 201
audiometer: device that measures hearing
auditory canal/auditory meatus: either of two passageways, the *external auditory canal* leading from the outer ear to the tympanic membrane or eardrum, and the *internal auditory canal* passing through the temporal bone to the brain, 76
auditory nerve/acoustic nerve: nerve consisting of the cochlear nerve and the vestibular nerve and connecting the inner ear with the brain, conveying the sense of hearing and of equilibrium, 76, 77, *77, 79*
aura: subjective, momentary sensory perception of an unusual nature that occurs just before the onset of an epileptic convulsion, 473
Aureomycin: trade name for the antibiotic tetracycline
auricle: atrium
auscultation: diagnostic procedure of listening, as to sounds in the chest with a stethoscope, *442, 443*
automated medical screening, 167
automobiles, exhaust, as pollutant, 359–362, *360, 560*
autonomic nervous system: network of nerves originating in the spinal column, and including the sympathetic and parasympathetic nervous systems, that control and stimulate the functions of body tissues and organs not subject to voluntary control, such as the heart or stomach, 27, 28, *28*, 41
and breathing, 59
and carbon dioxide level, 58
and digestive sphincters, 48
and gallbladder, 51
and hypothalamus, 66
and senses, 71
avocados, nutrients in, 309
avocation, need for, 266–269
axial skeleton: skeleton, axial
axillary: underarm
axon: cylindrical fiber in neurons carrying impulses away from the cells, 28, 29, *29*, 30, 73

B

baby foods, *109*
baby-sitters, 224, 227, 258
baby teeth/deciduous teeth/milk teeth: the first temporary set of human teeth, 20 in all, which begin to appear about the age of six months and are usu. complete by the end of the second year, 109
bacillary dysentery: a usu. acute form of dysentery caused by bacilli, 527–528
bacillus (*pl., bacilli*): any of a class of straight, rod-shaped bacteria having both beneficial and disease-causing effects, 440
pathogenic, 364
back, problems in aging, 207
backaches, 415, *415*
in pregnancy, 150
tips for avoiding, 207
backbone: spinal column

back pain, causes of, 459–460
bacteria (*sing., bacterium*): one-celled microorganisms that come in three varieties—bacillus, coccus, and spirillum—and that range from the harmless and beneficial to the virulent and lethal, *436,* 439
and antiseptics, 446
in dental plaque, 96
in gingivitis, 428
in large intestine, 56
and lymph, 39
and meningitis, 476
and teeth, 97
in tuberculosis, 547
bacterial endocarditis: *endocarditis*
bacterial growth and odor, 381
bacterial infections of skin, 396–397
badminton, 170
bag of waters: amniotic fluid
balance, 76
body, and shoes, 174
impairment of, 592
organ of, *77, 78*
site of, 26
baldness/alopecia: common hereditary condition of males marked by a gradual loss of hair on the crown of the head until only a fringe remains around the sides and in the back, often called *male pattern baldness*, 178–179, 386–387, *386*
from curling irons, 383
and heredity, 127
male pattern, 178, *179*, 386
patchy/alopecia areata: sudden but usu. temporary loss of hair in patches, 178
from sebaceous cysts, 398
bananas, nutrients in, 310
Banting, Frederick, 574
barber's itch: sycosis
barbiturate: any of a class of drugs derived from barbituric acid that depress the central nervous system, used medically as sedatives and sleeping pills and in the treatment of epilepsy and high blood pressure, and illicitly to counteract the effects of stimulant drugs, 140, 421, 655–657
abuse of, 656–657
consumption of, *648*
dangers of, 140–141
legitimate use of, 655–656
poisoning, 688
barium enema: enema in which a barium mixture is used to visualize the inner walls of the large intestine by X ray, used to detect cancer and other diseases
barium sulfate: an insoluble barium compound used to facilitate X-ray pictures of the stomach and intestines, 539
baroreceptors/barostats: sensitive nerve cells that respond to changes in blood pressure and may help to regulate it, 514
barostats: baroreceptors
Basal Body Temperature/BBT: accurate measure of body temperature taken under uniform conditions, used to determine a woman's day of ovulation, 144
basal caloric state, 329, 330
basal cell cancer, 200

basal ganglia: group of nerve cells embedded in the cerebral hemisphere, the largest part of the human brain
  in Parkinson's disease, 474
basal metabolic rate test, *444*
basal metabolism: the minimum energy, measured in calories, that the body needs to maintain essential vital activities when it is at rest
basal thermometer: thermometer scaled in tenths of degrees instead of fifths, used by women to determine the time of ovulation
bathing and muscle tone, 89
bath oil, 380
baths, types of, 379
BBT: Basal Body Temperature
beaches, polluted, 364
beans, nutrients in, 305, 306
beard, growth of, 387
bed clothing in care of sick, 447
bed rest
  prolonged, 167, 180
  in rheumatic fever, 517
bedwetting: enuresis
beef, *310, 311*
  chart, 300
  nutrients in, 299–300, 301
beer, 632
beets, nutrients in, 306
behavior and praise, 231
  regulation of, 26–27
Behrman, Dr. Howard T., 387
Bell, Sir Charles, 470
belladonna: plant with purple-red flowers whose leaves and roots yield a number of poisonous alkaloids used in medicine
  in Parkinson's disease, 475
Bell's palsy: facial paralysis due to lesion of the facial nerve, 470–472
belonging, need for, 274
Benamid, 452
benign: mild or nonmalignant, and responding to treatment
Benzedrine: amphetamine
benzine, as poison, 688
beriberi: disease of the peripheral nerves characterized by partial paralysis and swelling of the legs, caused by the absence of B complex vitamins
Berlin, Dr. Cheston M., 661
Best, Charles, 574
betatron, *620*
beverages
  alcoholic: alcoholic beverages
  carbonated, nutrients in, 319
bicarbonate of soda and oil fires, 679
biceps muscle, *15*
bicuspids, *5*
bicycle exerciser, *498*
bicycling, *131*, 170, 198
bile: bitter, viscid alkaline fluid used in digestion, esp. of fats, that is secreted by the liver and stored in the gallbladder, 51, 53, 55, 522
  black, *54*
  yellow, *54*
biliary tract: duct that conveys bile.
bilirubin: pigment found in bile, 537
Binoctal, 656
biodegradable: capable of being broken down, as a chemical compound, by microorganisms
biological death: death of the brain,

following clinical death, 293. Compare *clinical death.*
biomicroscope/slit lamp, *206, 586*
biopsy: excision of tissue or other material from a living subject for clinical and diagnostic examination
  muscle, 479
birth abnormalities: birth defects
birth canal: passageway formed by the cervix and vagina through which a fetus passes in the birth process, 243
birth control: the regulation of conception by employing preventive methods or devices, 250–255, *251, 252*
  information for teen-agers, 241, 244–245
  methods of, *142, 143*
birth date, prediction of, 155
birth defects, 153, 445
  and chemicals in food, 368
  and LSD use, 661
  and marihuana, 665
  in pelvic area, 457
  and rubella, 114, *115*
  skeletal, 448
  of skull, face and jaw, 465
  and smoking, 149
  and thalidomide, 147
birthmark: mark or stain existing on the body from birth, 401
  vascular: hemangioma
birth process, *160, 161*
biscuits, nutrients in, 313
bite, improper: malocclusion
black eye, 466
blackheads, 128, 398, *399*
black lung disease: form of pneumoconiosis common in coal miners and caused by constant exposure to coal dust, 563–564, *563*
black-outs, 30
bladder: elastic membranous sac near the front of the pelvic cavity, used to store urine temporarily, 81, 83, 595
  and autonomic nervous system, *28*
  cancer of, 356
  female, *83, 602*
  infection of: cystitis
  inflammation of: cystitis
  loss of control, 30
  male, *84, 242, 605*
  tumors in, 604
bleaching
  of hair, 385
  of unwanted hair, 388
bleeders: hemophiliacs
bleeding, 669–672
  control of, *670, 671, 672*
  functional, 572
  of gums, 429
  irregular, 252
  nosebleed, 427
  severe, 668, 670
  as sign of miscarriage, 154
  as symptom, 442
  See also *hemophilia, hemorrhage.*
blepharoplasty: surgical technique to correct congenital defects in the eyelids or to alter their size or shape, 178, 407
blindness and glaucoma, 586
blind spot, *73*, 206
  and optic nerves, 73
blinking, *76*

blister: small rounded sac, esp. on the skin, containing fluid matter, often resulting from injury, friction, or scalding, *422*
blood: blister containing blood from broken capillaries, often resulting from a pinch or other injury, 422
  in chicken pox, 117
  on feet, 422
  water, 422
blistering in sunburn, 417
blood, 33–34, 484
  alcohol concentration in, 635–636
  analysis, 443
  and bone, interchange of materials, 10
  cholesterol content, 297
  clotting of, 36
    and calcium, 11
  components of, 34–37
    made in bones, 3
  diseases of, 484–494
  irradiation of, *493*
  normal smear, *36*
  oxygen-poor, 57
  pumping of, 40
  purified by kidney, 81
  reoxygenation of, 41
  Rh factor, 152
  in spinal fluid, 444
  tests on, 36–37
  type O, and peptic ulcer, 530
  in urine, 443
  venous, 40
  whole, clot of, *34*
    fractionation of, *38*
blood bank techniques, *487*
blood cells, manufacture and turnover, 38–39
  movement through capillaries, 39
  proportions of, 36
  red/red corpuscles/erythrocytes, 10, 35, *36*, 484, 488
    diseased, *493*
    diseases of, 487–492
    excess: polycythemia
    lifespan of, 38
    and Rh factor, 152
    size of, 39
  white/white corpuscles/leukocytes, 35–36, *36*, 443, 484
    diseases of, 492–494
    manufacture of, 38
blood count: examination of blood components, used in diagnosis. A *complete blood count* reveals the size, shape, and number of white and red cells and platelets in a cubic millimeter of blood. A *differential blood count* determines the percentage of leukocytes and other cells, 37, *488*
  complete/CBC, 443
blood group/blood type: classification of the blood, commonly designated AB, A, B, and O, based on the specific generic differences in the composition and chemical properties of the blood, 37
blood-letting in polycythemia, 491
blood loss, shock caused by, 685
blood poisoning/septicemia: introduction of virulent bacteria into the bloodstream, usu. from a local infection such as a boil or wound, and marked by chills, fever, and fatigue

normalities and obtain blood samples, 518

cardiac insufficiency, 520

cardiac massage: emergency procedure consisting of the application of rhythmic pressure on the chest in order to compress the heart and start it beating again, 674–675

cardiac muscle: the striated but involuntary muscle of which the heart is composed, 13, 41, 56

cardiac problem and danger of isometrics, 172

cardiac sphincter: ring of muscle at the entrance of the stomach, or cardia, that opens to allow food to enter from the esophagus, *44*, 49, *49*, 522, *525*

in achalasia, 525

cardiac X-ray series: chest X rays taken after the patient has swallowed an opaque liquid such as barium sulfate

cardiologist: physician specializing in the diagnosis and treatment of heart disease

cardiology: the branch of medical science dealing with the heart, its physiology and pathology

cardiopulmonary resuscitation, external, 510

cardiovascular disease/heart disease: disorders affecting the heart and blood vessels, *501*

and cholesterol, 343

and noise pollution, 373

See also *heart disease.*

cardiovascular specialist: physician specializing in the diagnosis and treatment of diseases of the heart and blood vessels

caries: dental caries

carotene: orange or red crystalline pigment converted to Vitamin A in animal metabolism, 379

carotid artery: either of two major arteries of the neck supplying blood to the head, *32, 33*

carpal: pertaining to the bones of the carpus, or wrist, *9*

carpus: the wrist

carrier: person who is immune from infection of specific disease-causing bacteria that his body carries and that can be transmitted to others who are not immune, 440

and muscular dystrophy, 480

of sickle-cell trait, 490

typhoid, 529

carrots, nutrients in, 306

cartilage: tough, elastic supporting tissue, 8, 11

and muscle function, 14

cartilage plate/epiphysis: extremity of a long bone, originally separated from it by cartilage but later consolidated with it by ossification, 126

slipped, 457

cartilage rings, 60

casts, plaster, 455

catalyst: substance or agent that causes a chemical reaction while remaining stable, such as an enzyme or hormone in the human body

hormones as, 65

cataract: the gradual clouding and opacity of the lens of the eye, lead-

ing to impaired passage of light and loss of vision, 206, 586

senile: cataract affecting elderly people due to degenerative changes in the lens

surgery for, *587*

in unborn child, 152

cathartic: medicine for purging the bowels, 431

as cause of constipation, 207

caudal: situated at the tail end or bottom; posterior

caul: membrane (*amnion*) surrounding the fetus if it is unruptured and intact about the baby's head at delivery, 159

cauliflower, nutrients in, 306

cautery, chemical: chemosurgery

cavities: dental caries

CBC: complete blood count. See *blood count.*

cc: cubic centimeter

cecum: blind pouch or cavity open at one end, esp. the cavity below the ileocecal valve that forms the first section of the large intestine, *49*, 52, 55

celery, nutrients in, 306

cell body, *29*

cells

in cervical cancer, *621, 622*

malignant, *610*

normal, *610*

oval, 699

sense receptor, 71

taste: taste buds

cellular death, 293

cellular metabolism, waste products of, 82

cellular therapy: treatment for the process of aging in which a person is injected with cells from healthy embryonic animal organs with the idea that the animal cells from the particular organ injected will then migrate to the same organ in the aging body and reactivate it, 287

cellulose, 56

cementum: the layer of body tissue developed over the roots of the teeth, 4, *5*

central nervous system: the portion of the nervous system that contains the brain and spinal cord and controls voluntary action and movement, 14, 24, 27–28

and aging, 166

and alcohol, 141, 636, 643

and amphetamines, 652, 655

and caffeine, 184

and cocaine, 655

and drugs, 138

narcotics, 657

and heroin, 658

inflammatory conditions, 444

and obesity, 325

cephalhematoma: swelling under a newborn baby's scalp, that usu. dissolves within a few weeks, 100

cereals, whole grain, 347

cerebellum: large section of the brain located below and behind the cerebrum, consisting of a central lobe and two lateral lobes, and which coordinates voluntary muscle movements, posture, and equilibrium, 26, *26*, 65

cerebral arteriogram: an X-ray picture of the brain used to investigate brain damage, esp. after a hemorrhage or stroke, and made by injecting opaque dye into the blood vessels serving the brain and X-raying them

cerebral arteriosclerosis: degenerative changes in the arteries of the brain

cerebral cortex: the cells and fibers that look like a convoluted layer of gray matter and that cover the cerebral hemisphere of the brain, *26, 79*

in Parkinson's disease, 474

cerebral hemisphere: one of the two halves into which the brain is divided

cerebral hemorrhage: hemorrhage into the cerebrum of the brain or within the cranium, 497

cerebral palsy: inability to control movement caused by nonprogressive brain damage resulting from a prenatal defect or birth injury, 470, *471*

cerebrospinal fluid/CSF: the clear, colorless fluid that surrounds the brain and spinal cord, 24, 463, 469

analysis of, 444

in meningitis, 476

cerebrospinal meningitis: inflammation of the membranes that cover the brain and spinal cord

cerebrovascular: of or relating to the vessels supplying blood to the brain

cerebrum: the upper anterior part of the brain, consisting of two hemispherical masses which constitute the chief bulk of the brain in man and is assumed to be the seat of thought and will, 24

lobes of, 26

cervical cancer, 621, *621*

cervical cap: contraptive device made usu. of soft plastic which fits over the cervix, 253

cervical spine: cervical vertebrae

cervical vertebrae/cervical spine: the top seven vertebrae of the backbone, which are located in the neck and support the head, 6, *7*

cervix: neck of the uterus, 243, *243*, *244*, *571*

dilation in labor, 159

incompetent, 154

removal of: hysterectomy, total

cestode: tapeworm

Chafetz, Dr. M. E., 646

chafing: inflammation of two opposing skin surfaces, caused by warmth, moisture, or friction, 393

chamber

anterior, of eye, 75

of heart, 40

posterior, of eye, 75

champagne, 632

chancre: primary syphilitic lesion resembling a sore with a hard base, 442, 524, 607

change, attitude toward, 265

change of life: menopause

changes

effect on children, 234

physical, in middle age, 165–167

chapping: condition where skin is irritated, cracked, or roughened,

circumcision and cervical cancer, 623
cirrhosis: condition associated with excessive drinking in which there is an abnormal formation of connective tissue and a wasting of the tissue of the liver, 536–537
and alcohol, 637
clavicle: the bone connecting the shoulder blade and breastbone; the collarbone, 3, 6, *7*
cleanliness, and acne, 399
cleansing cream, 379, 380, 381
cleft lip/harelip: genetic defect in which the upper lip is not completely joined, 119, *403*, 404, 465
cleft palate: genetic defect in which the hard palate is not completely joined, 119, *403*, 403–404, 465
climacteric
  female: menopause
  male: in men, the psychological equivalent of the menopause, characterized by forgetfulness, depression, and declining sexual interest, 182–183
clinical death: cessation of respiration and heartbeat, 293. Compare *biological death.*
clinics, hearing aid, 201
clitoris: small, erectile organ of the female in the front part of the vulva
clonic: of or characteristic of clonus
clonic phase: the period during a grand mal epileptic convulsion when spasms of rigidity and relaxation (or jerking) occur in rapid succession, 473
clonic spasm: *spasm*
clonus: muscular spasm characterized by rapid alternation of contraction and relaxation. Compare *tonus.*

matter or obtain tissue for diagnosis

curette: small instrument, usu. resembling a spoon or scoop with sharpened edges, used in curettage

curling irons, electric, 383

Cushing's syndrome: excess of hormones secreted by the adrenal cortex, characterized by weakness, purple streaks in the skin, and a moon face, 570

cuspids, 5

cusp of tooth, 5

custard, baked, nutrients in, 298

cuticle: 1. epidermis. 2. crescent of toughened skin around the base of a nail, 18.

cyanosis: disordered circulatory condition due to inadequate oxygen supply in the blood and causing a livid bluish color of the skin

cyanotic: bluish in color due to cyanosis

cyclamates: sodium cyclamate

cyclopropane in childbirth, 161

cypress vats in whisky making, 634

cyst: saclike mass containing liquid or semisolid material
sebaceous, 398

cystic duct: duct that carries bile from the gallbladder to the juncture with the hepatic duct, where the common bile duct is formed

cystic fibrosis: hereditary disease of infants and young children marked by cysts, excessive fibrous tissue, and mucous secretion, 153

cystitis: inflammation of the bladder, characterized by a burning sensation when voiding, frequent need to urinate, and sometimes blood in the urine, 83, 435, 602

cystoscope: device used to view the interior of the bladder after being inserted in the urethra

D

dairy foods, 130, 194

dance, modern, 134

D and C: dilation and curettage

dandruff: condition marked by itching and flaking of the skin, esp. of the scalp, 385

Data-Phone, 507, 511

dates, nutrients in, 310

dating, steady, 240

db: decibel

DBI/phenformin: drug that stimulates the production of insulin in the pancreas, 580

DDT, 368–369

deafness, 201–203, 593–594
from loud music, 374
mixed, 201
from on-the-job noise, 373
from snowmobile noise, 375
and sound, 370–371
in unborn child, 152

Dearborn, Dr. Lester W., 287

death
fear of, 293
five major causes of, 501
in middle years, 272–273
stages of, 293

See also *biological death, clinical death.*

death rates, 501
from air pollutants, 358
breast cancer, 614
cancer, 609
colon-rectum cancer, 619
heart disease, 500, 502, 506
from heroin abuse, 659
lung cancer, 612
and obesity, 325
oral cancer, 625
skin cancer, 623
and tuberculosis, 545
uterine cancer, 621

decalcification/bone atrophy: the loss of lime or calcium salts from the bones or teeth, 448

decibel/db: unit for measuring the intensity of sound, 370

deciduous teeth: baby teeth

decision-maker: ego

defecation: the discharge of feces, 522

defibrillator: device that sends a jolt of electricity into the heart muscle in order to stop fibrillation and get the heart back to normal rhythm, 508

deficiency diseases, nutritional, 319–320

deformity
facial, after Bell's palsy, 472
in hemophilia, 486
from joint injuries, 453

degenerative: characterized by deterioration or change from a normally active state to a lower or less active state, esp. of body tissue, as in a disease process

dehydration, 82

delirium tremens/DTs: violent form of delirium characterized by nausea, confusion, crawling sensation on the skin, and hallucinations caused esp. by rapid lowering of blood alcohol levels in very heavy drinkers, 643

delivery
approach to, 155–158
normal, 159

delivery date, calculation of, 156

deltoid muscle, 14

dementia: mental deterioration resulting from an organic or functional disorder, 478
presenile/Alzheimer's disease: mental degeneration (dementia) resulting from functional or organic disorder, as cerebral arteriosclerosis, that occurs in middle age, 478

Demerol: meperidine

demyelination: gradual loss of myelin, resulting in paralysis, numbness, or other loss of nerve function, 29

dendrites: short, gray filaments in neurons that conduct impulses toward the cell body, 28, 29, 30

dental care, prepaid, 211

dental caries/cavities: ulceration and decay of teeth, 136, 175–176, 467, 524

dental checkups, 93

dental floss: strong, silky filament for cleaning between the teeth, 98, 190

dental hygiene for hemophiliacs, 487

dental service, home care, 211

dental surgeon: oral surgeon

dentin: the hard calcified substance that forms the body of a tooth, 4, 5
in tooth decay, 175–176, 467

dentist: one who specializes in the diagnosis, prevention, and treatment of disease affecting the teeth and their associated structures

dentistry: the branch of medical science that concerns the study, diagnosis, prevention, and treatment of diseases of the teeth, gums, and associated structures

denture(s): frame of plastic or other material adapted to fit the mouth and containing one, several, or a complete set of artificial teeth to replace natural teeth that have been lost, 176, 190–192, 190, 191, 468
care of, 191–192
cleaning of, 192
fitting of, 191
ill-fitting, 428
immediate, 192
implant, 191
partial, 176
and periodontal disease, 95

denture brush, 192

deodorants, 381

Department of Health, Education and Welfare, Public Health Services, National Institutes of Health, 474

dependence: *drug dependence*

depilatory: chemical product capable of removing or loosening hair, 127
chemical, 388

depressant: drug or other substance that reduces or calms the physiological processes of body or mind, 655–657. Compare *stimulant.*

depression, 219
and physical activity, 189

dermabrasion: the removal of layers of skin by planing with an abrasive tool to dispose of wrinkles or skin blemishes, 177, 177, 201

dermal: of or relating to the skin

dermatitis: inflammation of the skin, 391, 391
contact: dermatitis caused by a hypersensitive reaction to external contact with a substance or material, 105, 385, 391
stasis, 200

dermatologist: physician specializing in the diagnosis and treatment of disorders of the skin, 394

dermatology: the branch of medical science dealing with disorders of the skin

dermis/corium/true skin: the inner layer of the skin, which contains blood vessels, nerves, connective tissue, sweat glands, and sebaceous glands, 18, 19, 19, 378, 378

desensitization, 413

desert rheumatism: coccidioidomycosis

Desoxyn: methamphetamine

desserts, nutrients in, 298

detached retina/separated retina: eye disorder in which the membrane at the back of the eye (retina) is separated from its bed, as by being torn, thus impairing vision, 586–587

digestive tract: parasites in, 439
  troubles in, 427–431
digitalis: the dried leaves of foxglove, containing several glycosides, often used as a heart tonic
in congestive heart failure, 520
dilate: to become larger, as the pupil of the eye in diminished light
dilation and curettage/D and C: enlarging the opening into the uterus and the scraping of the uterus with a curette, 155

dimethyltryptamine: DMT
dinner
  low-calorie menus, 331
  low-fat, 349
  low-sodium, 340
  minimal residue, 351
diphtheria: respiratory, bacterial disease marked by the formation of a false membrane that obstructs breathing, 117, 440
in pregnancy, 152
diphtheria antitoxin, *117*
diplopia, 484
disagreement, ways of expressing, 217–218
discharge from body opening, 89
discipline, of children, 230–233
  agreement of parents on, 260
disclosing tablets: tablets which, after being chewed, leave a temporary stain on plaque remaining on teeth after brushing, 98
disease(s)
  causes of, 437–440
  childhood, 114–119
  food-borne, 343, 345
  hereditary and congenital, 444–445
  occupational, 355–357, 563
  secondary, 568
  spread of, 440
  See also specific diseases.
disinfectants: germicides
disk(s)
  intervertebral, 6
  removal of, 464
  slipped/herniating disk: painful displacement (herniation) of one of the fibrous disks of the spinal column between two vertebrae, such that it presses against nerves and may cause sciatica, 415, 460
dislocation(s): the partial or complete displacement of one or more of the bones at a joint, 453–454
  correction of, 455
  joint, 11
  elbow, *453*
  hip, 457
disorders, internal, and skin, 16
distal: relatively remote from the center of the body, or from a point considered as central. Compare *proximal.*
distal muscles: the muscles of the extremities (the hands and the feet)
distillation: separation of the more volatile parts of a substance from the less volatile by boiling and condensing the vapors into separate liquids
diuresis: excessive excretion of urine, 596
diuretic(s): substance stimulating the secretion of urine
  in congestive heart failure, 520
  in gout, 421
  in hypertension, 515
  in nephrosis, 602
diverticula (*sing., diverticulum*): pouches or sacs opening off the large intestine, 531, *531*
diverticulitis: inflammation of diverticula in the digestive tract, esp. in the colon, 531
  and diet, 341

diverticulosis: the presence of diverticula in the digestive tract, 531
divorce, 270–271
  and early marriage, 247
dizziness, 30
DMT/dimethyltryptamine: synthetic hallucinogen, 662
DNA molecule: model of, *612*
Doll, Dr. Richard S., 609
Dolly (*slang*): methadone
Dolophine: methadone
DOM/STP: synthetic hallucinogen, 662
dominance, eye, 75
Donora, Pennsylvania, inversion, 358, 558
donor centers, *37*
donors, blood, *37*
  "universal," 37
dopamine: chemical compound found in the brain, needed in the synthesis of norepinephrine and epinephrine, 475
Doriden: glutethimide
dorsal: toward, near, or in the back. Compare *ventral.*
double vision/diplopia: condition in which a single object is perceived as two images due to inability to coordinate focusing of the eyes, 484
douching: flushing of a body part or cavity, esp. the vagina, with water as a means of cleansing
  as birth control method, 254
doughnuts, nutrients in, 317
downs/downers/goof balls (*slang*): barbiturates or other drugs that depress the central nervous system, 655–657
DPT injection: injection to provide immunity against diphtheria, pertussis (whooping cough), and tetanus, 104, 109, 113–114, 117, *117,* 118
drainage system for lymph, 39
dreamer (*slang*): morphine
dreams as key to subconscious, 219
drinking
  intelligent, 185
  problem defined, 641
  tips on avoidance of, 185
drinking habits, *628, 629*
drinking trends, 628–629
driving and alcohol, 185, 635, 638–639, *639, 640*
drooling, 470, 471
dropsy: former term for edema, esp. when caused by cardiac insufficiency
drowning, 675–676
drug(s): 1. any substance other than food that changes or has an effect on the body or mind, 649–666. 2. narcotic drug, 649
  abuse, 651–652
  as allergens, 413
  antihypertensive, 515
  antismoking, 183
  cholesterol-reducing, *504*
  in labor pains, 160
  over-the-counter, 649–650
  prescription, 650–651, *651*
  self-prescribed, 650
  use of. 138
drug addicts and serum hepatitis, 537
drug dependence: physical or psychological accommodation to the periodic or continuous presence of a

digestive, 50, 55
and muscle chemistry, 479
in obstructive-airway disease, 563
pancreatic/pancreatic juice, 51
ptyalin, 45
role of, 58
epidemic: 1. (*adj.*) affecting many in a community at once, as a disease. 2. (*n.*) the temporary prevalence of a disease in a community or throughout a large area, 437
epidemiologist: physician specializing in epidemiology
epidemiology: the branch of medical science concerned with the study and prevention of epidemic diseases
epidermis/cuticle: the outer, non-vascular layer of the skin, overlying the dermis, 18, *19*, 30, 377, *378*
epididymus, *570*
epigastric: pertaining to the upper middle part of the abdomen
epigastric pain, 532
epiglottis: the leaf-shaped plate of cartilage at the base of the tongue that covers that trachea during the act of swallowing, *44, 47*, 48, 60, *60*
epilepsy: chronic nervous disorder characterized by sudden loss of consciousness and sometimes by convulsions, 472–474, 695
diagnosis of, *472*
idiopathic, 473
treatment of, 474
Epilepsy Foundation of America, 474, 695
epinephrine: adrenaline
epiphysis: cartilage plate on the extremity of a long bone, 126
slipped: the slipping or dislocation of the end of a bone (epiphysis), as of the femur at the hip joint, 457
episiotomy: incision made during labor to enlarge the vaginal area enough to permit passage of the baby, 162
epithelial: pertaining to the epithelium
epithelium: membranous tissue that lines the canals, cavities, and ducts of the body, as well as all free surfaces exposed to the air
Equanil: meprobamate
equilibrium. See *balance.*
erection: enlarged and firm state of the penis when sexually stimulated, 242
erysipelas: acute bacterial skin infection characterized by bright red patches, 397
erythremia: polycythemia vera
erythrocyte/red blood cell/red corpuscle: cell found in the bloodstream, often lacking a nucleus, the carrier of hemoglobin, 10, 35, 484
esophagoscope: device inserted into the esophagus to permit its inspection
esophagus: the tube through which food passes from the mouth to the stomach, *44, 47, 47*, 48, *49*, 60, *60*, 522, 525–526, *525*
diverticulum of, *531*
foreign bodies in, 529
inflammation of, 526

estrin, 154
estrogen: any of several hormones found in the ovarian fluids of the female which promote growth of secondary sex characteristics and influence cyclical changes in the female reproductive system, 67, 70, 125, 571
deficiency in menopause, 180
excess, 572
in ovulation, 146
replacement therapy, 572
ethanol: ethyl alcohol
ethchlorvynol/Placidyl, 657
ether in childbirth, 161
ethinamate/Valmid, 657
ethmoid bone: sievelike bone at the base of the skull behind the nose, 80
ethnic groups and tuberculosis, 545
ethyl alcohol/grain alcohol/ethanol: product of the distillation of fermented grains, fruit juices, and starches, used in beverages and having intoxicating properties, 627, *627*
etiologist: physician specializing in studying the causes of disease
etiology: 1. the cause or causes of a disease, 437. 2. the branch of medical science dealing with the causes of disease.
eunuch: in males, the failure at puberty to develop secondary sex characteristics due to disorder or removal of testicles, 570
Eustachian tube: passage connecting the middle ear to the upper throat which equalizes air pressure on both sides of the eardrum, 77, *77, 79*
infection of, 590
obstruction of, 435, 542, 591
examination, neurological, 469
excrete: to eliminate, as waste matter, by normal discharge from the body
excretion: 1. the act of excreting. 2. the body's waste matter, as sweat, urine, and feces.
skin as organ of, 18
exercise, 91–92, *167, 168, 169, 170, 171, 172, 173*
for arthritis, 206, 449, 450, *450*
and bowel action, 430
and circulation, *512*
combined with reducing diet, 328
in epilepsy, 474
for feet, 174
as habit, 327
and heart attack, 512
and heart disease, 204
and hernia prevention, 16
lack of, 416
in later years, 196, 197–200
maximum level, 133
in middle years, *92*, 167–173
as substitute for smoking, 183
teen-age boys, 132–134
teen-age girls, 134
in weight reduction, 330
exercise program, 133, 134
exocrine gland: any of various glands, such as mammary or sebaceous glands, having ducts that carry their secretions to specific locations, 65, 566. Compare *endocrine gland.*

exophthalmic goiter: *hyperthyroidism*
expectorate: discharge from the mouth, as saliva or phlegm
expiration, *59, 540*
extension: state of being extended or straightened
of limbs, 15
extensor: muscle whose function is to extend or straighten a part of the body, 14–15
external cardiac massage: *cardiac massage*
external cardiopulmonary resuscitation: ECPR
extremities, 421–425
eye(s), 71, 72–76, *73*
in aging, 206
and autonomic nervous system, *28*
blood-shot, 490
color of, 379
common troubles of, 433–434
crossed/strabismus, 119–120, 121
in infancy, 105
surgery for, 403
diseases of, 584–589
drainage network, 76
effect of auto exhaust, *560*
farsighted, 121
focusing machinery of, 72
makeup for, 382
and muscular dystrophy, 481
nearsighted, 121
selection-rejection monitors for food, 45
supporting structures, and service units of, 75–76
eyeballs, movements of, 75
eye charts, *585*
eyeglasses
for children, 120–121
for correcting myopia, *584*
eyeground: the inner side of the back of the eyeball, 582
eyelids, 75
in Bell's palsy, 472
cosmetic surgery on: blepharoplasty
inflammation of: sty
eye muscles, 14
eye patch for strabismus, 403
eyestrain: disorder caused by excessive or improper use of the eyes and characterized by fatigue, tearing, redness, and a scratchy feeling in the eyelids, 414, 433–434
eye teeth: the upper canine teeth

F

face
birth defects, 465
injuries to, 466–467
face lift: rhytidoplasty
facial canal: Fallopian canal
facial nerve, paralysis of: Bell's palsy
facial plasty: rhytidoplasty
fainting: brief loss of consciousness, 427, 695
in heat exhaustion, 417
in neurogenic shock, 685
Fallopian canal/facial canal: bony canal in the skull, 471
Fallopian tubes: the pair of tubes connecting the ovaries and the uterus, through which the egg must pass at the time of ovulation, 243, *243, 244, 571*

fibrous, 96
forbidden in acne, 399
and hangover, 186
hazards from, 366–369
high-calorie, 187
and hives, 392
importance of, 295
iron-rich, 490
molecules, breaking down, 53
and morning sickness, 149
natural, 349
nutrients in (table), 298–319
organic, 346–347, 349
  stores, *349*
passage through stomach, 49
prepared, 367
protein, 296
psychological aspects, 350–353
shopping for, 193
solid, for infant, 301
storage of, 345
symbolic aspects, 353
food additives, 345–346, *345*
Food and Drug Administration/FDA,
  346, 650, 655
and liquid silicone, 406
food chain: the relationship of organisms considered as food sources or
  consumers or both, as the relationship of a flowering plant to a bee
  to a bird
food debris, 96, 97
  removal of, 98
food poisoning: digestive disorder
  marked by nausea and vomiting,
  caused by bacteria found in decaying or rancid food, 440, 536
food tube: esophagus
foot doctor: podiatrist
force breathing, 59
forces, balance of: Yin and Yang
forearm movement, muscle action in,
  15
foreign bodies
  in alimentary tract, 529
  in eye, 588
  and white blood cells, 36
forensic medicine/forensic pathology:
  subspecialty of pathology dealing
  with the various aspects of medicine and the law
forensic pathology: forensic medicine
foreplay, sexual, 249
foreskin: the loose skin (prepuce)
  covering the head of the penis
formula for newborns, 103–104, *104*
Fort, Dr. Joel, 649
Foster Grandparent Program, 281
foundation creams, 382
fovea: shallow rounded depression in
  the retina, directly in the line of
  vision at a point where vision is
  most acute, 72, *73*
fracture: break in a bone, 11, 682. See
  *closed fracture, complete fracture,
  incomplete fracture.*
  depressed, 465
  of facial bones, 466
  healing of, 454–456
  kinds of, 453
  in later years, 10
  in osteogenesis imperfecta, 448
  pubic, 458
  rib, 464
  skull, 465–466
  spinal, decompression of, 464
  spontaneous, *453*

treatment of, 455–456
frame sizes and weight, 321
Framingham Study, 198
frankfurters, nutrients in, 303
frauds in health aids, 215
freckle: small, brownish or dark-
  colored spot on the skin, 400
freezing of skin: cryosurgery
frequencies, sound, 371
frequency, urinary, 595
Freud, Sigmund: Austrian neurologist
  (1856–1939) who founded psychoanalysis and shaped the course of
  modern psychiatry, 218–219, *218*
friction, reduction of, in joints, 14
friends, older, of teen-agers, 238–239
frigidity: sexual unresponsiveness in
  women, 249–250, 264
Froehlich's syndrome: failure of secondary sex characteristics to develop in males due to anterior
  pituitary disease, 570
frontal lobes, 26
frontal lobotomy: rarely performed
  surgical operation of cutting into
  the frontal lobes of the brain to
  alter behavior
frostbite: partial freezing of a part of
  the body, esp. of the extremities or
  ears, 393, 419–420
fructose/levulose: very sweet crystalline sugar
  to prevent hangover, 186
fruit cocktail, nutrients in, 310
fruits, fresh, *187*, 194
  nutrients in, 309
frustration, 262
FSH: follicle-stimulating hormone
functional hypertension: hypertension, essential
fundus: the rounded base or bottom
  of any hollow organ
fungus (*pl., fungi*): any of a group of
  plants including the mushrooms,
  molds, yeasts, and various microorganisms, some of which cause diseases in human beings, 106, 395, 439
  and respiratory diseases, 549
fungus infections, 395–396
  of oral cavity, 524
furniture polish, as poison, 688
fuse: electrical safety device that
  interrupts a circuit when current
  becomes too strong
fusion
  spinal, 464
  for scoliosis, 461
  for slipped disk, 460
  of spinal joints: spondylitis

G

galactosemia: hereditary condition
  affecting infants who lack an enzyme that converts galactose (a
  sugar) into glucose in the blood
gallbladder/cholecyst: small pear-
  shaped pouch situated beneath the
  liver that serves as a reservoir for
  bile, *44, 49, 51, 55*, 522
  diseased, 538, *538*
  removal of, 55
gallstone(s): solid substance formed
  in the gallbladder that can obstruct
  the flow of bile and prevent the
  digestion of fats, 55, 538

and diet, 341
and jaundice, 537
games
  of children, *86, 226*
  as exercise, 198
  in middle age, 168–170
gamete: either of two mature reproductive cells, an ovum or sperm
  cell
gamma globulin
  in measles, 114
  and Rh factor, 152
gamma rays, *493*
ganglion (*pl., ganglia*): 1. cluster of
  nerve cells outside of the central
  nervous system, 30. 2. cyst of a tendon, as on the wrist.
gangrene: death of tissues in a part
  of the body, caused by lack of
  adequate blood supply, 456, 497
  danger in frostbite, 419
  in diabetes, 497, 583
garbage, burning of, *356*
garbage cans, noise levels, *373*
garden clubs, 277
gardening, 198, 276–277, *277*
gas, asphyxiation by, 686
gaseous exchange, in respiration, *57,
  61, 62*
gases, anesthetic, in childbirth, 161
gasoline, as poison, 688
gastric analysis: extraction and study
  of gastric juices
gastric juice: the acid fluid secreted
  by the glands lining the stomach,
  containing several enzymes
gastric ulcer: ulcer of the mucuous
  membrane of the stomach, 50. See
  also *peptic ulcer.*
gastritis: inflammation of the stomach, 429–430, 532
  acute: sudden, sharp attack of gas-
    tritis
  chronic: recurrent and persisting
    attacks of gastritis
  toxic: gastritis caused by the swal-
    lowing of a poisonous substance
gastrocamera, *529*
gastroenteritis: inflammation of the
  mucous membrane that lines the
  stomach and intestines, 430
gastroenterologist: physician specializing in the diagnosis and treatment
  of gastrointestinal disorders
gastroenterology: the branch of medical science dealing with the study
  of the stomach and intestines and
  the disorders affecting them
gastrointestinal disorders, 522–539
  and diet, 341
  emotional, 353
  treatment of, 539
gastrointestinal series: GI series
gastrointestinal symptoms, 442
gastrointestinal tract or canal: alimentary tract or canal
gastroscope: device that allows inspection of the interior of the
  stomach
gelatin dessert, nutrients in, 319
gene: hereditary unit contained within a chromosome and associated
  with specific physical characteristics
  transmitted from parents to offspring, 127, 445
general practitioner/GP: physician
  whose training is not specialized

and includes some preparation in pediatrics, surgery, and obstetrics and gynecology, thus enabling him to care for an entire family

generation gap, 245

genetic counselor: specialist, usu. a physician, who counsels couples on the probability of genetic disorders occurring in their offspring

genetic factors and congenital defects, 152–153

genitalia: genitals

genital itch in diabetes, 576

genitals/genitalia: the reproductive organs
  cleansing of, 89
  female, 84
  male, 84–85
  size of, 126

genitourinary tract: urinogenital tract

genus: class or category of plants and animals ranking next above the species, as the genus *Homo* in *Homo sapiens*

Georgia alcoholic treatment program, 645

geriatrics: branch of medicine dealing with diseases and physiological changes associated with aging and old people

German measles: rubella

germ-fighting of lymph nodes, 39

germicide: disinfectant or other agent capable of killing disease germs, 441, 446
  as poison, 688

gerontologists, 189

gerontology: scientific study of the processes and phenomena of aging

GI: gastrointestinal

giantism: gigantism

gigantism/giantism: disorder due to oversecretion of somatotrophin by the pituitary gland and resulting in excessive growth, 66

Gillsberg, Dr. Bjorn, 368

gin, 634

gingival: pertaining to the gums

gingivitis: inflammation of the gum tissues, 190, 428

girdle, maternity, 150

girls
  attitude to parents, 228–230
  exercise goals, 134
  future outlook for, 236
  puberty in, 122–125

GI series/gastrointestinal series: X rays of the esophagus, stomach, and intestines utilizing an opaque substance swallowed by the patient, 539

gland(s): any of various organs that secrete substances essential to the body or for the elimination of waste products. See also under *endocrine system.*
  adrenal, *64*, 67–69, 136, 566, 569–570
  ductless: glands, endocrine
  endocrine, 64–71
    diseases of, 566–583
    role of, 65
    roles in aging, 166
  exocrine, 65, 566
  lacrimal, 76, *76*
  lymph, 64
  mammary, 65
  mucus, 65

olfactory, 80

parathyroid, 70, 566, 573

parotid, 45, 116
  inflammation of, 524

pineal/pineal body, 70–71

pituitary/hypophysis cerebri/pituitary body, *26*, *64*, 65, *66*, 123, 566, *567*
  anterior/hypophysis, 566–568
    hypofunctioning, 567
  posterior, 572–573

prostate, 67, 85, 126, *242*, 243, 604–605
  in aging, 208–209
  cancer of, 605
  enlarged, 208
    benign, 604
  inflammation of: prostatitis

salivary, *44*, 45, *47*, 522, 524

sebaceous, 19, *19*, 65, *378*, 381, 382
  blocking of, 398
  and chapped skin, 418
  of hair, 21
  location of, 378
  overactive, 127–128
  of skin, 22

sublingual, 45

submandibular: submaxillary

submaxillary/submandibular gland, 45

sweat, 19, *19*, 22–23, 65, *378*, 381
  location of, 378
  in temperature regulation, 23, 377
  swollen, 114, 116

thymus, 70–71
  in myasthenia gravis, 484

thyroid, *64*, 69–70, 566, *567*, 568–569

glandular fever: mononucleosis, infectious

glare and eyestrain, 434

glaucoma: disease of the eye characterized by increased pressure on the eyeball and leading to loss of vision if untreated, 76, 206, 586

glomerules, 81

glomeruli (*sing., glomerulus*): tiny tufts of capillaries in the kidneys through which the blood passes in the filtering of wastes, *82, 600*
  inflammation of, 599–600

glomerulonephritis: inflammation of the glomeruli, 600

glossitis: inflammation of the tongue, characterized by a bright red or glazed appearance, 429

glossopharyngeal nerve: the nerve that supplies sensation to the throat and rear of the tongue, *27*

gloves, rubber, 446

glucagon: hormone produced by the islets of Langerhans in the pancreas, 69

glucose/blood sugar: sugar found normally in blood and abnormally in urine, as in the case of diabetes mellitus, 58, 353
  and liver, 53
  metabolism in diabetes, 574
  production of, 575
  tests, personal, 581

tolerance test/GTT: test that determines the rate at which glucose in the blood is reduced, or metabolized, used as an indicator of chemical diabetes or a prediabetic condition, 583

glucosuria: condition, as diabetes mellitus, in which the urine contains glucose. See also *renal glucosuria.*

glutethimide/Doriden, 657

glycerin: glycerol

glycerol/glycerin: sweet, oily alcohol, one of the components of natural fat, 296

glycogen: animal starch usu. stored in the liver for conversion to glucose when the body needs energy, 574
  in liver, 53
  in pregnancy, 155

glycosuria: *glucosuria*

goiter: enlargement of the thyroid gland, often due to lack of iodine in the diet, 70, 569
  exophthalmic: *hyperthyroidism*

Goldfarb, Dr. Alvin I., 293

golf, 168

gonad(s): male or female sex gland; ovary or testicle, 70, 566
  female, 571–572
  male, 570–571
  maturation of, 125

gonadotrophic hormone/gonadotrophin/gonadotropin: any of three hormones that stimulate the gonads and are secreted by the anterior pituitary gland, 70, 125

gonioscope: specialized ophthalmoscope for examining the angle between the cornea and the iris

gonococcus: parasitic bacterium that can cause gonorrhea, 439, 608

gonorrhea: contagious venereal disease transmitted by sexual contact, 245, 608

goof balls (*slang*): barbiturates

goose flesh, 21

gout: metabolic disease characterized by painful inflammation of a joint, as of the big toe, and an excess of uric acid in the blood, 421, 451–452, *452*
  and alcohol, 637

Government Printing Office, 277
  Superintendent of Documents, 284, 324

GP: general practitioner

Graafian follicles: small sacs in the ovaries that contain the developing ova, 67

grain alcohol: ethyl alcohol

grain products, nutrients in, 313

grand mal: major epileptic seizure, characterized by falling, loss of consciousness, and spasmodic jerking of the arms and legs, 473, 695. Compare *petit mal.*

grandmother, role of, 265

granulocytes: neutrophils

grapefruit, nutrients in, 310

grapefruit juice, nutrients in, 310

grape juice, nutrients in, 311

grapes, nutrients in, 311

grass (*slang*): marihuana

gray matter: *cortex*

green soap, tincture of, 385

greenstick fracture: incomplete fracture, with the bone bending on the unbroken side, more common in children than adults, 453, 454

grippe: influenza

ground: connection which conducts electricity between an electric circuit and earth

grounding: installing a ground

growing years, importance of diet, 312

growth
of five-year-old, 111
spurt before menarche, 123

growth hormone/growth-stimulating hormone/somatotrophin: hormone secreted by the posterior lobe of the pituitary gland that stimulates growth, 66, *66, 568*
excess production of, 567–568

growth-stimulating hormone: growth hormone

GTT: glucose tolerance test

"guard hairs": vibrissae

Guild, Dr. Warren R., 185

guilt, function of, 218, 232–233

guilt feelings
of children, *232*
of working mothers, 256

gum(s)
care of, 93–98
disease: periodontal disease
inflammation of: gingivitis
massage of, 98

gunshot accidents: firearm accidents

gynecologist: physician specializing in gynecology, often an obstetrician as well, 84, 144
and late menarche, 123

gynecology: the branch of medical science that deals with the care and treatment of women and their diseases, esp. of the reproductive system

H

H (*slang*): heroin

hair, 20–21, 382–385
and aging, 200
body, 388
care of, *383*
cleansing of, 89
color of, 384–385
curling of, 382–383
drying, 385
excess, 179
removal of, 127, 387–389
as extension of skin, 18
on fire, first aid for, *678*
general care of, 385–387
graying of, 384
ingrown, 387
setting lotions, 383
straightening, 383–384
texture of, 382–384
transplant: the surgical grafting of hair-bearing skin from the back or sides of the scalp onto bald areas of the head 179, 408
unwanted: hirsutism
washing of, 93, 385
See also *skin and hair.*

hair curlers and baldness, 386

hairdresser, professional, *383*

halitosis: offensive mouth odor, usu. caused by poor oral hygiene, 429, 524

Hall-Stone ring, *252*

hallucinogen: drug or chemical capable of inducing hallucinations, 139, 660–662

hallucinogenic: capable of producing hallucinations

hamburger patties, nutrients in, 299

hammer/malleus: the outermost of the three ossicles of the middle ear, the bone between the eardrum and the anvil, 76, 78, *79*

hammer toe: clawlike deformity of a toe, 175

handball, *92*

hands
bones of, 3, *9*
joints of, 9, *9*
washing of, 89, *380*
of children, 112

hangnail: piece of skin partially torn loose from the root or side of a fingernail, 425

hangover: headache, nausea, dizziness, and other after-effects of excessive alcoholic consumption, an allergic reaction to alcohol, or emotional stress while drinking, 636–637
prevention of, 186
treatment of, 186

"hangup," amphetamine, 654

harelip: cleft lip

hashish: hallucinogenic substance more potent than marihuana, obtained from the leaves and flowers of the Indian hemp plant, 663, *663*

hatter's disease: chronic mercury poisoning, common among hatters in former times because of their use of mercury in preparing felt, 356

hay fever: allergic rhinitis

hay-fever season, *552*

head
blows to, 466
injuries, 465–466
wounds, 684

headache: pain or ache across the forehead or within the head, 30, 262, 413–415, *414.* See also *tension headache.*
acupuncture in treatment of, *704*
sick: migraine

healing, slow, as symptom, 207

healing process and fractures, 454

health, and condition of skin and hair, 377

health insurance, 211–212
and alcoholism, 643

Health Insurance Institute, 212

Health Insurance Plan study, 198

hearing, 76, 590, *590*
area of brain, *26*
loss of, 201–203, 591
mechanism of, 78–79
organ of, 77
threshold of, 370, 371

hearing aids, 201–203, *202, 203,* 594, *594*
for children, 121
National Health survey on, 201

hearing problems in children, 121
caused by rubella, *593*

heart, 31–33
abnormalities: heart disease, congenital
artificial aortic valve, insertion of, *503*
and autonomic nervous system, *28*
circulation of blood, *40*
functioning of, 444
interaction with lungs, 56
location of, 31, *31,* 41

musculature of, 41
rubber parts for, *517*
structure and performance of, 40–42

heart-assist device, *517*

heart attack
coronary thrombosis, 499, 506, 692
emergency care, 509–510, 692–693
and exercise, 197–198
prevention of, 510–512
risk factors, 510
and smoking, 183
statistics on, 500
symptoms of, 508

heartbeat, 41–42
and calcium, 11
disturbance of, 508
and marihuana, 138
rapid: tachycardia
and regular exercise, 134

heart block: lack of coordination in the heartbeat of the atria and ventricles, often causing unconsciousness and other symptoms (Stokes-Adams syndrome), 521

heartburn, during pregnancy, 148–149

heart disease/cardiovascular disease, 91, 137, *183,* 500–521, *501*
atherosclerotic, 416
congenital, 500–502, 518–520
hypertensive: impairment of heart function due to persistent hypertension, 500
in later years, 203–205
as major killer, 31
and obesity, 325

heart failure: inability of the heart to pump enough blood to maintain normal circulation
congestive: heart failure resulting from the inability of the heart muscle to keep a sufficient supply of blood in circulation, resulting in congestion or swelling of the tissues, 337, 520

heart-lung machine, *505, 506*
miniature, 520

heart murmur: abnormal sound heard in the region of the heart
in rheumatic heart disease, 517–518

heart muscle, failure of, 508–509

heart patients and sexual activity, 285–286

heart surgery, 506
advances in, 31

heart valves, artificial, *516*

heat
for arthritis, 206
in earache, 434

heat cramps: muscle spasms resulting from loss of salt due to excessive sweating

heat exhaustion/heat prostration: weakness or fainting as a result of prolonged exposure to heat, caused by a decreased blood supply to the heart and brain and an increased supply to the skin, 417–418, 680

"heat flush," 23

heat-pressing of hair, 383

heat prostration: heat exhaustion

heat rash: prickly heat

heatstroke: sunstroke

Heine-Medin disease: poliomyelitis

helmet in contact sports, *467*

helminth: parasitic worm that invades the intestines, most often via food or water, 534

hemal: of or relating to blood

and puberty, 123
replacement therapy, 181, 572
sex, 70, 124
thyroid: thyroxin
thyroid-stimulating/TSH, 67
thyrotropic, *66*
transported by blood, 34
and undescended testicles, 126
hormone treatment, and aging, 287
horn cells, anterior, in poliomyelitis, 476
horny layer of epidermis: stratum corneum
horse (*slang*): heroin
hosiery, proper fit of, 174
hospitalization, children and, 233–234
hospital stay under Medicare, 211
hotels, retirement, 290
hot flashes, 572
housekeeper, and care of newborn, 101
housemaid's knee: chronic inflammation of the bursa in front of the knee due to pressure from constant kneeling or injury, 423
housewife, average, 248
housework, and working mothers, 257
Housing and Urban Development Agency/HUD, 290
housing for later years, 288, 289
housing projects, public, *291*
HUD: Housing and Urban Development Agency
human fats, liver build-up of, 53
Human Sexual Inadequacy, 263
Human Sexual Response, 263, 285
humerus: the long bone of the arm from elbow to shoulder, 7, 9, 15, *15*
humpback: *kyphosis*
hunchback: *kyphosis*
hunger, constant, 207
hunger headache, 415
husband
attitude to menopause, 181
impotent, 263–264
of working wife, 256
hydradenitis suppurativa, *396*
hydrocarbons as pollutants, 359, 360
hydrocele: localized accumulation of fluid, esp. surrounding the testicles in the scrotum
hydrocephalus: accumulation of cerebrospinal fluid within the brain
hydrochloric acid, 50
in anemia, 490
in pernicious anemia, 489
hydrogenation: the subjection of a material to hydrogen, as the process by which unsaturated fats are solidified
hydrogen atoms in saturated fats, 297
hydrogen peroxide
in bleaching hair, 385, 388
in cleaning ears, 435
hydronephrosis: enlargement of the kidneys with urine due to an obstruction of the ureter, 604
hydrophilic: having an affinity for water, as the soft contact lens
hydrophilic lenses: contact lenses, soft plastic
Hydrophilic Ointment USP XVL, 201
hydrophobia: rabies
hydrotherapy for arthritis, 206
hygiene
of eye, 76
oral, 97

personal, 89, 441
of children, 112
in pregnancy, 147
Hyman, Dr. Harold T., 186
hymen: thin membrane usu. partially covering the entrance of the vagina in virgins
imperforate, 124
hyperacusis: abnormal and sometimes painful acuteness of hearing, 471
hyperfunction: disorder of an endocrine gland, characterized by excess secretion of a hormone
hyperglycemia: abnormally high amount of sugar in the blood, 580
hypermetropia: farsightedness
hypermetropic: farsighted
hyperopia: farsightedness
hyperopic: farsighted
hypertension/high blood pressure: excessively high blood pressure, sometimes caused by a disease (secondary hypertension) and sometimes not (essential hypertension), 42, 83, 91, 262, 416, 513, 514
with atherosclerosis, 497
and cadmium, 365
as cause of heart disease, 500
causes of, 514
chronic: essential hypertension
control of, 502
and diet, 337
effect of noise, 373
essential/chronic hypertension/functional hypertension: hypertension, or high blood pressure, that is not a symptom of disease and has no known cause, 426, 514–515
and heart attack, 511
and heart disease, 512
in kidney failure, 598
malignant: form of essential hypertension with an acute onset and rapid rise in pressure, 515
and oral contraceptives, 251
in pregnancy, 149
secondary: hypertension arising as a consequence of another known disorder, 514
and sexual activity, 286
symptoms of, *427*
hypertensive heart disease: heart disease, hypertensive
hyperthyroidism: abnormal and excess activity of the thyroid gland, resulting in oversecretion of thyroxin and an abnormally high metabolism, characterized by fatigue, weight loss, rapid pulse, intolerance to heat, and sometimes by protruding eyes (in which case the disorder is called *exophthalmic goiter*), 69–70, *568*, 569
hypnosis in childbirth, 162
hypnotic: tending to produce sleep
hypoallergenic: less likely to produce an allergic reaction
hypochondria: extreme anxiety about one's health, usu. associated with a particular part of the body and accompanied by imagined symptoms of illness
hypofunction: disorder of an endocrine gland, characterized by too little secretion of a hormone

hypoglycemia/low blood sugar: abnormally small amount of glucose in the blood, which can lead to insulin shock, 353, 579
hypoglycemic drug: drug intended to reduce the amount of glucose in the blood by stimulating the release of insulin from the pancreas
oral, 580
hypophysis: *pituitary gland*
hypophysis cerebri: pituitary gland
hyposensitization: program for desensitizing allergy patients by injecting them with progressively larger doses of pollen or other allergens to build tolerance levels, 554
hypotension: excessively low blood pressure
hypothalamus: region of the brain below the thalamus, important in regulating the internal organs and associated with the functioning of the pituitary gland, *28*, 65–66, 125, 566
and infertility, 142
hypothermia: artificially low body temperature produced by gradually cooling blood, used to slow metabolism and reduce tissue oxygen need so that heart and brain can withstand short periods of interrupted blood flow during surgery, 520
hypothyroidism: deficient functioning of the thyroid gland, resulting in undersecretion of thyroxin and an abnormally low metabolism, characterized by lack of energy, thick skin, and intolerance to cold, 69, 568–569
hysterectomy: surgical procedure in which the uterus is completely removed, 180, 572
radical: surgical removal of the uterus, cervix, ovaries, and Fallopian tubes, 180–181
total: surgical removal of the uterus and cervix, 180
hysterogram: X-ray examination of the uterus and surrounding areas, 146

I

ice cream, 130, 194
nutrients in, 298
ice milk, 194
nutrients in, 298
ice skating, *172*
id: the concealed, inaccessible part of the mind, the seat of impulses that tend to fulfill instinctual needs, 219
identification: mental process, often unconscious, by which a person associates with himself the attributes of another with whom he has formed an emotional tie, *229*
with parent, 228–230
identification of diabetics, *580*
identity, search for, 237–238
idiopathic: (of diseases) originating spontaneously or of unknown cause
ileocecal valve: the valve between the ileum of the small intestine and the cecum, the first section of the large intestine, *49*, 52, 55

knees, injuries to, 454
Knudsen, Dr. Vern, 369
Koch, Larry J., 374
Koch, Robert, 548
kyphosis: backward curvature of the spine characterized as a humpback or hunchback, 461, 462

L

labeling and drugs, 650
labor, in childbirth, 158–163
  dry, 159
  stage three, 163
  stage two, 159–160
laboratories, underground, 653
laboratory tests in diagnosis, 443
labyrinth: the winding passages of the inner ear, 78, 592
lacrimal gland: tear-producing gland over the eye
lactogenic hormone/LTH/luteotrophic hormone/luteotrophin/luteotropin/prolactin: hormone secreted by the anterior lobe of the pituitary gland that stimulates the production of milk in the mammary glands, *66*, 67, 164
Lamaze, Dr. Ferdinand: French physician who pioneered in the development of a natural childbirth technique, 162
lamb
  chart, 302
  nutrients in, 301, 302
laminated glass: shatterproof glass, as in automobile windshields, consisting of two sheets of tempered glass with a sheet of plastic between
Langerhans: islets of Langerhans
language development, 226
lanolin
  and chapped skin, 418
  for dry skin, 380
  and hangnails, 425
laparotomy: surgical procedure for examining or treating the female reproductive organs within the abdominal cavity, 146
larvae, hookworm, *535*
laryngeal cartilage, *47*
laryngitis: inflammation of the mucous membranes of the larynx, causing the voice to become hoarse or disappear altogether, 433
  chronic: permanently hoarse voice resulting from thickened, toughened mucous membrane in the larynx, due to too many attacks of laryngitis
laryngologist: physician specializing in the diagnosis and treatment of disorders of the throat
laryngology: the branch of medical science concerned with the study and treatment of the throat and related areas
larynx/voice box: the organ of voice in humans and most other vertebrates, consisting of a cartilaginous box in the upper part of the trachea across which are stretched vocal cords whose vibrations produce sound, 48, 60, *60*
  in laryngitis, 433
laser radiation, 357

lateral: relating to or directed toward the side
laws and alcohol problems, 645–646
laxative: substance that has the power to loosen the bowels, as milk of magnesia, 167, 431, 526
lead, 365
  in auto exhausts, 361
  as pollutant, 359
lead poisoning, 360–361
leaflet: flap of a heart valve, 516
  synthetic substitutes, 517
learning
  habit of, 188
  and identification with parent, 229
  in later years, 283
left-handedness in infant, 109
leftovers, 196
leg, shortening of, 457
Legg-Perthes' disease: inflammation of the bone and cartilage in the head of the femur (thigh bone), 457
legislation to control noise, 374
legs
  bowed, 448, 449
  care of, in pregnancy, 151
  problems with, 421–423
  relief of tension in, 172
leisure activities
  for later years, 274–282
  in middle years, 266–269
lemonade concentrate, nutrients in, 311
lens: biconvex transparent body behind the iris of the eye that focuses entering light rays on the retina, *73*, 74, 75
lesion: any abnormal change in an organ or tissue caused by disease or injury
  primary, of syphilis, 607
lettuce, nutrients in, 307
leukemia: form of cancer involving the blood and blood-making tissues, characterized by a marked and persistent excess of leukocytes, 443, 492–493, 611, *612*
  lymphocytic: form of leukemia characterized by uncontrolled over-activity of the lymphoid tissue
leukocyte/white blood cell/white corpuscle: white or colorless cell found in the bloodstream important in providing protection against infection, 35–36, *36*, 484, 492–494
leukopenia: abnormal reduction in the number of leukocytes in the blood, 493
levodopa: medicine used in treating the symptoms of Parkinson's disease, 475
levulose: fructose
LH: luteinizing hormone
libido: the instinctual craving or drive behind all human activities, esp. sexual, the repression of which leads to neurosis
  male, 570
library, public, *278*
Librium: chlordiazepoxide
lice, head, 385–386
lidocaine: chemical used as a local anesthetic, 508
life expectancy, alcohol and, 637–638
lifetime care facilities, 290–291

ligament(s): band of tough, fibrous connective tissue that binds together bones and provides support for organs, 14
  as braces, *15*
  and fallen arches, 421
  joint-capsule, tearing of, 453
  strained, 460
  torn, 450
ligation: the act of tying or binding up, as an artery. See also *tubal ligation.*
light
  for reading, *434*
  sensitivity, 114
light control, and focusing, 74
lightening: during the last few weeks of pregnancy, a shift in fetal pressure from the upper abdomen to the pelvic region as the head of the fetus moves toward the birth canal, 157
lighter fluid, as poison, 688
lighting, improper, and eyestrain, 434
lignite tar industries and skin cancer, 356
limbs of nephron, *600*
lipase: enzyme that breaks down fats, 50
Lippes Loop, *252*
lip reading/speech reading, 203
lips, and selection or rejection of food, 43
Lipscomb, Dr. David M., 375
lipsticks, 382
liqueurs, 633
liquid intake, importance of, 430
liquor laws, 639
listening habits, and hearing loss, 201
literature, educational, 284
liver: large, glandular organ situated just under the diaphragm on the right side, that processes blood and regulates its composition, as by storing sugar and releasing it in assimilable form (glucose), and that secretes bile, *44*, *49*, 52–55, 64
  cirrhosis of, 441
  disease, 536–538
    and acupuncture, 698
    and diet, 337
  functions of, 53
  inflammation of: hepatitis
  position of, *31*, *43*
  as producer of red blood cells, 38
  regeneration, capacity for, 55
liver (food), nutrients in, 301
liver spots/chloasma: yellowish brown patches that appear on the skin, 400
loans, for senior housing, 290
lobe(s): rounded or protruding section or subdivision, as of an organ of lung, 61
  occipital, 74
  of pituitary, anterior, 65, 66–67
  of pituitary, posterior, 65–66
  See also *cerebrum, lobes of.*
lobotomy: *frontal lobotomy*
lockjaw: tetanus
locomotion in cerebral palsy, 470
loins: the part of the body between the lower rib and the hip bone
London smog, 358, 558
loneliness, *286*
lordosis: abnormal inward curvature of the spine, 150, 460

lordotic posture: posture characteristic of some women in late pregnancy, in which the shoulders are slumped, the neck bent, and the lower spine curved forward to bear the weight of the fetus

Los Angeles smog, 360

"Lou Gehrig's disease": sclerosis, amyolotrophic lateral

low blood sugar: hypoglycemia

LSD/lysergic acid diethylamide: colorless, odorless, tasteless drug produced synthetically that causes the user to experience hallucinations, 139, 660–661

LTH: lactogenic hormone

lubricating fluid in bursas, 14

lubrication of eye, 76
in Bell's palsy, 472

lumbago: pain in the lower back, 8, 459

lumbar: pertaining to or situated near the loins

lumbar puncture: spinal tap

lumbar region of spine, 6, 7, 8

luncheon
fattening, *416*
low-calorie menus, 331
low-fat, 349
low-sodium, 340
minimal residue, 351

lung(s), 34, 59, 61–62, 540
air sacs in emphysema, *562*
and autonomic nervous system, *28*
collapsed, 61
disease of, 555–565
external appearance of, *60*
and fractured ribs, 464
fungus disease of: histoplasmosis
of heavy smoker, *613*
interaction with heart, 56
interior of, *60*
position of, *31*
pumping of blood to, 40
removal of, 61–62
structure of, 61
surface area, 62

lung cancer, 137, 183, 356, 562, 612–614
absence of pain in, 61
and air pollution, 560
and smoking, *183*

lung disease
black, 356
white: byssinosis

lung tissue, *541*
of coal miner, *563*
in emphysema, *561*
of heavy smoker, *556*

lunula: the living part of the nail, the pale, half-moon shape at the nail base, 21

luteinizing hormone/LH: a hormone secreted by the anterior lobe of the pituitary gland that stimulates a Graafian follicle to release an ovum during each menstrual cycle and converts the follicle into corpus luteum, *66*, 67

luteotrophic hormone: lactogenic hormone

luteotrophin: lactogenic hormone

luteotropin: lactogenic hormone

lye, as poison, 688

lymph: transparent fluid resembling blood plasma that is conveyed through vessels (lymphatic vessels) and lubricates the tissues, 39–40
circulation of, 39–40

lymphangiogram: the visualization by X ray of lymph nodes after injection of an opaque fluid

lymphatic: pertaining to or conveying lymph

lymphatic system, 39–40

lymph gland: lymph node

lymph node/lymph gland: one of the rounded bodies about the size of a pea, found in the course of the lymphatic vessels, that produce lymphocytes, 39, 64
enlarged, 114

lymphoblast: young cell that matures into a lymphocyte

lymphocyte: variety of leukocyte formed in the lymphoid tissue, 36, 38, 39, 492
in mononucleosis, 494

lymphocytic leukemia: leukemia, lymphocytic

lymphoid: pertaining to lymph or to the tissue of lymph nodes

lymphoma: abnormal (neoplastic) growth of lymphoid tissue, symptomatic of various diseases, as lymphocytic leukemia or Hodgkin's disease, 611

lymph vessels, 39–40

lysergic acid diethylamide: LSD

Lysol, 446, 447
as poison, 688

lysozyme: enzyme present in tears that is destructive to bacteria, 76

M

M (*slang*): morphine

macaroni, nutrients in, 317

macrobiotics: the idea, Oriental in origin, that an equilibrium should be maintained between foods that make one active (Yang) and foods that make one relax (Yin), 349

macrocephalic: individual with macrocephaly

macrocephaly: excessive head size, 465

macula: spot or discoloration. See also *macula lutea, senile macula degeneration.*

macula lutea: yellowish area in the retina related to color perception and marked by most acute vision

magnesium in teen-age diet, 130

magnesium trisilicate, 530

mainlining: injection of heroin directly into a vein, 140, 658

Majzlin Spring, *252*

makeup: cosmetics

malaise: feeling of being run-down, listless, uncomfortable, weary, and generally unwell, 543

malaria: disease caused by certain animal parasites transmitted by the bite of the infected anopheles mosquito, causing intermittent chills and fever
in pregnancy, 152

male pattern baldness: *baldness*

males, and heart attacks, 506

malignant: so aggravated as to threaten life, usu. resistant to treatment, and often having the property of uncontrolled growth, as a cancer

malleus: hammer

malnutrition: nutritional deficiency, as of essential proteins, vitamins, or minerals, causing impairment of health and certain specific diseases, 317, 319–320, 524
causes of, 319–320
in obesity, 320

malocclusion: faulty closure of the upper and lower teeth, 428, 435

mammography: specialized X-ray examination of the breasts, 616

mammoplasty: surgical procedure to augment the size of the breasts, 406

mandible, *7*

manganese, 298

manipulation technique in acupuncture, 700

Mao Tse-tung and medical techniques, 705

margarine, nutrients in, 318

marihuana: the dried leaves and flowers of the hemp plant (*Cannabis sativa*), which if smoked in cigarettes or otherwise ingested can produce distorted perception and other hallucinogenic effects, 138–139, *138, 662,* 662–665, *665*
effects of, 664
smokers, *664*

marriage, 246–260
early, 246–247
postponement of, *236*
problems in, *271*
See also *divorce, separation.*

marriage counselor, 248

marrow: either of two types of soft, vascular tissue found in the central cavities of bones—*red marrow,* which produces red blood cells, and *yellow marrow,* composed mainly of fat cells
red, 10, 38
yellow, 10

Massachusetts General Hospital, 645

massage, foot, 174

mass media, influence of, and teen-agers, 240

mastectomy: surgical removal of the breast
radical: surgical removal of the breast, underlying chest muscles, and lymph glands in the armpit, 617
simple, 619

master gland: pituitary gland

Masters, Dr. William H., 263, 264, 285

mastitis: inflammation of the breast, 164

mastoplasty: surgical procedure to reduce the size of the breasts, 406

masturbation: the touching or rubbing of the genitals for sexual pleasure and usu. orgasm
infantile, 219
in later years, 286–287
and teen-agers, 241
maturity, emotional, 218
and increased pressures, 262

Maugham, Somerset, 287

maxilla, *7*

MD: muscular dystrophy

M.D.: Doctor of Medicine

mead, 628

meal(s)
home delivered, 211, *289*
nutritious, *90*
one-dish, 196

musculoskeletal system: the human body's network of muscles and bones

myasthenia gravis: chronic disease characterized by muscular weakness and general and progressive exhaustion, 483–484, *483*

myelin: semisolid fatlike sheath that surrounds the axon of a neuron, 29, *29*

myelogram: X ray of the spinal cord obtained by the injection of a radio-opaque liquid material into the spinal cord area

myelography: technique of recording myelograms and the science of interpreting them, 464, 470

Myerson, Bess, 367

myocardial infarction: the process of congestion and tissue death (necrosis) in the heart muscle caused by an interruption of the blood supply to the heart, 41, 506

myocardium: the muscular tissue of the heart, 41

myoneural junction defect, 483

myopathy: any abnormality or disease of the muscles, 480

myopia: nearsightedness, 121, *584*, 589

myopic: nearsighted

myotonia: disorder characterized by increased rigidity or spasms of muscle, 482–483

myotonia congenita: congenital disease characterized by temporary muscle spasms and muscle rigidity, 482

myotonic dystrophy: chronic, progressive disease characterized by weakness and wasting of muscles, cataracts, and heart abnormality, 482–483

N

naprapathy: the treatment of disease by the manipulative correction of ligaments and connective tissues

narcolepsy: disease in which the patient is overcome by drowsiness or an uncontrollable desire for sleep, 652

narcotic: 1. any of various substances, such as morphine, codeine, and opium, that in medicinal doses relieve pain, induce sleep, and in excessive or uncontrolled doses may produce convulsions, coma, and death, 657–660. 2. inducing sleep.

narcotics smugglers, *658*

nasopharyngeal: pertaining to the nasopharynx

nasopharynx: the upper part of the pharynx above and behind the soft palate

natural foods: foods processed minimally, although not necessarily organically grown, 349

navel/umbilicus: the depression at the middle of the abdomen where the umbilical cord of the fetus was attached, 100, 163

nearsightedness/myopia: inability to see distant objects clearly, 121, *584*, 589

Necator, 535

neck vertebra: vertebra, cervical

necrosis: death of a group of cells, tissue, or a part of the body

needle biopsy: the excising of a tissue sample for biopsy by means of a long needle

nematode: any of a class of roundworms, many of which, such as the hookworm or pinworm, are intestinal parasites in man and other animals, 535

neoplasm: any abnormal growth of new tissue, as a tumor, which may be benign or malignant

neoplastic: of or characteristic of neoplasms

nephric: renal

nephritis/Bright's disease: inflammation of the kidneys, 117, 599–601
  symptoms of, 600–601

nephrologist: physician specializing in the diagnosis and treatment of diseases of the kidney

nephrology: branch of medical science dealing with the structure, function, and diseases of the kidney

nephron: one of the basic filtration units of the kidney, consisting of Bowman's capsule, a glomerulus, and tubules, 81, *81*, 82, *82*, 600

nephron units, *595*

nephrosis/nephrotic syndrome: disease of the kidneys characterized by degenerative lesions of the renal tubules and loss of protein (albumin) through the urine, 601–602

nephrotic syndrome: nephrosis

neurologist: physician specializing in the care and treatment of the nervous system, 469

neurology: the branch of medical science that deals with the nervous system

neuron: nerve cell with all its processes and extensions, such as the axon and dendrites, 24, 28–30, *29*
motor: horn cells, anterior

neuropathologist: physician specializing in neuropathology

neuropathology: the branch of medical science that deals with the study, diagnosis, and treatment of diseases of the nervous system

neurosis/psychoneurosis (*pl., neuroses*): mental disorder having no organic cause and less severe than psychosis

neurosurgeon: physician specializing in surgery of the nervous system

neurosurgery: the branch of medical science that deals with the treatment of disease of the nervous system by means of surgery
in Parkinson's disease, 475

neurosyphilis: syphilis of the brain and spinal cord, 607–608

neurotic: 1. one who has a neurosis. 2. of or relating to neurosis.

neurotoxic: 1. (of certain poisonous snakes) transmitting venom that directly affects the nervous system and brain of the toxified animal, 691. Compare *hemotoxic*. 2. causing destruction or damage to nerve tissue.

neutrophil/granulocyte/polymorphonuclear leukocyte: granular leukocyte than than be stained with dyes that are neither acid nor alkaline (i.e., neutral), 36, 492, 493

nevus: birthmark or congenital mole

newborn
appearance of, 99–100, *99*
examination of, 163

Newman, Dr. Gustave, 285

New York City
air pollution in, 360
Department of Consumer Affairs, 367

New York Harbor, dead sea area, 364

nicotine: poisonous chemical with acrid taste contained in tobacco leaves, 136, 183–184

Niehans, Dr. Paul, 287

night, and eyesight, 72

nipples
care of, in breast feeding, 103
inverted, 406

nit: the egg of a louse or other parasitic insect, 385–386

nitrates, 367

nitrites, 367

nitrogen, in amino acids, 296

nitrogen dioxide: suffocating gas that is poisonous when inhaled, 559

nitrogen oxides, 359, 360

nitrogen salts, 82

nitroglycerin: colorless or pale yellow oily liquid used to treat angina pectoris, 504, 693

nitrosamines in fish, 367

nitrous oxide in childbirth, 161

nocturia: frequent urination during the night, 595

nocturnal emission/wet dream, 126, 240

node: 1. swelling or enlargement, as in an arthritic joint, or a firm, flattened tumor on a bone or tendon. 2. any knoblike part, as a lymph gland.

nodule: little node, 200

noise
defined, 369
protection against, 373–375
rising levels of, 373

noise pollution, 79, *354, 355, 368,* 369–375, *369, 370, 371, 372, 373, 374, 375*

Noludar: methprylon

noodles, nutrients in, 317

norepinephrine: hormone manufactured by the adrenal medulla that affects heart action and sympathetic nerve impulses

North American Association of Alcoholism Programs, 643

nose, 71, 72, 79–80
cleansing of, 89
cosmetic surgery on: rhinoplasty
as filter system, 63
reshaping of: rhinoplasty

nosebleed, 427

"nose brain": rhinencephalon

no-take: absence of any reaction to a vaccination, indicating that the person vaccinated has not developed an immunity and should be revaccinated

nucleus of cell, *29*

nuisance ailments, 409

numbness, 30
and demyelination, 29

nursery schools, 258–259, *259, 260*
and food, *352, 353*

nursing care
in nursing home, 213
See also *home nursing.*

nursing homes, 212–215
costs, 214–215
selection of, *213, 214*

nursing services, home care, 210–211

nutrient: substance that gives nourishment

nutrients
distributed by blood, 34
reconstituting, 53
tables of, 298–319

nutrition: all of the processes by which food is consumed, digested, absorbed, and assimilated by the body, 128–129
basic requirements, 295–299
in disease prevention, 441
and hair, 387

nutritional deficiencies, correction of, 320

nutritionist: specialist in the study of nutrition

nuts, nutrients in, 305

O

oatmeal, nutrients in, 316

obesity: excessive accumulation of body fat, 91, 330–332
and diabetes, 576, 583
and disease, 441
and exercise, 168
and health, 325–326

and hiatus hernia, 525
pinch test for, 186, 321–322, *322*
in pregnancy, 147
psychological consequences, 326–327

ob-gyn specialist: physician trained as an obstetrician and gynecologist, 144

objective: (of symptoms) of a kind that can be observed or measured by the examining physician through diagnostic techniques. Compare *subjective*.

obstetrician: physician specializing in obstetrics, often a gynecologist as well, 84, 144

obstetrics: the branch of medical science dealing with pregnancy and childbirth

obstructions
intestinal, 527
from round worms, 536
and strangulated hernia, 532
in windpipe, 676, *676*

obstructive-airway disease: condition characterized by the presence of chronic bronchitis and pulmonary emphysema, and involving damage to lung tissue and the bronchi, 560

obturator: special device inserted into a cleft palate to close it against the flow of air, 404

occipital: of or relating to the lower back part of the skull (occiput)

occipital lobe: the rear portion of each cerebral hemisphere which receives messages from the optic nerve, 26

occlusion: 1. the act of closing or shutting off so as to block a passage, as a blood vessel. 2. the manner of being shut, as the teeth of the upper and lower jaws.
study of, 94

occupational disease: disease(s), occupational

occupational hazard, noise as, 369
See also *disease(s), occupational.*

ocular: of or relating to the eye

oculist: ophthalmologist

odors, body, 93

Oedipal complex: repressed sexual attachment of son to mother, analogous to the Electra complex involving the daughter and father, 228

oil fires, 679

oil (fuel), low-sulfur, 358

oil glands: glands, sebaceous

oils
for dry skin, 380
nutrients in, 318

oil well, ruptured, *362*

ointment, lubricating, 393

okra, nutrients in, 307

Older Volunteers in the Peace Corps, 281

olfaction: the act, sense, or process of smelling

olfactory: pertaining to the sense of smell or the capacity to smell

olfactory cells, 45, 79

olfactory nerve: nerve, olfactory

oliguria: decreased production of urine

oncologist: physician specializing in the diagnosis and treatment of tumors oncology: the branch of medical science concerned with the study of tumors

onions, nutrients in, 307

open fracture: compound fracture

ophthalmologist/oculist: physician specializing in the care and treatment of the eyes

ophthalmology: the branch of medical science dealing with the structure, function, and diseases of the eye

ophthalmoscope: optical instrument for examining the interior of the eye

opiate: drug derived from opium, as morphine
  synthetic, 660

opium: narcotic drug obtained from the opium poppy from which morphine, codeine, heroin, and other drugs are derived, 657–658
  derivatives, 139, *657*
  poppy, *657*

oral cancer, 625

oral cavity, *47*, 522–524

oral health in later years, 190

oral irrigating devices, 98

oral surgeon/dental surgeon: dentist who specializes in oral surgery, *466*

oral surgery: the diagnosis and surgical treatment of diseases, injuries, and defects of the mouth and jaw

orange juice, nutrients in, 311

oranges, nutrients in, 311

orchitis: inflammation of the testicles, 116

organic foods: foods grown with the use of organic fertilizers only, such as compost or animal (not human) manure, and without the use of pesticides or herbicides, 346–347, 349

organisms
  arthritic-causing, 451–452
  as cause of disease, 439

organ of Corti: the true center of hearing within the cochlea of the inner ear, a complex spiral structure of hair cells, 77, 371

organs, vital, location in axial skeleton, 4

orgasm: the climax of the sexual act, normally marked by the male's ejaculation of semen and by relaxation of tension of both male and female, 249

orthodontia: orthodontics

orthodontics/orthodontia: the care and treatment of irregularities and faulty positions of the teeth, including the fitting of braces, 135–136

orthodontist: dentist specializing in orthodontics, 136

orthopedics: the branch of surgery dealing with the treatment and correction of deformities, injuries, and diseases of the skeletal system and its associated structures, as muscles and joints

orthopedic surgeon: orthopedist

orthopedist/orthopedic surgeon/orthopod: surgeon specializing in orthopedics, 458

orthopod: orthopedist

oscilloscope: instrument for visibly representing electrical activity on a fluorescent screen, 480
  in electromyography, 480

osseous: osteal

ossicle: one of the three small connecting bones of the middle ear, the hammer (or malleus), the anvil (or incus), and the stirrup (or stapes), that transmit sound from the eardrum to the cochlea, 3, 76, *77*

ossification: conversion into bone

ossify: to convert or be converted into bone

osteal/osseous: of or relating to bone

osteitis deformans: Paget's disease

osteoarthritis: chronic degenerative disease that affects the joints, 205, 450, 454, *456*
  in hip, 457

osteogenesis: formation and growth of bones
  imperfecta: condition in which bones are abnormally brittle and liable to fracture due to a deficiency of calcium 448

osteomyelitis: inflammation of the bone tissue or marrow, 11, 448–449
  spinal, 463

osteopath: physician trained in osteopathy

osteopathy: system of healing based on a theory that most diseases are caused by structural abnormalities that may best be corrected by manipulation

osteophyte(s): abnormal bony outgrowth
  in spinal arthritis, 461

osteoporosis: reduction in bone mass and increase in interior space, porosity, and fragility of bone, 448

otitis media: inflammation of the middle ear
  nonsuppurative: inflammation of the middle ear resulting from a blocked Eustachian tube and fluid collection in the middle ear, causing hearing damage, 591

otolaryngologist: physician specializing in the diagnosis and treatment of the ear, nose, and throat

otolaryngology: the branch of medicine dealing with the study and diseases of the ear, nose, and throat

otologist: one who specializes in the ear and its diseases, 201

otology: the branch of medical science dealing with the functions and diseases of the ear

otoplasty: surgical technique to correct protruding or overlarge ears or to build up or replace a missing ear, 408

otosclerosis: ear disorder resulting in hearing loss caused by the formation of spongy bone in the middle ear, 201, 591

otoscope: instrument used for examining the interior of the ear, *591*

outer ear: the external, fleshy part of the ear, including the auditory canal leading to the eardrum (tympanic membrane), 76
  spatial relationships of, *77*

ova: plural of *ovum*

ovarian: of or relating to the ovaries

ovarian dysgenesis: defective development of ovaries, 480

ovaries (*sing., ovary*): pair of female reproductive glands (gonads) that produce eggs (ova) and female sex hormones, *64*, 70, 243, *243*, *244*, *567*
  function of, *571*
  and hormone deficiencies, 154
  hyperfunction of, 572
  hypofunction, 571–572

overeating, 341
  emotional causes, 417

overweight, 91, 322–327, 416–417
  and back problems, 207
  and diabetes, 207
  in middle age, 186–187
  in pregnancy, 147
  prevention of, 327

oviduct, *148*

ovoid: egg-shaped

ovulation: the discharge of a mature egg cell (ovum) from the ovaries, occurring about once every 28 days at about the middle of the menstrual cycle, 70, 243, 244, 572
  and "the pill," 250
  and rhythm method, 253
  timing of, 142–143, 144

ovum/egg cell (*pl., ova*): female reproductive cell or gamete from which an embryo might develop if fertilized, 124, 243, *244*, *571*

oxygen
  blood as carrier of, 34
  and blood in lungs, 40
  in heart attack, *692*, 693
  and hemoglobin, 35
  necessity of, 539
  and red blood cells, 35
  requirements, 62–63
  transfer of, from blood to cell, 58
  in treatment of emphysema, 562

oxygen molecules, 57

oxygen starvation, 34

oxytocin: hormone secreted by the pituitary gland to help the muscles of the uterus contract during labor, 66, *66*, 162, 164

ozone: blue gas with a pungent odor that can be formed by the passage of electricity through the air, 360, 559

P

pacemaker
  artificial: electrically activated, battery- or nuclear-powered device used to stimulate normal heartbeat if the natural cardiac pacemaker fails to function, 41, *520*, 521, *521*
  cardiac: object or substance in the heart that regulates contraction of the heart muscle, or heartbeat, 520. See also *sinus node*.
  natural cardiac, 41
  nuclear, *521*

paddle ball, *171*

Paget's disease: 1. (osteitis deformans) chronic disease characterized by the softening and enlargement of the bones and usu. the bowing of the long, weight-bearing bones,

448. 2. cancerous disease of the breast marked by the inflammation of the areola and nipple.

pain(s), 441–442
  in bones, 11
  chest: chest pain
  in feet, 208
  in joints, 11
  labor, 159–162
  muscle, 16, 483
  pelvic, 252
  sacroiliac, 460
  thigh and groin, 457
  of unknown cause, 30
pain receptors, *29*, 71
pain threshold in noise pollution, 370
palate: the roof of the mouth
  hard: the bony part of the roof of the mouth, 47, *47*, 119
  soft/velum: the soft, muscular tissue at the rear of the roof of the mouth, *44*, 47, *47*, *60*
palpation: diagnostic procedure of feeling, pressing, or manipulating the body, 442–443
palpitation: rapid or fluttering heartbeat
palsy/paralysis: *Bell's palsy, cerebral palsy*
PAN: peroxyacl nitrate
panaceas and hangover, 186
pancakes, nutrients in, 316
pancreas: large gland situated behind the stomach and containing the islets of Langerhans that produce insulin and glucagon, and secreting pancreatic juice via small ducts to the duodenum, *44*, *49*, 55, 69, 572
  inflammation of, 116
pancreatic juice: secretion of the pancreas containing digestive enzymes, 51
pandemic: epidemic occurring over a very large area or worldwide, 437, 543
panic, acute marihuana, 139
Papanicolaou, Dr. George N.: developer of a test, called the *Pap smear* or *Pap test*, for detecting cancer of the cervix, 622
Papanicolaou smear: Pap smear
Papaver somniferum, 657
papillae (*sing., papilla*): tiny, nipple-shaped projections that cover the inner layer (dermis) of the skin and the surface of the tongue, 19–20, *20*
  renal, *81*, *595*
  of tongue, 46
papillary tumor: 1. papilloma. 2. malignant tumor of the bladder, so called because it is nipplelike in shape (Latin *papilla* means nipple).
papilloma/papillary tumor: benign tumor of the papillae of the skin, as a wart or corn
Pap smear/Papanicolaou smear/Pap test: method of early detection of cervical cancer consisting of painless removal of cervical cell samples, which are stained and examined, 181–182, *181*, 609, 622
Pap test: Pap smear
papule: pimple
paraldehyde for hangover, 186
paralysis
  and demyelination, 29

facial, 470
  infantile: poliomyelitis
  in poliomyelitis, 476
  in sickle-cell anemia, 490
  in spinal fracture, 463, 464
  in spinal osteomyelitis, 463
  in spinal tuberculosis, 462
  in spinal tumor, 463
  in stroke, 498
  from subdural hematoma, 465
paralysis agitans: Parkinson's disease
paranasal sinus: air cavity in one of the cranial bones communicating with the nostrils, 63
paraplegia: paralysis of the lower half of the body
parasite(s): animal or plant that lives in or on another organism (called the host), at whose expense it obtains nourishment, 439
  intestinal, 533–536
parasympathetic nervous system: the part of the autonomic nervous system that controls such involuntary actions as the constriction of pupils, dilation of blood vessels and salivary glands, and slowing of heartbeat, 28, *28*. Compare *sympathetic nervous system*.
parathormone, 70
parathyroid glands: four small endocrine glands near or embedded within the thyroid gland, usu. two per side, that regulate blood calcium and phosphorus levels, 70, 566, *567*, 573
parent(s)
  death of, *272*
  division of labor, 256–257
  of newlyweds, 246
  overprotective, 237
  and prevention of obesity, 327
  responsibilities, 260
  and sex education, 242
  single, 273
parental influence, and obesity, 324–325
parent-child relationships, 228–230
parenthood, 246–260
  decision for, 141
  guidelines for, 101–102
Parents Without Partners, Inc., 273
paresis: 1. partial paralysis. 2. general paralysis (*general paresis*) caused by degeneration of the brain as a result of syphilis.
parkinsonism: Parkinson's disease
Parkinson's disease/paralysis agitans/parkinsonism: chronic, progressive nervous disease characterized by muscle tremor when at rest, stiffness, and a rigid facial expression, 30, 474–475
parotid gland: either of two large salivary glands located below and in front of the ear, 45, 116
  inflammation of, 524
paroxysm: sudden onset of acute symptoms, as an attack or convulsions
parrot fever: psittacosis
particulate matter: fine particles in smoke that are dispersed by the wind and fall back to earth, 559
Pasteur, Louis, *436*
pasteurization, *436*

patch test: skin test for determining hypersensitivity by applying small pads of possibly allergy-producing substances to the skin's surface and hair dye, 385
patchy baldness: alopecia areata
patella: the kneecap
patent medicines, morphine in, 658
pathogen: disease-causing bacterium or microorganism, 440, *441*
pathogenic: disease-causing
pathologic: caused by or relating to disease
pathologic fracture: fracture that occurs spontaneously, as because of preexisting disease, without external cause
pathologist: physician or expert specializing in pathology
pathology: the branch of medical science dealing with the causes, nature, and effects of diseases, esp. disease-induced changes in organs, tissues, and body chemistry
patient-doctor relationships, 89, 293
Peace Corps, 281
peaches, nutrients in, 312
peanut butter, nutrients in, 305
pears, nutrients in, 312
peas, nutrients in, 305, 307
pedal: of or relating to the foot
pediatric dentist: dentist specializing in the care and treatment of the teeth of children
pediatrician: physician specializing in the care and treatment of children
pediatrics: the branch of medicine dealing with the care and treatment of children and their diseases
peer relationships in nursery schools, 258–259
Peking Medical College, 705
Peking Review, 702
pellagra: disease caused by a vitamin deficiency and characterized by gastric disturbance, skin eruptions, and nervous symptoms, 317
pelvic area, diagnosis of disorders, 457
pelvic girdle: the part of the human skeleton to which the lower limbs are attached, 4, 8
pelvis: 1. the part of the skeleton that forms a bony girdle or basin joining the lower limbs to the body, and consisting of the two hip bones and the sacrum. 2. the central area of the kidney from which urine drains into the ureter, 83.
  injury to, 458
penicillin: powerful antibacterial substance found in a mold fungus and prepared in several forms for the treatment of a wide variety of infections, *439*
  in dental surgery, 518
  in glomerulonephritis, 601
  in pneumonia, 544
  in scarlet fever, 117
  in syphilis, 608
penis: tubular male organ of sexual intercourse and excretion of urine, located at the front of the pelvis, 242
Pentothal: thiopental
peppers, nutrients in, 307
pep pills (*slang*): amphetamines

pepsin: enzyme secreted by the gastric juices of the stomach, 50

peptic ulcer: ulcer of the mucous membrane of the stomach (gastric ulcer) or small intestine (duodenal ulcer) caused by the action of acid juices, 529–530

perception as function of skin, 18

percussion: diagnostic procedure of striking or tapping the body with instruments or with the fingers, 443

pericardium: the membrane that surrounds and protects the heart, 41

peridental: periodontal

perimeter: device for determining peripheral vision

periodontal/peridental: situated around a tooth

periodontal disease/gum disease/pyorrhea, 94, 95, 176, 190, 428, 429, 467

periodontal membrane: membrane, periodontal

periodontia: periodontics

periodontics/periodontia: the branch of dentistry dealing with the diagnosis and treatment of periodontal (gum) diseases

periodontist: dentist who specializes in periodontics

periosteum: the tough, fibrous membrane that surrounds and nourishes bones, 10, 10, 14

peripheral nervous system: the nerves and ganglia outside the brain and spinal cord, 28

peristalsis: wavelike muscular contractions of the alimentary canal that move the contents along in the processes of digestion and excretion, 48, 522

peristaltic wave: the alternate contraction and relaxation of muscles in the alimentary canal in peristalsis, 48

peritoneoscopy: technique for examining the female reproductive organs within the abdominal cavity, 146

peritoneum: the serous membrane that lines the abdominal cavity enclosing the abdominal organs, 56

peritonitis: inflammation of the lining (peritoneum) of the abdominal cavity, 533

peroxyacl nitrate/PAN, 360

personality, area in brain, 26

perspiration: sweat

pertussis: whooping cough

pessary: any device worn within the vagina, as to remedy a displaced uterus or to prevent conception

pesticide residues, 346, 368–369

pesticides, 346

petit mal: minor epileptic seizure, with very brief loss of consciousness, 473–474, 695. Compare grand mal.

pets, allergic reaction to, 553

Peyer's patches: oval areas of lymphoid tissue in the intestine that manufacture lymphocytes, 38

peyote: the mescal cactus of Mexico or the powerful hallucinogenic drug obtained from its dried upper part (called buttons), 139, 662, 662

phalanges (sing., phalanx): the bones of the fingers or toes, 3, 9

pharmacist: one skilled in the compounding and dispensing of medicines

pharmacologist: expert in pharmacology

pharmacology: the science of the action of medicines, their nature, preparation, administration, and effects

pharyngitis: inflammation of the pharynx, commonly called a sore throat, 114, 411, 600

pharynx: the part of the alimentary canal between the palate and the esophagus, serving as a passage for air and food, 44, 47–48, 47, 49, 60

phenformin/DBI, 580

phenmetrazine/Preludin, 655

phenol: carbolic acid

phenylketonuria/PKU: inherited metabolic disorder that can cause mental retardation if not treated by a special diet soon after birth, 153

Phisoderm, 446

Phisohex, 446

phlebitis: inflammation of the inner membrane of a vein, 494–495

phlegm: viscid, stringy mucus secreted in abnormally large amounts, as in the air passages, 542

phlegmatic temperament, 54

phonocardiogram: graph recording the sounds produced by the heart, used to evaluate heart murmurs and other abnormal sounds

phosphates as pollutants, 363, 364

phosphorus in teen-age diet, 129–130

physical dependence: accommodation of the body to continued use of a drug, such that withdrawing the drug causes pronounced physical reactions (withdrawal symptoms), 140

physical examination, 88
for parenthood, 99

physical medicine: branch of medicine utilizing physical procedures, such as heat, cold, massage, or mechanical devices, to diagnose disease or treat disabled patients

physical therapist: specialist in physical therapy

physical therapy/physiotherapy: the treatment of disability, injury, or disease by external physical means, such as heat, massage, planned exercises, electricity, or mechanical devices, to restore function or aid rehabilitation
for arthritis, 450, 451
for cerebral palsy, 470, 471
for muscular dystrophy, 482
for poliomyelitis, 477
for stroke, 498, 499

physician(s): 1. any authorized practitioner of medicine. 2. one trained in medicine, as distinguished from surgery.
emergency services, 668, 669
in nursing homes, 213

physician-patient relationship, 89, 293

physiotherapy: physical therapy

pia mater: the delicate, vascular, innermost membrane of the three membranes that envelop the brain and spinal cord

picnicking, 274

piebald skin: vitiligo

pies, nutrients in, 316

pigment: substance that imparts coloring to tissue, 377
disorders, 400
in feces, 53
loss of, 200
in skin, 378–379

piles: hemorrhoids

"pill, the": contraceptives, oral

pill-popping, 654

pills
consumption of, 649
dependence on, 167
reducing, 332

pimple(s), 128, 398–399

pinch test: obesity, pinch test for

pineal body: pineal gland

pineal gland/pineal body: small, cone-shaped body of rudimentary glandular structure located at the base of the brain and having no known function, 70–71

pinkeye: acute, contagious conjunctivitis, marked by redness of the eyeball, 114, 433, 588

pins, for healing fractures, 454, 455, 458

pinworm: parasitic worm of the lower intestines and rectum, esp. of children, causing intense itching in the anal area, 535

pituitary body: pituitary gland

pituitary gland/hypophysis cerebri/pituitary body: small endocrine gland situated at the base of the brain, consisting of anterior and posterior lobes whose hormonal secretions stimulate the production of hormones in other glands and regulate vital body functions such as growth and metabolism, 26, 64, 65, 66, 123, 566, 567
anterior/hypophysis, 566–568
hypofunctioning, 567
posterior, 572–573

PKU: phenylketonuria

placebo: any harmless substance given to humor a patient or as a test in controlled experiments on the effects of drugs

placenta: the vascular structure in pregnant women that unites the fetus with the uterus, and through which the fetus is nourished via the umbilical cord, usu. expelled naturally immediately following birth (when it is called the afterbirth), 64
and carbohydrates, 155
development of, 153
expulsion of, 163

Placidyl: ethchlorvynol

plantar warts: warts on the soles of the feet, caused by a virus, 398

plaque: mucus containing bacteria that collects on teeth, 95, 96, 97, 98, 135, 190

plasma: the clear fluid portion of the blood, 35, 484

plasma proteins, 485

plastic surgeon: physician specializing in plastic or cosmetic surgery

plastic surgery: surgery that deals with the restoration or healing of lost, injured, or deformed parts of the body, mainly by the transfer of

colon (sigmoid) with the aid of a sigmoidoscope, 620

prodrome: symptom resembling a premonition that signals the onset of a disease or of an epileptic seizure, 473

profibrinolysin: the inactive precursor of fibrinolysin, an agent in the process of dissolving blood clots, 485

profile, health, 167

progesterone: hormone of the ovary that prepares the uterus for receiving the fertilized ovum, 67, 70, 125, 571, 572

prognathism: the condition of having a protruding jaw, esp. the lower, *405*

prognosis: prediction made by a doctor as to the probable course of a disease, 437

Prohibition era, 628, 639

prolactin: lactogenic hormone

prolapsed: slipped or moved from the usual place

proof: strength of alcohol in an alcoholic beverage, indicated by a proof number equal to twice the percentage of alcohol by volume (100 proof = 50% alcohol), 631

propanolol: drug that causes blood vessels to dilate, used in the treatment of angina pectoris, 504

prophylactic: tending to ward off or prevent, as disease or conception

prophylactic therapy in tuberculosis, 549

prophylaxis: treatment intended to prevent disease, as the cleaning of teeth
dental, 94

prostate gland: partly muscular gland in males at the base of the bladder around the urethra that releases a fluid to convey spermatozoa, 67, 85, 126, *242*, 243, 604–605
in aging, 208–209
cancer of, 605
enlarged, 208
benign: enlargement of the prostate gland resulting in difficulty in voiding and retention of urine in the bladder, 604
inflammation of: prostatitis

prostate trouble, 182

prostatic urethra/posterior urethra: the part of the male urethra that passes across the prostate gland

prostatitis: inflammation of the prostate gland, characterized by painful and excessive urination, 435
acute: severe, relatively uncommon form of prostatitis, marked by painful and excessive urination, high fever, and a discharge of pus from the penis

prosthesis (*pl., prostheses*)/prosthetic device: artificial substitute for a missing or amputated part, as an arm or leg, 456
aortic valve, *502, 503*

prosthetic device: prosthesis

protection as function of skin, 18, 93

protein(s): any of a class of highly complex organic compounds, composed principally of amino acids, that occur in all living things and form an essential part of animal food requirements
blood-clotting, 484
body, in emergency situation, 68
breakdown of, 50
defined, 296
and liver, 53
in pregnancy, 317
requirements, 295–296
sources of, *297*
in urine, 443

protein deprivation, 320

proteinuria: excretion of protein through the urine
in pregnancy, 149

prothrombin: the inactive precursor of thrombin, an agent in the process of forming blood clots, 485

protozoa (*sing., protozoon*): microscopic animal organisms that exist in countless numbers, including one-celled organisms and parasitic forms that cause malaria, sleeping sickness, and other diseases

proximal: relatively near the center of the body, or near a point considered as central. Compare *distal.*

proximal muscles: those muscles closest to the trunk of the body, such as the shoulder-arm and hip-thigh muscles

prune juice, nutrients in, 312

prunes, nutrients in, 312

pruritus: localized or general itching, 393
anal: intense itching in the area of the anus, 393, 431

pseudohypertrophic muscular dystrophy/Duchenne's muscular dystrophy: disease characterized by the enlargement and apparent overdevelopment (hypertrophy) of certain muscles, esp. of the shoulder girdle, which subsequently atrophy, *480*

psilocin, 662

Psilocybe mexicana, 662

psilocybin: derivative of the mushroom *Psilocybe mexicana,* which produces hallucinations in the user, 662

psittacosis/parrot fever: infectious disease of parrots and other birds that can be transmitted to humans and cause symptoms like those of influenza

psoriasis: a noncontagious chronic condition of the skin, marked by bright red patches covered by silvery scales, 399–400, 437

psychedelic drugs, 660

psychiatrist: physician specializing in psychiatry, 219, 220–221, *220*, 248
in menopause problems, 265

psychiatry: the branch of medicine that treats disorders of the mind (or psyche), including psychoses and neuroses

psychic determinism, 219

psychoanalysis: system of psychotherapy originated by Sigmund Freud for treating emotional disorders by bringing to the attention of the conscious mind the repressed conflicts of the unconscious, 218–219, *218*

psychoanalyst, 221

psychological block
and underweight, 333
and weight reduction, 328

psychological dependence: emotional desire or need to continue using a drug

psychologist: specialist in psychology, 221, 248

psychology: the science dealing with the mind, mental phenomena, consciousness, and behavior

psychomimetic: having properties capable of producing changes in behavior that mimic psychoses

psychomotor: having to do with muscular movements resulting from mental processes

psychomotor convulsion/temporal lobe convulsion: epileptic convulsion characterized by compulsive and often repetitious behavior of which the patient later has no memory, 473

psychoneurosis: neurosis

psychosis (*pl., psychoses*): severe mental disorder often involving disorganization of the total personality, with or without organic disease
and LSD, 661
and tranquilizers, 657

psychosomatic: pertaining to the effects of the emotions on body processes, esp. with respect to initiating or aggravating disease

psychotherapist: specialist in psychotherapy, 221

psychotherapy: the treatment of emotional and mental disorders by psychological methods, such as psychoanalysis, 221
in alcoholism, 645
group, for heroin addicts, 660

ptomaine: substance derived from decomposing or putrefying animal or vegetable protein, rarely the cause of food poisoning, which is usu. caused by bacteria such as Salmonella

ptosis: drooping of the upper eyelid, 484

ptyalin: enzyme in saliva that begins the chemical breakdown of starch, 45

puberty: period during which a person reaches sexual maturity and becomes functionally capable of reproduction, 70, 566
delayed, 124
growth pattern in, *122*
precocious: early menarche (first occurrence of menstruation), before the age of eight or nine, 123

puberty rites, 235

pubic: in the region of the lower abdomen

pubic hair, first appearance of, 113

pubis: the lower anterior part of the hip bone, *7, 8*

public housing, 290

pulmonary: of or relating to the lungs

pulmonary artery: artery, pulmonary

pulmonary emphysema: emphysema of the lungs. See *emphysema.*

pulmonary tree, branches of, *57*

pulmonary tuberculosis: *tuberculosis*

auricle: atrium
autonomic nervous system
 and breathing, 59
 and carbon dioxide level, 58
blood, oxygen-poor, 57
brain, breathing center of, 59
breath cycle, 62
breathing, frequency of, 62
bronchi, 60, 61
bronchial tubes, 61
bronchioles, 60, 61
capillaries, 57
carbon dioxide, 57
 need for, 58–59
 and oxygen exchange, 57
cartilage rings, 60
cilia, 63
description of, 56–63
diaphragm, 59
diseases of, 539–554
 and air pollution, 355, 356
 allergic, 550–554
 lung disease, 555–565
ducts, alveolar, 61
epiglottis, 60
esophagus, 60
expiration, 59
filter system, beyond the nose,
 63
force breathing, 59
gaseous exchange, 57, 61, 62
"guard hairs": vibrissae
hay fever, 63
heart, interaction with lungs, 56
hemoglobin, 57
infections, 410–412
inspiration, 59
larynx, 60
lung(s), 59, 61–62
 collapsed, 61
 diseases of, 555–565
 interaction with heart, 56
 lobes of, 61
 removal of, 61–62
 segments of, 61
 structure of, 61
 surface area, 62
 tissue, 62
lung cancer, 61, 137, 183, 356, 560,
 562, 612–614
medulla, function in breathing, 59
membranes, mucus-secreting, 63
 pleural, 61
minor ailments in, 431–433
moisture, essential role of, 57
mouth breathing, 63
muscles, breathing, 59
nasal cavity, 63
nose, filter system, 63
oxygen, requirements, 62–63
 transfer of, from blood to cell,
 58
oxygen molecules, 57
papillae of tongue, 46
pharynx, 60
pleura, 61
pleural cavity, 61
pleurisy, 61
pneumothorax, 61
 artificial, 61
pollution control in, 62
pulmonary tree, branches of, 57
respiration, one-cell level, 57–58
respiratory passages, upper, and
 common cold, 541
rib cage, 59

septum, 56
sinuses, paranasal, 63
spinal column and diaphragm, 59
trachea, 59–60, 432, 676–677
tuberculosis, 61
turbinates, 63
veins, pulmonary, 57
ventricle
 left, 57
 right, 56
vibrissae/"guard hairs," 63
voice, 60

responsibility, and adulthood, 237
rest, 92–93
 for arthritis, 206
rest-activity pattern in diabetes, 577
restorations, tooth, replacement of,
 175–176
resuscitation: mouth-to-mouth respiration
reticulum: network of cells or cellular
 tissue
retina: the inner membrane at the
 back of the eyeball, containing
 light-sensitive rods and cones which
 receive the optical image, 72, 73
 detached, 586–587
 in hypertension, 513
 in myopic eye, 584
retinoscope: special device for examining the retina
Retired Senior Volunteer Program,
 281
retirement, challenges of, 189
retirement housing, requirements of,
 290
rhesus factor: Rh factor
rheumatic fever: acute infectious disease chiefly affecting children and
 young adults, characterized by
 painful inflammation around the
 joints, intermittent fever, and inflammation of the pericardium and
 valves of the heart, 117
 and delayed puberty, 124
 and heart disease, 500, 502, 515–518
 symptoms, 515
 treatment of, 517
rheumatic heart disease: impairment
 of heart function as a result of
 rheumatic fever, 500
rheumatism: painful inflammation
 and stiffness of muscles, joints, or
 connective tissue
rheumatoid arthritis: chronic disease
 characterized by swelling and inflammation of one or more joints,
 often resulting in stiffness and
 eventual impairment of mobility,
 205, 449, 449
 juvenile, 450
rheumatoid spondylitis, 459
rheumatologist: physician specializing in rheumatology
rheumatology: subspecialty of internal medicine concerned with the
 study, diagnosis, and treatment of
 rheumatism and other diseases of
 the joints and muscles
Rh factor: protein present in the
 blood of most people (called Rh-
 positive) and absent from others
 (called Rh-negative). Under certain conditions the blood of a pregnant Rh-negative woman may be

incompatible with the blood of her
 fetus, 37, 152, 491–492
rhinencephalon/"nose brain": the
 part of the brain controlling the
 sense of smell, 80
rhinitis: inflammation of the mucous
 membranes of the nose
 allergic/hay fever: 63, 550, 551–552,
 554
rhinoplasty: plastic surgery of the
 nose, 178, 404, 404
Rh-negative: Rh factor
Rh-positive: Rh factor
rhythm method: birth control method whereby sexual intercourse is
 avoided during the period of ovulation in the menstrual cycle, 253–254
rhytidoplasty/face lift/facial plasty:
 plastic surgery to eliminate facial
 wrinkles, 178, 406–407, 407
rib(s), 3
 congenital absence of, 464
 extra neck, 464
 floating, 6
 number of, 4
rib cage: thoracic cage
riboflavin/vitamin B_2: member of
 the vitamin B complex, found in
 milk, green leafy vegetables, eggs
 and meats
rice
 brown, 347
 nutrients in, 317
rickets: early childhood disease characterized by softening of bones and
 consequent deformity, caused by
 deficiency of vitamin D, 318, 449
rickettsiae (sing., rickettsia): parasitic microorganisms transmitted to
 humans by the bites of infected
 ticks, lice, and fleas, and causing
 Rocky Mountain spotted fever,
 Q fever, rickettsial pox, and typhus,
 440
rickettsial: caused by or pertaining to
 rickettsiae
rickettsial disease: any of the diseases, as typhus or Rocky Mountain spotted fever, caused by rickettsiae
rickettsial pox: infectious disease
 (rickettsial disease) transmitted by
 mites which infest mice, and characterized by fever, chills, rash,
 headache, and backache, 440
ringworm/tinea: contagious fungus
 disease of the skin, hair, or nails
 marked by ring-shaped, scaly, reddish patches of skin, 395, 439
riser: floor-to-ceiling steam pipe
Ritalin: methylphenidate
rock music, and hearing loss, 375
Rocky Mountain spotted fever: infectious disease (rickettsial disease)
 transmitted by the bite of certain
 ticks and characterized by fever,
 chills, rash, headache, and muscular
 pain, 440
rod: one of many rod-shaped bodies
 in the retina of the eye, sensitive to
 faint light and peripheral objects
 and movements, 72. Compare cone.
Roentgen, Wilhelm, 443
roentgenogram: X-ray photograph
roentgenologist: physician specializing in the diagnosis and treatment

of diseases with the application of X rays

roentgenology: the branch of medical science dealing with the properties and effects of X rays

rolls, nutrients in, 317

root canal: the passageway of nerves and blood vessels in the root of a tooth leading into the pulp, 4, *5*

root canal treatment, 176

root of tooth, *5*

Rose Water Ointment, USP XVI, 201

roughage: food material containing a high percentage of indigestible constituents

roundworm/ascaris: parasitic nematode worm, as the hookworm and pinworm, whose eggs hatch in the small intestines, 536

rowing, 170

rubber cement, as poison, 687

rubber pants, and infants, 106

rubella/German measles: contagious viral disease benign in children but linked to birth defects of children born of women infected in early pregnancy, 114–115, *115*, 445, 518

and deafness, 593

and hearing defects, *593*

vaccine, *88, 151*

in pregnancy, 151

rubeola: measles

Rubin, Dr. Isadore, 285

Rubin's test: tubal insufflation

rum, 634

running, 198

Rupp, Dr. Ralph R., 374

rupture: 1. any breaking apart, as of a blood vessel. 2. hernia.

rust removers, as poison, 688

S

Sabin vaccine: live polio vaccine taken orally to immunize against polio, 104, 109, 118

saccule, *78*

sacroiliac: pertaining to the sacrum or the ilium, or to the .places on either side of the lower back where they are joined

sacroiliac joints, 460

sacroiliac point, 8

sacrum: bone in the lower spine formed by the fusing of five vertebrae, constituting the rear part of the pelvis, 7, 8

saddle block: form of anesthesia used esp. for childbirth, in which the patient is injected in the lower spinal cord while in a sitting position, 161

safety, in nursing homes, 214

safety glass: glass strengthened by any of various methods to reduce the likelihood of the glass shattering upon impact

Saf-T-Coil, *252*

St. John's University, marihuana research, 665

St. Vitus's dance: chorea

sake, 633

salad dressings, nutrients in, 318

salicylic acid in collodion, for removal of corns, 423

saliva: fluid secreted by the salivary glands in the mouth that lubricates

food and contains an enzyme (ptyalin) that begins to break down starch, 45, 80, 524

lack of, 429

salivary glands: glands located in the mouth which secrete saliva, *47*

Salk, Dr. Jonas, 477

Salk vaccine: dead polio virus taken by injection to immunize against polio

Salmonella: genus of aerobic bacteria that cause food poisoning and other diseases, including typhoid fever, 440

Salmonella food poisoning, 536

Salmonella typhosa: rod-shaped bacteria that cause typhoid fever, 528

salt: sodium chloride

salting out: the injection of a saline solution into the amniotic fluid to induce labor and thus terminate a pregnancy, 155

salt tablets, 417

sanatorium rest cure, of tuberculosis, 548

sanguine disposition, *54*

sarcoma: malignant tumor that arises in the connective tissue (bones, cartilage, tendons), 611

saturated: (of fats) tending to increase the cholesterol content of the blood

sausage, nutrients, 303

scabies/the itch: contagious inflammation of the skin caused by a mite and characterized by a rash and intense itching, 396

scag (*slang*): heroin

scalp, 24

care of, 93

sebaceous glands in, 93

scapula: shoulder blade

scarlet fever: contagious disease caused by streptococci and characterized by a scarlet rash and high fever, 117

scar reduction, 408

schedule in diabetes, 581

Schlemm, canals of, 76

schoolboy (*slang*): codeine

school lunches, *314*

Schwartz, Dr. Alfred, 188

sciatica: pain along the sciatic nerve, 415, 459

sciatic nerve: nerve of the lower spine that traverses the hips and runs down the back of the thigh of each leg

sclera: the firm outer coat of the eye continuous with the cornea, visible as the white of the eye, *73, 75*

sclerose: to harden and thicken, as tissue

sclerosis: abnormal thickening and hardening of tissue, as of the lining of arteries

amyolotrophic lateral/"Lou Gehrig's disease," 29

multiple, 29, 30

scoliosis: spine, lateral curvature

scopolamine in childbirth, 161

screws inserted in fractures, *455*

scrofula: tuberculosis of the lymph nodes, esp. of the neck

scrotum: pouch that contains the testicles, 85, 126, 570

cancer of/"soot-wart," 356

scurvy: disease characterized by livid spots under the skin, swollen and bleeding gums, and prostration, caused by lack of vitamin C, 317

seasickness: *motion sickness*

seat belts and pregnancy, 150

sebaceous cyst: hard, round, movable mass contained in a sac, resulting from accumulated oil from a blocked sebaceous gland duct

sebaceous gland: gland within the dermis that secretes oil (sebum) for lubricating the skin and hair, 19, 65, 381, 382

blocking of, 398

and chapped skin, 418

of hair, 21

location of, 378

overactive, 127–128

of skin, 22

sebum: fatty lubricating substance secreted by the sebaceous glands, 22

secondary disease: disorder of a target gland caused by an excess or deficiency of a stimulating hormone supplied by the anterior pituitary gland

security, need for, 274

sedative: medicine for allaying irritation or nervousness, 421, 426, 433, 435

poisoning, 688

sedentary activity, *324*

seeing, centers for, 26

seizures: convulsions

selenium, 366

self-diagnosis, and medications, 650

self-expression

importance in middle years, 266–268

need for, 274

self-medication, 167, 186

in diabetes, 579

semen: thick, whitish fluid containing spermatozoa that is ejaculated by the male at orgasm, 126, 243

examination, 144–145

semicircular canals: three fluid-filled tubes of the inner ear that govern the sense of balance and communicate with the vestibular nerve, 78, *78, 79*

seminal vesicle: one of two small pouches on either side of the prostate gland that serve to store spermatozoa temporarily, 67, 85, 126, *242*, 243, 254

senile macula degeneration: visual defect affecting the elderly, 206

senile purpura: small hemorrhages in the skin of older people, 200

sensations, and skin, 18

sense(s)

and aging process, 188

balance, 76, 78, *592*

defined, 71–72

diseases of the eye and ear, 584–594

hearing, 72, 76, *592*

organs of, 71–80

sight, 26

smell, 26, 45, 72, 80

taste, 72, 79

touch, 18, 72

in fingertips, 20

See also *ear, eye.*

sensory area of brain, *26*

sensory messages, 469

sensory neurons, *29*

stroke/apoplexy: attack of paralysis caused by the rupture of an artery and hemorrhage into the brain, or by an obstruction of an artery, as from a blood clot, 205, 497, 512
  rehabilitation for, *498*
  therapy for, *204, 205*
study groups, 269
sty: small, inflamed swelling of a sebaceous gland on the edge of the eyelid, 433
subconscious, role of, 218–219
subcutaneous injection: an injection given in the subcutaneous tissue beneath the skin
subcutaneous tissue: layer of fatty tissue below the skin (dermis) which acts as an insulator against heat and cold and as a shock absorber against injury, 18, 19, *19, 378*
subjective: (of symptoms) of a kind that only the patient is aware of. Compare *objective*.
sublingual gland: either of a pair of salivary glands located beneath the tongue, 45
submandibular gland: submaxillary gland
submaxillary gland/submandibular gland: either of a pair of salivary glands located under each side of the lower jaw, 25
sucking, as infant need, 223
Suffolk County, Long Island, water pollution in, 363
sugar
  in blood, 443
  and tooth decay, 468
  in urine, 443, 574, 576
sugars, 45, 296
  nutrients in, 318
suggestion therapy, 398
sulfa drug: any of a group of organic compounds used in the treatment of a variety of bacterial infections
sulfonylurea: drug used to treat diabetes, 580
sulfur, in teen-age diet, 130
sulfur dioxide, *359,* 559
  and headache, 414
  as pollutant, 358
sunburn, 417
sunlight
  and aging of skin, 200, 379
  lack of, and rickets, 449
  and psoriasis, 400
sunscreens, 201
sunstroke/heatstroke: condition marked by an acutely high fever and the cessation of perspiration, caused by prolonged exposure to heat and sometimes leading to convulsions and coma, 418, 680
suntan, cause of, 20
suntan lotions, 417
superego: largely unconscious element of the personality, regarded as dominating the ego, for which it acts principally in the role of conscience and critic, 219
superior vena cava: the large vein that brings blood from the upper part of the body to the heart, *32, 40, 40*
suppository: solid, usu. cylindrical medicated preparation that lique-

fies from heat after insertion in a body cavity, as the rectum or the vagina
suppuration: the formation of pus
surgeon: physician who specializes in the diagnosis and treatment of disease by means of surgery
surgery: the branch of medicine dealing with the correction of disorders or other physical change by operation or manipulation
  and acupuncture, 702
  for appendicitis: appendectomy
  for breast cancer, 617, 619
  for cervical cancer, 623
  for colitis, 533
  for colon-rectum cancer, 620–621
  for congenital heart disease, 502
  coronary artery, 505–506
  cosmetic, 178, 402–408
  for detached retina, 587
  for diverticulosis, 531
  elective, 403
  eye, *587*
  heart, *519*
  in hemophiliacs, 487
  for hernia, 532
  for kidney tumor, 604
  and obesity, 326
  open-chest, acupuncture in, 702
  open-heart, *505,* 519-520
  for older skin conditions, 201
  oral, *94,* 468
  plastic, 402–408, 467
  prostate, 209
  for prostatic cancer, 605
  for prostatic enlargement, 604
  and rheumatic fever 517
  for ulcer, 530
surgical: of or relating to surgery
surgical diathermy: electrosurgery
suture: 1. to sew together cut or separated edges, as of a wound, to promote healing. 2. the thread, wire, gut, etc., used in this process.
suture line: line formed by the edges of the separate bones of a baby's skull, 4
swallowing, 47–48
  difficulty in, 526
sweat/perspiration, 23, 381
  evaporation of, *22*
sweat gland: any of numerous glands that secrete sweat, found almost everywhere in the skin except for the lips and a few other areas, 19, 22–23, 65, 381
  location of, 378
  in temperature regulation, 23, 377
sweet potatoes, nutrients in, 308
sweets
  and dental health, 96
  nutrients in, 318
swelling
  of feet and ankles, 204, 208
  as symptom of kidney problem, 602
swimmer, assistance to, *675*
swimming, *135,* 169, 198
  and menstruation, 124
swordfish, and mercury, 365–366
sycosis/barber's itch: bacterial infection of the hair follicles, marked by inflammation, itching, and the formation of pus-filled pimples, 397
sympathetic nervous system: the part of the autonomic nervous system that controls such involuntary ac-

tions as the dilation of pupils, constriction of blood vessels and salivary glands, and increase of heartbeat, 28, *28.* Compare *parasympathetic nervous system.*
symptom: change in one's normal feeling or condition of well-being, indicating the presence of disease, 437
  subjective, 441–442
symptomatic: having observable symptoms of a disease or condition. Compare *asymptomatic.*
Synanon: organized live-in community of drug addicts in which group psychotherapy is used to encourage rehabilitation, 660
synapse: the junction point between two neurons, across which a nerve impulse passes from the axon of one neuron to the dendrite of another, *29,* 30
syndrome: set of symptoms occurring at the same period and indicating the presence or nature of a disease
synovia/synovial fluid: viscid, transparent fluid secreted as a lubricating agent in the interior of joints and elsewhere
synovial aspiration/synovial fluid exam: laboratory analysis of synovia, withdrawn from joints by needle, in order to diagnose gout or certain forms of arthritis
synovial fluid: synovia
synovial fluid exam: synovial aspiration
syphilis: contagious venereal disease transmitted by sexual contact and congenitally to offspring of infected mothers, 440, *606,* 607–608
  and arteritis, 494
  latent, 607
  and oral lesions, 524
  secondary stage of, *606, 607*
  tertiary, 607
  untreated, 245
syringes, insulin, *578*
syrup, nutrients in, 319
systole: the instant of peak pumping action of the heart, when the ventricles contract and blood is impelled outward into the arteries, followed immediately by relaxation (diastole), 42
systolic pressure: measure of blood pressure taken when the heart is contracting, the higher of the two figures in a reading, 513

T

table tennis, 170
tachycardia: abnormally rapid heartbeat, 426–427, 490
  paroxysmal: attacks of abnormally rapid heartbeat (tachycardia) that begin and end abruptly, 427
tail, lost, of man, 4
Taiwan, water pollution in, 365
T and A operation/adenotonsillectomy, 120
tangerines, nutrients in, 313
Taoism, and acupuncture, 697
tapeworm/cestode: any of various worms with segmented, ribbonlike bodies, often of considerable length,

that are parasitic on the intestines of humans and other vertebrates, 534

eggs, *534*

tar derivatives in psoriasis, 400

target gland: any of the endocrine glands that function when stimulated by hormones secreted by the anterior pituitary, as the thyroid, adrenal cortex, testicles, or ovaries

tarsal: any of the bones of the tarsus, or ankle, *9*

tarsus: ankle

Task Force on Research Planning in Environmental Health Science, 355, 368

taste bud: one of the clusters of cells in the tongue that contain receptors for discriminating salt, sweet, sour, or bitter tastes, 45, 79

bitter, 47
number of, 46
salty, 47
sour, 47
sweet, 47

taste sensation in Bell's palsy, 471

TD/tetanus-diphtheria toxoid, 113

tea, 184

teachers and sex education, 241–242

tears, 76, *76*

teen-agers
as baby-sitters, 258
See also *age groups, teen-agers.*

teeth, 4–6, *44*
adult, *5*
artificial, 468
See also *dentures.*
of baby, 109
care of, 93–98, 468
in middle age, 175–176
in teen years, 135–136
cleaning of, *97*, 429
positions of, *46*
primary, 111
replacement, 176
role in digestion, 45–46
treatment of, 467–468
and vitamin deficiencies, 524

teething: process by which new teeth break (erupt) through the gums in infants and young children, 106, *107*

teething biscuits, 109

television
and child, 111–112
and eyestrain, 434

temperament, and body humors, *54*

temperance movement, 628

temperature
basal, 253–254
body, 447
controlled by skin, 377
and marihuana, 138
internal, maintenance of, 23
and ovulation, 144
rectal, of infant, 107
skin, in breast cancer, 617
and skin blood vessels, 22
and smoking, 137
in sunstroke, 418

temperature control as function of skin, 18

tempered glass: safety glass that has high resistance to blunt objects and breaks by crumbling into small fragments instead of shattering

temporal lobe convulsions: convulsions, psychomotor

tendinitis: inflammation of a tendon, 424

tendon: band of tough, fibrous connective tissue that binds a muscle to another part, as a bone, and by means of which muscular force can be exerted on other parts of the body, 14, *14*

inflammation of: tendinitis

tendon sheath, inflammation of: tenosynovitis

tennis, 168–169

tennis elbow: pain in the outer side of the elbow joint, usu. caused by a too vigorous twisting motion of the hand that strains a tendon or inflames a bursa, 424

tenosynovitis: inflammation of the sheath that covers a tendon, 425

tension
discharged through play, 226
exercises for, 171
feelings of, 262
and impotent anger, 263
and infertility, 141–142
muscle, 207
relieved by food, 353
and sexual problems, 265
and working wife, 256

tension headache: severe headache induced by tension, which causes unconscious constriction of head and neck muscles, 414

Terramycin: trade name for the antibiotic tetracycline

testes: testicles

testicle(s)/testis (*pl., testes*): one of a pair of male reproductive glands (gonads) that produce spermatozoa and male sex hormones, situated in a pouch (scrotum) at the base of the penis, 64, 70, 85, 125, 126, 242, *242, 567, 570*
hyperfunction, 571
hypofunction, 570–571
inflammation of: orchitis
undescended, 126, 571

testicular failure, 182

testis: testicle

testosterone: male sex hormone manufactured in the testicles, 70, 570

tests
fertility, 144–146
laboratory, 88
urine, 581

tetanus/lockjaw: acute bacterial infection usu. introduced through a puncture wound, leading to muscle spasms, esp. of the jaw muscles, and often fatal, 117–118, 670
in pregnancy, 152

tetanus-diphtheria toxoid: TD

tetany: nerve disorder characterized by muscle spasms and sometimes convulsions, caused by too little calcium in the blood, 70

tetracycline: crystalline powder isolated from a soil bacillus that forms the base of several antibiotics, including Aureomycin and Terramycin

tetrahydrocannabinol/THC: principal compound of cannabis (hashish or marihuana), believed to be the active ingredient, 664

thalamus: round mass of gray matter at the base of the brain that trans-

mits sensory impulses to the cerebral cortex

thalidomide, 147, 153

THC: tetrahydrocannabinol

therapeutic: designed or tending to heal or to cure disease

therapist, reputable, 221

therapy: treatment of a disease by a prescribed method or medicine, 437

thermogram: measurement of the surface temperature of a region of the body, such as the breast, with an infrared sensing device, 617, *617*

thermometers, 446

thiamine/vitamin B_1: vitamin found in cereal grains, green peas, liver, egg yolk, and other sources, and also made synthetically, that protects against beriberi

thighbone, 8
fracture, *458*

"Thinking About Drinking" (pamphlet), 647

thiopental/Pentothal, 656

thirst, as symptom, 207

thoracic: of or relating to the thorax, or chest cavity

thoracic cage/rib cage, *59, 60,* 520
disorders of, 464–465
in pneumothorax, 565

thoracic lymph duct, 40

thoracic spine: thoracic vertebrae, 6

thoracic surgeon: surgeon specializing in thoracic surgery, having to do with the chest cavity

thoracic surgery: branch of surgery having to do with the chest cavity and its organs, the heart and lungs, and large blood vessels

thoracic vertebra: vertebra, thoracic

thorax: chest, 540, *540*

Thorazine, 186

thoughts, and guilt feelings, 218, 232–233

threadworms/nematodes, 535

throat, *79*
sore: *pharyngitis*

throat infections, 120

thrombin: enzyme present in the blood that reacts with fibrinogen to form fibrin in the process of clotting, 485

thrombocytes: platelets

thromboembolism: obstruction of a blood vessel by a blood clot (thrombus) that has broken away from the place where it was formed, 251

thrombophlebitis: formation of a blood clot (thrombus) in the wall of an inflamed vein (phlebitis), 495, 564

thromboplastin: substance found in blood platelets that helps to convert prothrombin into thrombin in the clotting process, 485

thrombosis: formation of a blood clot (thrombus) in a blood vessel, resulting in the partial or complete blocking of circulation, 497. See also *coronary thrombosis.*

thrombus: stationary blood clot within a blood vessel, 499, 506
in stroke, 497

thrush: fungus infection in the mouth, esp. of infants, characterized by white patches that become sores, 524

thymectomy: surgical removal of the thymus, 484

thymus: glandlike lymphoid organ located near the base of the neck, believed to play a role in the body's immunological responses, *64,* 70–71, *567*

thyroid activity in pregnancy, 153–154

thyroid gland: endocrine gland located at the neck just below the larynx, extending around the front and to either side of the trachea (windpipe), and secreting the hormone thyroxin, which is vital to growth and metabolism, *64,* 69–70, 566, *567,* 568–569

thyroid pills, 69, 332

thyroid-stimulating hormone/TSH: hormone secreted by the anterior lobe of the pituitary gland which stimulates the production of hormones in the thyroid gland, 67

thyroxin: hormone secreted by the thyroid gland, vital to growth and metabolism, 69–70, 568
deficiency of, 568–569
in goiter, 569

tibia: the shin bone, the inner and larger of the two bones of the lower leg, *7*
fractured, 456

tics, 30

tinea: ringworm

tingling sensations, hand and arm, 150

tinnitus: ringing, buzzing, hissing, or clicking sound in the ears, not caused by external stimuli, 201, 435, 592

tints, hair, 384–385

tipping, in nursing homes, 215

"tired mother syndrome," 372

tissue(s)
bone, types of, 10
brain, 24
connective, in leg bone, *10*
death of: gangrene
gum, 95
heart, 41
interior bone, 11
kidney, reserve capacity of, 81
living, bone as, 3
lung, 62
muscle, atrophy of, 16
subcutaneous/underskin, 18, 378

tissue impairment, and alcohol, 637

tobacco, effects of, 137

tobacco tar in cigarettes, *557*

toe, big, in gout, 452
See also *hammer toe, stiff toe.*

toenails
brittle, 208
cutting of, 208
health of, 391
ingrown, 175, 208

toilet training, 110–111, 225, 526

tolerance: the ability of the body to adjust to increasingly larger doses of a drug through habitual use, 140

tomato juice, in hangover prevention, 186

tongue, 14, *44, 47,* 72, 79–80
coated, *428,* 429
inflammation of: glossitis
role in digestion, 46–47
sense receptors on, 79

tongue, beef, nutrients in, 303

tonic: of or characteristic of tonus

tonic phase: the period during a grand mal epileptic convulsion when the body is rigid, 473

tonic spasm: *spasm*

tonometer: device for measuring pressure, as of the eyeball

tonsil: either of two small, round, lymphoid organs at each side of the back of the throat, 120

tonsillectomy: surgical removal of the tonsils, 120

tonsillitis: inflammation of the tonsils

tonus: muscular spasm characterized by persistent contraction. Compare *clonus.*

tooth
extraction of, *94*
structure of, *5*
See also *teeth.*

toothache, 176
acupuncture in, *704*

toothbrush, 97
electric, 98, *98*

tooth decay, *96*
prevention of, 468

toothpaste, fluoride, 96

touch, 18, 20, 72

touch receptor, *19, 378*

tourist offices, foreign, 276

tourniquet: bandage or other material tied tightly to constrict an artery to stop bleeding, 671–672, *672*

toxemia of pregnancy: metabolic disorder of pregnant women, characterized by a rise in blood pressure, swelling of tissues, weight gain, and headaches (pre-eclampsia) and sometimes by convulsions and loss of consciousness (eclampsia), 149–150, 317

toxic: 1. caused by or having to do with a toxin or poison. 2. poisonous.

toxin: any of a group of poisonous compounds produced by animal, vegetable, or bacterial organisms, 536

trabecula (*pl., trabeculae*): strand of connective tissue, as in a bone, *10*

trachea/windpipe: the passageway for air from the larynx to the lungs, *44, 47,* 48, 59–60, *60,* 69
irritation to, *432*
obstruction in, 676–677

tracheostomy/tracheotomy: emergency surgical procedure of cutting into the trachea, 529
in croup, 121

tracheotomy: tracheostomy

traction: subjection of muscle or a fractured part to a pulling force, as by a system of weights and pulleys, 455
for slipped disk, 460
weight, 457

tranquilizer: drug with a calming or sedative effect, 265, 421, 426, 433, 435, 655, 657
in alcoholism, 645
consumption of, *648*
for hangover, 186

transfusions, blood, 37, *37*
early, *486*
and hepatitis, 537
in purpura, 487

transplants, 293
heart, 506
kidney, 599, *599*
See also *hair, transplant.*

transverse colon: the section of the colon leading from the ascending colon and extending horizontally across the abdomen beneath the liver and stomach

trauma: 1. any injury or wound to the body. 2. severe emotional shock.
to the eye, 587–588

travel, *276*
in later years, 275–276
in middle years, 269

tremors, 30
in Parkinson's disease, 474

triceps muscle, *15*

trichina: Trichinella spiralis

Trichinella spiralis/trichina: the parasitic worm that causes trichinosis, 535

trichinosis: disease caused by a parasitic worm (Trichinella spiralis) that enters the body via undercooked or raw meat, esp. pork, invading the intestines and muscles and provoking gastrointestinal symptoms initially and muscle stiffness and pain later, 535

triglyceride: glycerol compound containing one to three acids

trimester: period of three months, used to identify the progress of a pregnancy, which consists of three such periods

trip (*slang*), hallucinogenic, 660

trivalent: pertaining to a form of the Sabin polio vaccine in which each dose gives protection against three strains of polio, 118. Compare *monovalent.*

tropical diseases, 528

true skin: dermis

trust, basic, 223

trypanosomiasis: sleeping sickness

trypsin: enzyme in the pancreatic juice that breaks up proteins for digestion

TSH: thyroid-stimulating hormone, 67

tubal insufflation/Rubin's test: the injection of carbon dioxide gas, or sometimes ordinary air, into the uterus to check for obstructions in the Fallopian tubes, 145–146

tubal ligation: the tying or binding of a tube, esp. of the Fallopian tubes as a method of sterilization

tubercle: small nodule or tumor formed within an organ, as that produced by the bacillus causing tuberculosis

tubercle bacillus: rod-shaped bacterium that causes tuberculosis, *545,* 547

tuberculin: liquid containing substances extracted from weakened (attenuated) tubercle bacilli, used as a test for tuberculosis

tuberculin test: skin test for determining whether tuberculosis bacteria are present, used esp. for children, 548, *549*
for infant, 109

tuberculosis: infectious, communicable disease caused by the tubercle

Illustration
Credits

FEDERAL HEALTH PROGRAMS SERVICE

Operation of the Federal Health Programs Service includes the U.S. Public Health Service Hospital and Clinic system, the Division of Emergency Health Services, the Division of Federal Employee Health and the Medical Programs of the U.S. Bureau of Prisons, the U.S. Coast Guard, and the Office of Federal Employees' Compensation. In addition, the HSMHA Employee Health Program on Alcoholism was initiated during 1972.

PHS Hospitals and Clinics

The hospitals and clinics continued their efforts toward increasing efficiency in providing high quality comprehensive health care to those who may receive treatment at PHS facilities; among these are: American seamen, officers and enlisted men of the U.S. Coast Guard and their dependents, military personnel and their dependents, and Federal employees who are injured on the job or become ill as a result of their work.

Eight general hospitals are located in Baltimore, Boston, Galveston, New Orleans, Norfolk, San Francisco, Seattle, and on Staten Island, N.Y. A hospital for leprosy patients is located in Carville, Louisiana. In addition, 30 outpatient clinics and 236 contract physicians' offices are maintained.

Patient loads for the hospitals and clinics followed the downward trend of the past decade. There were 34,465 hospital admissions and 1,761,558 outpatient visits recorded during the year. As a result of this trend of declining inpatient workloads, the hospitals are operating at less than maximum capacity. The facilities have, on the other hand, become important community health resources in many areas. Recognizing this potential for increasing the value of these facilities to the communities and to assure maximum utilization, the Department continued studies, begun the year previous, to determine the feasibility of converting the hospitals from Federal to local control. Such conversion would give the communities greater latitude in using the present excess capacity of the hospitals to meet local needs. During the year, initial evaluation was made on the possibility of transferring PHS hospitals in Boston and San Francisco to community control and management.

Training

The hospitals and clinics, in support of their basic mission of patient care, continued to offer training in a wide variety of health careers ranging from post graduate physician education to the training of health aids and other medical support personnel. There were 254 physicians in residency or intern training during the year, and 118 of these completed their training. In addition, 37 dental interns completed training.

The Marine Physicians' Assistants School at the Staten Island PHS Hospital has been redesigned into a 12-month program and is now closer in scope to other Physicians' Assistant programs. This Staten Island program, begun as a Purser-Pharmacist Mate school to provide trained emergency medical manpower aboard ships which did not carry physicians, was the first of its kind and has trained 160 thus far.

The Orthopedic Assistant program, also at Staten Island, continued in cooperation with the Staten Island Community College of the City University of New York. This program is designed to prepare young men and women for careers as orthopedic assistants who will be responsible for medical duties under the direction of orthopedic surgeons. The course, recognized by the American Academy of Orthopedic Surgeons, consists of over 800 hours of medical training supplemented by 50 academic hours. Graduates will receive an associate in applied science degree from the City University of New York and a certificate of training from the Public Health Service. Training programs in other areas included hospital pharmacy, dietetics, medical record library science, medical and·X-ray technology, and nursing assistants. Many of these programs are carried out in cooperation with a wide variety of academic, community, and governmental agencies. Over 500 professionals and 1,500 allied health personnel received training during 1972.

Research

The hospital-clinic system conducted basic and clinical biomedical research as well as health services research as an integral part of the patient care program. During the year, 100 clinical research projects were being conducted. Steady progress continued throughout the year in research designed to develop new and more effective ways of rehabilitating patients with leprosy or other diseases where loss of sensitivity in the extremities leads to bone resorption and crippling.

Scientists at Carville (Louisiana) PHS Hospital have developed a technique whereby slipper-sox which have been im-

pregnated with microspheres of dye can be used to determine pressure points in shoes for people with insensitive feet. People ordinarily know when shoes don't fit. They feel tight. It hurts to walk and blisters form quickly. People with diseases such as leprosy or diabetes, however, may lose these warning signs or feedback mechanisms of pain and discomfort. In these, tight shoes may quickly lead to blisters, ulcers, infection, and permanent damage.

Carville's technique is based on making microspheres of dye that will burst at pressures which might cause irritation or blisters of the skin. Thus, a color change replaces pain as a feedback mechanism which enables patients to get a perfect fit for insensitive feet. Work is also continuing at Carville on the use of the armadillo as an experimental animal for leprosy research. Heretofore, no satisfactory experimental model has been available for investigation of leprosy on a systemic or cellular level. A Carville scientist, in collaboration with the Gulf South Research Institute, succeeded in infecting an armadillo with lepromatous leprosy in 1971. Three more were infected in 1972.

As in the past, the multi-hospital cooperative study of renal disease and hypertension, a definitive study in this area, continued to make noteworthy contributions to the understanding of these important causes of disability and death. Progress was also made in studies in the use of whole-body radiation in the treatment of cancer and the effects of simulated weightlessness on body metabolism and heart and circulatory function.

Other Medical Programs

The health of Federal prisoners is a legal responsibility of the Public Health Service. FHPS personnel assigned to the Medical Program, Bureau of Prisons, Department of Justice, provide medical, surgical, psychiatric, dental, and related care for over 22,200 prisoners in 30 medical facilities throughout the nation. Nineteen of these facilities have become fully accredited by the Joint Commission on Accreditation of Hospitals. The U.S. Coast Guard Medical Program provided comprehensive health services at both shore and floating units to active and retired Coastguardsmen and their dependents. In addition, PHS officers were assigned to the Office of Federal Employees' Compensation of the Department of Labor, to the Peace Corps, and the Cuban Refugee Program.

HSMHA Employee Health Program on Alcoholism

This program was established under section 201, Title II, Public Law 91-616, to provide an alcohol abuse, alcoholism prevention, treatment and rehabilitation program for all HSMHA's civilian employees. A model program was set up in FHPS to deal initially with 14,000 Federal employees in the Washington-Baltimore area. The model program began as a detection, referral, and treatment program for employees serviced by seven employee health units. The initial goal is to provide training for supervisors on all levels in the alternatives and resources available for dealing with employees who have problems with alcohol. In addition, the program has begun a "hot line" service for alcoholic problems, has established a publication to give authoritative information and to promote understanding of the alcoholic, and, in conjunction with agency personnel officials, has sought to clarify policies affecting the employees who have drinking problems.

Division of Federal Employee Health

The Division of Federal Employee Health augmented preventive occupational health care and consultative programs for Federal employees during FY 1972.

The heads of Federal Departments, under P.L. 79-658, may provide health services to employees under their jurisdiction limited to treatment of on-the-job illness, selected examinations, referral to private physicians and dentists, and preventive programs relating to health, only after consultation with the Public Health Service. The Division also operates reimbursable health units for the delivery of such services, where possible.

Comprehensive surveys of health needs and required facilities were provided to 58 agencies desirous of implementing employee health services during the fiscal year.

New DFEH health units were established in Atlanta, Georgia; Detroit, Michigan; St. Louis, Missouri; Buffalo, New York; Durham, North Carolina; and Seattle, Washington. By June 30, 1972, a total of 91 health units were in operation offering a full range of services to 160,000 Federal employees.

Taken from the 1972 Annual Report of the Public Health Service

Physical Fitness

One of the most important health studies of our time was started by the National Institutes of Health back in 1949. The population of an entire community was put under continuous scrutiny by a team of doctors who recorded the daily habits of thousands of men and women. For nearly a quarter of a century, the citizens of Framingham, Massachusetts, have been observed at work, at play, and in the home. They have been measured and weighed repeatedly, their food analyzed, their cigarettes counted, blood pressure checked, and so on, without interfering with the normal life styles of the individuals.

The Framingham Study

Results of the Framingham Study of a generation of a typical American community reveal certain patterns between a way of life and the most common cause of death, which is cardiovascular disease. The links between the American way of life and the American way of death were found to be too many cal-ories, mainly in the form of saturated fats and sugar, too many cigarettes, and too little exercise. Dr. William B. Kannel, Medical Director of the Framingham Study and a member of the Harvard Medical School faculty, reported that the most sedentary, or least active, men had about three times the heart attack risk as the most physically active. The rate of risk of cardiovascular disease seemed to be generally proportional to the degree of obesity, resulting from too many calories. The use of cigarettes was found to be associated with all manifestations of cardiovascular disease. One other link, which is still being explored, is high blood pressure.

The Framingham Study of the adult lives of some 5,000 subjects confirms what most doctors had suspected for many years—that physical activity helps counteract the effects of overweight, diets rich in fats and sugar, blood pressure, and similar factors. Dr. Kannel's report added another explanation: physical exercise probably helps extend the life and health of even those people with

Art and caption material reprinted from Field & Stream Guide to Physical Fitness.
Illustrations by Alex Orr. Copyright © 1970 by Holt, Rinehart and Winston, Inc.
Reprinted by permission of Holt, Rinehart and Winston, Inc.

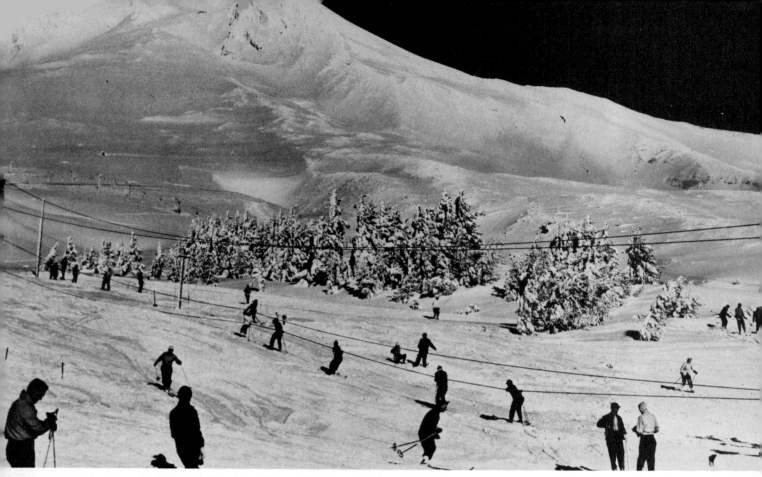

Participating in outdoor winter recreation has an energizing effect. Thousands visit the slopes of Mount Hood in northern Oregon annually—to ski, toboggan, and take photographs.
—*U.S. Forest Service (Hugh Ackroyd)*

cardiovascular disease by developing collateral circulation. In other words, a person who might otherwise develop heart trouble because of a diminished blood supply in his coronary arteries can forestall that threat to his life by physical exercise which promotes the increased flow of blood through alternate blood vessels.

There is a valuable lesson in the Framingham Study for every reader of this book: daily exercise, which requires no greater investment than a more efficient use of free time, can extend your life and retard certain organic diseases of the heart and blood vessels—diseases that account for more than half of the "natural" deaths in America each year.

Winter Exercise

If you are a typical American adult, the chances are that you are a "fair weather athlete." Although some men and women enjoy a hike through the freshly fallen snow to an outdoor ice skating rink, or an occasional visit to a ski run, too many individuals use the period between Indian summer and the return of spring as a time to take things easy, and indoors. That television producers save their best shows for the fall and winter months suggests that their careful surveys find most families indoors at that time. Sales of phonograph records and tape cassettes reach a peak as winter advances. And despite the let down in physical activity, the long periods of relaxed entertainment seem to stimulate tremendous appetites for high-carbohydrate goodies like potato chips, pretzels, candy, beer, and soft drinks. This seasonal irony is compounded by the fact that autumn usually is marked by an increasingly heavy schedule of cocktail parties, business or club lunches, dinner parties, and holiday feasts that may stretch through several days.

The Value of Physical Fitness

The ancient Greek physician Hippocrates may have established the first rule of physical fitness some 2,400 years ago. He outlined what he called the Law of Use which governs the living organism: "That which is used develops; that which is not used wastes away." Modern medical practice still follows that Hippocratic concept in preventive medicine as well as in the rehabilitation of surgical patients. Dr. Harry J. Johnson, Chairman of the Medical Board of the Life Extension Institute, expresses the Hippocratic Law of Use this way: "Life itself is movement. Even the developing embryo moves and stretches within the uterus by the fifth week of life — long before the mother becomes aware of it. And what does the mother say when she feels the first detectable stirring? She says she 'feels life.' "

After the birth of the baby, doctors have found that the mother recovers more quickly from the effects of childbirth if she gets out of bed and into action as soon as possible instead of lying in bed for a week or more to recuperate. The baby, during its hours of wakefulness, is in almost continuous motion—crawling, grasping, walking, running, jumping; the joy of activity continues in most normal children until adulthood.

There are exceptional people who almost literally keep moving throughout adult life. For example, Senator William Proxmire of Wisconsin is a strong advocate of jogging and regularly runs from his place of residence to his office on Capitol Hill. President Truman kept newsmen panting at his heels during his brisk morning walks. Individuals in all walks of life who spend a good deal of time in an office recognize the importance of daily exercise.

When Dr. Leonard Larson was president of the American Medical Association, he explained the importance of exercise in developing greater strength, stamina, endurance, and recuperative powers of the human body. "During exercise," said Dr. Larson, "the muscles need more oxygen and food. The blood circulates faster to meet the needs of the muscles and to carry off wastes. Body cells increase so that muscles gain strength and flexibility. There also is improved neuromuscular coordination."

Everyday Emergencies

A frequently overlooked fringe benefit of physical fitness is an improved ability to

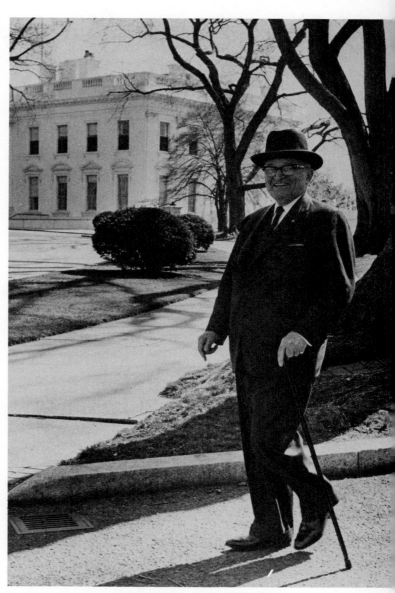

President Harry Truman thrived from the tonic effect of his invigorating 30-minute early morning walks.
—UPI Compix

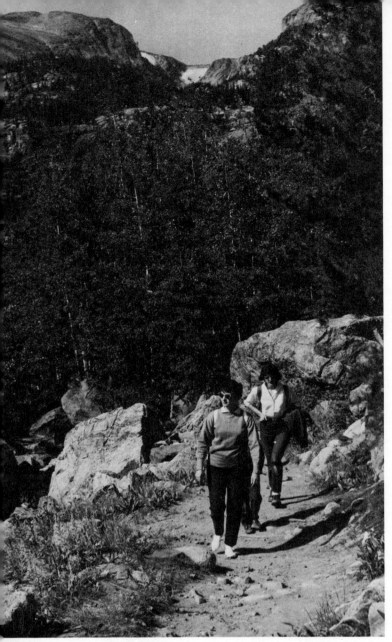

Hiking is a delightful pastime and an exhilarating experience. These hikers are enjoying nature during a leisurely, refreshing walk in the Rocky Mountains.
—*National Park Service*

survive everyday emergency situations that create a sudden demand for physical strength and endurance, which in turn require greater than normal performance by the heart and blood vessels, lungs, nerves, and muscles. This was illustrated during a meeting of physicians to discuss the health hazards of flying. The medical director of one of the major airlines was asked if he had any records of passengers on his airline dying of a heart attack. "Yes," the medical director replied matter-of-factly. "Last year, seven of our passengers died of heart attacks. But not while they were flying. In each case, the passenger was running down a corridor to catch a flight when he collapsed and died." Each of the victims, it must be assumed, was "out of condition," perhaps a bit paunchy and flabby from lack of exercise, and unable to meet the ultimate test of fitness: the sudden demand on the body's organs to meet a brief modern emergency of running with suitcase in hand to reach the airline counter before the gates closed.

Running for a plane, running for a bus, running for a commuter train, pushing a stalled car, carrying an air conditioner up a flight of stairs—these are civilization's equivalents of the primitive human's battles with wild animals or hand-to-hand combat with tribal rivals. But the primitive man probably had a better chance for survival in an emergency because he maintained muscle, heart, and lung strength and endurance through the daily demands of his prehistoric life style.

Vigorous Recreational Activities

The alpine lakes of the mountains of Idaho were once stocked with trout that were carried there in milk cans strapped to the backs of husky college boys. Some years out of college and softened by sedentary jobs, the same individuals, burdened only by sack lunches and fishing rods, had to stop several times for their "second wind" when they returned recently to the same lakes. There are still duck hunters who travel each autumn to a hilltop on the California-Oregon border; it is a favorite hunting ground for waterfowl that skim over the hill which separates two lakes on the Pacific Flyway. To reach the hilltop, the hunters have to scale a thousand feet of slippery lava rocks, and many drop out along the trail because of dizzy spells, painful leg cramps, and other discouraging symptoms. The peak bears the nickname of "Cardiac Ridge."

The point here is that true physical fitness involves more than a few easy or specialized exercises. A man can be a championship weight-lifter with the physique of Mr. America, but he may not be able to compete in running, swimming, or other sports activities unless he has developed and maintained strength and endurance in the heart, lungs, and muscles used for functions other than weight-lifting. Conversely, an individual who considers himself in good physical condition because he has been jogging for the past two years might be unable to lift a portable TV set. The goal for anyone seeking an exercise program should be all-around physical fitness, with good heart and lung conditioning in addition to muscular strength.

Weight Control and Exercise

While no single set of exercises will guarantee physical fitness, neither will exercise alone control an overweight problem—although the Framingham Study has suggested a complementary relationship between exercise and weight control. The catch is that it takes a lot of exercise to get rid of a pound of fat. It would require, for example, about 90 minutes of swimming to burn up the calories you gain by eating a 450-calorie piece of chocolate layer cake; for most people, it would be easier to control weight by skipping the cake.

One pound of body fat is equivalent to about 3,600 calories of food. That amount of fat is about equal to a food intake of ten calories a day over a period of a year. In other words, you can add or lose a pound of fat by altering your diet by approximately ten calories a day. A three-inch cookie averages about 120 calories, slightly more than the amount of calories in ten medium potato chips. Translated into weight-control terms: if you eat one cookie a day beyond your body's normal food requirements—or ten potato chips more—you should gain about 12 pounds in a year. Or if you regu-

larly munch on such goodies, you should be able to reduce your weight by approximately 12 pounds a year simply by eliminating one cookie per day, or its equivalent.

Calorie Consumption During Normal Activities

An average human body needs about 1,500 calories a day just to survive; it burns about one calorie per minute in maintaining such simple body functions as breathing, keeping the body temperature at a normal level, and so on. A person who spends most of his time sleeping or watching TV doesn't need much more than a calorie per minute of food energy. A person who operates an electric typewriter for an hour requires only about 20 calories more for that period of work than a sleeping person. Driving a car for one hour might increase the body's need for calories by about 100 more than the amount needed for sleeping; one tablespoon of mayonnaise or a half-dozen saltine crackers will provide enough calories for one hour of driving.

By matching the calories in snack foods with the calorie needs of the human body for such low levels of inactivity as driving a car, watching TV, or operating an office machine, it is easy to see how pounds of

Operating an office machine burns up few calories. Sedentary workers should be careful to avoid snacks containing the extra calories that cause overweight.
—*Santa Fe Railway*

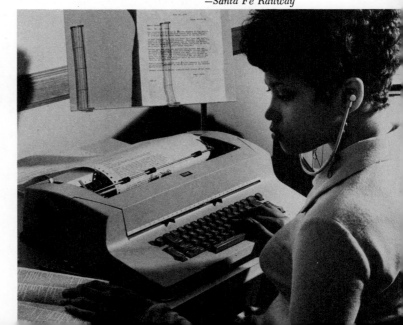

body fat can accumulate within a short period of time.

Even walking, which is considered a mildly active way of utilizing calories, burns only three calories per minute above the basic needs of the body. So you would need to walk two hours to burn an extra 360 calories—the equivalent of a slice of cherry pie. The next time a friend assures you that you can burn up the calories in a piece of fruit pie by walking back to the office after lunch, make the friend promise to walk with you because it will require six miles of walking.

Lack of Exercise and Weight Gain

Nevertheless, it is better to walk for two hours after eating a piece of pie than to remain inactive after adding hundreds of excess calories to your body's fuel supply— if you can't resist the temptation to add the calories—because there *is* a relationship between weight control and exercise. Some people apparently gain weight even though they eat no more than their friends and relatives who remain slim. Careful studies made of obese people who ate only small or average amounts of food—in some cases as few as 1,800 calories a day—showed that they were simply less active than their slim friends and relatives who consumed the same amount of calories.

In one instance involving students, motion pictures were taken of the obese youngsters working out with their classmates in physical education classes. The investigators discovered by watching the movies that the overweight students were in effect faking the exercise routines; that is, they did not play enthusiastically, but merely went through the motions.

What about the need for fat deposits in the body as a source of energy? The answer is that while fat is indeed a rich source of energy for the body, the human body chemistry is geared to convert protein to energy, if needed. But the body is not equipped to build protein molecules from fat. As for sugar in the diet, the body gets all it needs from carbohydrates in fruits, vegetables, and other food sources.

Planning Your Own Physical Fitness Program

Any weight control program in connection with physical fitness improvement should be tailored to your individual needs and directed by a physician. Only your doctor knows for sure about your individual nutrition needs, and no two individuals are precisely alike. The same rule applies to physical conditioning: you could have a hidden bodily deficiency that would not cause problems in a sedentary life style. But a sudden strenuous program of jogging, calisthenics, or other athletic activity could be enough to push you over the brink. After an examination, the doctor can recommend a tailored approach to physical conditioning —a program that will permit certain types of exercise but restrict or eliminate others. There are so many methods of exercise available today that an effective program can be built around any individual physical problems.

Exercises Keyed to Age

Age ordinarily is one factor in determining which exercises are more suitable for an individual, although everybody knows people who seem young at 60 and others who appear to be old at 30. The general rule for determining whether it is safe to begin an exercise program is this: if you are still in your 20s and have passed a standard physical examination within the past year, it should be safe to begin a progressive program of conditioning without further examination. But if you are over 30 years of age, you should have passed a complete physical examination that included an electrocardiogram within the past 90 days.

If you are over the age of 50, you can still begin a physical fitness program, but it should be a medically supervised program.

For the over 50 group, the doctor may advise that certain activities, such as jogging and competitive sports, be restricted or eliminated. Jogging can be damaging to the spine in persons beyond the age of 40 and can aggravate signs of arthritis. But walking, golf, swimming, bicycling, and exercising on a stationary cycle are alternate types of exercising for the past-middle-age set.

Fitness and Mental Health

In addition to the physical benefits gained by exercise, Dr. Ernest Simonson of the University of Minnesota Medical School found in a study of 10,000 persons that physical activity can be a definite aid to mental health. Typical comments by his subjects reflect that they "feel more alive" when they exercise. Dr. Simonson reported after analyzing the improved mental health of his subjects: "It is common logic that if one feels better, his attitude toward others will be more congenial. When one is in a cordial, happy frame of mind, he will likely make wiser decisions, and his world in general will look better."

The late Dr. William Menninger, one of the world's foremost experts on mental health, explained that

Good mental health is directly related to the capacity and willingness of an individual to play. Regardless of his objections, resistances; or past practice, an individual will make a wise investment for himself if he will budget some of his time each day for his play—and take it seriously.

Dr. Menninger added that play provides an outlet for instinctive aggressive drives that enable a person to "blow off steam." Physical activity, he said, is a necessary supplement to daily work.

At the Beginning

Two things to remember in planning your own physical conditioning program are:
• Tailor the exercises and sports to your own needs and interests. If you have wanted

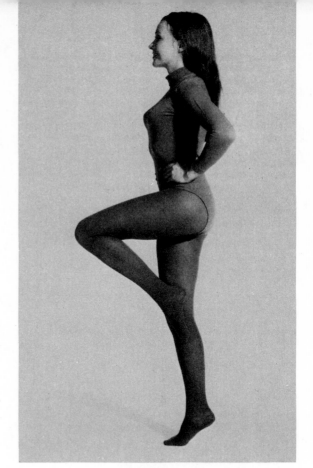

Exercise produces a healthful tone in mind and body.
—*Ewing Galloway*

to ride a bicycle, or learn water skiing, or take regular fishing trips, this is your opportunity to begin.

• Follow a progressive program in which you start at the bottom and improve gradually over a period of weeks or months. Don't expect overnight miracles, and be willing to cut back on the pace of your workouts if you find the going tough; you may be pushing yourself too fast. Your goal is to improve your own physical condition to the highest level feasible for your age and other possible limiting factors. Don't expect to set any new world records; just try to do the best you can—for your own health.

Warm-up exercises: The easiest place to begin your exercise program is in your own home, with the kind of warm-up exercises that you performed each day in high school. The main difference is that you will be on your own, unless you can find a friend or family member to participate in the workouts. You can do your own counting.

1 BEND AND STRETCH

Starting position: Stand erect, feet shoulder-width apart. *Action:* Count 1. Bend trunk forward and down, flexing knees. Stretch gently in attempt to touch fingers to toes or floor. Count 2. Return to starting position.

Note: Do slowly, stretch and relax at intervals rather than in rythm.

2 KNEE LIFT

Starting position: Stand erect, feet together, arms at sides. *Action:* Count 1. Raise left knee as high as possible, grasping leg with hands and pulling knee against body while keeping back straight. Count 2. Lower to starting position. Counts 3 and 4. Repeat with right knee.

3 WING STRETCHER

Starting position: Stand erect, elbows at shoulder height, fists clenched in front of chest. *Action:* Count 1. Thrust elbows backward vigorously without arching back. Keep head erect, elbows at shoulder height. Count 2. Return to starting position.

4 HALF KNEE BEND

Starting position: Stand erect, hands on hips. *Action:* Count 1. Bend knees halfway while extending arms forward, palms down. Count 2. Return to starting position.

5 ARM CIRCLES

Starting position: Stand erect, arms extended sideward at shoulder height, palms up. *Action:* Describe small circles backward with hands. Keep head erect. Do 15 backward circles. Reverse, turn palms down and do 15 small circles forward.

6 BODY BENDER

Starting position: Stand, feet shoulder-width apart, hands behind neck, fingers interlaced. *Action:* Count 1. Bend trunk sideward to left as far as possible, keeping hands behind neck. Count 2. Return to starting position. Counts 3 and 4. Repeat to the right.

7 PRONE ARCH

Starting position: Lie face down, hands tucked under thighs. *Action:* Count 1. Raise head, shoulders, and legs from floor. Count 2. Return to starting position.

8 KNEE PUSHUP

Starting position: Lie on floor, face down, legs together, knees bent with feet raised off floor, hands on floor under shoulders, palms down. *Action:* Count 1. Push upper body off floor until arms are fully extended and body is in straight line from head to knees. Count 2. Return to starting position.

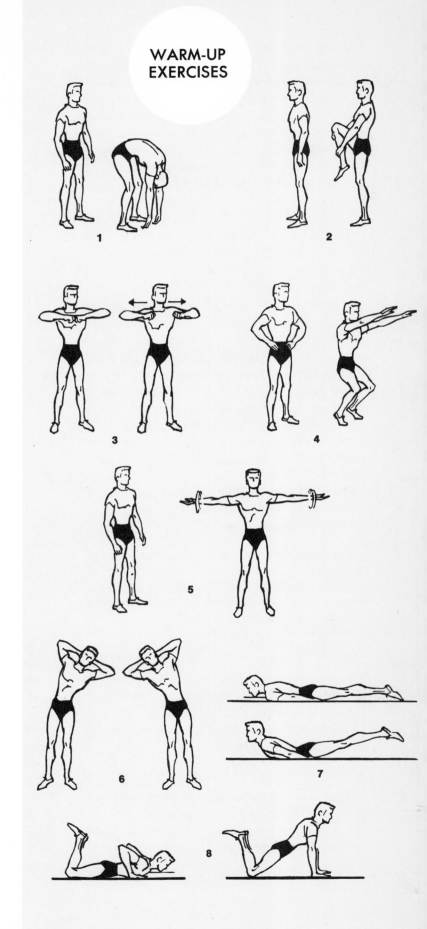

WARM-UP EXERCISES

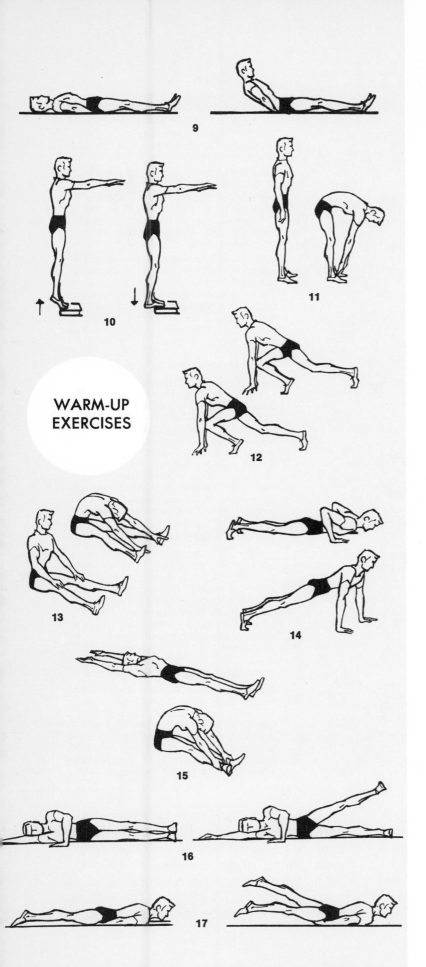

WARM-UP EXERCISES

9 HEAD AND SHOULDER CURL
Starting position: Lie on back, hands tucked under small of back, palms down. *Action:* Count 1. Tighten abdominal muscles, lift head and pull shoulders and elbows up off floor. Hold for four seconds. Count 2. Return to starting position.

10 ANKLE STRETCH
Starting position: Stand on a stair, large book or block of wood, with weight on balls of feet and heels raised. *Action:* Count 1. Lower heels. Count 2. Raise heels.

11 TOE TOUCH
Starting position: Stand at attention. *Action:* Count 1. Bend trunk forward and down keeping knees straight, touching fingers to ankles. Count 2. Bounce and touch fingers to top of feet. Count 3. Bounce and touch fingers to toes. Count 4. Return to starting position.

12 SPRINTER
Starting position: Squat, hands on floor, fingers pointed forward, left leg fully extended to rear. *Action:* Count 1. Reverse position of feet in bouncing movement, bringing left foot to hands and extending right leg backward—all in one motion. Count 2. Reverse feet again, returning to starting position.

13 SITTING STRETCH
Starting position: Sit, legs spread apart, hands on knees. *Action:* Count 1. Bend forward at waist, extending arms as far forward as possible. Count 2. Return to starting position.

14 PUSHUP
Starting position: Lie on floor, face down, legs together, hands on floor under shoulders with fingers pointing straight ahead. *Action:* Count 1. Push body off floor by extending arms, so that weight rests on hands and toes. Count 2. Lower the body until chest touches floor.
Note: Body should be kept straight, buttocks should not be raised, abdomen should not sag.

15 SITUP (ARMS EXTENDED)
Starting position: Lie on back, legs straight and together, arms extended beyond head. *Action:* Count 1. Bring arms forward over head, roll up to sitting position, sliding hands along legs, grasping ankles. Count 2. Roll back to starting position.

16 LEG RAISER
Starting position: Right side of body on floor, head resting on left arm. *Action:* Lift left leg about 24″ off floor, then lower it. Do required number of repetitions. Repeat on other side.

17 FLUTTER KICK
Starting position: Lie face down, hands tucked under thighs. *Action:* Arch the back, bringing chest and head up, then flutter kick continuously, moving the legs 8″-10″ apart. Kick from hips with knees slightly bent. Count each kick as one.

WARM-UP EXERCISES

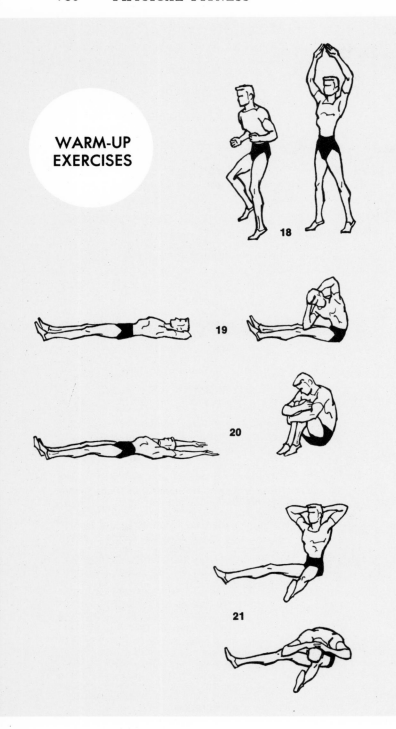

18 CIRCULATING ACTIVITIES

WALKING—Maintain a pace of 120 steps per minute for a distance of 1 mile. Swing arms and breathe deeply.

ROPE—Skip or jump rope continuously using any form for 30 seconds and then rest 30 seconds. Repeat 2 times.

RUN IN PLACE—Raise each foot at least 4" off floor and jog in place. Count 1 each time left foot touches floor. Complete the number of running steps called for, then do specified number of straddle hops. Complete 2 cycles of alternate running and hopping.

STRADDLE HOP—Starting position: At attention. *Action:* Count 1. Swing arms sideward and upward, touching hands above head (arms straight) while simultaneously moving feet sideward and apart in a single jumping motion. Count 2. Spring back to starting position. Two counts in one hop.

19 SITUP (FINGERS LACED)

Starting position: Lie on back, legs straight and feet spread approximately 1' apart. Fingers laced behind neck.
Action: Count 1. Curl up to sitting position and turn trunk to left. Touch the right elbow to left knee. Count 2. Return to starting position. Count 3. Curl up to sitting position and turn trunk to right. Touch left elbow to right knee. Count 4. Return to starting position. Score one situp each time you return to starting position. Knees may bend as necessary.

20 SITUP (ARMS EXTENDED, KNEES UP)

Starting position: Lie on back, legs straight, arms extended overhead.
Action: Count 1. Sit up, reaching forward with arms encircling knees while pulling them tightly to chest. Count 2. Return to starting position. Do this exercise rhythmically without breaks in the movement.

21 SITTING STRETCH (ALTERNATE)

Starting position: Sit, legs spread apart, fingers laced behind neck, elbows back.
Action: Count 1. Bend forward to left, touching forehead to left knee. Count 2. Return to starting position. Counts 3 and 4. Repeat to right. Score one repetition each time you return to starting position. Knees may be bent if necessary.

The purpose of the warm-up exercises is to increase the blood flow to the muscles and gradually limber up the body. And a warm-up period of at least 20 minutes should be used before any strenuous exercise. Otherwise, you may experience strains and sprains, or worse. It is quite possible to rupture a tendon or injure a joint by starting with certain strenuous exercises without a preliminary warm-up period. Also, remember to taper off a workout period with mild muscular activity, such as walking, until breathing and body temperature have returned to normal levels.

The warm-up exercises include body benders, situps, pushups, bend and stretch, ankle stretch, knee lifts, straddle hops, walking, running-in-place, and rope-skipping workouts, among a wide assortment of calisthenics. You can select from the assortment of warm-up exercises illustrated on pp. 778–780 those that are best suited to your own situation. If you live in a house or apartment where you are likely to irritate other occupants by running in place or skipping rope, you can find other exercises that stimulate the general body circulation. But if you have facilities, such as a basement or garage, or a ground-floor bedroom where there is room for straddle hops or rope skipping, the exercises that provide the better range of action should be followed. Most of the exercises can be done in a small area; airline personnel investigating a strange thumping in a jet aircraft at 30,000 feet altitude one morning discovered a passenger running in place in the rest room.

Although no special equipment is necessary, don't hesitate to invest in a few items of gym equipment—dumbbells, weights, a stationary cycle, or whatever you think you need to help you in your own fitness program. For the cost of one or two days in a hospital, you can buy enough exercising equipment to keep yourself out of the hospital for several years.

Muscle soreness: You can expect some muscular soreness for the first two or three weeks of the toughening stage of physical conditioning, particularly if you have shunned exercise for several years. Later on, as you progressively increase the work load on your body you may experience some stiffness or soreness. Usually this is only a warning sign that you are moving up the fitness scale too quickly. On the other hand, if the muscle soreness is relatively mild and goes away overnight, you can assume that

you are not overdoing the exercise routine.

If your muscles and joints appear to suffer from the exercise load, simply slow down to an easier pace and work back up the scale again at a more gradual rate. By working at your own pace, with only the goal of improving your muscular strength and endurance, you can build a lot of flexibility into your fitness program. You don't have to compete with others; if you need an extra day or week to advance from one stage to the next, take the extra time. It's your own conditioning routine, and the suggested benchmarks or guidelines for the accompanying exercises can be adapted to your own needs.

The Indoor Exercise Program

Based on the U.S. Army's 6–12 conditioning project, the Indoor Exercise Program on pp. 782-793 includes six sets of exercise routines. Each set requires 12 minutes a day to complete. Each of the sets, from I to VI, is in turn divided into three levels of activity. They are labeled A, B, and C. The entire program, therefore, is designed to provide a progressive scale of physical conditioning for 12 minutes a day over a period of 18 weeks. You should begin at the C-level of set I and follow that routine for the first week. At the start of the second week, you progress to the B-level exercise routine of set I, and to the A-level routine at the beginning of the third week. Then, assuming that you follow the schedule according to its original design, you advance to the C-level routine of set II of the 6–12 exercises at the start of the fourth week, and so on.

The progression guides accompanying each table of 6–12 exercises represent suggested goals for healthy males. Women generally are not expected to match the suggested pace, although some may be able to do so. To follow the progression guide of Table I, read the first vertical column of numbers under the word *Exercises*. Under Exercise 1, in the age group of 17–29, are the numbers 15, 13, and 11. These numbers show the repetitions of Exercise 1 to be completed within two minutes, the number indicated at the bottom of the column. The beginner in that age group should attempt to complete 11 side straddle exercises within two minutes, or at least he should work toward that primary goal. He also should try to complete 14 of the modified pushups in 1 minute, 12 situps in 1 minute, and so on. If he can accomplish the C level goals in the first week, he progresses to the B level goal of 13 side straddle exercises within two minutes, 16 modified pushups, 13 situps, and so on. You will note that the total of the minutes suggested for the various exercises is 12 regardless of the age group or exercise level chosen. The greatest amount of time is allocated to running in place, and the number of steps ranges from a beginning level of 30, or six per minute, for men over 60 to a maximum of 250, or

TABLE I
PROGRESSION GUIDE

AGE GROUP	LEVEL	EXERCISES 1	2	3	4	5	6
17	A	15	18	14	15	15	250
to	B	13	16	13	13	13	235
29	C	11	14	12	11	11	215
30	A	13	14	12	13	13	200
to	B	11	13	11	11	11	185
39	C	9	12	10	9	9	165
40	A	11	11	10	11	11	150
to	B	9	10	9	9	9	135
44	C	7	9	8	7	7	120
45	A	9	8	8	9	9	100
to	B	7	7	7	7	7	90
49	C	5	6	6	5	5	80
50	A	7	6	6	7	7	75
to	B	5	5	5	5	5	70
59	C	3	4	4	3	3	60
60	A	4	5	4	4	4	50
and	B	3	4	3	3	3	40
over	C	2	3	2	2	2	30
Minutes for each exercise		2	1	1	1	2	5

1. Side straddle, arms overhead and straight, palms facing.

   — Turn trunk to the left and bend forward over the left thigh, attempt to touch the fingertips to the floor outside the left foot, keep the knees straight. Alternate the movement to the opposite side.

   — Down and up to one side is one repetition.

2. Kneeling front rest, hands shoulder width apart. The weight is supported on the knees and by the arms.

   — Bend elbows and lower body until chest touches the floor. Keeping knees on the floor, raise body by straightening the arms.

   — Down and up is one repetition.

3. Supine position, fingers interlaced and placed behind the head.

   — Maintaining the heels on the floor, raise the head and shoulders until the heels come into view. Lower the head and shoulders until fingers contact the floor and head rests on the hands.

   — Up and down is one repetition.

4. Body erect, feet slightly spread, fingers interlaced and placed on rear of neck at base of the head.

   — Bend the upper trunk backward, raise the chest high, pull the elbows back, and look upward. Keep the knees straight. Recover to the erect position, eyes to the front.

   — Bending backward and recovery is one repetition.

5. Body erect, feet spread less than shoulder width, hands on hips, elbows back.

   — Do a full knee bend, at the same time bend slightly forward at the waist. Touch the floor with the extended fingers, keeping the hands about six inches apart. Resume the starting position.

   — Down into the touch position and return to the starting position is one repetition.

6. Run in place, lift feet 4 to 6 inches off floor. At the completion of every 50 steps do 10 "Steam Engines." Repeat sequence until the required number of steps is completed.

   — Count a step each time left foot touches the floor.

   Steam Engines - Lace the fingers behind the neck and while standing in place raise the left knee above waist height, at the same time twist the trunk and lower the right elbow to the left knee. Lower the left leg and raise the right leg touching the knee with the left elbow thus completing the movement to that side. Continue to alternate the movement until the sequence is completed.

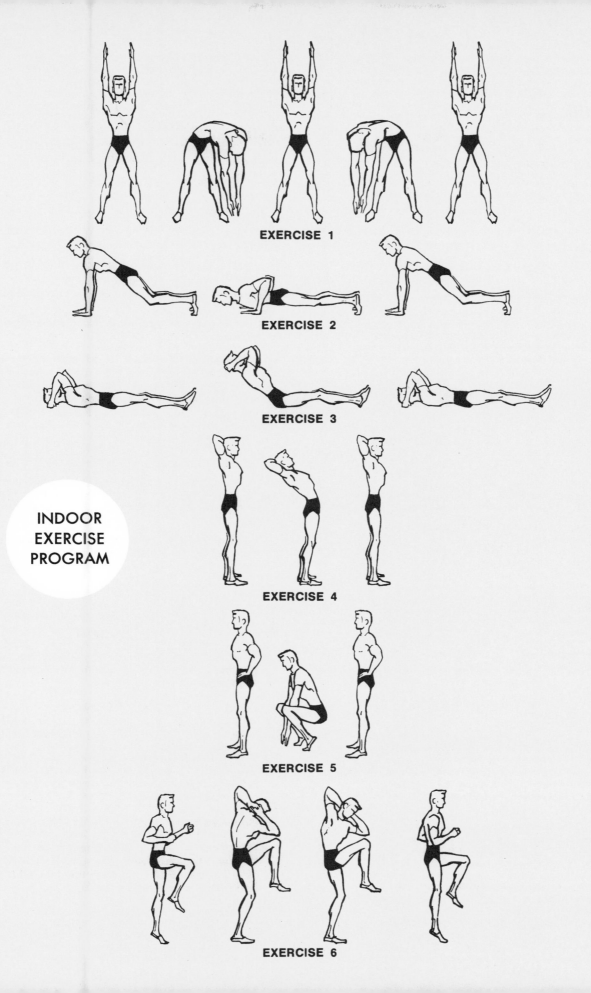

EXERCISE 1

EXERCISE 2

EXERCISE 3

INDOOR
EXERCISE
PROGRAM

EXERCISE 4

EXERCISE 5

EXERCISE 6

50 per minute, for a young man in good condition.

Adapting the Program to Meet Your Needs

There is considerable flexibility in adapting this program to suit your own physical abilities, whether you are a man or woman. Each individual is as different in his physical strength and endurance as his fingerprints or other traits. The important thing about these sets of exercises is that most normal adults can perform most or all of them at one of the beginning levels, and with that beginning level as a benchmark the individual can gradually follow the progression guidelines to a higher level of fitness.

Some individuals may already be in such good condition that they can work up to the A-level of Table VI at the ninth week instead of the 18th week without any of the

TABLE II
PROGRESSION GUIDE

AGE GROUP	LEVEL	EXERCISES					
		1	2	3	4	5	6
17 to 29	A	17	17	17	9	19	300
	B	15	15	15	8	17	270
	C	13	13	13	7	15	245
30 to 39	A	15	15	15	8	17	235
	B	13	13	13	7	15	210
	C	11	11	11	6	13	190
40 to 44	A	13	13	13	7	15	175
	B	11	11	11	6	13	155
	C	9	10	9	5	11	135
45 to 49	A	11	11	11	6	13	125
	B	9	9	9	5	11	110
	C	7	7	7	4	9	100
50 to 59	A	9	9	9	5	11	95
	B	7	7	7	4	9	85
	C	5	5	5	3	7	75
60 and over	A	6	7	7	4	9	70
	B	5	5	5	3	7	60
	C	4	4	4	2	5	50
Minutes for each exercise		1	1	1	1½	1½	6

1. Wide side straddle, arms overhead and straight, palms facing.

   — Bend at the knees and the waist, swing the arms down, and reach between the legs as far as possible. Look at the hands. The thighs are parallel to the floor during the bend. Recover to the starting position with a sharp movement.

   — Down and up is one repetition.

2. Front leaning rest position with body straight from head to heels.

   — Bending at the waist and keeping the knees locked, jump forward to a jack-knife position bringing the feet as close to the hands as possible. With the weight on the hands, thrust the legs to the rear resuming the front leaning rest position.

   — Up into the jack-knife position and return to the front leaning rest position is one repetition.

3. Supine position with arms straight overhead, palms facing.

   — With a sharp movement sit up, bringing the heels as close to the buttocks as possible and the knees to the chest. Swing the arms in an arc overhead to a position outside the knees and parallel to the floor. To recover swing the arms overhead keeping them straight. At the same time move the legs forward until they are straight.

   — Sitting up and returning to the supine position is one repetition.

4. Feet spread more than shoulder width apart, fingers laced behind the neck and elbows are back.

   — Bend forward at the waist vigorously, then twist the trunk to the left, then to the right and return to the erect position.

   — Keep the knees locked and back straight.

   — Bend forward, twist left, twist right, and return to the erect position is one repetition.

5. Bend forward at the waist, grasping the right toes with right hand, left toes with left hand, knees are slightly bent.

   — Walk forward retaining this position.

   — Count a repetition each time a foot contacts the floor.

6. Run in place, lift feet 4 to 6 inches off floor. At the completion of every 50 steps do 10 "Heel Clicks" Repeat sequence until the required number of steps is completed.

   — Count a step each time left foot touches the floor.

   Heel Clicks - Jump upward about 12 inches and bring the heels together. Before landing on the floor, separate the feet 15 to 18 inches. Immediately upon contact with the floor repeat the jump and heel click.

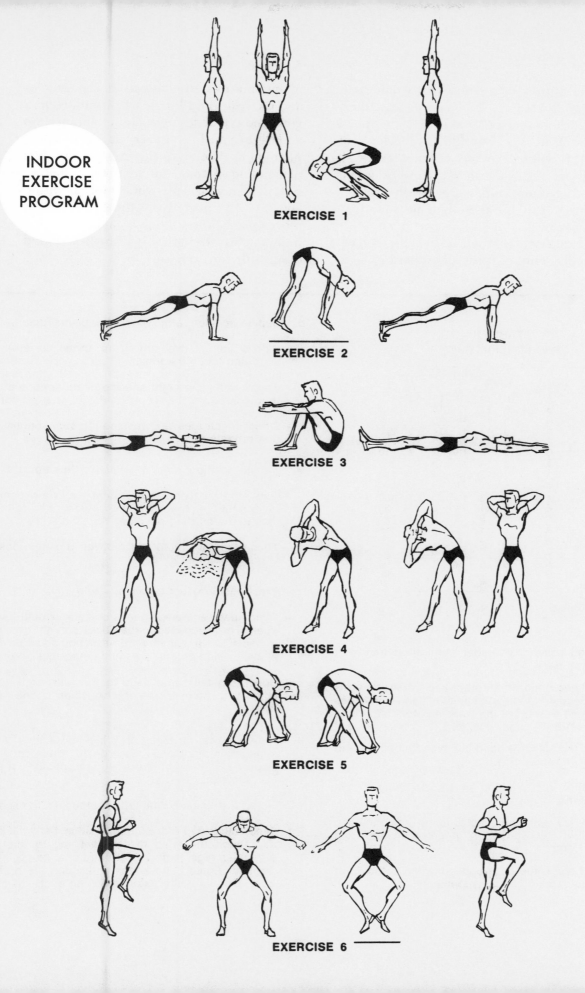

EXERCISE 1

EXERCISE 2

EXERCISE 3

EXERCISE 4

EXERCISE 5

EXERCISE 6

muscle stiffness or soreness that would indicate too fast a rate of advancement. Others may feel more comfortable if they spend two or three weeks at the C or B-level of Table I before moving to another level. There are no fixed rules to this program; the progression guides are merely suggestions that can be altered to fit your personal needs.

But don't go through the exercises half-heartedly. One purpose of exercising is to maintain a modest overload on the muscles and the heart and lungs, which builds up a good reserve of strength and endurance. So you have to push a bit every day to make the plan work; if some of the exercises are less demanding of your muscles and circulatory system than your daily work responsibilities, you may be wasting your time. A man who moves pianos for a living would do little to improve his strength by lifting six-pound dumbbells for exercise.

TABLE III
PROGRESSION GUIDE

AGE GROUP	LEVEL	EXERCISES 1	2	3	4	5	6
17 to 29	A	10	19	19	16	10	350
	B	9	17	17	15	9	315
	C	8	15	15	14	8	280
30 to 39	A	9	17	17	14	9	270
	B	8	15	15	13	8	240
	C	7	13	13	12	7	210
40 to 44	A	8	15	15	12	8	200
	B	7	13	13	11	7	180
	C	6	11	11	10	6	160
45 to 49	A	7	13	13	10	7	150
	B	6	11	11	9	6	135
	C	5	9	9	8	5	120
50 to 59	A	6	11	11	8	6	115
	B	5	9	9	7	5	105
	C	4	7	7	6	4	95
60 and over	A	5	9	9	7	5	90
	B	4	7	7	6	4	80
	C	3	5	5	4	3	70
Minutes for each exercise		1½	1	1	1½	1	6

1. Feet spread less than shoulder width apart, hands on hips, elbows back.

   — Do a full knee bend, trunk erect and thrust the arms forward. Recover to the erect position, and with knees locked, bend forward at the waist and touch the toes and recover to the erect position.

   — Down into the full knee bend, recover, touch toes and recover is one repetition.

2. Front leaning rest position with body straight from head to heels.

   — Lower the body until the chest touches the floor, keep body straight. Recover by straightening the arms and raising the body.

   — Down and touch the floor and recovery to the front leaning rest position is one repetition.

3. Supine position, arms overhead, palms facing.

   — With a sharp movement sit up, thrust the arms forward and touch the toes.

   — Keep the legs straight and the heels in contact with the floor.

   — Sit up, touch toes, and resume the supine position is one repetition.

4. Supine position, arms overhead, palms upward.

   — Raise the legs and swing them backward over the head until toes touch the floor. Recover by returning legs to the starting position.

   — Touch toes overhead and recover to supine position is one repetition.

5. Erect position, feet together.

   — Bend knees and place hands on floor, shoulder width apart. Thrust legs to the rear, body straight from head to heels. Move legs forward assuming squat position, elbows inside of knees. Assume erect position.

   — Down into full squat, legs to the rear, back to full squat and return to the erect position is one repetition.

6. Run in place, lift feet 4 to 6 inches off floor. At the completion of every 50 steps do 10 "Knee Touches." Repeat sequence until the required number of steps is completed.

   — Count a step each time left foot touches the floor.

   Knee Touches - From a stride position, bend the knees and touch the knee of the rear leg to the floor, straighten legs, jump upward and change position of the feet. Again bend knees and touch the opposite knee. Continue alternately touching each knee.

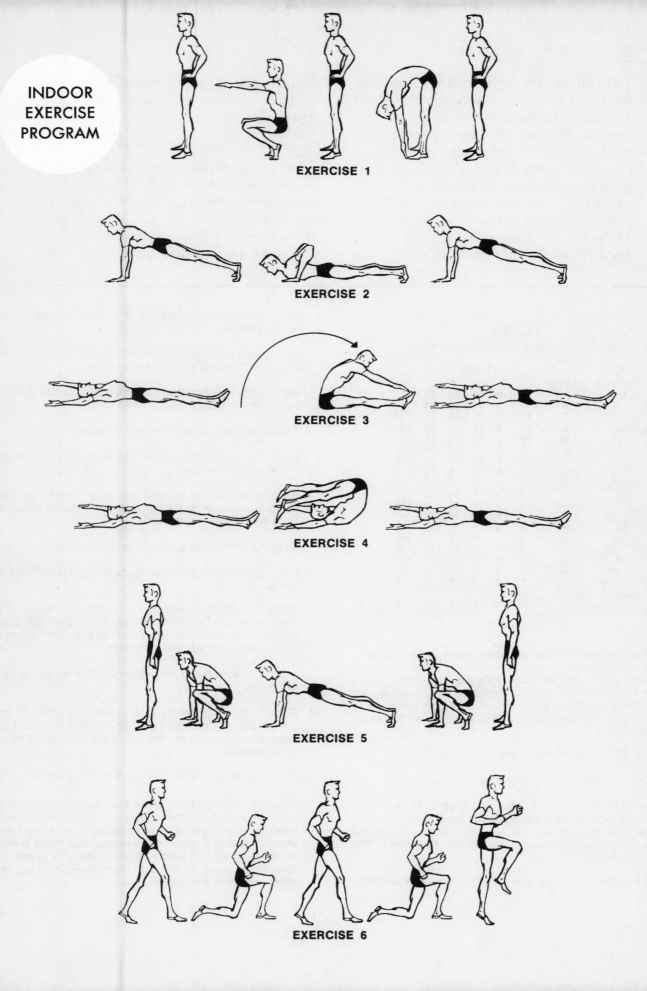

INDOOR EXERCISE PROGRAM

EXERCISE 1

EXERCISE 2

EXERCISE 3

EXERCISE 4

EXERCISE 5

EXERCISE 6

On the other hand, there are people over the age of 45 who should be cautious about advancing beyond set IV of the Indoor Exercise Program. If they experience discomfort at the C-level of set V, they should drop back to the A-level of Table IV. This program is designed to fit all sorts of individual needs and abilities; some individuals probably should not advance beyond the Table III set of exercises. If there is any question about the level at which you should taper off your personal progressive program, discuss the matter with your doctor.

Maximum Performance Plateau

The rate of improvement in your physical condition will seem to be quite rapid at first, then increase slowly as you reach a plateau about halfway through the 18-week program. You can tell when you have reached your peak performance because you will

TABLE IV
PROGRESSION GUIDE

AGE GROUP	LEVEL	EXERCISES 1	2	3	4	5	6
17	A	12	9	12	24	25	400
to	B	11	8	11	22	23	380
29	C	10	7	10	21	21	360
30	A	11	8	11	23	23	305
to	B	10	7	10	21	21	290
39	C	9	6	9	20	20	275
40	A	10	7	10	20	21	225
to	B	9	6	9	18	18	215
44	C	8	5	8	16	16	205
45	A	8	6	8	16	16	175
to	B	7	5	7	14	14	165
49	C	6	4	6	12	12	155
50	A	6	5	6	13	13	135
to	B	5	4	5	11	11	130
59	C	4	3	4	10	10	120
60	A	5	4	5	10	10	100
and	B	4	3	4	9	9	95
over	C	3	2	3	8	8	90
Minutes for each exercise		1	2	1	1	1	6

1. Erect position, hands at sides, feet spread slightly.

— Bend knees, incline trunk forward, and place hands on floor between legs. Straighten knees, keeping feet in place and fingers touching floor. Again bend knees and resume the first position. Recover to the erect position.

— The above sequence is one repetition.

2. Erect position, hands at sides, feet together.

— Bend knees, place hands on floor between legs. Thrust legs to the rear. Execute two complete push-ups and then thrust the legs forward bending the knees with arms between the knees. Recover to the erect position.

— The completion of all eight counts is one repetition.

3. Back position with arms out to sides and legs raised to the vertical.

— Lower legs to the left, raise legs to the vertical, lower to the right, again raise to the vertical.

— Keep legs together and the head and hands in contact with the floor throughout the exercise.

— The above sequence is one repetition.

4. From back position, raise legs with heels 10 to 12 inches from the floor.

— Spread legs as far as possible, close them together. Continue to open and close legs until required repetitions have been completed.

— Opening and closing legs in one repetition.

5. Front leaning rest position, body straight from head to heels.

— Bend the left knee and bring the left foot as far forward as possible, return left leg to original position. Repeat movement with the right leg. Continue exercise alternating left and right legs.

— A leg thrust forward and returned to the rear is one repetition.

6. Run in place, lift feet 4 to 6 inches off floor. At the completion of every 50 steps do 10 "Jumping Jacks." Repeat sequence until the required number of steps is completed.

— Count a step each time left foot touches the floor.

Jumping Jacks - Feet spread shoulder width apart, arms extended overhead. Jump upward, bring heels together and at same time squat to a full knee bend position, bring the arms downward and place hands on the floor elbows inside of knees, directly under the shoulders. Jump to the side straddle and swing the arms sideward overhead.

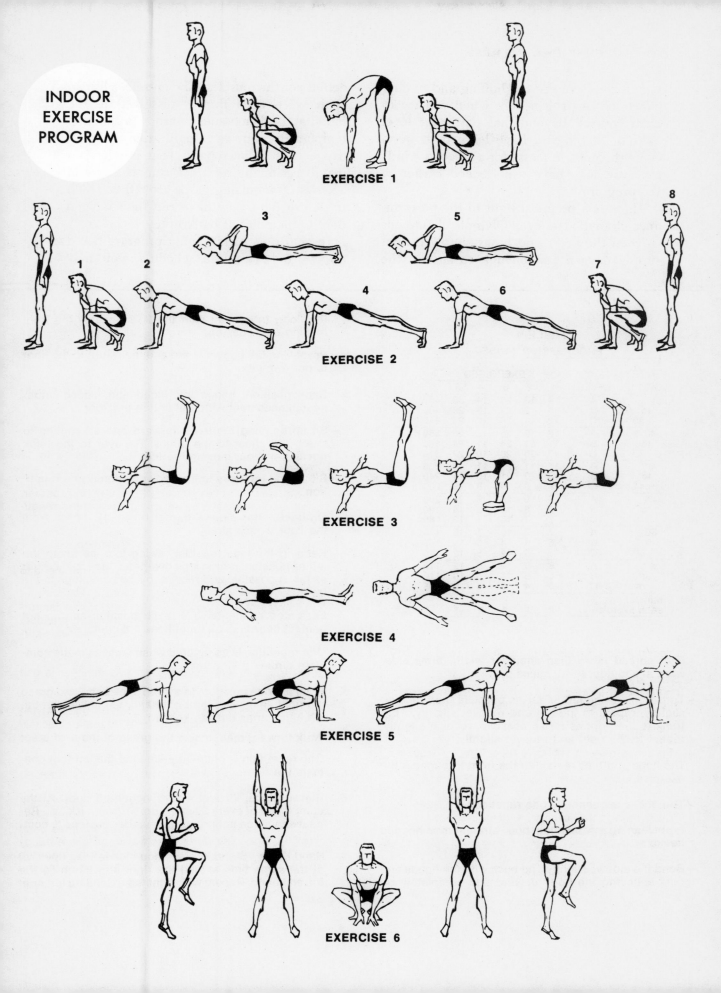

INDOOR
EXERCISE
PROGRAM

EXERCISE 1

EXERCISE 2

EXERCISE 3

EXERCISE 4

EXERCISE 5

EXERCISE 6

begin to experience the huffing and puffing effects of an oxygen debt when you try to push yourself beyond that particular level —even though you have learned to overcome the need to pause for a "second wind" that you may have experienced earlier in the program.

There is a practical limit to the performance of anybody—even Olympic champions —when the heart and lungs simply cannot supply oxygen fast enough to sustain the activity of the muscles. The muscle cells can "borrow" oxygen that is dissolved in the blood and other tissues in order to function temporarily, but eventually that debt of oxygen has to be repaid. That is why you may occasionally see track stars collapse in a series of agonizing gasps after they reach the finish line: they have run their oxygen debt to the point of bankruptcy.

In your own conditioning program based on the 6–12 exercise schedule, you may

TABLE V
PROGRESSION GUIDE

AGE GROUP	LEVEL	EXERCISES					
		1	2	3	4	5	6
17	A	14	13	28	14	30	450
to	B	13	12	27	13	28	430
29	C	12	11	26	12	26	410
30	A	12	12	25	12	26	350
to	B	11	11	24	11	24	330
39	C	10	10	23	10	22	310
40	A	11	11	23	11	23	250
to	B	10	10	21	10	21	240
44	C	9	9	19	9	19	230
45	A	9	9	20	9	20	200
to	B	8	8	18	8	18	190
49	C	7	7	16	7	16	180
50	A	7	7	16	7	16	170
to	B	6	6	14	6	14	155
59	C	5	5	12	5	12	140
60	A	6	6	12	6	12	115
and	B	5	5	11	5	10	110
over	C	4	4	9	4	9	105
Minutes for each exercise		2	1	1	2	1	5

1. Feet spread more than shoulder width, arms sideward at shoulder level, palms up.

— Turn trunk to the left as far as possible then recover slightly, repeat to the left and recover slightly. Turn trunk to the right as far as possible, recover slightly, repeat to the right and recover slightly.

— The head and hips remain to the front throughout the exercise.

— The above sequence is one repetition.

2. Front leaning rest position, body straight from head to heels.

— Bend the elbows slightly and push with the hands and toes bouncing the body upward and completely off the floor. In contact with the floor resume the front leaning rest position.

— Propelling the body upward and the return to the floor is one repetition.

3. Back position, hands interlaced and placed under head, knees bent with feet flat on the floor.

— Sit up bending the trunk forward and attempting to touch the chest to the thighs. Recover to the back position without moving the feet.

— Sit up and recovery to the back position is one repetition.

4. On back, arms sideward, feet raised 12 inches from the floor, knees straight.

— Keeping the legs together, swing legs as far to the left as possible, swing legs overhead, then to the right as far as possible and recover by swinging legs to the front.

— Legs stop momentarily at each position and do not contact floor until all repetitions are complete.

— One repetition is completed when legs make the complete circle.

5. From a stride position do a deep knee bend and grasp the right ankle with the right hand, left ankle with the left hand, arms outside knees.

— Walk forward maintaining the grasp of the ankles.

— One repetition is counted each time the left foot contacts the floor.

6. Run in place, lift feet 4 to 6 inches off floor. At the completion of every 50 steps do 10 "Hand Kicks." Repeat sequence until required number of steps is completed.

Hand Kicks - Stand in place and kick left leg upward, at the same time extend the right arm touching the toe and hand. Repeat with right leg extending left arm.

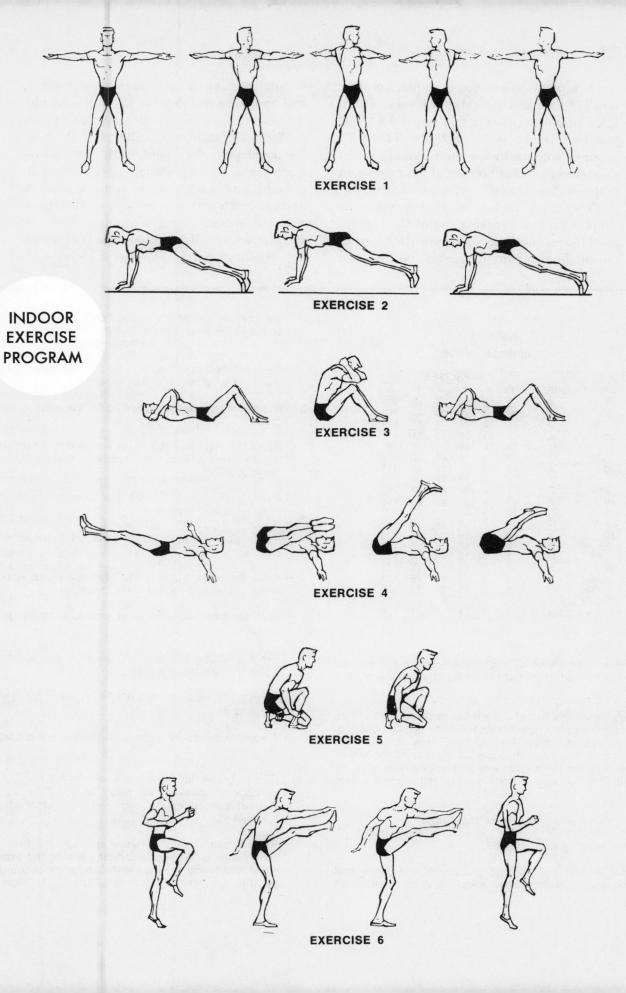

INDOOR EXERCISE PROGRAM

EXERCISE 1

EXERCISE 2

EXERCISE 3

EXERCISE 4

EXERCISE 5

EXERCISE 6

reach a point where, for example, you can do all of the exercises at the A level of Table V without experiencing an oxygen debt, but you can't make it through the Table VI routines without huffing and puffing. Then you will know that you are at your personal plateau of maximum performance. But you don't quit exercising at that point; you simply continue working out at the highest level that is comfortable for you. If you drop out of the program after reaching the level of your maximum performance your physical condition will deteriorate within two or three weeks.

There are still goals ahead and skills to be developed after you reach your maximum performance plateau—development of strength and endurance for participation in certain sports or improvement of the function of special muscle groups used in athletic activity. Rope skipping, a traditional conditioning exercise, always a favorite of

TABLE VI
PROGRESSION GUIDE

AGE GROUP	LEVEL	EXERCISES 1	2	3	4	5	6
17	A	17	15	32	32	35	500
to	B	16	14	30	30	33	480
29	C	15	13	28	28	31	460
30	A	15	13	30	30	31	400
to	B	14	12	28	28	29	380
39	C	13	11	26	26	27	360
40	A	13	10	27	27	27	310
to	B	12	9	25	25	25	285
44	C	11	8	23	23	23	265
45	A	11	9	23	23	23	250
to	B	10	8	21	21	21	230
49	C	9	7	19	19	19	210
50	A	9	8	19	19	19	200
to	B	8	7	17	17	17	190
59	C	7	6	15	15	15	175
60	A	8	7	15	15	17	140
and	B	7	6	13	13	15	130
over	C	5	5	10	10	12	120
Minutes for each exercise		2	1	1	1	1	6

1. Feet spread shoulder width apart, left fist clenched and overhead, right fist clenched at waistline in rear of body.

   — Simultaneously thrust the left fist as far to the right as possible and the right fist as far to the left as possible. Recover and repeat. Reverse the hands with the right fist above the head and the left in rear at the waistline. Repeat the movement to the opposite side by thrusting the upper body to the left with the arm motion.

   — The above sequence is one repetition.

2. Front leaning rest position.

   — Bend elbows slightly and push with the hands and toes bouncing the body upward and completely off the floor. At the height of the bounce, clap the hands and quickly return them to a position directly under the shoulder to catch the body weight.

   — Push off the floor, clap hands, and return to the front leaning rest position is one repetition.

3. Back position, arms extended to the side at 45 degrees.

   — Raise the legs and the trunk into a V position bringing the trunk and legs as close as possible. Return to back position.

   — Raising the legs and trunk and recovery to the back position is one repetition.

4. Prone position with hands clasped in small of the back.

   — Arch the body, holding the head back and rock forward, relax and repeat the movement.

   — Arch the body, rock forward, and relax is one repetition.

5. From a sitting position lift the hips supporting the body on the hands and feet.

   — By moving the arms and legs walk on all fours either forward or backward.

   — A repetition occurs each time the left hand contacts the floor.

6. Run in place, lift feet 4 to 6 inches off floor. At the completion of every 50 steps do 10 "Pike Jumps." Repeat sequence until required number of steps is completed.

   Pike Jumps - Jump forward and upward from both feet, keeping the knees straight. Swing the legs forward and touch the toes with the hands at the top of each jump.

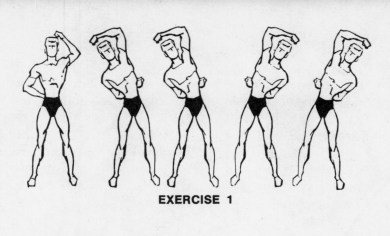

EXERCISE 1

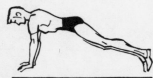
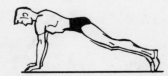

EXERCISE 2

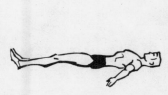
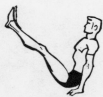
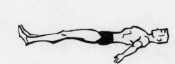

EXERCISE 3

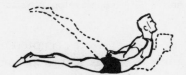

EXERCISE 4

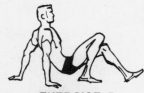

EXERCISE 5

INDOOR
EXERCISE
PROGRAM

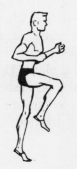
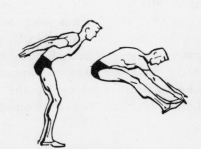
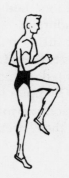

EXERCISE 6

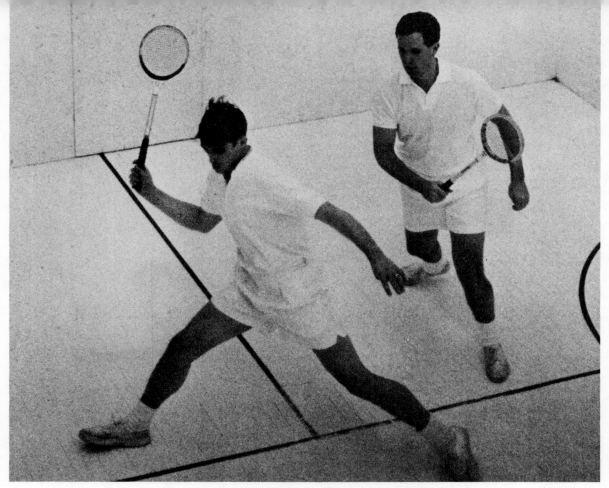

Squash is a lively, invigorating indoor sport requiring the stamina, alertness and agility that develop physical fitness.

professional boxers in training, is an example of an athletic activity that requires a high level of coordination, muscular function, and heart-lung performance to do well. Anyone who has tried high-speed rope skipping for more than three minutes without missing a jump knows it is more than a playground game; in fact, such a test has been used by the army in training soldiers for combat duty.

Weight Lifting

Another special method of developing strength and endurance is weight lifting practice. Weight lifting may be one of the oldest known sports that utilizes equipment; youths who wanted to participate in the ancient Greek Olympics of nearly 2,750 years ago were required to lift a heavy iron weight to prove their strength before they were accepted into the ritual. Weight lifting as a formal competitive sport was popular in Europe for many generations, but it did not attract much attention in North America until the 1930s when the United States organized its first weight lifting team for Olympic competition.

Exercising With Barbells

Although competitive weight lifting generally is considered a masculine activity, there is no reason why women could not work out with barbells if they wanted to do so. Body weight is not necessarily a factor; U.S. championship weight lifting has a minimum body weight class of 114.5 pounds while A.A.U. competition is held in a 123-pound body weight class. However, most women probably are not interested in developing the muscle groups that would benefit from lifting barbells. The type of

Exercise 1, Squat Dosage—6 repetitions, 50 pounds (commonly called the flatfoot deep knee bend). Place the bar upon the shoulders. Stand with feet about 18 inches apart. Keeping the feet flat, lower the body into the low squat position. Come erect and repeat. Exhale as you lower into the squat position and inhale as you come up.

Exercise 2, Waist Bender Starting dosage—6 repetitions, 40 pounds. Assume the standing position with the bar across the shoulders, feet shoulder-width apart. Bend forward at the waist until the upper body is parallel to the ground; return to the starting position. Each time you return to the upright position will constitute one repetition.

Exercise 3, Curl Dosage—6 repetitions, 40 pounds. Grasp the barbell with the palms facing to the rear and assume the standing position, feet shoulder width apart. With the barbell held in front of the hips, flex the elbows and lift the weight until the bar touches the upper chest. Lower the barbell back to the hip level position. Inhale deeply with the upward movement and exhale on the downward movement. Each time the bar touches the chest will constitute one repetition.

Exercise 4, Side Bender Starting dosage—6 repetitions per side, 40 pounds. Assume the standing position, feet shoulder width apart, with the bar across the shoulders. Bend to the left as far as possible and return to the starting position. Repeat six times and then execute the same procedure to the right for six repetitions.

Exercise 5, Standing Press Starting dosage—6 repetitions, 45 pounds. Grasp the bar with the palms facing forward and assume the starting position. Curl the weight to the upper chest position. Inhale deeply and press the bar upward to an overhead position. Exhale as you lower the bar to the chest position. Each time the bar is pressed upward constitutes one repetition.

Exercise 6, Upward Row Starting dosage—6 repetitions, 40 pounds. Grasp the bar, hands close together, palms to the rear, and assume the standing position. Starting with the bar held in front of the hips, flexing the elbows and the shoulder girdle muscles, lift the bar straight up to an overhead position. Inhale deeply as you lift the bar. Exhale as you lower the bar to the hip position. Each time the bar returns to the hips will constitute one repetition.

Exercise 7, Shoulder Curl Starting dosage—6 repetitions, 25 pounds. Grasp the bar palms down, and assume the standing position. Keeping the elbows locked, curl the bar, pivoting the arms at the shoulders until the bar is in an overhead position and as far to the rear as possible. Return the bar in the same manner to the hip position. Each time the bar returns to hip position constitutes one repetition.

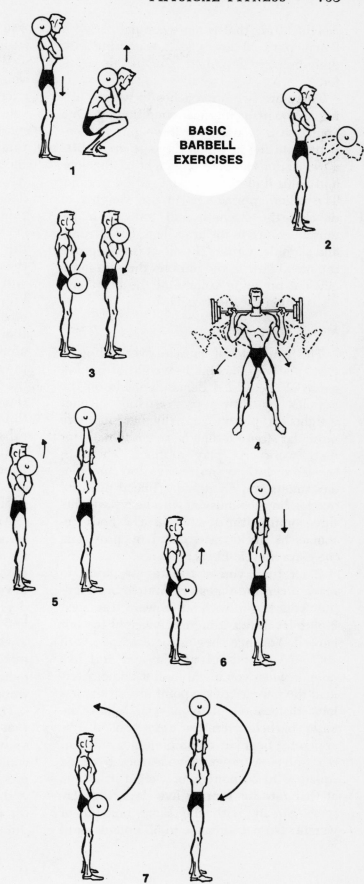

BASIC BARBELL EXERCISES

weight lifting that is more compatible with female physical fitness goals, exercising with dumbbells, is described later in this chapter.

There are two approaches to weight lifting as a part of physical conditioning. One approach is to use barbell weights in competitive lifting in which the participant lifts a tremendous amount of weight off the floor and holds it aloft for a brief period of time. The other approach is to use weights to develop the strength and tone of major muscle groups in the arms, legs, back, trunk, and shoulder girdle. The effect is to improve the blood flow to the muscles through more efficient pumping volume of the heart and distribution by the capillaries.

Muscle Overload

The principle of muscle overloading is particularly applicable in weight lifting because of the added demands made on the muscles by lifting progressively heavier weights. A person normally has no more muscular strength than he seems to need for daily work and play routines. There is, therefore, little or no reserve for emergencies unless you create an artificial need by overloading the muscles with heavy weights three or four times a week. The body responds to the extra demand by providing the extra muscle fibers.

Each time you stimulate the body to reach a certain plateau of muscle overloading, you begin working toward the next higher level by adding more weight to your barbell. You may begin, for example, with 40 to 50 pounds of weight and add five pounds when you are able. But do not overload the muscles to the point of a strain or a joint dislocation. Also, as you follow the basic barbell exercises described in this appendix, begin at the minimum number of repetitions. After you have learned to do six squats with 50 pounds of weight, continue at that rate for four or five days, then try seven squats with the same amount of weight. Do not advance to 55 pounds until

you can handle 10 or 12 at the starting weight level.

Warm-up exercises: As mentioned above, you should go through a period of warm-up exercises before you begin a weight-lifting routine. Another factor to remember is that most weight-lifting exercises require postural control—which means you must hold the back straight during the lifting phase. Always squat to grasp the barbell from the floor; the bend-and-stretch technique could result in a serious back injury.

Other tips for weight lifting: Begin with the feet spread about 12 inches apart and the toes under the bar; otherwise the bar will tend to swing toward the feet when the lift movement begins. For most barbell exercises, grasp the bar overhand with the thumbs hooked under the bar; keep the arms spread apart by at least the width of the shoulders. For performing curls, reverse the hold with an underhand grip and the thumbs hooked above the bar. Breathe through the mouth and inhale as you lift; exhale on the return movement. Keep the weight evenly distributed between the hands.

Exercising With Other Weights

Another type of weight lifting is performed with dumbbells. There are at least ten different exercises that can be executed with these small, inexpensive weights to develop muscles from the waist to the shoulders and arms. Like the barbell exercises and the 6–12 program, they should be followed in a progressive order. Start with the minimum number of repetitions and advance gradually by adding one or two repetitions per week.

Dumbbells are somewhat deceptive in that they appear easy to handle when first viewed on the counter of a sporting goods store. And a pair is no heavier than a bag of groceries. But when the exercise routines with dumbbells are followed according to directions, you will discover muscles you didn't know you had.

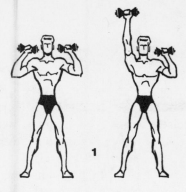

BASIC DUMBBELL EXERCISES

exercise 1

To develop shoulders and the back of the arm. Hold dumbbells at shoulder height. Push bells overhead to a full extension with the palms forward. Lower the bell back to the shoulder. Alternate right and left arm. Inhale as you push weight to full extension. Exhale as you lower the weight to the shoulder. **Repetitions:** first week—8. second week—10. third week—12.

exercise 2

To develop the front of the upper arm. Hold dumbbells at arm's length parallel to the feet. Curl the weight to the shoulder, rotating the bell as the biceps contract. Lower the bell back to the starting position, reversing the rotation. Contract the triceps (back of the arm) to insure a full extension. This is done only after the bell has reached the starting position. Keep the bell under control as you lower it. Alternate right and left arms. Inhale as you curl the weight. Exhale as you lower the weight. **Repetitions:** first week—8. second week—10. third week—12.

exercise 3

Curl weight until forearm is parallel to the floor. Return to the starting position. Repeat required number of repetitions. Curl bells to the shoulders. Lower weight until forearm is parallel to the floor. Return to the shoulder position. Repeat required number of repetitions. Lower bells to the starting position and curl required number of repetitions through full range of movement. Curl both bells at same time. **Repetitions:** first week—4 each movement. second week—5 each movement. third week—6 each movement.

exercise 4

To develop the back of the upper arm. Hold dumbbells above and back of each shoulder by pointing the elbows up and holding them close to the head. Hold the elbows in place and extend the weight overhead by contracting the triceps. Lower the weight to the starting position. Alternate right and left arm. Inhale as you push weight to full extension. Exhale as you lower the weight to the shoulder. **Repetitions:** first week —8. second week—10. third week—12.

exercise 5

To develop the shoulders. Use the standing position, holding the bells at arm's length in front of the thighs with the palms to the rear. Raise the bells to the shoulder, keeping the weight close to the body as the elbows go up and out. Lower the weight to the starting position, keeping the weight under control. Inhale as the weight goes up. Exhale as the weight goes down. **Repetitions:** first week—12. second week—14. third week—16.

exercise 6

To develop the shoulders. Use the standing position. Place the feet at shoulders' width apart, bending the knees a little more than usual. Roll the hips back slightly. Hold the bells at arm's length in front of you. Now, raise both bells laterally rotating the arms so the back of the hands come together on completion of the contraction. Keeping the bells under control, lower them to the starting position. Elbows should be slightly bent to avoid strain. **Repetitions:** first week—6. second week—8. third week—10.

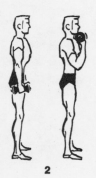

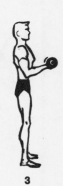

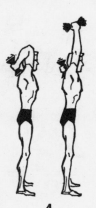

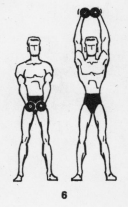

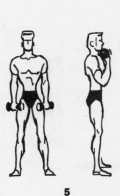

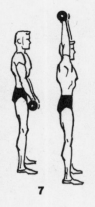

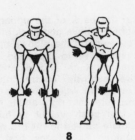

BASIC DUMBBELL EXERCISES

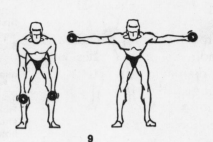

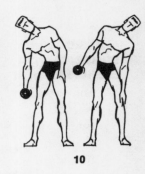

7

8

9

10

exercise 7

To develop the shoulders. Use the standing position holding the bells at arm's length with the palms to the rear. With the elbows slightly out of locked position, raise the bells overhead without rotating the arm. Return to the starting position. Inhale as you raise weight over head. Exhale as you lower weight to starting position. **Repetitions:** first week—6. second week—8. third week—10.

exercise 8

To develop the upper back. Stand with feet at shoulders' width apart. Bend the knees and lean forward until the trunk is parallel to the floor. Hold the bells at arm's length directly below the shoulder. Raise the bells, alternately to the shoulder by driving the elbow up and to the rear. Inhale as you pull weight up. Exhale as you lower the weight to the starting position. **Repetitions:** first week—12. second week—14. third week—16.

exercise 9

To develop the upper back. Stand with feet at shoulders' width apart. Bend the knees and lean forward until the trunk is parallel to the floor. Hold the bells at arm's length directly below the shoulders. Extend the arms laterally until they are parallel with the floor. Return to the starting position and repeat. Inhale as the bells are extended laterally. Exhale as the bells are lowered to the starting position. **Repetitions:** first week—6. second week—8. third week—10.

exercise 10

To exercise the waist. Stand with the feet shoulder width apart. Hold one bell in the right hand at arm's length by the right thigh. Do not bend forward or backward, but lean to the right, lowering the bell below the right knee. Now, lean to the left touching the left hand below the left knee. Repeat the desired number of repetitions. Change the bell to left hand to exercise the right side of the waist. Inhale as weight rises. Exhale as weight goes down. **Repetitions:** first week—15. second week—20. third week—25.

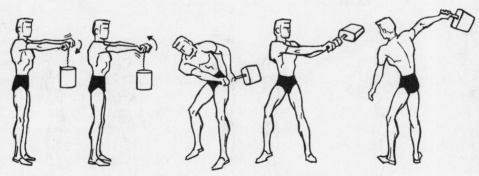

Twist Grip   **War Clubs**

Still other weight-lifting exercises designed to develop specific muscles are the war club swings and the twist grip. The war club weighs approximately 20 pounds and consists of a handle about 14 inches long and one inch in diameter attached to the weight. It is swung in circles with one or two hands or swung as a hatchet or a baseball bat. It is intended to improve the function of muscle groups in the trunk, back, and shoulders, but provides fringe benefits for the arms and waist also.

The twist-grip exerciser, which is used to develop muscles of the arms and hands, can be made at home from such simple objects as a foot-long piece of pipe, a length of rope, an empty container, and about 20 pounds of cement. The rope is attached to the pipe at one end and the other end is attached to the weighted container. By holding the pipe at arm's length and turning the pipe in the hands, the weight is raised and lowered, using alternately an underhand and overhand grip on the pipe.

Isometrics

Still another method of developing specific muscle groups is known as isometrics. Although isometrics was once popularized as an easy way to exercise, most physical fitness experts agree that there is no such thing as an easy exercise. This opinion applies especially to isometrics; if isometric exercises are performed according to the rules, they can be as difficult as any other kind of exercise. In fact, most isometric exercises should not be performed by an individual who has not been examined by a physician first. The effects of straining some muscle groups while holding the breath can prove dangerous for a person whose heart is not in good condition.

The term isometrics is used to describe a technique in which the muscle is contracted without moving the body part involved, and the muscle is held in contraction for about ten seconds before it is relaxed. Isometrics

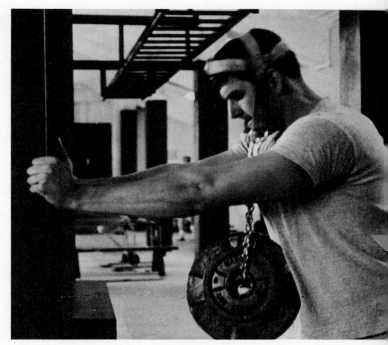

This athlete is doing a neck strengthening exercise.
—IPS

also are called static exercises, as contrasted with dynamic exercises or isotonic muscle activity in which the muscles not only contract but flex and extend extremities. Some exercise routines may include both isometrics and isotonics; in weight lifting, isometric muscle contractions are used to grasp the weight at the floor and to hold the weight in an overhead position but an isotonic contraction is involved in moving the weight through a curl or press between the isometric phases.

It should be understood that a specific isometric exercise generally is designed to develop only one specific group of muscles. To get the comparable benefits of a warm-up series of exercises and a 6–12 program you would have to perform a very large number of different isometric exercises to involve all of the body's muscles that need daily exercising. Also, they do not provide the aerobic effect of the more active exercise routines. *Aerobics* refers to the kind of physical activity that requires maximum or nearly maximum effort for at least four minutes in order to get the heart and lungs, as well as the muscles, involved in the conditioning effects. In other words, a ten-second isometric muscle contraction is not likely to require the kind of bodily effort that creates an oxygen debt.

Yet isometrics do have a place in physical conditioning, as one unit of an overall exercise effort that also includes warm-up routines and calisthenics, with perhaps a little running or jogging as well. Briefly, the best way to perform isometric exercises is to inhale deeply just before you start the muscle contraction. Hold your breath while you exert the greatest possible effort in muscle contraction. At that point the muscle should begin to quiver from the strain of the contraction. Hold the contraction for at least five seconds, longer if the exercise requires; use a watch with a sweep second hand for timing. Then relax the muscle and exhale.

Most isometric exercises can be performed with little or no equipment; although special equipment is available for some exercises, many can be performed by using a desk, wall, or door jamb as an immovable object against which you can exert the force of your muscle contractions.

Exercises for Women

Physical conditioning programs for women are essentially the same as for men, although women are more likely to be conscious of bulging muscles that seem to produce bodily proportions they may regard as unattractive. However, there are exercise routines that can have the effect of balancing proportions. Running and cycling, for example, tend to favor development of the muscles from the hips downward. Weight lifting or other exercises designed to develop the muscles from the waist up can be used to advantage by women who want to reshape that part of the body. On the other hand, exercises that tend to develop musculature where it is unwanted can be avoided. Particularly recommended for women who plan

to be mothers are exercises that strengthen the abdominal and back muscles.

Basic exercises for women include running or jogging, bending and twisting at the waist, situps, and modified pushups, as well as standing on the toes while stretching the arms upward. Special exercises for enhancing the female figure can begin with a series of bustline exercises. One is an isometric press that starts with the palms of the hands facing together, fingers clasped and pointed upward, and arms close to the chest. Inhale deeply and push the hands against each other with maximum effort. Hold the breath while pressing and continue for seven seconds. Then relax, exhale, and repeat the exercise. Two other exercises are performed while lying flat on the floor with a weight in each hand; dumbbells, bricks, or books can serve as weights. Start with weights in

The bicycle exercise is beneficial to hips and thighs.
—*Ewing Galloway*

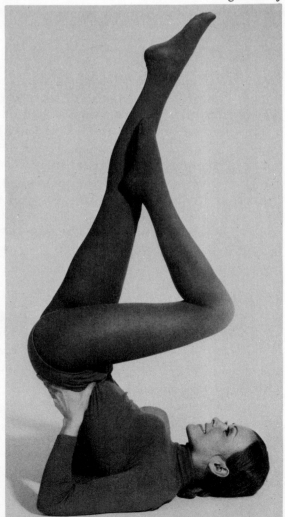

FOR THE BUSTLINE

1 The Press

Starting position: Stand or sit erect. Clasp hands, palms together, close to chest. Action: Press hands together hard and hold for 6-8 seconds. Repeat three times, resting briefly and breathing deeply between repetitions.

2 Pullover

Starting position: Lie on back with arms extended beyond head. Hold books or other objects of equal weight in hands. Action: Count 1—Lift books overhead and down to thighs, keeping arms straight. Count 2—Return slowly to starting position. Repeat 3-6 times.

3 Semaphore

Starting position: Lie on back with arms extended sideward at shoulder level. Hold books or other objects of equal weight in hands. Action: Count 1—Lift books to position over body, keeping arms straight. Count 2—Lower slowly to starting position. Repeat 3-6 times.

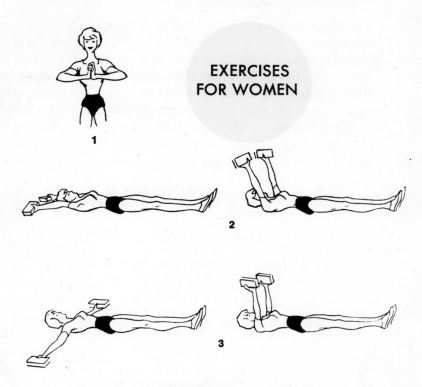

EXERCISES FOR WOMEN

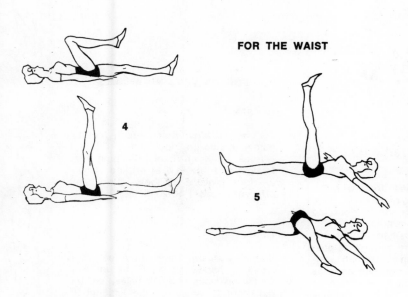

FOR THE WAIST

4 Knee Lifts

Starting position: Lie on back with knee slightly bent, feet on floor and arms at side. Action: Count 1—Bring one knee as close as possible to chest, keeping hands on floor. Count 2—Extend leg straight up. Count 3—Bend knee and return to chest. Count 4—Return to starting position. Repeat 5-10 times, alternating legs during exercise.

The double knee lift is done in the same manner, raising both legs at the same time. Do 5-10 repetitions.

5 Crossover

Starting position: Lie on back, arms extended sideward, palms down. Action: Count 1—Raise right leg to vertical position and move slowly to left until almost touching floor. Keep arms, head and shoulders on floor. Count 2—Return to starting position. Counts 3 and 4—Same action to other side. Do 5-10 repetitions.

hands, arm stretched back over the head with backs of the hands on the floor. Next raise both arms without bending the elbows and move the weights overhead and down to the floor at the hips. While counting to yourself for rhythm, return to the original position and repeat the exercise. The second is a variation of the previous exercise, with the weights being lifted straight overhead from a starting position of the arms extended sideward at shoulder level. But don't bend the elbows.

Cycle-type exercises and ballet stretches are recommended for hips and thighs. Ballet stretches can be performed from a standing position, with one hand on the hip and the other holding onto a steady object such as a chair. Another exercise for the hips and thighs is patterned after the "cheerleader" position. While kneeling on the floor, hands on hips and back straight, bend backward as far as is comfortable without bending the back or moving the knees. Return to the starting position and begin again.

Among the suggested exercises for calves and ankles is the rocker. With feet together and hands on hips, legs straight, rock back on your heels with toes off the floor. Then rock back with your weight on the toes and the heels off the floor.   KNA

FOR HIPS AND THIGHS

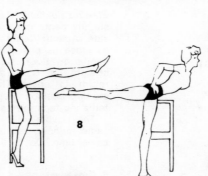

6 Cheerleader

Starting position: Kneel on floor, back straight, hands on hips. Action: Count 1—Bend backward as far as possible, keeping knees on floor and body straight. Count 2—Return to starting position. Repeat 10-15 times.

7 Bicycle

Starting position: Lie on back with hips and legs supported by hands. Action: Simulate bicycle pumping action with legs. Pump 50-100 times.

8 Ballet Stretch

Starting position: Stand erect with left hand resting on back of chair for support. Action: Count 1—Raise right leg sideward as high as possible. Count 2—Return to starting position. Count 3—Swing right leg forward as high as possible. Count 4—Return to starting position. Count 5—Swing right leg back as high as possible. Count 6—Return to starting position. Do 5-10 repetitions, then repeat exercise with left leg.

9 Two-Way Stretch

Starting position: Kneel with hands on floor, back straight. Action: Count 1—Arch back, bend head down and bring left knee as close as possible to chin. Count 2—Lift head high and extend left leg as far backward and up as possible. Repeat 6-10 times with each leg.

EXERCISES FOR WOMEN

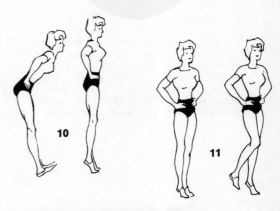

FOR CALVES AND ANKLES

10 Rocker

Starting position: Stand erect, feet together, hands on hips. Action: Count 1—Rock back on heels, keeping legs straight and raising toes off floor. Count 2—Rock forward on toes, lifting heels off floor. Repeat 10-20 times.

11 Hop

Starting position: Stand erect, feet close together, hands on hips. Action: Hop lightly on both feet 50 times, on the right foot 25 times, on the left foot 25 times, on both feet 50 times.

12 Stemwinder

Starting position: Stand erect, left foot lifted clear of floor. Action: Rotate left foot in small circles 20 times. Repeat with right foot.

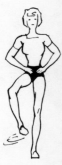

THESAURUS OF MEDICAL TERMS

Key Word	Adjective	Study	Specialist	Major Disorders
allergy	allergic	allergology	allergist, allergologist	respiratory and skin disorders, e.g. asthma and contact dermatitis
anesthesia	anesthetic	anesthesiology	anesthesiologist	
blood	hemal	hematology	hematologist	anemia, leukemia, hemophilia
blood vessels	vascular	angiology	vascular surgeon	varicose veins, phlebitis
bone	osteal, osseous	orthopedics	orthopedist, orthopedic surgeon, orthopod	back disorders, fractures, trauma
brain *See* nervous system.				
cancer *See* tumor.				
causes of disease	etiologic, etiological	etiology	etiologist	
chest cavity	thoracic	thoracic surgery	thoracic surgeon	lung cancer, tuberculosis, emphysema
children	pediatric	pediatrics	pediatrician	all diseases children are subject to
colon and rectum	proctologic, proctological	proctology	proctologist	hemorrhoids, cancer of the rectum or colon
cosmetic surgery *See* plastic surgery.				
diet	nutritive	nutrition	nutritionist	malnutrition, obesity
digestive tract	gastroenteric	gastroenterology	gastroenterologist	digestive difficulties, ulcers, gallstones, inguinal hernia
disease	pathologic, pathological	pathology	pathologist	
ear	otologic, otological	otology	otologist	hearing or equilibrium disorders
ear, nose, and throat	otolaryngological	otolaryngology	otolaryngologist, ENT specialist	hearing or equilibrium disorders, laryngitis, upper respiratory infections
endocrine glands *See* glands.				
epidemics (geographical distribution of disease)	epidemic, epidemical	epidemiology	epidemiologist	forms of cancer, cholera, influenza
eye	ophthalmic	ophthalmology	ophthalmologist, oculist	glaucoma, cataract, detached retina
foot	pedal	podiatry, chiropody	podiatrist, chiropodist	arch troubles, bunions, ingrown toenails
gastrointestinal tract (GI tract) *See* digestive tract.				
general medicine			general practitioner (GP)	
genital tract (female) *See* reproductive system (female).				
genital tract (male) *See* urinogenital tract (male).				
glands (endocrine)	glandular	endocrinology	endocrinologist	diabetes, hyperthyroidism, hypothyroidism
hair *See* skin and hair.				
heart	cardiac, coronary, cardiologic, cardiological	cardiology	cardiologist, cardiovascular specialist	angina, coronary thrombosis (heart attack), atherosclerosis, hypertension